Tidy's Physiotherapy

Twelfth edition

Tidy's Physiotherapy

Twelfth edition

Ann Thomson MSc, BA, MCSP, DipTP
Vice Principal, School of Physiotherapy, Middlesex Hospital, London

Alison Skinner BA, MCSP, HT, DipTP
Senior Lecturer, School of Physiotherapy, Middlesex Hospital, London

Joan Piercy BA, FCSP, DipTP, DipPE
Formerly Head of School of Physiotherapy, North East London Polytechnic and London Hospital School of Physiotherapy, London

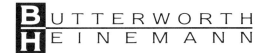
BUTTERWORTH
HEINEMANN

Butterworth–Heinemann Ltd
Linacre House, Jordan Hill, Oxford OX2 8DP

 PART OF REED INTERNATIONAL P.L.C.

OXFORD LONDON BOSTON
MUNICH NEW DELHI SINGAPORE SYDNEY
TOKYO TORONTO WELLINGTON

First published by John Wright & Sons Ltd 1932
Second edition 1934
Third edition 1937
Fourth edition 1939
Fifth edition 1941
Sixth edition 1944
    Reprinted 1945
Seventh edition 1947
Eighth edition 1949
Ninth edition 1952
Tenth edition 1961
Eleventh edition 1968
    Reprinted 1973, 1974, 1976, 1978, 1982, 1983, 1986, 1987
Twelfth edition 1991
    Reprinted 1991

© Butterworth–Heinemann Ltd 1991

British Library Cataloguing in Publication Data

Tidy, Noel Margaret
    Tidy's Physiotherapy — 12th ed.
    1. Medicine. Physiotherapy
    I. Title   II. Thomson, Ann   III. Skinner, Alison
        IV. Piercy, Joan
    615.82

    ISBN 0 7506 1346 7
            0 7506 0273 2 Butterworth–Heinemann International Edition

Library of Congress Cataloguing in Publication Data

Thomson, A. M. (Ann M.)
    Tidy's Physiotherapy — 12th ed./Ann Thomson, Alison Skinner,
Joan Piercy
    Rev. ed. of: Tidy's Massage and remedial exercises in medical and surgical
conditions/edited and rev. by J. O. Wale. 11th ed. 1968.
    Includes bibliographical references
    ISBN 0 7506 1346 7
    1. Massage-Therapeutic use. 2. Exercise therapy.
    I. Skinner, A. T. (Alison T.)   II. Piercy, Joan.   III. Tidy,
        Noel Margaret. IV. Title.   V. Title: Physiotherapy.
    [DNLM: 1. Exercise Therapy. 2. Massage. WB535 T482t]
    RM721.T455 1990
    615.8'2-dc20
    DNLM/DLC   89-21547
    for Library of Congress   CIP

Printed and bound in Great Britain by Thomson Litho Ltd,
East Kilbride, Scotland.

Preface

In keeping with Miss Tidy's theme in her preface to the first edition, the authors have aimed at providing a general textbook for students and recently qualified physiotherapists. In the eleventh edition, Miss Wale aimed to concentrate on the basic principles of physical treatment in relation to pathology, and the medical and surgical techniques employed. Since the last revision the practice of physiotherapy has developed considerably and we have tried to take this into account. This edition is designed to enable the reader to identify patients' problems by the application of anatomy, physiology, pathology and behavioural science and to provide guidelines as to how physiotherapy can solve or alleviate these problems.

In some areas there are fairly precise treatment programmes which are based on empirical evidence and provide the inexperienced physiotherapist with a secure starting point. In other areas advice and guidelines are much more general, as dictated by co-morbidity and multiple problems of the patient. Physiotherapy is increasingly appropriate in primary health care and physiotherapists are becoming first-contact practitioners. Therefore there are guidelines to help the physiotherapist make decisions on programmes of treatment, advice and prevention. The text is based on the experience of senior clinicians, together with that of the authors, for the benefit of the reader. The authors recognize that there is no substitute for clinical practice in developing the broad spectrum of skills required from the competent physiotherapist.

The chapters have been renamed and reorganized. Those on neurology have been updated to take account of the changing patterns of these diseases. There is additional information on soft tissue injuries, diseases and disorders of the skin, obstetrics and gynaecology, and care of the elderly, whilst the coverage of other conditions such as systemic and bone diseases has been condensed. A major change has been the inclusion of Appendices I–IV which emphasize the skills of physiotherapy.

The authors are very grateful to many friends and colleagues for theier help and support with the completion of this work. In particular we would like to thank the following:

For contributing chapters 25 and 26, Mrs Myrtle Collins BA, MCSP formerly of the Middlesex Hospital. For creating the illustrations with infinite patience, Mrs Angela Christie. For various photographs; Orthopaedic Department, The Royal London Hospital (Chapter 4); Miss Cathie Hewitt (formerly University College Hospital) (Chapter 16); Ms Ann Levick of Seton Health Care Group plc (Chapter 18); Mrs Grace Skinner (Chapter 27); Mrs Jill Pickard (Chapters 6, 11, Appendix II); Hillingdon Hospital, Paediatric Department, Mrs Pam Scott (Chapter 7); For typing the text, Miss Mary Archer, Mrs Jean Oliver, Miss Evelyn Coggins, Miss Jo Rendle, Miss Helen Walkington, Miss Anne Maitland. For providing information and guidance, Miss Brenda Williams (Chapter 3, 4, 5); Miss Gill James (Chapters 12, 13, 14); Mrs Alison Sherwin (Chapters 12, 13, 14, 15); Miss Geraldine Watkins (Chapter 6); Miss Jackie Gealer (Chapter 8); Mrs Alison Stiles (Chapter 17); Mrs Sheila Harrison (Chapter 18); Mrs Ann Reed (Chapter 21); Mrs Penny Robinson (Chapter 22); Mrs Shirley Gordon (Chapters 25, 26); Mrs Jennifer Newman (Chapter 27); Mrs Marna Hawkins (Appendix IV).

For general encouragement, especially in our hours of despair, Miss E. M. Coggins, Principal, The Middlesex School of Physiotherapy and our colleagues of the same school together with our friends at Wyke Green Golf club; Mr Baker of John Wright and Mrs Sylvia Hull of Butterworths.

We would also like to acknowledge the work of Miss Cicely Browning, formerly Principal of the Prince of Wales Hospital School of Physiotherapy, who contributed much of the text on neurology, fractures and dislocations for this edition in the early 1980's. Due to the delay in completion of some other parts of the book it became necessary to update these sections.

A.T.
A.S.
J.P.

Publisher's note

The use of 'she' and 'he' in this book to refer to physiotherapist and patient respectively is for convenience only. No sexual stereotyping is implied.

Contents

Chapter 1

Introduction

Society and the environment are undergoing continual change, and health care providers have a constant challenge to rise to the demands placed upon them. In 1976, the Department of Health and Social Security (DHSS) published *Prevention and Health – Everybody's Business*. In 1978 at Alma-Ata in the Union of Soviet Socialist Republics, the World Health Organisation (WHO) declared: 'The existing gross inequality in the health status of the people particularly between developed and developing countries is politically, socially and economically unacceptable and is, therefore, of common concern to all countries'. The goal of the WHO is 'Health for all by the year 2000'. In the United Kingdom a report entitled *The Nation's Health – A Strategy for the 1990s*, edited by Alwyn Smith and Bobbie Jacobson, was published in 1988 and sets out many recommendations for health promotion. Furthermore, a National Fitness Survey was launched in February 1990.

The above initiatives are relevant to all health carers, and physiotherapists should play an important part in many of these developments.

Over the years the patterns of diseases have changed both within individual countries and throughout the world. Some diseases have been eradicated or reduced in severity as the result of improved health care and education. For example, there are no cases of smallpox and fewer epidemics of anterior poliomyelitis in the world today as the result of vaccination programmes, and cases of tuberculosis have declined owing to a combination of drugs, vaccination and health education. New or improved drugs have altered disease patterns as in the use of antibiotics to combat infection, and anti-inflammatory drugs for alleviating symptoms in some rheumatic diseases. However, the inequality of health provision means that some countries have not had the same degree of success in reducing disease as others. Despite improvements in health care some diseases such as the acquired immune deficiency syndrome (AIDS) have developed, and certain bacteria and viruses have become resistant to some drugs.

There are other reasons for changes in disease and injury patterns such as alterations in the environment which may be natural or man made. Increases in population and increasing affluence in some countries may lead to the development of other health problems, for example the greater volume of road traffic has increased the number of road accidents and consequent injuries despite improved education in accident prevention; a greater percentage of people develop coronary heart disease; more people participate in sporting activities, resulting in more sports injuries. On the other hand, preventive measures and health education have been successful in reducing the incidence of some diseases and injuries. For example, the campaign to stop people smoking has led to a decrease in the numbers developing lung cancer, and safer work practices have decreased the number of people injured in heavy industrial work. These are but a few of the changes that have taken or are taking place with consequent effects on the rehabilitation services. The alterations in medical technology and improved health care have in some instances increased the demands on the physiotherapy profession and in others decreased them. More physically and mentally handicapped children survive and people have a longer life expectancy. These together with developments in cardiac and transplant surgery, neurosurgery and some other surgical procedures all place further demands on the physiotherapy services. However, improved anaesthetics and surgical skills, including the use of day surgery, have decreased the risk of some post-operative complications and reduced the demand for physiotherapy in general surgery.

There have been a number of policy changes in the health service which have altered the way in which physiotherapy services are organized. Community care has increased with the consequent need for physiotherapy. The community physiotherapist helps to monitor patients who have been discharged from hospital to ensure that they are maintaining the level of physical activity reached on leaving hospital and to ensure that they are progressing towards optimal or full independence if possible. She may see patients in the community for advice and/or treatment, and this may include guidance and advice to relatives or other carers. The advent of direct general practitioner referrals has increased the demand for physiotherapy, particularly in outpatient departments. Although the demand on the physiotherapy services may often be increased by these changes they should improve the effectiveness of delivery.

The role of the physiotherapist has altered to meet the above changes and demands. The physiotherapist is recognized as a health professional to whom other health professionals will refer patients for assessment and advice (Department of Health and Social Security, HC 77(33). – Relationships between the medical and Remedial Professions). The physiotherapist will decide on whether treatment is required and if so what treatment, how it should be altered and progressed, and when it should be terminated. The physiotherapist is part of the health team concerned with the overall management of the patient and consequently must understand the roles of the other health care professionals. She must be able to communicate with them so that physiotherapy is appropriate and complementary to the total management. This management must be seen in the context of other services which may be required.

Physiotherapy includes assessing the patient, planning and implementing the treatment programme, evaluating, and then altering the treatment as the result of the evaluation. An assessment includes an examination, and the consequent clinical decision about whether treatment is appropriate and if so the aims, and the objectives that may be achieved. The examination identifies the problems presented by the patient as the result of his disease or injury. Also it considers other factors that could affect these problems, for example the age of the patient, his attitude and response to the disease or injury, his home conditions, and his work. The physiotherapist must understand the social, cultural and environmental factors as these may affect the ultimate requirements of each patient with regard to home, work and leisure. When planning the treatment the techniques must be carefully selected

to fulfil the aims and objectives, and then evaluated and changed as necessary. There is no regimen or recipe of techniques that can be applied to any one condition, as disease and injury do not run the same course in every patient.

The skill of the physiotherapist lies in the ability to gain the cooperation of the patient, to make a good assessment, to select the appropriate techniques, to implement and evaluate the treatment plan effectively thus leading the patient towards complete or optimal indepedence. Thus the physiotherapist is involved in a complex decision-making process in order to give an effective treatment which considers the whole patient and his environment.

The terms 'techniques' and 'skills' need to be defined as they are used in various parts of this book. The term 'technique' is generally used in describing a particular procedure relating to a specific method of treatment. For example: axial sling suspension is one of the techniques used as part of the overall technique of sling suspension, effleurage is one of the massage techniques, hold/relax/repeated contractions/slow reversals are proprioceptive neuromuscular facilitation techniques (PNF), cross fire technique is a procedure used when applying short-wave diathermy, and so on. Some techniques require skill in the placing of the apparatus whereas others require skill in the actual physical handling of the patient as with massage or PNF. A technique must be performed skilfully to be effective. A competence in the performance of techniques forms part of the assessment/examination procedure in giving a licence to practise. However, a physiotherapist will continue to improve her skill during her professional work, also she may acquire further techniques and skills in some specialities, and some physiotherapists may develop new techniques. These aspects can be seen in any profession involving manual skills.

The skilled performance of a technique is not the only skill required by a physiotherapist, and it is the ability to combine a number of skills that makes a good physiotherapist and will result in effective treatment (Figure 1.1).

Research has been slow to develop in the field of physiotherapy and so many of the skills and techniques in use have not been evaluated. In earlier days when physiotherapists found a skill or technique to be successful in the treatment of a number of patients it was retained, whereas others judged to be ineffective were discarded. Today physiotherapists who have a knowledge of research method and those who have carried out research may question the criteria on which some of these judgements were made. Nevertheless some skills and techniques have undoubtedly been of immense value to patients, and it would be wrong to discard these simply because they have not been subjected to any form of analysis. A critical and analytical

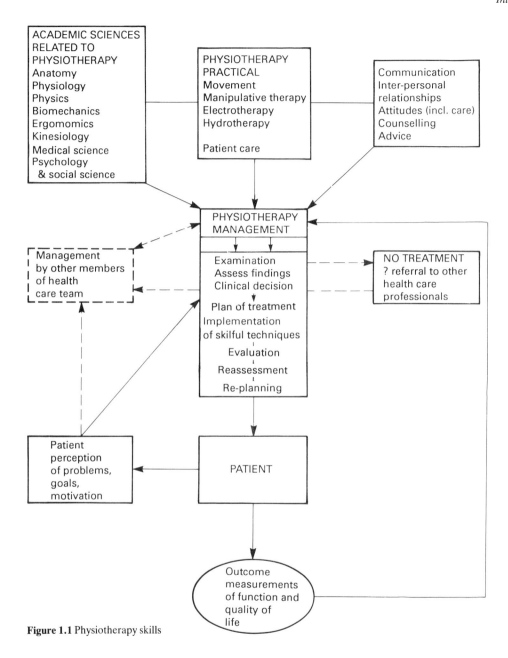

Figure 1.1 Physiotherapy skills

approach will help in the present and future evaluation of physiotherapy.

In order to justify the use of physiotherapy as an essential part of the total management of a patient the physiotherapist must be able to demonstrate the effectiveness and efficiency of the treatment.

Research takes time to develop and is often difficult when the treatment forms part of the total management of the patient. A major problem in physiotherapy research is the number of factors that may affect the outcome of a treatment – for example, the psychological and social problems linked with the illness or injury, interpersonal relationships between therapist and patient, the communication skills of the therapist, the motivation of the patient, the severity of the disease or injury and the prognosis.

An essential contribution to future research is the need for physiotherapists to collect data in a form that can be used when analysing the effectiveness of treatments and the efficiency of physiotherapy services.

Chapter 2

Causes of disease

Definition

A disease implies an abnormal state of the body and may concern the structure and/or function of a part or the whole. It may be a temporary condition affecting the person in which case there will be a return to normal structure and function, as with the common cold. Alternatively the person may be left with a permanent disability, as for example an amputation of the leg for a severe injury.

Some diseases remain permanently throughout the life of the person, either causing death or increasing incapacity. Atherosclerosis may be present over a number of years and then death may occur suddenly owing to a coronary thrombosis. Multiple sclerosis may be present for 20 years or more with the patient becoming increasingly disabled, but it may not be the actual cause of death.

The results of disease that leave some abnormality can be described in a number of ways depending on the disease and its effect on the person. The terms usually used are impairment, disability and handicap. These terms are often used interchangeably but they have different connotations and it is useful to define them, particularly in relation to disability and handicap:

1. *Impairment* – A defect in structure and/or function, or a loss of part of the body.
2. *Disability* – Loss or reduction of functional ability.
3. *Handicap* – The person is disadvantaged by their disability.

An impairment does not necessarily result in a disability, for example a person with short sight may have this corrected with spectacles or contact lenses and therefore see as well as a person with normal sight. However, without spectacles the person would be disabled and handicapped. The loss of a single tooth does not usually affect the ability to eat. The loss of the tip of the little finger might have no effect on the function of the hand but the loss of the thumb would result in disability and possibly handicap. A person who is disabled is not necessarily handicapped. For example, someone who has had a leg amputated is disabled although he may be able to walk and take part in some sporting activities. The extent of his activities will depend on the level of the amputation, age, general health and previous ability and motivation. Some disabilities are not obvious; for example, a person who has a back problem with constant pain will not be able to undertake normal activities and yet there is no visible disability.

Handicap is a more difficult term to define as it depends on a number of factors. The man with a lower limb amputation and who can walk with a prosthesis may not be disadvantaged if he has a sedentary job, but if he was a manual worker he would be handicapped. However, this term is more complicated if you consider in what way the person is disadvantaged – is it work, leisure activites, home life? The man with the amputation who was not handicapped for work may be handicapped in relation to his leisure activities if he previously played rugby at county or international level. It is not within the scope of this book to discuss these definitions further, but it is important that the student is aware of the problems when planning rehabilitation programmes.

Classification

Disease falls into two main categories – congenital and acquired.

Congenital

These are diseases that are present at birth.

Inherited

These may be autosomal dominant or recessive, the former giving Huntington's chorea, for example. There are sex linked diseases such as Duchenne muscular dystrophy and haemophilia.

Genetic abnormalities of chromosomes

These may be inherited or there may be an accidental abnormality. Down's syndrome falls into this group and there is an error in the genetic material transmitted by one of the parents but the error does not exist in the cells of the parent.

Developmental abnormalities acquired *in utero*

If the mother develops rubella this may affect fetal development. Certain drugs, such as thalidomide, given during pregnancy can affect development.

Acquired

A large number of diseases fall under this heading, and they can be grouped as follows:

1. *Infection* – This includes diseases due to bacteria, viruses, parasites, worms and fungi. The last three are not very common in the United Kingdom and are not included in this text.
2. *Injury* – Trauma may cause damage to any of the structures in the body, fractures of bone, dislocations of joints, soft-tissue structures such as ligaments, tendons and muscle, peripheral vessels and nerves. Head injury may cause neurological damage, fractured ribs may puncture the lung. Apart from trauma there are other physical causes of damage to the body. For example, excessive heat can cause burns, excessive cold may result in frostbite, damage may occur following radiation with ultraviolet light or irradiation with X-ray. Certain chemical substances may be toxic and affect the tissues either by surface contact, absorption through the surface, inhalation, or taken with food or drink. This group should include the adverse effects due to some drugs.
3. *Degeneration* – Degenerative changes can occur in various tissues in the body, and sometimes this may be due to circulatory disease and ischaemia. Osteoarthritis is a degenerative disease affecting articular cartilage but the cause is unknown.
4. *Dietary deficiencies or excesses* – Inadequate diets either in amount or proportion can cause disease.

Excess cholesterol has been suggested as one of the factors causing atherosclerosis although there is no conclusive evidence. Lack of vitamins and minerals can be responsible for various diseases, for instance lack of vitamin D may result in rickets or lack of vitamin C may give scurvy. However, with modern knowledge many of these are preventable.

5. *Other causes of disease* – Some diseases do not fall readily under the above headings because the cause is unknown. Certain conditions of the circulatory system fall under this heading; for example, atherosclerosis may be partly due to incorrect diet but other factors have been suggested such as stress, inadequate exercise and smoking. Diseases with no known causation may be termed idiopathic, as for example idiopathic scoliosis.

Infection

This is one of the chief sources of human disease and so a brief description of the micro-organisms involved is included.

Bacteria

These are microscopic living organisms that exist all round us, in the air we breathe, in the soil, in the animate and inanimate objects with which we are in daily contact. They fall into two main groups – pathogenic and non-pathogenic. The pathogenic bacteria are those that cause disease, and they subdivide into the following groups:

1. *Bacilli* – These are rod shaped and may form threads or chains. An example of a disease caused by this group is tuberculosis caused by the tubercle bacillus.
2. *Cocci* – These are spherical organisms and may be arranged in bunches. The staphylococcus and streptococcus are examples of this group.
3. *Spirochaetes and protozoa* – These are responsible for a range of infections, including dysentery, malaria and syphilis.

Bacteria multiply asexually by binary fission.

Viruses

These organisms are so small that they are invisible under normal microscopy. They will pass through a membrane filter and range from about 20–300 nm in size compared with bacteria which are about 1–20 μm. They have the power to enter specific cells from which they multiply and cause signs of disease. They can then escape to other cells and extend the infection. All viruses contain nucleic acid, either DNA or RNA. The DNA viruses cause such diseases as smallpox, herpes simplex, Epstein–Barr and hepatitis B, while the RNA viruses may cause colds, rubella or measles. AIDS is another viral disease caused by the human immune-deficiency virus (HIV).

Methods of entry and body defence

1. *Direct contact or contagion* – This may occur by touching an infected body or object and entry is via the skin, through the pores or hair follicles. Alternatively infection may be via an abrasion.
2. *Inhalation* – Organisms are breathed in and gain access to the tissues through the respiratory tract.
3. *Ingestion* – Organisms can be taken in with food and reach the tissues via the digestive tract.
4. *Sexual transmission* – Organisms may be transmitted by sexual intercourse when one partner is infected. The HIV virus may gain access to the body in this way.
5. *Blood transfusion* – This is another method of entry and is a particular danger in the case of haemophiliacs, a number of whom have been infected with the HIV virus from a blood transfusion.

The main defence of the body is the reticulo-endothelial system, the leucocytes in the blood, areas of lymphoid tissue such as the tonsils and adenoids, lymph glands and lymph tissue in the digestive tract. Some of the lymphocytes, the neutrophils and monocytes, are phagocytic and so ingest dead cells and bacteria. Others are responsible for long-term defence and immunity through the production of antibodies (immunoglobulins) in response to the presence of an antigen. The cells in the body also produce a substance called interferon which is an antiviral substance.

Unfortunately, the immune defence system can occasionally go wrong and some elements of the defence mechanism will react against parts of the body. This seems to occur with allergies and is a possible cause of rheumatoid arthritis.

Treatment

Antibiotics – These can be used to treat some infections. The most famous antibiotic, which was first used clinically in about 1940, is penicillin. Since then many others have been developed.

Anti-viral agents – Ribavirin has been used successfully in an aerosol spray for the treatment of bronchiolitis and pneumonia. Interferon has been used in treating shingles and chicken pox.

Vaccines – A vaccine is a less virulent form of the virus. When a person is vaccinated with the attenuated virus it stimulates the body to produce antibodies and these will protect the person if they come in contact with the virus. For example, the Salk vaccine has almost eradicated anterior poliomyelitis in countries that have developed an adequate vaccination programme.

Immunization – This is a passive method of protecting the body. The person is injected with a serum containing the required antibodies to protect them against a particular infection. For example, there is immunization against tetanus, diphtheria, whooping cough and others. Some of these can be combined and given in one injection.

Inflammation

This is the reaction that occurs in the body tissues as the result of an injury or irritant. If the severity of the injury causes destruction of tissue (necrosis) then the inflammatory reaction will occur in the surrounding area. The inflammatory process is defensive and is an attempt to remove the irritant, debris and dead cells. It also prepares the way for repair.

An inflammatory condition is indicated by the addition of the suffix '-itis', hence tonsillitis, bronchitis, appendicitis and so on.

Acute inflammation

Pathological changes

Vascular

The initial reaction is a momentary vaso-constriction which may be the result of direct mechanical stimulation. This is followed by dilation of arterioles, capillaries and venules due to the action of a chemical mediator and in the case of the arterioles by the axon reflex. The dilation of the vessels allows more blood to flow to the area (hyperaemia), which is followed by a slowing of the blood flow (stasis). There is an increased permeability of the vessel walls which allows fluid to pass into the tissues and thus increases the viscosity of the blood.

Normally the cellular constituents of the blood lie in the axial stream but the slowing of the blood flow allows the larger white cells to fall away and they adhere to the walls of the blood vessels (margination). Some of the leucocytes migrate into the surrounding tissues and are concerned with defending the body against the infection, or results of injury.

Tissues

A number of changes take place in the tissues at the site of the damage. There is a proliferation of connective tissue cells. The exudation of fluid (transudate) from the vessels helps to dilute the toxins and this may lessen or prevent further tissue damage. If the transudate is rich in fibrinogen it may clot and form a network of fibrin which may prevent further spread of infection. The lymphocytes produce antibodies which combat infection and the phagocytic leucocytes the dead bacteria and cells or other foreign material. The resulting debris is carried in the transudate to the adjacent lymph vessels.

Lymph

As the tissues become swollen with the increased fluid this is absorbed into the surrouding lymph vessels and carried to the lymph nodes where any foreign matter is further exposed to the action of phagocytic cells and antibodies.

The basic principles of these changes of inflammation are the same in whichever tissue it occurs, but the proportion of these changes varies. For example, in serous membranes a larger amount of protein-rich fluid is produced.

Clinical features

Pain – This is usually present because the exudate presses on the surrounding tissues but this can be variable in degree depending on whether the inflammation is occurring in a confined space or in loose tissue. Also pain may depend on the virulence of the organism or the severity of the injury. It will depend on the number of pain nerve endings in the affected tissue.

Redness – If the inflammatory reaction is near to the surface then the redness of the skin will indicate the underlying hyperaemia.

Heat – The active hyperaemia will cause a local rise of temperature.

Swelling – The increased exudation will cause swelling which will be apparent in superficial reactions. The amount of fluid will depend on the extent and severity of the inflammatory reaction and the type of tissue affected.

Loss of function – A number of factors can affect function. Pain can limit movement particularly if it affects the structures around the joint or muscle tissue. Swelling round a joint may limit movement or increased exudation of a serous membrane may affect the underlying organ, as with pleurisy which will affect respiration. In some instances there will be no loss or very little loss of function, as for example with a scratch.

General inflammation

In some cases when there is a virulent organism it may gain access to the whole body via the blood and lymphatic system and give rise to a general septicaemia. The changes are similar to those of a local inflammation but they are widespread. The patient feels and is very ill with a rise in body temperature. Antibiotics have decreased the gravity of such conditions.

Chronic inflammation

This may occur when there is a mild reaction to the injury or irritant. Minor trauma may be insufficient to produce an acute reaction or the defence system of the body may be more effective. Chronic inflammation may follow an acute reaction when the defence of the body is insufficient to allow resolution and there is a persistent low-grade infection or irritant. The changes depend on the tissues affected but there is usually a greater increase of fibrous tissue. Exudation is less in some cases but in others, such as chronic bronchitis, there may be increased secretion of mucus.

Termination of inflammation

There are a number of ways in which the reaction can terminate and these will depend on the cause of the inflammation, the defence system of the body and the particular tissues affected.

Resolution – In this method the exudate is absorbed and the debris is removed by the phagocytes and enzymes. Following this activity the tissue returns to normal. If the infection is mild or the irritant removed this may occur quickly. In the case of a severe infection, which is dealt with by the defence system of the body or outside intervention, resolution can still occur but the process will be slower.

Fibrosis – Fibrous tissue may be formed as a result of the reaction, particularly when there is a chronic inflammation. This may take the place of normal tissue, or form adhesions between normal tissues, and so affect function.

Suppuration – As a result of a pyogenic infection toxins are produced which cause the death of some cells which are then liquefied. This liquefied material, plus inflammatory exudate, living and dead polymorphs, and bacteria constitutes pus. If the pus is contained within the tissue it forms an abscess. Unfortunately this provides an ideal medium for the growth of bacteria and production of toxins leading to further necrosis of tissue. Pressure builds up in the abscess and pus may extend into the surrounding tissues thus spreading the infection to other sites.

Necrosis – This is death of tissue cells. It has been mentioned as occurring in an inflammatory reaction, and if it affects a small area resolution may occur. However, with extensive areas of necrotic tissue this cannot happen and then bacterial infection may lead to gangrene (decay of tissue).

Healing of a skin wound

Healing depends on whether there is a clean cut (or incision) and very little tissue loss or there is a greater degree of tissue destruction. In the former instance healing is by primary union (first intention) while in the latter healing is by secondary union (second intention).

Primary union

The following events occur:

1. *Blood clot* – This fills the gap and acts as a protective cover.
2. *Inflammatory reaction* – This is mild and occurs during the first 24 hours. There is exudation of fluid, invasion of the area by macrophages which ingest and digest fibrin, red cells and other debris.
3. *Epithelial bridge* – Squamous epithelium grows across the gap and then the layers of skin hypertrophy.
4. *Dermis and subcutaneous tissue* – There is formulation of granulation tissue. This is accompanied by revascularization and the reforming of lymph channels.
5. *Fibrous tissue* – This forms to unite the cut edges of the wound.

Normal skin is formed after about 14 days and continues to develop but it is devoid of hair follicles, sweat and sebaceous glands.

Secondary union

The basic pattern of healing is similar to that for primary union except that there is tissue loss and a greater gap to be filled. A larger amount of scar tissue is formed which is avascular. Gradually the scar tissue tends to contract, pulling on surrounding tissues.

Factors affecting healing

Blood supply – A good supply is essential for healing. An inadequate supply will slow the healing process and if there is a lack of blood to the area more tissue will die and this will result in the formation of more scar tissue.

Infection – This will delay healing and may cause further damage to the tissues.

Irritation – Persistent irritation will slow healing. Sometimes rough handling or the removal of a dressing can break down the granulation tissue.

Type of tissue – Some tissues are capable of regeneration and will re-form after disease or injury. However, certain important tissues cannot reproduce and amongst these is nerve tissue within the brain and spinal cord. Recent research has shown that some of the white fibres in the spinal cord may be capable of regeneration given favourable conditions.

Chapter 3

Introduction to fractures

Definition

An interruption in the continuity of the bone which may be a complete break or an incomplete break (crack).

Classification

There are two main types of fracture and various subdivisions which are named according to the position of the fractured parts of the bone.

Closed fracture

This type indicates that there is no communication between the external surface of the body and the fracture (Figure 3.1).

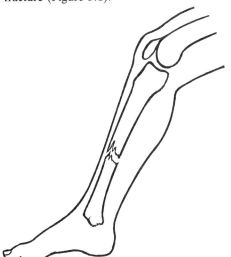

Figure 3.1 Closed fracture

Open fracture

There is a communication between the fracture and the skin (Figure 3.2). This could occur because the displacement of the bone ends has caused one or both to pierce the skin, or because an external force has pierced the skin, soft tissues, and fractured the bone. This type of fracture is an additional cause for concern because of the possibility of infection.

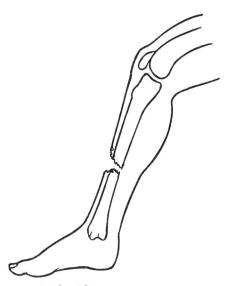

Figure 3.2 Open fracture

The position of the parts of the bone may indicate the nature of the injury. A torsional force is likely to give a spiral fracture (Figure 3.3), whereas a direct blow could give a transverse (Figure 3.4) or oblique (Figure 3.5) fracture depending on the angle of the force and whether the limb is fixed or moving. Longitudinal force tends to result in compression or crush fractures (Figure 3.6). In some instances there are a number of fragments of bone and this is termed a comminuted fracture (Figure 3.7). Types of fracture may also relate to age or disease. In young children the bones are still relatively malleable and so fractures are more likely to present as an incomplete fracture known as a greenstick fracture (Figure 3.8), or in the case of a longitudinal force as a compression fracture. The bones of the elderly are often more brittle (osteoporotic) and fracture with relatively little force as can occur in a fractured neck of femur.

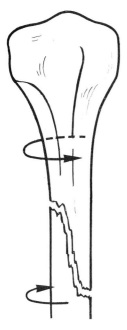

Figure 3.3 Spiral fracture

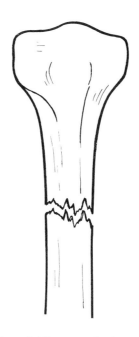

Figure 3.4 Transverse fracture

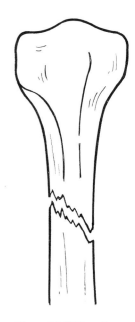

Figure 3.5 Oblique fracture

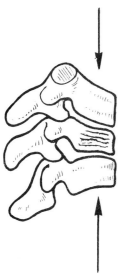

Figure 3.6 Compression fracture

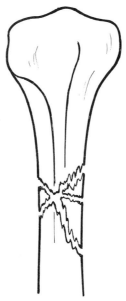

Figure 3.7 Comminuted fracture

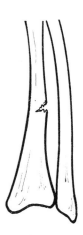

Figure 3.8 Greenstick fracture

Causes

Trauma

Most fractures are due to some form of injury. This might be a direct blow with considerable force as may occur in a motor accident, falling from a height, or a weight falling on a hand or foot. Other fractures may be caused by indirect violence such as falling on an outstretched hand which could fracture the lower end of the radius, or a foot caught in a hole when running which could give a torsional force resulting in a fractured tibia and fibula. Stress or fatigue fractures are caused by repeated minor trauma which can occur after walking long distances and often affect one or more metatarsals. These fractures are usually confined to the lower limbs and can affect the fibula or tibia as well as the metatarsals, depending on the type of activity.

Pathological fractures

These fractures occur as the result of disease that affects the composition of the bone, making it liable to fracture often as the result of a relatively trivial injury. There are a number of such diseases but those most commonly seen are carcinoma – either metastic or osteogenic sarcoma, osteogenesis imperfecta (fragilitas ossium), Paget's disease and infection affecting the bone.

Clinical features

Immediately after the fracture

The features will vary depending on the cause and nature of the injury. If the injury is severe or there are multiple injuries the patient could be unconscious. In other cases such as fatigue fractures, some impacted or crack fractures the patient may be able to use the limb although complaining of pain.

Generally the following features will be present:

1. *Shock* – This will vary according to the extent of the injuries, the position of the fracture(s), the age of the patient and the circumstances of the trauma.
2. *Pain* – This will also vary according to the circumstances mentioned in (1).
3. *Deformity* – This will be noticeable when there is displacement of the bone fragments.
4. *Oedema* – This will be localized immediately after the injury and then gradually become more extensive.
5. *Marked local tenderness* – This may be an important feature in an injury that appears to be trivial.
6. *Muscle spasm*.

7. *Abnormal movement and crepitus* – No attempt should ever be made to elicit these as it might result in further damage.
8. *Loss of function* – This may be complete in severe injuries but some activity may be possible when the injury is less severe such as a fatigue fracture, some impacted or crack fractures.

Following reduction and fixation

1. *Pain* may continue for a variable amount of time depending on the injury and associated problems to soft-tissue structures.
2. *Oedema* – This may be a problem in achieving adequate fixation. It may be necessary to apply a temporary plaster or splint and then re-apply the plaster as soon as the swelling has reduced. In fractures of the limb bones oedoma may be apparent below the level of the plaster and it is necessary to elevate the limb, exercise the fingers or toes not enclosed in plaster and perform static contractions of the muscles within the plaster.
3. *Loss of function* – This will be variable depending on the particular fracture and type of fixation.

After removal of the fixation

Sometimes normal function can be regained very quickly with little help required from the physiotherapist, whereas in other cases there are a number of problems, for which intensive treatment may be required, as follows:

1. *Pain* – In some instances this may be due to a fear of movement causing pain rather than actual pain. It could be due to stretching of adhesions or to complications such as Sudeck's atrophy.
2. *Oedema* – The swelling should have been reduced while the patient was in plaster. However, once the plaster has been removed the weak muscles may not provide adequate support or pumping action on the veins in which case swelling may reappear.
3. *Limitation of joint movement* – The joint may be stiff due to the formation of adhesions or because of swelling. Movement may also be limited because of weak muscles in which case it will be possible to move the joint passively through range. If the fracture has affected the joint surface this may cause limitation of movement which it may not be possible to regain.
4. *Weak muscles* – There will be a loss of power in muscles which have not been used, or not properly used, for several weeks. In some instances this may be quickly regained with normal use but where this is impossible a rehabilitation programme will be required.

5. *Loss of function* – In lower limb fractures mobility will depend on the nature of the fracture. It may be possible to resume walking during the period of fixation with a walking plaster, splint or bandage depending on the fracture. Alternatively the patient may have to commence walking by non-weight bearing for the affected leg using crutches, progressing to partial weight bearing using crutches, or a frame or sticks and eventually to full weight bearing. Some patients, particularly the elderly, may be permitted to start with partial weight bearing. A person with a sedentary job may be able to return to work with crutches whereas a manual worker or athlete could not do so.

In upper limb fractures – Full movement may be regained in a relatively short time or may take many weeks depending on the severity of the injury and the extent of the disability when the fixation is removed. Both in upper and lower limb fractures there may be complications due to soft-tissue damage particularly of nerve tissue which may greatly increase the time required to gain full or optimum function.

Healing of fractures

Healing starts immediately after the fracture has occurred and is a continuous process. In order to explain the process clearly it can be taken through five stages. Two or more of these stages can be seen to be taking place at the same time in different parts of the fracture site.

1. *Stage of haematoma* – As a result of the tearing of blood vessels at the time of the injury a haematoma is formed at the fracture site. A very small portion of bone immediately adjacent to the fracture dies and is gradually absorbed.
2. *Stage of sub-periosteal and endosteal cellular proliferation* – There is a proliferation of cells from the deep surface of the periosteum adjacent to the fracture site. These cells are precursors of the osteoblasts and form round each fragment of bone. At the same time cells proliferate from the endosteum in each fragment and this tissue gradually forms a bridge between the bone ends. During this stage the haematoma is gradually absorbed.
3. *Stage of callus formation* – The proliferating cells mature as osteoblasts or in some instances as chondroblasts. The chondroblasts form cartilage and this is found in varying amounts at a fracture site but is not essential to healing. The osteoblasts lay down an intercellular matrix of collagen and polysaccharide which then become impregnated with calcium salts thus forming the immature bone called callus or woven bone. This

is visible on X-ray and gives evidence that healing is taking place.
4. *Stage of consolidation* – Osteoblastic activity results in the change of primary callus to bone which has a lamellar structure and at the end of this stage union is complete. This new bone forms a thickened mass at the fracture site and obliterates the medullary cavity. The amount of this new bone varies for a number of reasons. It tends to be more extensive if there has been a large haematoma or it has been impossible to obtain exact apposition of the bone fragments.
5. *State of remodelling* – The lamellar structure is changed and the bone is strengthened along the lines of stress. The surplus bone formed during healing is gradually removed and eventually the bone structure appears very similar to the original (Figures 3.9–3.13). In children healing is usually very good and it is difficult to see the fracture site on a radiograph. However, in adults there is usually a permanent area of thickening which might be felt or even seen in a superficial bone.

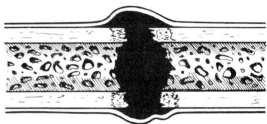

Figure 3.9 Haematoma

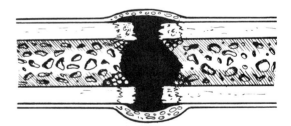

Figure 3.10 Periosteal and endosteal proliferation

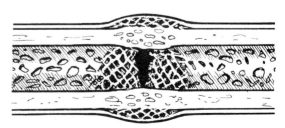

Figure 3.11 Callus formation

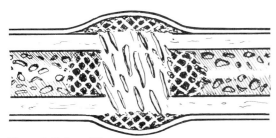

Figure 3.12 Consolidation

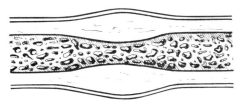

Figure 3.13 Remodelling

Healing of cancellous bone

This follows a different pattern from that described above because of its structure. As with compact bone a haematoma is formed but as there is no medullary cavity the second stage differs. The cancellous structure gives a greater area of contact between the fragments of bone and penetration of the bone-forming tissue is facilitated by the open arrangement of trabeculae as it grows out from both fragments. The osteogenic cells lay down intercellular matrix which is then calcified to form woven bone. Then the process of remodelling continues to form the cancellous bone.

Union of fractures

The time taken for a fracture to unite is highly variable and depends on many factors, as follows:

1. *Type of bone* – Cancellous bone heals rather more quickly than compact bone. Healing of long bones depends on their size so that bones of the upper limb unite earlier (3–12 weeks) than those of the lower limb (12–18 weeks). The femur may often take 4–5 months to heal.
2. *Classification of fracture* – It is easier to obtain good apposition with some fractures than others. This may depend on the initial position of the fragments before reduction and the effect of muscle pull on the fragments.
3. *Blood supply* – A good blood supply is essential for normal healing to take place.
4. *Fixation* – Adequate fixation prevents impairment of the blood supply which may be caused by

movements of the fragments. It also maintains the reduction thus preventing deformity and consequent loss of function.
5. *Age* – Union of a fracture is quicker in young children and consolidation may occur between 4 and 6 weeks. Age makes little difference to union in adults unless there is accompanying disease.

Delayed union – This indicates that healing is taking longer than would normally be expected.

Non-union – In this case there are distinct pathological changes and radiological evidence of non-union. There appears to be no callus formation and the fractured ends of bone become dense and the outline clear cut. The gap between the bone fragments may be filled with fibrous tissue and form a pseudo-arthrosis.

Complications

Infection – This may occur in an open fracture as organisms can gain entrance via the open wound. A superficial infection may be dealt with and cause no problems but if the infection should penetrate to the fracture area it could cause osteomyelitis and lead to delayed or non-union.

Avascular necrosis – A lack of blood supply to part of a bone will cause it to die (necrosis). This can be a complication of certain fractures when one fragment is deprived of its blood supply. Bone gains its blood supply by the soft-tissue structures attached to it or by intra-osseous vessels. In certain instances one part of the bone is very dependent on the intra-osseous vessels for its blood supply, and if this is interrupted because of a fracture avascular necrosis may occur. It can occur in fractures of the neck of the femur leading to avascular necrosis of the head and in fractures of the scaphoid bone where the proximal pole may be affected. This may be a cause of non-union of the fracture and as the fragment usually includes an articular surface it will lead to osteo-arthritis.

Mal-union – This may occur if there is poor alignment of the fragments and the resulting deformity could affect function. Overlapping of the fragments could lead to shortening and this would affect function particularly if it occurred in the lower limb. Angulation or rotation of the fragments may impair function because of the altered mechanics.

Joint disruption – If the fracture extends to the joint surface and there is displacement it may not be possible to achieve perfect alignment of the fragments and this could lead to restriction of joint movement. Disruption of the joint surface may lead to later development of osteo-arthritis.

Adhesions – These may be intra-articular and/or periarticular. The intra-articular adhesions may occur when the fracture extends into the joint surface and there is a haemarthrosis. If this is not absorbed fibrous adhesions may form within the synovial membrane. Periarticular adhesions may occur if oedema is not reduced and it is allowed to organize in the tissues. This will lead to adhesions forming between tissues such as the capsule and ligaments resulting in joint stiffness. This is less of a problem now that new techniques of fixation allowing early mobilization have been developed.

Injury to large vessels – These consist of haemorrhage due to tearing of large vessels or occlusion. If a large artery is occluded in such a position as to cut off practically the whole blood supply to the limb this may lead to gangrene or if there is a partial occlusion an ischaemic contracture may develop. These injuries must be dealt with as an emergency by the surgical team. Thrombosis of veins may occur in the neighbourhood of the fracture. This is manifested by the sudden development of a cramp-like pain in the part, by an increase of swelling, and by marked tenderness along the line of the vein. Anything that appears to be abnormal in the circulatory system must be reported to the surgeon immediately.

Injuries to muscle – Muscle fibres may be torn or the muscle ruptured as a result of the injury and this will cause additional bleeding and swelling. Tendons may be severed particularly in the case of open fractures or sometimes there may be a rupture following a fracture. Surgical intervention is usually necessary to repair a rupture.

Injuries to nerves – A nerve may have been injured at the time the fracture occurred. If the nerve is severed then there will be immediate paralysis and anaesthesia of the parts supplied by it and surgery will be required to repair the nerve. However, if the nerve is not severed recovery can be expected although the time taken will vary depending on whether it is an axonotmesis or a neuropraxia.

Sudeck's atrophy – This is a complication which may occur after the fixation is removed and is usually seen in relation to fractures of the lower end of the radius or more rarely in fractures around the ankle. The patient complains of severe pain on attempting movement, and the hand is swollen. The skin appears shiny and the hand feels cold. It usually responds to physiotherapy but recovery is slow and may take several months. Fortunately this complication is comparatively rare.

Injury to viscera – This may be a complication particularly of fractures of the pelvis or thorax.

Principles of management

First aid

The principal aim of anyone dealing with a fracture or possible fracture is to prevent any further damage occurring. Thus the patient should not be moved unless the first aider is qualified to deal with the situation. In the case of severe injuries it is necessary to ensure that the airway is clear. Apart from this the patient should be kept as warm as possible until skilled medical help arrives. The patient should not be given anything to drink as it may be necessary to give an anaesthetic on arrival at hospital.

Principles of treatment by the surgeon

The initial treament will depend on the extent of the injuries. In severe cases there may be other problems that take priority over treatment of the fracture: shock, bleeding, maintenance of the airway and ventilation, and possibly other injuries.

The surgeon will aim to obtain good reduction and alignment of the fracture, followed by immobilization that is sufficient to promote good healing and restoration of function.

Reduction

This is not always necessary even when there is some displacement. However, when there is poor alignment of the fragments or the relative positions of the joints above and below the fracture are lost as a result of the angulation or rotation, or there is a loss of leg length, then reduction is usually necessary. Radiographic examination is used to ascertain the exact position of the fragments before and after reduction.

Closed reduction – The fracture is manipulated by the surgeon under a general or in some instances a local anaesthetic.

Reduction by traction – In certain fractures such as the shaft of the femur there may be considerable displacement due to the injury and to muscle spasm and in order to reduce this and relieve the spasm it may be necessary to maintain traction for a period of time by weights or screws. This reduction may be obtained under an anaesthetic or by a long period in bed.

Open reduction – Very careful consideration is given to a case by the surgeon before undertaking an open reduction. However, it may be necessary to prevent complications and possibly to deal with damage to soft-tissue structures, blood vessels or nerves.

Immobilization

The objectives of immobilizing a fracture are to maintain the reduction, to promote healing and to relieve pain. In some fractures where there is no likelihood of displacement fixation may not be necessary.

Methods of immobilization

External splinting

The standard method is still plaster of Paris (Figure 3.14) which is easy to apply and cheap to use. However, it has the disadvantage of being heavy and must be kept dry. Plastics are now used for fixing some fractures because of their light weight, and also they are impervious to water. They are more costly than plaster of Paris and this prevents them being used more widely. Other methods of fixation include strapping, bandages, malleable strips and aluminium or wire.

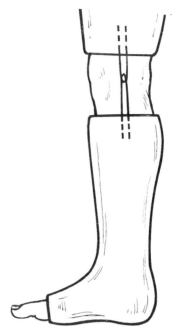

Figure 3.15 Functional bracing

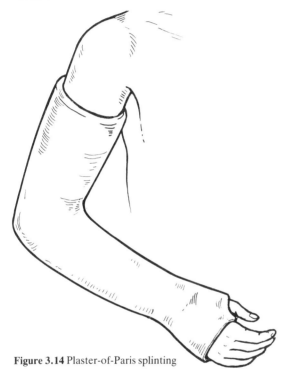

Figure 3.14 Plaster-of-Paris splinting

It has been found unnecessary to fix some fractures as rigidly as in the past and an example of this is cast bracing (functional bracing) following a fractured shaft of femur. After an initial period in traction the patient is placed in a cast brace (Figure 3.15). This is made of plaster of Paris but with hinges incorporated at the knee to allow movement. This has reduced the problem of stiff knees that occurred due to prolonged immobilization. Another benefit of allowing movement of joints, provided that it does not stress the fracture site, is that it may promote union by improving the blood supply.

Another method of external splinting used when there is extensive damage, particularly in fractures of the tibia, is to use an external frame. Nails are placed transversely into the bone and fixed externally on a vertical plate (Figure 3.16). Prolonged

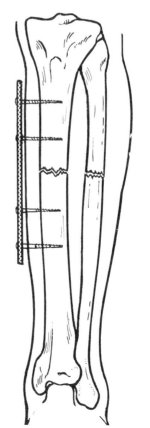

Figure 3.16 External splinting

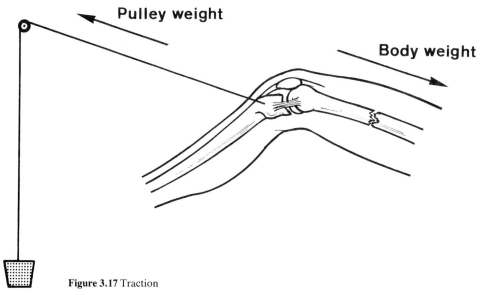

Pulley weight

Body weight

Figure 3.17 Traction

traction may be necessary to maintain the reduction of some fractures particularly the femur, tibia, and some cervical spine injuries (Figure 3.17).

Internal fixation

If it has been necessary to use open reduction then the surgeon will probably choose internal fixation as this has the advantage of allowing the patient greater mobility. The fracture can be fixed by an intramedullary nail, plates and screws, compression plates and screws or wiring. Occasionally a bone graft and screws may be used, particularly in cases of delayed or non-union (Figures 3.18 and 3.19).

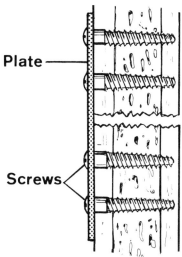

Plate

Screws

Figure 3.18 Screws and plate

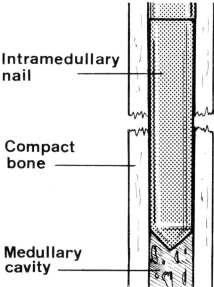

Intramedullary nail

Compact bone

Medullary cavity

Figure 3.19 Intramedullary nail

Physiotherapy management

This can be divided into management during immobilization and then after removal of fixation.

The physiotherapist must be careful to avoid anything that might delay repair or lead to non-union. Thus it is essential that the principles of fractures outlined in the earlier part of this chapter are understood and that discussion takes place with a member of the surgical team to ascertain the need for any particular precautions. No apparatus should be interfered with unless removal for treatment is allowed, and if so it must be correctly reapplied and the fracture site carefully supported while it is off. The physiotherapist must be aware of the possible complications and report any untoward signs or symptoms.

Physiotherapy during immobilization

The aims during this period are as follows:

1. Reduce oedema – It is very important to do this as quickly as possible to prevent adhesion formation. It will also help to decrease the pain.
2. Assist the maintenance of the circulation to the area – active exercise either by static or isotonic muscle activity will help to maintain a good blood supply to the soft tissues and aid the reduction of swelling and prevent the formation of adhesions.
3. Maintain muscle function by active or static contractions.
4. Maintain joint range where possible.
5. Maintain as much function as allowed by the particular injury and the fixation.
6. Teach the patient how to use special appliances such as crutches, sticks, frames and how to care for these or any other apparatus.

The physiotherapist must assess the patient and the situation in order to decide on the treatment required. It is not always necessary to treat a patient throughout this stage provided that the patient can be taught to do his own exercises and is as independent as the circumstances will allow. The patient must appreciate what is required and be motivated to carry it out. The physiotherapist is responsible for monitoring the patient through this stage. If it is necessary to continue treatment this may be in the ward for an inpatient but outpatients may either be treated in a physiotherapy department or at home if there is a domiciliary service. Good treatment at this stage may prevent some of the problems that can occur when the fixation is removed.

Swelling should be reduced by elevating the limb and by active or static contractions of muscles thus minimizing the formation of adhesions and consequent stiff joints. Muscles that cannot produce movement of a joint because of the fixation and do not work statically will waste very rapidly. However, isometric or isotonic contractions performed correctly and repeated often enough will prevent excessive wasting. Encouraging functional activity when possible also helps reduce the rehabilitation time after the fixation is removed.

Patients must understand the importance of their treatment and physiotherapists must understand the problems and requirements of each patient.

Physiotherapy after the removal of fixation

The physiotherapist carries out an assessment of the patient and then formulates a plan of treatment. Although certain clinical features can be expected after a particular fracture they will appear in different degrees in each patient and in some cases may not be present. Every patient presents different problems apart from the injury and these may relate to age, family, work, leisure and the psychological reactions of the individual. These must all be taken into account in planning a programme of treatment and evaluating progress so that changes may be made as appropriate.

The aims of treatment relating to the fracture will include:

1. To reduce any swelling.
2. To regain full range of joint movement.
3. To regain full muscle power.
4. To re-educate full function.

Swelling

Swelling should not be a great problem if exercises and general activities have been carried out during the immobilization period. However, it may be a problem in the lower limb if the muscles are very weak and there is a loss of joint range as both factors will prevent an adequate pump action on the veins. Any oedema must be reduced as quickly as possible as this will hinder active movement and lead to the formation of adhesions thus extending the rehabilitation period.

Range of joint movement

Before attempting to regain any decreased range of movement the physiotherapist must have examined the patient to determine the reason for the loss of range. It could be due to pain, oedema, adhesions or weak muscles. If there has been a disruption of the joint surfaces this may preclude a return to full range.

Muscle power

The building of muscle power will depend on gaining maximal activity of the muscles and using them in all actions – prime movement, antagonist, fixator and associated movements with other muscle groups.

Full function

In the majority of cases it should be possible to regain full function but if not the physiotherapist must aim to gain the optimum function, and the extent of this will depend on the complications preventing full recovery. Planning must also take into account the needs of the patient in relation to home, work and leisure. In preparing a patient to return to work the physiotherapist needs to appreciate that the patient may have to work all day and know what type of work is involved – heavy labouring, industrial work on a production bench requiring repetitive movements of the hand or foot or both, or office work which can require a variety of different activities. Similarly home and leisure activites must be considered so that the patient is fully rehabilitated.

Physiotherapy techniques

These are given in Appendix 1 and must be carefully selected following the assessment of the patient. The physiotherapist must evaluate each treatment and change the techniques as required. Treatment should be intensive, particularly in the final stages of rehabilitation, but always within the capability of the patient. This is a difficult judgement to make and requires skill in selecting the appropriate techniques and deciding how they should be carried out. For example, with movement techniques the physiotherapist must judge carefully how many times each exercise should be performed and whether assistance or resistance is required.

Other members of the team

The physiotherapist is a member of the rehabilitation team. The membership of this team can change according to the stage of treatment and the physiotherapist must liaise and work with the other members throughout the rehabilitation period. Initially if the patient is in hospital the members of the team will include medical staff, nurses and radiographers. Once the patient returns home other members of the health care professions may be needed to support and/or treat the patient. These could include a district nurse, health visitor, occupational therapist and social worker. Vocational training for a change in occupation may be necessary and the disablement resettlement officer may give assistance with regard to future employment.

Chapter 4

Fractures

Fractures of the upper extremity	*Fractures of the vertebral column,*
Fractures of the lower extremity	*thorax and pelvis*

This chapter will not include descriptions of all fractures but will deal with those in which physiotherapy management is important or there are complications that the physiotherapist should know about.

Fractures of the upper extremity

Fractures of the hand and fingers

Fractures of the phalanges or metacarpal bones can result in deformity and/or stiffness of joints which can be very disabling, and so it is important that there is careful management to produce the optimum result.

Phalanges

The surgeon will endeavour to gain good reduction and fixation but it is also important to keep the period of immobilization as short as possible if a good result is to be obtained and this is usually about 3 weeks. The position of the fixation will vary depending on which phalanx or phalanges are fractured and on the stability of the reduced fracture. This can be very important in relation to regaining function of the hand and the surgeon has to decide on the priorities in each case. In certain unstable fractures internal fixation may be the method of choice but if external fixation is used a rolled gauze bandage may be placed in the palm and the finger placed over this with flexion at the metacarpo-phalangeal joint and as near extension as possible at the interphalangeal joints. In stable fractures a Garter strap splint may be used which fixes the injured finger to the adjacent finger and gives some support while encouraging movement (Figure 4.1).

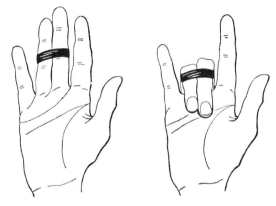

Figure 4.1 Garter strap splint applied to sound and damaged fingers to assist movement of the latter

Metacarpals

The main problem for physiotherapy management are crush injuries which may cause fractures of the metacarpals with resultant pain and oedema.

Complications

The principal complication of these fractures is stiff joints and this can be very disabling for many upper limb activities. Apart from this there could be severe soft-tissue damage which could affect muscles, blood vessels and nerves.

Physiotherapy management

It is essential to reduce the swelling as quickly as possible to prevent the formation of adhesions and consequent stiffness. Mobility of unaffected joints must be maintained, and it is important to ensure

19

that all joints of the arm are moving through full range as a fall on the hand may have caused soft-tissue damage round other joints. As soon as the fixation has been removed intensive treatment must be given to regain movement and function. In some cases this needs intensive daily treatment whereas in others movement returns quickly and it is sufficient for the physiotherapist to instruct the patient in a home programme and to monitor progress as necessary. The patient may also be having treatment from the occupational therapist and it is important that the two therapists should discuss the problems and have an integrated plan of treatment.

Fracture of the scaphoid

This fracture tends to occur in young adults as the result of a fall on the outstretched hand. It may be overlooked either because the person considers it to be a strain and does not attend a doctor or the fracture may not be visible on the initial radiograph. In the latter case the arm is usually placed in plaster as a precaution and radiographed again after a couple of weeks.

Complications

Healing is often slow in this fracture and in some instances there may be non-union. If the fracture occurs through the waist of the bone the blood supply to the proximal part of the bone will be impaired and avascular necrosis may develop. A long-term effect may be the development of osteoarthritis.

Physiotherapy management

Treatment is not usually required but the physiotherapist should be aware of the possible complications if treatment is necessary.

Fractures of the forearm bones

These may occur in the radius or ulna alone or both bones. If both bones are fractured this may be the result of direct violence, or indirect violence such as a fall on the outstretched hand when spiral fractures are likely to occur. The resulting displacement may be difficult to correct and in some instances may need an open reduction. Accurate reduction is very important because a loss of the normal relationship between the two bones may result in impairment of rotation and consequent loss of function. Fixation is usually by a full-length plaster with elbow at a right angle and this is retained for approximately 6 weeks. In children the damage may not be so severe and they may sustain a greenstick fracture with minor

angulation which normally will heal without any complications.

Fractures of the lower part of the radius are very common, particularly in the elderly, usually caused by a fall on the outstretched hand. This may result in the typical dinner-fork deformity due to the backward displacement of the lower end (Colles' fracture) (Figure 4.2). After reduction the wrist may

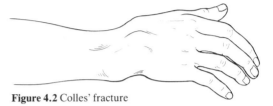

Figure 4.2 Colles' fracture

be immobilized with a complete plaster from just below the elbow to the hand ending just above the proximal crease on the palm or alternatively a plaster slab. The position of the wrist and whether or not there is a complete plaster will depend on the pattern of the displacement. If there is gross swelling it may be necessary to use a plaster slab and then a complete plaster when the swelling has reduced. Fixation is usually maintained for 4–6 weeks.

Fractures of the upper end of the radius are less common and tend to occur in younger people following either a direct blow or a fall on the outstretched hand which causes a fracture through the head of the radius. Fractures of the ulna alone are not as common as those of the radius. A fracture of the upper end of the ulna may occur in conjunction with a dislocation of the head of the radius and this may require open reduction.

Complications

The problems of fractures through the radius and ulna have already been mentioned, with the possibility of cross-union or a loss of the normal relationship between the two bones. This would impede pronation and supination and impair normal activities of the hand and arm.

There are a number of complications that can occur with fractures of the lower end of the radius although these are rare considering the numbers of fractures dealt with in a fracture clinic. Stiffness in the wrist and fingers can be a problem if the swelling is not reduced while the wrist is immobilized. Stiffness can also occur in the shoulder as it could be injured when the person falls but this might not be apparent at the time of the fracture. Occasionally there can be a rupture of the extensor pollicis longus and this occurs 4–8 weeks after the fracture. A late complication can be that of Sudeck's atrophy. Median neuritis can also be a complication if displacement causes stretching or compression of the nerve.

Physiotherapy management

During immobilization – The physiotherapist should see these patients as soon after reduction as possible. There is likely to be a considerable amount of swelling in the fingers and the patient may be reluctant to move them because of pain. This swelling must be reduced and movement of the fingers and arm be encouraged otherwise adhesions may develop and the rehabilitation programme after the removal of the fixation will be prolonged. It is also important to see that movement of the shoulder is not limited as it is difficult to mobilize in the elderly and this would affect the use of the hand as well as other activities of the arm. The physiotherapist must assess the patient and continue treatment until the swelling has been reduced and the patient is using the arm as normally as possible within the limits of the fixation. If the patient has understood the importance of the exercises and can carry on without supervision then there is no need to continue treatment. However, as many of the patients are elderly they may need to be monitored or treated over a longer period.

After removal of fixation – If the fracture has healed normally and without any residual deformity, the swelling has been reduced, and the patient has been using the arm during the immobilization period, then recovery may occur very quickly. However, there may be stiffness of the wrist and fingers and loss of supination at the radio-ulnar joints which, accompanied by weakness of muscles, requires a longer period of rehabilitation. With the elderly the emphasis must be on the restoration of function for the activities of daily living. However, many elderly patients are very active and the physiotherapist must consider the needs of each patient whether it may be driving a car, gardening, playing golf or any other activity.

Fractures of the upper arm

Fractures of the condyles of the humerus

These fractures are found mainly in children as a result of a fall. A supracondylar fracture is the commonest type and requires very careful management because of the possible complications. After reduction the arm may be immobilized in one of the following ways depending on the type of fracture:

1. Plaster with the elbow at approximately 90° or a little more and extending from below the shoulder down to the wrist or hand. The plaster should be cut so that it is possible to feel the radial pulse at the wrist.
2. A posterior slab plus a collar and cuff.
3. A collar and cuff.

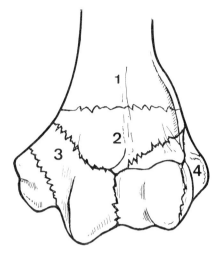

Figure 4.3 Lower end of humerus to show common fracture sites (left side, anterior aspect). 1 = Supracondylar fracture; 2 = Y-shaped fracture of condyles; 3 = medial condylar fracture; 4 = lateral condylar fracture

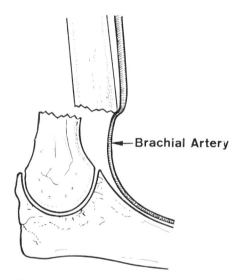

Figure 4.4 Supracondylar fracture of the humerus

Some fractures of the condyles may extend on to the articular surfaces and thereby cause additional problems (Figure 4.3).

Complications

One of the most serious complications that can occur is damage to the brachial artery which could be severed or contused (Figure 4.4). Therefore a very careful watch must be kept on the circulation and the patient will probably be kept in hospital for at least 24 hours. Impairment of the circulation requires emergency treatment as occlusion can lead to irreversible effects within a few hours. If the circulation is not restored Volkmann's ischaemic contracture may develop. This affects the flexor muscles of the forearm which are replaced by fibrous tissue which contracts and produces flexion of the wrist and fingers (Figure 4.5). The skin and nerves will also be affected by the diminished blood supply. In such cases it is not possible to regain normal function and it may be necessary to carry out some reconstructive surgery followed by a rehabilitation programme to regain optimum function.

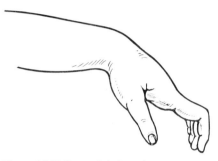

Figure 4.5 Volkmann's ischaemic contracture

Another problem that can develop is post-traumatic ossification (sometimes known as myositis ossificans). If there is a severe injury some of the periosteum may be torn from the bone resulting in bleeding and the formation of a haematoma. Osteoblasts can invade this blood clot and new bone will develop. It can also occur as the result of forced extension of the elbow when movement is limited following a fracture. First indications that this is developing may be pain and loss of movement. The elbow should be rested in a sling or collar and cuff for about 3 weeks to allow the haematoma to be absorbed. If this does not occur and bone is formed it may be necessary to remove the bone tissue surgically.

If deformity develops at the elbow such as a cubitus valgus this may cause a stretch on the ulnar nerve which may require surgical intervention with a transposition of the nerve from the posterior to the anterior aspect of the elbow.

Fractures that extend onto the articular surfaces and cause disruption of the joint may cause a permanently stiff elbow, lead to the development of osteoarthritis, or both.

Physiotherapy management

Normally children mobilize quickly after the removal of fixation and treatment may not be

necessary, particularly if the parents are aware of the care needed in regaining movement and do not attempt or allow any forced extension at the elbow. However, sometimes it is helpful for the physiotherapist to teach the child simple free exercises with one or both of the parents present so that they can monitor and encourage the child and report back if necessary. If the child is very active it is sometimes helpful to keep the arm under the shirt or blouse for the first few days and allow the child to use that arm when the activity can be supervised. When the parents are not able to understand what is required or cannot supervise the activity then it may be preferable for the child to attend for physiotherapy.

Fractures of the shaft of the humerus

These fractures usually occur in the middle third of the bone and may be due to direct or indirect violence (Figure 4.6). Direct violence may give a transverse or oblique fracture which may or may not be displaced and sometimes presents as a comminuted fracture. Displacement may also be effected by muscle pull, and if it is below the insertion of Deltoid the upper fragment will be moved laterally. Indirect violence tends to give a rotational force resulting in a spiral fracture and this usually heals more quickly than a transverse fracture.

Fixation will depend on the stability of the fracture. In stable fractures the fixation can be minimal and consist of a sling alone or with a posterior slab from below the shoulder to the wrist with the elbow at 90°. If the fracture needs greater fixation a complete plaster from the shoulder to the wrist or hand may be applied. The above methods do not fix the shoulder and in very unstable fractures it may be necessary to fix the shoulder with a plaster spica or by extending the previous type of plaster over the superior aspect of the shoulder. In certain cases internal fixation is used with an intramedullary nail or plates and screws.

Union of these fractures usually occurs in 6–8 weeks or possibly earlier with a spiral fracture.

Complications

Because the fracture usually occurs in the middle part of the shaft the radial nerve may be affected as it winds through the sulcus. The injury may compress the nerve and give a neuropraxia or if it is stretched it may result in an axonotmesis. Normally these will recover spontaneously although an axonotmesis will take longer as degeneration of the nerve has occurred within the sheath. In an open fracture the radial nerve may be severed resulting in a neurotmesis and this will have to be sutured.

Delayed or non-union can be complications but are not very common.

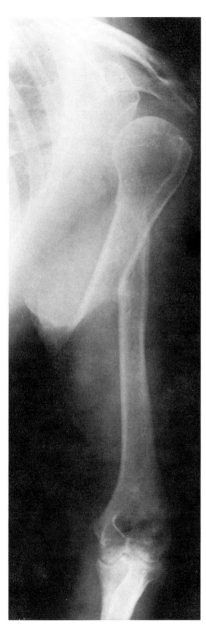

Figure 4.6 Radiograph showing fracture of shaft of humerus

Physiotherapy management

During immobilization the treatment will depend on the type of fixation and whether shoulder movements are allowed. Finger movements and static contractions for muscles working over the immobilized joints should be started at once and continued throughout this period. If the patient is able to do these on his or her own there is no need to attend the department until the fixation is removed. However, if shoulder movements are started early the patient may need help from the physiotherapist. These may start with assisted active movements and change to free active when the patient has sufficient muscle power to do this and is not experiencing any pain. The movements of abduction and rotation should be left till last.

After removal of fixation – Once the fracture has consolidated the patient should be reasssessed and treatment started to regain full range movement of the shoulder girdle, shoulder joint and elbow. Muscle power must be built up by progressive exercises although care must be taken at the beginning of this stage not to stress the fracture site. The rehabilitation programme must take into account the work and other needs of the patient. Intensive daily treatment is ideal but if the patient is able to return to work before the programme is completed then attendances may need to be reduced. Some patients are quite capable of continuing their own programme at home.

Fractures of the upper extremity of the humerus

There are two fractures in this group which are of particular importance to the physiotherapist: fracture of the greater tuberosity and fracture of the surgical neck. Fractures of the greater tuberosity are usually caused by a fall on the shoulder and can occur at any age. If there is no displacement fixation is unnecessary but the patient may be given a sling or a collar and cuff to relieve the pain. This should be discarded as soon as possible and normal movement encouraged.

Fractures of the surgical neck usually occur in elderly people as the result of a fall on the outstretched hand. There may or may not be displacement of the fragments but in a large number of cases the fragments are impacted. Displaced fractures, and particularly those occurring in the elderly, are not usually reduced for a number of reasons:

1. Lack of good alignment does not affect union.
2. It is preferable to avoid surgery in the elderly unless essential.
3. Early movement is important to avoid a stiff shoulder.

Complications

A stiff shoulder in the elderly can be a serious problem as it may require a long period of treatment and even then function may be impaired. A fractured greater tuberosity may lead to a painful arc syndrome particularly if there is a thickened area of bone on the greater tuberosity which interferes with abduction. A complication of a fractured surgical neck may be damage to the axillary nerve resulting in a neuropraxia or axonotmesis.

Physiotherapy management

Early mobilization is the keynote to the treatment of these fractures to prevent the development of a stiff shoulder. Movement should be started as soon as the pain has decreased enough to allow the patient to move. Treatment should always be geared to functional movements so that the patient may become independent as soon as possible.

Fractures of the clavicle and scapula

These fractures seldom require physiotherapy unless complications lead to a restricted range of movement in the shoulder girdle or shoulder joint and muscle weakness.

Fractures of the lower extremity

The bones of the lower limb are mostly weight-bearing and so fractures may cause a loss of mobility as the patient may be unable to walk or may need to use crutches, sticks or a frame. If an elderly person is unable to walk for any length of time this may seriously affect their chance of becoming independent again. Independence should be regarded as a priority and this may affect the choice of methods of reduction and fixation. Similarly with young people mobility may be important because of their work but also it may be essential to regain full-range movement and muscle power in order to do their work whereas with the elderly this may not be necessary to gain functional independence.

Fractures in the foot

The phalanges and metatarsals are most likely to be fractured by a heavy object falling on the foot. This will also cause soft-tissue damage and consequently swelling is likely to be severe. These fractures do not as a rule require reduction or immobilization. However, a below-knee walking plaster is usually applied for fractures of the metatarsals to relieve pain and enable the patient to walk. If swelling is severe the patient will need to rest in bed with the leg elevated for a few days.

Another type of fracture that occurs in the metatarsals is a stress fracture often known as a 'March' fracture. It is caused by repeated minor trauma such as may arise from prolonged walking particularly on hard surfaces and usually in someone who is unaccustomed to walking long distances. It is

usually a crack fracture affecting the shaft or neck of the second or third metatarsal. No fixation is required but a walking plaster may be applied if the pain is severe.

Physiotherapy management

During immobilization – If a below-knee walking plaster is applied the physiotherapist will teach the patient to walk correctly in the plaster. When there is swelling the patient should be taught how to position the limb when sitting or lying down and which exercises to practise while in plaster.

After removal of fixation – Treatment is not always necessary but the muscles supporting the arches of the foot are probably weak and the patient should be taught the appropriate exercises. It is necessary to ensure that there is a correct walking pattern.

Fractures of the calcaneum

Usually this fracture occurs as the result of a fall from a height onto the feet, fracturing the calcaneum on one, or sometimes both feet. It may well be accompanied by a fracture of one of the lower thoracic or upper lumbar vertebrae.

Minor crack fractures can be dealt with by applying a below-knee plaster to relieve pain and pressure on the calcaneum and retaining it for 2–3 weeks. Severe compression fractures are a greater problem and there is some controversy about the best method of dealing with them. The standard method is to elevate the limb on a Braun's frame (Figure 4.7) for 3–4 weeks and then weight bearing may not be permitted for a further few weeks. Mobilization must be started during the above period. Some orthopaedic surgeons favour reduction of the fracture, but so far there does not seem to be any evidence to suggest that one method is more effective than the other.

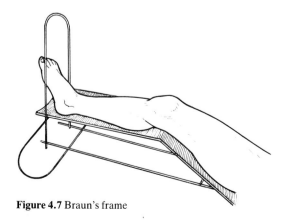

Figure 4.7 Braun's frame

Complications

Stiffness may occur for two reasons: (1) because of the development of periarticular and intra-articular adhesions, and (2) because of disruption of the articular surfaces.

Osteoarthritis may develop as a result of the disruption of the joint surfaces.

Physiotherapy management

The emphasis is on the reduction of the oedema and mobilization. If the patient is kept in bed and the limb elevated as described above movements should start for the hip and knee and be followed by movement of the ankle and toes as soon as the pain has decreased sufficiently to allow this. Movements of inversion and eversion will not be attempted at this stage.

Once the patient is allowed to weight bear it is important to re-educate gait as well as concentrating on strengthening muscles and regaining range of movement in the ankle and foot. It may not be possible to regain any movement at the mid-tarsal joints and the patient will have to learn to adapt to this loss of movement. The arches of the foot will probably have flattened and this may be the result of weak muscles, deformity of the foot, or both. In the former case the muscles can be stengthened but if the latter is the case the arches will not re-form. The patient may continue to have persistent pain and tenderness for a long time after the fracture has healed and it is difficult to relieve. The physiotherapist may help by advice on footwear and the use of mol foam pads to relieve pressure on a painful area.

Fractures around the ankle

The common fractures in this region affect the lower ends of the tibia and fibula and are often associated with dislocation of the ankle. Usually they occur as the result of a twisting force or sometimes from a vertical compression force. The types of fractures can be described according to the nature of the injury causing them and seem to fall into five main categories as shown below (Figure 4.8).

In fractures without displacement a below-knee walking plaster may applied for 3–6 weeks. When there is displacement it is important for the surgeon to try to ensure that reduction establishes the normal relationship at the ankle joint, and then a below-knee plaster is applied and retained for 8–10 weeks. If reduction cannot be attained by manipulation and plaster immobilization it may be necessary to have an open reduction and use a screw or screws to maintain a good position of the fragments followed by immobilization in a below-knee plaster.

FRACTURES RESULTING FROM ABDUCTION AND/OR LATERAL ROTATION FORCE

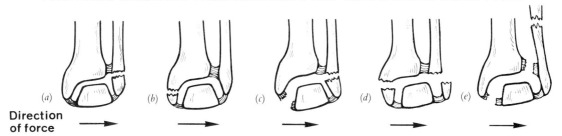

FRACTURES RESULTING FROM ADDUCTION FORCE

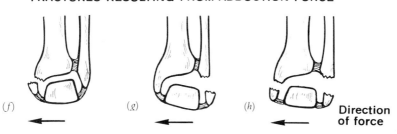

Figure 4.8 *Fractures resulting from an abduction/lateral rotation force:* (*a*) fracture of lateral malleolus; (*b*) avulsion fracture of medial malleolus; (*c*) fracture of lateral malleolus, rupture of medial ligament, and lateral shaft of talus; (*d*) fracture of lateral and medial malleoli and lateral shift of talus; (*e*) tibio-fibular diastasis – rupture of tibio-fibular and medial ligaments, fracture of shaft of fibula, and lateral shift of talus.

Fractures resulting from an adduction force: (*f*) fracture of medial malleolus; (*g*) avulsion fracture of lateral malleolus; (*h*) fractures of lateral and medial malleoli plus medial shift of talus

Complications

Limitation of movement in the ankle joint and foot could result from peri-articular and intra-articular adhesions or from disruption of the articular surfaces. The latter may also lead to the later development of osteoarthritis.

Physiotherapy management

During immobilization – Initially the aim is to reduce the oedema and if the patient is not hospitalized he should be told to keep the limb elevated for most of the day. Some movements can be started immediately, such as hip and knee movements in the lying position which will assist the reduction of the swelling as well as maintaining the movement at these joints. Toe movements and static contractions of the muscles working over the ankle joint should be started as soon as the pain will allow them. The time at which weight bearing is allowed in the plaster is variable depending on the extent of the injury and the reduction of swelling. Sometimes the patient may start non-weight bearing with crutches progressing to partial and then full weight bearing. The physiotherapist must teach the patient how to use crutches if they are necessary and ensure that the other exercises are being carried out.

After removal of fixation – Fractures with no displacement will mobilize quickly and need very little physiotherapy, if any. However, those that have had displacement and been immobilized for a longer period may present with a stiff ankle and foot. The physiotherapist must assess the range of movement in these joints and the strength of the muscles working over them and select the appropriate techniques for mobilizing and strengthening. There may be flattening of the arches supporting the foot, and the muscles supporting them must be strengthened. Fractures around the ankle with soft-tissue damage can be unstable owing to loss of proprioception and this should be re-educated using a balance board.

Fractures of the shafts of the tibia and fibula

These fractures are common and can occur at all ages, either as a result of direct or indirect violence. Often they are open fractures either because of the direct violence or because the tibia is very close to the surface and the fragments may extrude through the skin. Direct violence, commonly due to a road accident, is likely to give an oblique or transverse fracture with the fragments displaced. It may be comminuted and further complicated by soft-tissue damage. Fractures caused by a rotatory force, such as may occur in skiing, are usually spiral and the

fractures of the two bones are at different levels. In displaced fractures the tibia must be reduced and any soft-tissue damage attended to as a priority.

Fixation will depend on the type of fracture and the amount of soft-tissue damage. In closed fractures or those where the fracture is stable after reduction the leg may be encased in a long plaster from the thigh to just above the toes with the knee slightly flexed and the ankle at a right angle. Usually the patient can start walking with crutches non-weight-bearing within a few days. Later a rocker or plaster boot may be applied so that the patient can walk on the plaster but the time at which this occurs will depend on the surgeon. Alternatively a functional brace with a hinge at the ankle may be used and this has the advantage of allowing more movement and a better walking pattern. If there is a lot of soft-tissue damage and consequent swelling a split plaster may be applied and the leg placed on a Braun's frame. This is replaced with a long leg plaster once the swelling has decreased. Another method that is used to immobilize this fracture is external splinting which may be used when there is a risk of infection (Figure 4.9). Sometimes internal fixation is used with either an intramedullary nail or plate and screws. Union of these fractures normally takes 3–4 months.

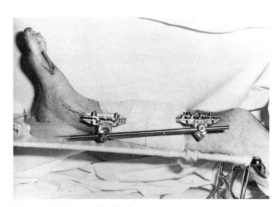

Figure 4.9 External splinting

Fractures of the tibia or fibula alone are not very common. The tibia can be the site of a stress fracture due to repeated minor trauma probably associated with sport. If the fibula is fractured it may be complicated by a rupture of the inferior tibio-fibular ligament.

Complications

Infection – This is a possible complication as many of these are open fractures. Fortunately the problem is less serious these days with the advent of antibiotics and better care of the wound and soft tissues.

Vascular impairment – This can occur due to damage to a blood vessel or a plaster which is too tight. Great care must be taken by all concerned with the management of these patients to watch for any circulatory deficiency.

Delayed or non-union – Occasionally these fractures are very slow to heal or there may even be non-union.

Physiotherapy management

During immobilization

The first priority is to reduce swelling especially when there has been severe soft-tissue damage. If the patient is in hospital with the leg elevated the physiotherapist must encourage toe and hip movements and static contractions of the muscles round the ankle and knee. As soon as the patient is allowed to walk a correct gait should be taught whether it be non-weight bearing or partial weight bearing with crutches, or later in a walking plaster, or in a functional brace. It is very important that the patient continues the exercises throughout the immobilization period. This may be on their own if the physiotherapist is satisfied that they are being carried out.

After the removal of fixation

An intensive programme of treatment will probably be required to regain full function. Oedema may occur in the lower leg because of muscle weakness and this must be reduced quickly using techniques suitable for the particular patient and with emphasis on movement. Initially the programme will include a larger number of non-weight-bearing exercises and then progressing to partial and full weight bearing as the patient gains range of movement and muscle power. Ideally the patient should attend daily but if this is not possible because they are working or it is too long a distance to travel, or it is an elderly patient then it may be necessary to accept fewer attendances. If the patient is not able to attend as often as is thought necessary then it is very important to gain the cooperation of the patient to undertake a home programme. Patients who are going back to heavy manual work, which involves walking or repetitive leg movements, or who undertake competitive sport will require to have an intensive final stage rehabilitation programme to gain full range, muscle power and endurance for their particular needs. If circumstances allow and facilities are available it may be better for these patients to attend a special rehabilitation centre where they can either be resident or attend daily.

Fractures around the knee

These include fractures of the tibial condyles, the patella and the femoral condyles.

Injury to the tibial condyles usually affects the lateral condyle and may comprise either a comminuted compression or a depressed plateau fracture. In the former case reduction is not usually attempted and early mobilization is encouraged. Depressed plateau fractures require reduction to try to achieve a good articular surface. Following this type of injury the patient may be kept in bed for 3–4 weeks with the knee protected by a posterior plaster shell. Active movements including the knee should be started during this period. Once the patient is allowed to walk they may require some support such as a cast brace, crutches or sticks.

Fractures of the patella can be caused by a direct blow on the knee or a sudden violent contraction of the quadriceps. The former tends to cause a crack or comminuted fracture whereas the latter may produce a transverse fracture. Following a crack fracture the leg is immobilized in a plaster cylinder for about 3 weeks and then active exercises are given to regain full function. Internal fixation may be required if there is separation of the parts and this will be followed by immobilization for about 2 months. If the chances of regaining a smooth contour of the articular surfaces is low then the surgeon may decide to excise the patella as this results in very little loss of function and is preferable to a stiff knee or to developing osteoarthritis, particularly in the elderly patient.

Fractures of the femoral condyles are not very common but a supracondylar fracture occurs more frequently and usually as the result of considerable violence. The patient may be placed in continuous weight traction for approximately 6 weeks and then if union is beginning the leg may be placed in a cast brace and partial weight bearing started. Sometimes open reduction and internal fixation may be used and this has advantages for the elderly and the young as it allows early weight bearing.

Complications

Stiff knee – This could occur as the result of adhesions or because of disruption of the articular surfaces in fractures of the tibial condyles or patella.

Osteoarthritis – This may occur as a late complication following disruption of the articular surfaces.

Genu valgum – This may develop following depression of the lateral tibial condyle.

Physiotherapy management

Haemarthrosis may be a problem after fractures of the tibial condyles and the patella and if this is tense it will probably be aspirated and bandaged firmly. However, the swelling that occurs as a result of a synovitis will gradually absorb and may be assisted by static contractions of the quadriceps and hamstring muscles. If other soft-tissue structures are damaged there may be further swelling in which case the limb should be elevated to assist drainage.

Tibial condyles – Although the patient is on bed rest for a few weeks following compressed fractures exercises are started as soon as possible. Initially toe, ankle and hip movements are carried out with a back slab to support the knee. Static contractions for the quadriceps and hamstrings are commenced and followed by assisted active and then free active knee movements as soon as the pain will allow. Once the patient is allowed up the physiotherapist must teach him or her to use any appliances such as a cast brace, crutches, or sticks and then re-educate a correct gait when the patient is fully weight bearing.

Fractures of the patella – The patient should be taught to do static contractions for the muscles working over the knee although the surgeon may not permit quadriceps contractions for a week or more after excision of the patella. After removal of the plaster cylinder the programme should concentrate on regaining full-range movement of the knee, full muscle power and a normal gait.

Supracondylar fractures – If the patient is in traction active movements for the toes and ankle can be started at once with static contractions for the quadriceps and gluteal muscles. Once the fracture is stable the surgeon may permit knee movements to be started, probably after 2–3 weeks. The physiotherapist must take particular care in dealing with the traction and see that it is left in the correct position. The patient may have a cast brace fitted at 4–6 weeks and walking may be allowed partial weight bearing. The physiotherapist will be able to continue with non-weight-bearing leg exercises and should be able to gain a good range of knee movement before the cast brace is removed and full weight bearing can begin. Final rehabilitation will depend on the assessment and must be linked with the age and needs of the particular patient.

Fractures of the shaft of the femur

These fractures are usually the result of severe violence and may occur at any part of the shaft, and may be of any type – transverse, oblique, spiral and may be comminuted. Usually there is marked displacement with overlap of the fragments which could lead to shortening if this is not corrected. The angulation will depend partly on the injury and partly on muscle spasm pulling the fragment in the direction of the attached muscles. These fractures are often reduced by continuous traction with balanced suspension which is maintained for at least

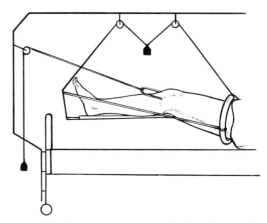

Figure 4.10 Continuous traction with balanced suspension for fractured shaft of femur

6–12 weeks (Figure 4.10). The time will depend on the type of fracture and method of management. If the fracture is uniting and the surgeon considers it a suitable method of treatment a cast brace may be fitted at approximately 6 weeks, and partial weight bearing may be started. For children under the age of 3 'gallows' traction may be used (Figure 4.11). An alternative to traction is the use of an intramedullary

TRACTION FOR CHILD WITH FRACTURED SHAFT OF FEMUR

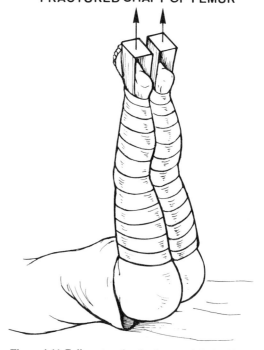

Figure 4.11 Gallows traction for fractured shaft of femur

nail which can either be performed by the closed technique whereby the nail is passed through the greater trochanter and down the shaft or by open reduction and inserting the nail through the fracture site. The closed method is preferable as there is less risk of infection.

Complications

Other injuries – These are likely to occur because of the severity of the injury and may include damage to an artery or nerve, or simultaneous dislocation of the hip.

Infection – As this fracture is often an open fracture there is a risk of infection.

Delayed or non-union – Occasionally a complication of this injury.

Mal-union – If the overlap of the fragments is not reduced or there is redisplacement this can occur with consequent shortening of the femur.

Stiff knee – This is a likely complication particularly if the fracture is near the joint and also when the period in traction is prolonged. The use of the cast brace has helped to decrease this problem.

Physiotherapy management

During immobilization the treatment will depend on the type of fixation and whether there are any other injuries. If the patient has continuous traction applied to the leg the aim of the physiotherapist is to try to minimize the problems that can arise from prolonged immobilization. Exercises for the toes and ankle along with static contractions for the gluteal muscles can be started at once, and it is important to watch for any complications that might arise as the result of damage to arteries or nerves. As soon as the pain has decreased the patient should be taught to do static quadriceps and hamstring contractions. Knee movements can be started in traction although the amount of knee flexion is usually restricted to about 60°. If a cast brace is to be fitted the physiotherapist must prepare the patient for walking partial weight bearing on crutches. During the period in the brace exercises can be continued and muscle power should be improved by increasing the numbers of repetitions for each exercise and performing the movements against gravity when the muscles are strong enough. Once the fixation has been removed the rehabilitation programme must be geared to the problems of the individual patient and their needs.

When the fracture has been fixed internally with an intramedullary nail mobilization can occur more quickly and this can be important with elderly patients. The patient is usually on bed rest for approximately 2–3 weeks but can undertake active leg exercises. Following this the patient will start walking partial weight bearing and progress to full weight bearing once the surgeon is satisfied that the reduction is satisfactory and that union is progressing normally, and the physiotherapist is satisfied that there is adequate muscle power and range of movement.

If the patient has an open reduction the physiotherapist must assess for any post-operative complications. Young children immobilized in a 'gallows' traction tolerate this well and will move around and give themselves adequate exercise and after the removal of the fixation they usually mobilize very quickly. The physiotherapist should assess them in the ward and again when the fixation is removed in case any treatment is required.

Fracture of the upper end of the femur

Trochanteric fractures nearly always occur in the elderly as the result of a fall. In view of the need for early mobilization operative fixation by a compression screw plate, or a nail plate, is the method of choice. The patient is nursed free in bed and is up partial weight bearing in 2–3 days. Occasionally when operative treatment is not practical continuous traction may be used but it has the disadvantage of a long period of bed rest.

Fractures of the neck of the femur – This is a common injury in the elderly and is often due to a trivial injury such as a stumble on an uneven pavement. The reason that this may result in a fracture is because the bone is osteoporotic in many elderly people. The resulting fracture is usually displaced with lateral rotation of the shaft so that the leg will be laterally rotated in comparison with the other limb. Occasionally the fragments are impacted in slight abduction and the patient may be able to get up and walk after the injury. The impacted fracture may be treated conservatively with rest in bed for 2–3 weeks followed by partial weight bearing. The displaced fractures will need operative fixation and the usual method is to excise the head and do a replacemnt arthroplasty using one of the metal prostheses available (Figure 4.12). This is the method of choice because of the danger of avascular necrosis and also the patient can mobilize quickly. An alternative method of fixation is a compression screw plate but if avascular necrosis of the head occurs then it means a second operation.

Complications

Avascular necrosis – This can occur as the blood supply to the head of the femur may be impaired following a fractured neck of femur.

Non-union – This can occur as the result of avascular necrosis or if there is inadequate immobilization.

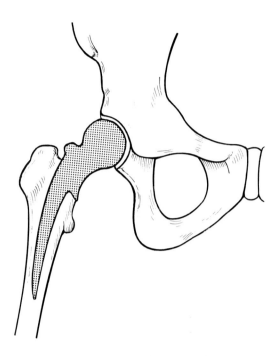

Figure 4.12 Replacement of the femoral head

Osteoarthritis – A later complication due to disruption of the articular surfaces.

Physiotherapy management

As most of these fractures occur in the elderly the main priority of treatment is to regain function and independence as quickly as possible. Following internal fixation for a trochanteric fracture the patient should have active exercises for the leg and be encouraged to move about in bed. As the patient has had surgery the physiotherapist must assess the chest and try to prevent any complications. Once the patient is allowed to walk partial weight bearing the physiotherapist must choose a suitable aid – crutches or a frame – and concentrate on gaining independence.

Physiotherapy will be similar for a fractured neck of femur following a replacement arthroplasty. Once the patient is independent enough to return home domiciliary physiotherapy is important to assess whether the patient can cope at home. Follow-up visits will be needed to ensure that the patient is managing alone or if there are relatives that they know how to help if required. The number of visits will depend on the needs of the patient, for some one may be sufficient whereas others may require a number of visits.

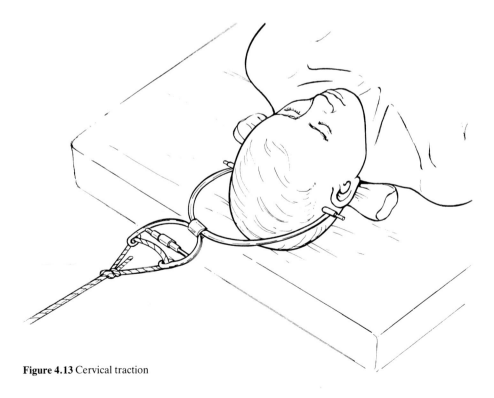

Figure 4.13 Cervical traction

Fractures of the vertebral column, thorax and pelvis

Fractures of the vertebral column

Fractures of the cervical spine are potentially the most dangerous as transection of the spinal cord at this level is likely to be fatal. If the patient survives with neurological damage it could result in a tetraplegia. Injuries of this type may occur as the consequence of a fall on the head from a height, such as may occur from young people diving from a height into water that is too shallow. Compression fractures are the least dangerous as they are the least likely to damage the spinal cord although if osteoarthritis develops there may be pressure on the nerve roots. These are usually treated by rest in a plaster or plastic collar for about 2 months. Fractures that occur with subluxation or dislocation can cause a complete or incomplete lesion of the spinal cord, although remarkably in some instances there may be no damage to the cord or only transient problems due to bruising or oedema. Usually this type of fracture is reduced with skull traction which is maintained until the fracture is stable, and then the patient may be fitted with a collar (Figures 4.13 and 4.14).

Fractures occurring in the thoracic and lumbar regions are the result of either a vertical force causing a compression injury to the vertebrae, or a flexion rotation injury which may give a fracture dislocation. In the latter case there is the likelihood of damage to the spinal cord or the cauda equina resulting in a paraplegia. Fixation is not required for compression injuries and the patient is nursed free

in bed for 1–3 weeks and then allowed up. Fracture dislocations with no nerve damage are reduced and have internal fixation because of the risk of any further displacement damaging the spinal cord or cauda equina in the lumbar region. At one time fracture dislocations that had caused a paraplegia were left without reduction, but the current treatment is by reduction and internal fixation as it is difficult to know the extent of the neurological damage at first.

Complications

Neurological damage – The extent of the disability will depend on the level of the lesion and whether it results in a complete or incomplete transection of the spinal cord or cauda equina.

Physiotherapy management

The management of patients with a tetraplegia or paraplegia is dealt with in Chapter 20 under Diseases of the Nervous System.

Patients who have had fractures in the cervical region uncomplicated by any neurological disease may suffer from considerable pain and stiffness in the neck for a long time after the initial injury. Some older patients may have had minor symptoms of cervical spondylosis prior to the injury and these symptoms may be exacerbated afterwards. The physiotherapist must assess the patient carefully before deciding on a suitable treatment plan to relieve the pain, improve the range of movement and strengthen the muscles. It is necessary to consider the posture of the patient and to find suitable positions for sleeping, sitting and working which will relieve the pain.

Compression fractures in the thoracic and lumbar vertebrae can be treated while on bed rest with techniques to relieve the pain caused by the muscle spasm. As the pain decreases the patient can be taught to do static contractions for the abdominal and back muscles, followed by active movements in the pain-free range. Once the patient is up and has been discharged from hospital a more vigorous rehabilitation programme can be started in the physiotherapy department. Many of the patients suffering this type of injury undertake heavy manual work such as mining or building and the injury occurred at work. In order to return to work they must have recovered full function and be strong enough to undertake the work. Thus an intensive programme of rehabilitation is required not only to mobilize and strengthen the back but for the whole body. If possible these patients should attend a special rehabilitation centre where they can have a full daily programme geared both to the individual needs of the patient and to their work.

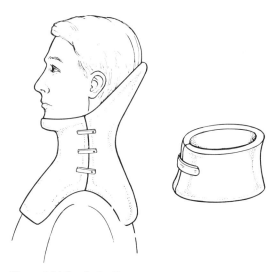

Figure 4.14 Cervical collars

Fractures of the thoracic cage

Fractures of the ribs can occur by direct violence or sometimes spontaneously as the result of a forced respiratory movement as in laughing or coughing. These fractures heal easily and the main problem is pain which will restrict normal breathing. Fractures that pierce the pleural cavity and possibly the lung are serious and it may be necessary to insert a drain in the pleural cavity to remove any air or fluid.

Severe injuries that fracture the sternum and/or cause multiple fractures of ribs can result from direct violence which may occur in a road accident or similar trauma.

Complications

Pulmonary problems – Following simple fractures these can occur if the patient is unable to obtain full expansion as a result of pain and pneumonia may develop, particularly in the elderly. Fractures that pierce the pleura and/or lung tissue can lead to complications such as pneumothorax, haemothorax, surgical emphysema or paradoxical respiration.

Physiotherapy management

The majority of simple fractures will not require any physiotherapy, but if there is a risk of pulmonary complications developing breathing exercises should be given to ensure full use of the thorax and expansion of the lungs. Pain may prevent full movement and it may be necessary to give the patient an analgesic or local anaesthetic prior to treatment.

Severe chest injuries may need the attention of both the orthopaedic and thoracic surgeons and the patient is likely to be in the intensive therapy unit, particularly if a tracheostomy is required. Physiotherapy management for patients in the intensive therapy unit is dealt with in Chapter 13. The emphasis must be on removing any secretions and regaining full expansion of the lungs.

Fractures of the pelvis

The majority of pelvic fractures are caused by direct violence occurring from falls or blows, or in the case of the severer forms by crushing. Apart from the shock sustained by the patient at the time of the injury, or from damage to the pelvic organs, the injury is rarely dangerous and if displacement occurs it may be minimal because of the support afforded to the bone by the numerous muscles and ligaments attached to its surface.

The pelvic ring may be described as consisting of two segments, the anterior or pubic portion which protects the pelvic organs and provides for the attachment of the muscles of the lower extremity, and the postero-lateral or iliac portion which transmits the weight of the body to the legs. An isolated fracture in either segment is not as a rule serious unless it is complicated by damage to the internal organs. The same is true of double or even multiple fractures in the anterior segment provided that there is no fracture or dislocation in the iliac segment. But if there are two or more fractures or dislocations with at least one in each segment then the displacement may be considerable. It is brought about both by the causative force and by the pull of the muscles passing from the spine to the pelvis or femur. For fractures with little displacement complete immobilization is not necessary and usually the patient is rested in bed for 1–3 weeks and then allowed to get up. When the pelvic ring is severely disrupted then reduction and fixation is necessary. If it is possible to reduce the displacement manually then fixation may be by means of a plaster spica but otherwise another method of external fixation may be used (pins through the iliac bones and fixed to a transverse bar).

Complications

There may be injuries to the bladder or urethra and possibly to other tissues within the pelvis. Osteoarthritis may be a late complication if there has been disruption of the acetabulum at the time of the injury.

Physiotherapy management

For fractures where there is little displacement and the patient is on bed rest exercises should be given to the legs. If there is some pain when weight bearing is allowed the patient may require crutches, sticks or a frame until this has decreased and it will be necessary to re-educate gait. Physiotherapy management for patients with displaced fractures and some type of fixation will be similar but progress will be much slower. If the patient is in a plaster spica then it will be necessary to teach static contractions for the leg and trunk muscles. Once the fixation has been removed the patient is likely to require a programme to regain the full range of movement in the joints of the leg and trunk and to re-educate walking.

Chapter 5

Dislocations

A *dislocation* of a joint occurs when the articular surfaces are completely separated from each other so that all apposition is lost (Figure 5.1).

Subluxation occurs when the articular surfaces are partially separated but there is still some part of each surface in contact (Figure 5.2).

The main cause of either dislocations or subluxations is trauma. Congenital malformation of the joint surfaces can occur and this could result in dislocation, as for example in a congenital dislocation of the hip. Dislocations can also occur when there is extensive muscle paralysis around a joint, for example in the shoulder of a patient with a hemiplegia when there is no return of muscle power around the shoulder. Subluxations can occur in patients suffering from rheumatoid arthritis when

there is destruction of joint surfaces and soft-tissue changes. Some joints are more likely to dislocate than others because of their anatomical structure, and this is particularly so in the case of the shoulder.

Many traumatic dislocations are associated with fractures and a number of these were mentioned in the previous chapter: fracture dislocation of the elbow, fracture dislocation of the ankle and fracture dislocation of the vertebrae. Usually dislocations due to trauma are accompanied by severe soft-tissue damage due to stretching or tearing of the structures around the joint. Ligaments may be partially or completely ruptured and may need surgical repair. Muscles, tendons, synovial sheaths and cartilage may also be damaged.

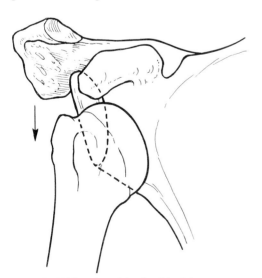

Figure 5.1 Dislocation of the shoulder joint

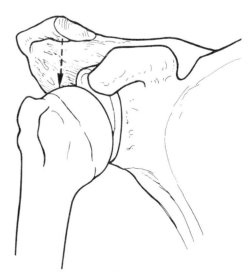

Figure 5.2 Subluxation of the shoulder joint

Traumatic dislocations

Clinical features

These will depend on whether there is a subluxation or dislocation as the clinical features arising from the former will be less obvious.

At the time of injury

1. Immediately there is an intense sickening pain which is often worse than that experienced with a fracture. The patient is conscious of a tearing sensation which differs from the sensation of breaking or snapping of a bone occurring with a fracture.
2. Deformity – this may be very obvious with a dislocation as the normal contour of the joint may be changed. However, there may be occasions when the deformity is not discernible or there is an accompanying fracture which may cause the dislocation to be overlooked.
3. Loss of function – the patient will not be able to move the limb.

Later features

1. *Swelling* – This occurs as the result of the tearing of the soft-tissue structures and the consequent inflammatory reaction. Exudation from an inflammatory reaction within the joint capsule will be serofibrinous and enhances the risk of adhesions.
2. *Bruising (ecchymosis)* – This is due to the extravasation of blood from the injured vessels.
3. *Stiffness* – If adhesions develop this could create a problem in regaining function.
4. *Muscle weakness* – This will occur in muscles around the joint and possibly in the rest of the limb if it is immobilized for any length of time.

The dislocations and subluxations described below are those that occur fairly commonly and where the physiotherapy management may be important.

Shoulder joint

This is a common dislocation in adults and can occur as the result of direct violence or, more frequently, indirect violence. The latter, which may occur due to a fall on the outstretched hand, tends to produce an anterior dislocation in which the head of the humerus is displaced forward and then lies in the infraclavicular fossa just below the coracoid process (subcoracoid dislocation). The former may be the result of a direct blow on the front of the shoulder, or sometimes the consequence of an epileptic convulsion, which may produce a posterior dis-location whereby the humeral head is displaced backwards and may come to lie below the spine of the scapula in the infraspinous fossa (subspinous dislocation). The dislocation is reduced as soon as possible as apart from the intense pain and loss of function further damage could result from prolonged stretching of the tissues. Further management will depend on the age of the patient. An elderly patient will have the arm rested in a large arm sling or a collar and cuff for a few days, whilst a young patient may have the arm bandaged to the chest for 2–3 weeks because of the danger of recurrent dislocation.

Complications

Axillary nerve lesion – This is more likely to occur with an anterior than a posterior dislocation and results in paralysis of deltoid and loss of sensation over a small area on the upper lateral aspect of the arm. This could be due to stretching causing an axonotmesis or to pressure resulting in a neuropraxia. The latter will recover within a few weeks but the former will take longer because degeneration will have occurred.

Associated fracture – Dislocation may be accompanied by a fracture of the greater tuberosity.

Recurrent dislocation – In some instances the damage caused by the dislocation does not heal and redislocation may occur. Once this happens further dislocations are likely and with the increasing frequency the initiating injury may be very slight. The damage involves the capsule being torn from the anterior rim of the glenoid cavity and the articular surface of the head of the humerus is dented postero-laterally. Recurrent dislocation occurs more often in the young probably because the initial trauma has been more severe and if they continue to take part in sports or are very active a minor injury may cause a further dislocation. In cases where redislocation is frequent and it upsets the normal activities of the person then surgery is advised. There are several surgical procedures but those commonly used are the Putti Platt whereby the subscapularis muscle is shortened to limit lateral rotation, and the Bankart which comprises reattaching the capsule to the rim of the glenoid cavity.

Physiotherapy management

This will differ according to the age of the patient.

Elderly patients

The mechanism causing the dislocation could be relatively trivial as the muscles may be weaker in the older person and the rotator cuff may not give the same stability to the shoulder joint as in a younger person. In such cases the soft-tissue damage may not be as extensive and treatment should start the day after the dislocation has been reduced. For the first day or two treatment should concentrate on moving the fingers, wrist, elbow and shoulder girdle. It is important to gain the cooperation of the patient and help them to relax. Sometimes heat and massage may help to achieve relaxation and enable the patient to begin gentle movements of the shoulder. Because of the nature of the injury it is usually easier to start with flexion/extension and leave rotation till last. The emphasis must be on regaining range of movement and function, as many elderly people will develop a stiff shoulder if they are not mobilized early. In the first few days following the injury it may be necessary to help the patient with axillary care until she can manage on her own. If the physiotherapist is the only health care professional seeing the patient in the early stage it is important to see that she can manage the activities of daily living on her own or with help from relatives. Otherwise it may be necessary to ask for support from the social services.

It may not be possible to regain full range of movement in the shoulder joint but this does not matter provided that the patient can perform all the functional activities that are required.

Young patients

There is not the same risk of developing a stiff shoulder in the young as in the elderly and so the shoulder may be kept bandaged to the chest for 2–3 weeks to allow healing of the soft tissues. This may help to lessen the chance of recurrent dislocation if there is not too much damage. During this time the patient can be taught to do static contractions for the muscles around the shoulder. Once the bandage has been removed the physiotherapist may find that the range of movement is quite good, in which case it is important to strengthen the adductors and medial rotators. Final rehabilitation will depend on the needs of the individual and some patients may need little or no treatment. However, patients returning to physical activity, whether work or competitive sport, may require an intensive programme with particular emphasis on developing muscle power throughout the range of movement.

In both of the above groups of patients the physiotherapist should ensure that there is active contraction of deltoid in the first few days of treatment. If there is an axillary nerve lesion, particularly an axonotmesis, then the physiotherapist will be concerned with re-educating the deltoid.

Patients who undergo surgery for a recurrent dislocation may have the shoulder immobilized for 3–4 weeks depending on the particular procedure and the surgeon. After this the patient will require a rehabilitation programme to regain range of movement, muscle power and full function. Because of the nature of the repair it may not be possible to regain full lateral rotation but it is unlikely to impede the activities of the patient.

Acromio-clavicular joint dislocation or subluxation

This may occur as the result of a fall on the shoulder and is a fairly common injury in contact sports, particularly rugby. A dislocation usually involves tearing of the conoid and trapezoid ligaments and consequently there is marked displacement. Internal fixation may be required to hold the joint in position until the ligaments heal, approximately 6–8 weeks. A subluxation is unlikely to rupture the ligaments and it is usually sufficient to support the arm in a sling for a couple of weeks.

Physiotherapy management

Following a subluxation the patient may not need any treatment apart from advice on when to move and how to progress movements. But after a dislocation and internal fixation the patient may need a more carefully supervised programme for the shoulder joint and shoulder girdle.

Elbow joint

Dislocation of the elbow joint usually occurs as the result of a fall on the outstretched hand, the ulna and radius being displaced posteriorly or postero-laterally. It is a common injury in children and also occurs in adults. There may be an accompanying fracture but the dislocation and associated soft-tissue injuries are the more important. The dislocation is reduced and the arm is rested in a posterior plaster slab with the elbow at approximately 90° for about 3 weeks. Sometimes a complete plaster is used but the posterior slab is preferable as swelling within the plaster could cause compression on vessels.

Complications

Vascular – As mentioned in Fractures (Chapter 4), around the elbow there is a danger of damage to the brachial artery which could result in a Volkmann's ischaemic contracture if the circulation is not restored before irreparable damage has occurred.

Nerve injury – This was also mentioned in Chapter 4.

Stiffness – Intra- and periarticular adhesions can make it difficult to regain full range of movement.

Post-traumatic ossification – see Fractures of the upper arm (page 22).

Physiotherapy management

This is similar to the treatment described for fractures around the elbow. Immediately after the injury care must be taken to watch for any impairment of circulation, or any loss of sensation or muscle power that could result from nerve injury. Once the fixation has been removed the emphasis is on regaining the range of movement and muscle power. No passive stretching should be used and the physiotherapist must advise the patient, or in the case of a child the parents, about the type of activity that can be undertaken. A supervised programme is advisable if there is a marked loss of movement due to the formation of adhesions.

Metacarpo-phalangeal and interphalangeal joints

Subluxation in these joints may occur as the result of pathological changes in rheumatoid arthritis. The first metacarpophalangeal joint is the most likely of these joints to be dislocated by a hyperextension injury, although sometimes it may be the carpometacarpal joint. The dislocation is reduced and the thumb supported by strapping with early movement being encouraged.

Dislocation of an interphalangeal joint is usually caused by forced hyperextension. The dislocation is reduced and although no immobilization is required some form of support may help to relieve the pain and allow movement of the hand.

Physiotherapy management

Treatment may not be required unless there is marked swelling, in which case the patient should be advised to keep the arm resting with the hand above the level of the shoulder when he is sitting for the first few days. Active movements for the arm should be started at once, and finger movements as soon as the patient can tolerate doing them. If there is residual limitation of movement when the swelling has decreased then an intensive treatment programme may be necessary to regain full function.

Hip joint

Although the hip is a ball-and-socket type joint its structure is very different from that of the shoulder, being considerably more stable and protected by strong ligaments, and so dislocation is relatively uncommon. Direct violence such as a car or motorcycle accident is the most likely cause of injury. The person is probably in the sitting position and a direct blow on the front of the knee forces the thigh back resulting in a posterior dislocation of the hip. After the dislocation has been reduced the patient is placed in light traction for 3–6 weeks. Active movements are started as soon as the pain will allow and continued after the traction is removed if necessary.

Complications

Damage to the sciatic nerve – Following a posterior dislocation there may be pressure on the sciatic nerve resulting in a neuropraxia. Provided that the pressure is removed recovery will occur in a few weeks. However, if more extensive damage has occurred resulting in degeneration of the nerve fibres then the prognosis may be poor.

Associated injuries – This dislocation is caused by severe violence and there will probably be a fracture dislocation with a portion of the bone from the acetabulum being taken off by the force of the impact. There may be other fractures in the limb or other parts of the body.

Osteoarthritis – This may occur at a later stage if the dislocation has damaged the articular surface.

Physiotherapy management

During the period in traction the patient should do active exercises for the hip, knee and foot to regain range of movement and muscle power. Following removal of the traction the patient may commence walking, partial weight bearing progressing to full weight bearing as soon as possible. The amount of treatment required will depend on the problems of the individual patient and their functional requirements. Because of the nature of the injury it can affect all age groups and so their needs will vary.

Patella

The patella can dislocate either as the result of an injury or due to a congenital abnormality. In the former case the dislocation is reduced and the knee is firmly bandaged for a few days. In the latter case there is recurrent dislocation which tends to occur with greater frequency and more easily as time passes. As a rule it does not happen in young children but seems to start in adolescence and is more common in girls than boys. Surgery may be required and this comprises transposing the insertion of the quadriceps from the tibial tubercle to a position that is more medial and distal. Thus contraction of the quadriceps will tend to pull the patella more medially.

Complications

Patellofemoral arthritis.

Physiotherapy management

Following traumatic dislocation little treatment should be required apart from strengthening the quadriceps. In the instance of recurrent dislocation various techniques have been used to strengthen the quadriceps, particularly vastus medialis, in order to reduce the tendency to dislocate. However, it is likely that surgery may be needed and this would be followed by a physiotherapy programme to strengthen the quadriceps and regain function.

Chapter 6

Soft-tissue injuries

Introduction

Soft-tissue injury comprises damage to ligaments, muscles, tendons with synovial sheaths, fascia and intra-articular cartilage.

All of these tissues are injured when bones are fractured or joints dislocated. There are, therefore, principles of treatment which are common to all injuries. This chapter is directed at the management of injuries without fracture or joint dislocation.

Anatomy and physiology

Ligaments

These are comprised of white connective tissue which forms bands either inside or outside the capsule of a synovial joint. They are tough, inelastic and unyielding but flexible and pliant so that they direct, limit and control normal movement whilst enabling it. Ligaments are attached to and blend with the periosteum of bones. A ligament is taut at the limit of the movement it prevents but is not designed to withstand prolonged tension which can result in pain.

Skeletal muscles

These are contractile, extensible structures which both produce and control movements. Muscles are composed of muscle fibres supported by connective fibroid tissue. Fibres may be type I (red, slow) or type II (white, fast). Most muscles are composed of a mixture of the two types but postural muscles tend to have more type I and muscles producing rapid movements have more type II. The muscle fibres blend with tendons (teno-muscular junction) which in turn blend with the periosteum of bones (teno-periosteal junction). Where muscles do not have tendons, attachment to bones is by blending of the fibrous tissue (endomysium, perimysium, epimysium) with the periosteum. Muscles with extensive attachments are connected by broad, tough sheets of white fibrous tissue termed aponeuroses. Muscles may also be attached to ligaments, cartilage, fascia and skin. Muscle fibres vary in arrangement and direction which enables the muscle to produce the functions of joint movement and stability. The strength of a muscle depends on the number of muscle fibres. For example, pennate muscles have many muscle fibres attached along the length of a tendon giving strength but a restricted range of movement (e.g. deltoid muscle).

Tendons

These are tough white cords of fibrous tissue, which do not have any elasticity. They vary in length and thickness according to the site within the body. Most muscles have tendons at one end. A tendon may be enclosed in a synovial sheath to prevent friction and may be separated from neighbouring structures by a bursa. They are very strong structures and so are rarely ruptured but injuries occur at the attachment to bone or the teno-muscular junction.

Fascia

This is composed of connective tissue and consists of two layers: superficial and deep.

Superficial

This is loose fibro-areolar tissue consisting of bundles of white collagen fibres with some yellow elastic fibres. It contains tissue fluid, connective tissue cells and fat in varying quantities.

The functions are to:

1. Store food reserves, e.g. fat.
2. Maintain warmth.
3. Facilitate movement of the skin.
4. Support nerves and blood vessels passing to and from the skin.

It varies in thickness, being thicker on the lower abdominal wall, the sole of the foot and palm of the hand. It is looser on the dorsum of the foot and hand which is why oedema is common in these areas. It may contain muscles, e.g. platysma.

Deep

This consists of well-defined, tough sheets of white fibrous tissue, forming inelastic tight-fitting sheaths round muscles. It separates muscles from each other, binding them down and holding them in place, as well as providing additional means of attachment. It provides inelastic support for veins and lymph vessels. It is thickened in certain areas, e.g. the iliotibial tract and retinaculae round the wrist and ankle where it keeps tendons in position.

Nutrition

Ligaments, tendons and fascia receive nutrition from a few blood vessels. Muscles receive nutrition from blood vessels contained within the fascia forming the sheaths. None of these structures have a rich blood supply.

Injuries to ligaments

Definitions

Sprain, strain and rupture are terms used to denote injuries. Acute sprain of a ligament is caused by a sudden twisting or wrenching of a joint which results in overstretching of the ligament. It is associated with the muscles controlling the joint being momentarily off guard so that the ligament is subjected to the full force of the movement. Only some of the fibres are ruptured, the severity of the injury depending on the number of fibres affected. The joint remains stable but the quality of stability depends on the number of fibres remaining intact.

Chronic sprain of a ligament is caused by repetitive stretching from a minor force which may be due to bad postural habit or poor quality of movement.

Strain may be used as a term in the diagnosis of partially ruptured ligaments but is more commonly applied to muscle and tendon injuries. Complete rupture is disruption of all fibres of the ligament caused by a sudden, violent force such that the joint is unstable.

Pathology – healing of ligaments

Ligaments, having only fair vascularity, heal slowly. Since they have no specialized cells, repair is always by fibrous tissue. Completely ruptured ligaments must be sutured and protected for lengthy periods. Otherwise the fibrous tissue forms a weak union between the ends of the fibres. The danger then is that the ligament lengthens and does not perform its stabilizing and controlling functions. Sprained ligaments also heal by fibrous tissue. The degree of protection required during healing depends upon the severity of the injury. It is important to gauge the point at which mobility must be rehabilitated because the healing fibrous tissue may form adhesions. The danger then is that the ligament, being bound to neighbouring structures, is prone to further injury and the movement controlled by the ligament is painful and limited (Evans, 1980).

Acute sprains: clinical features

History – There is a history of injury which the patient can usually describe.

Pain – There is a sudden pain and feeling of nausea at the time of the injury. The intensity of pain reduces but can be reproduced if the causative movement is repeated. As healing occurs the pain becomes less constant and is reproduced only if the ligament is stretched.

Swelling – This occurs rapidly and is due to escaping of tissue fluid into the fascial spaces around the ligament. Later, inflammatory exudate is a component of the swelling. If the joint capsule is injured, synovial fluid may be present in the swollen area.

Bruising – Blood escapes from injured blood vessels into neighbouring tissues. The red blood cells break down, releasing constituent pigments which produce the various colours of bruising. The presence of plasmaprotein fibrinogen in tissue fluid is a disadvantage because fibrin is formed, producing consolidation of the tissue fluid. Chronic swelling can result if treatment is ineffective. If blood goes into a joint space there is a haemarthrosis which limits joint movement.

Loss of movement – Protective muscle spasm and pain limit joint movement.

Loss of function – A lower limb ligament injury will prevent use of the limb, especially in walking and running. An upper limb ligament injury makes many activities of daily living difficult, e.g. dressing, writing.

Chronic sprains: clinical features

History – There is recurrent minor injury which may or may not be known to the patient. It may be necessary for the physiotherapist to analyse activities or sport techniques to identify the cause.

Pain – This is a dull aching around the area of the injured ligament. It may be constant or intermittent, tends to increase with activities which move the joint controlled by the ligament and may be superimposed occasionally by sharp stabbing pain.

Swelling – There is often an area over the ligament which feels like thickened jelly and cannot be moved like the fluid swelling of acute injuries.

Loss of movement – The movement controlled by the ligament is equally limited both passively and actively.

Instability – If the ligament is subjected to frequent prolonged stretching, it becomes weakened and the joint becomes unstable. Instability may also be due to loss of proprioceptive input due to damage of the mechano-receptors.

Loss of function – Activities are impaired and the muscles producing the movements of the affected joints tire more readily. Following activity, the patient may feel stiff and sore in the affected part.

Complete ruptures

History – The patient reports a definite injury often with an audible snap. Sometimes it is described like a kick or blow over the site of the rupture.

Pain – Sometimes there is little or no pain immediately after the injury but usually there is severe, sickening pain. The intensity reduces over the first few days, with treatment.

Swelling – A large amount of swelling forms rapidly, indicating gross tissue damage.

Bruising – This occurs as in acute sprains.

Loss of function – There is severe loss of function of the affected limb, e.g. weight bearing is impossible with a lower limb injury.

Treatment of ligaments

Acute injuries

Early management of an acute injury is very important in relation to the long-term outcome. The main aims as soon as the injury has occurred are as follows:

1. To enable healing to take place.

2. To reduce the risk of further injury.
3. To minimize swelling.

The important themes are, therefore rest, support, cold, compression and controlled exercise.

The main aims as healing takes place are:

1. To prevent adhesion formation.
2. To strengthen the muscles related to the ligament.
3. To re-educate proprioception.
4. To restore full mobility of the ligament and corresponding joint.
5. To restore the patient's confidence.
6. To restore the patient to full functional activity.

The main themes are therefore active exercises, manual and mechanical resistance, manipulative procedures, electrical procedures such as ultrasound, pulsed electromagnetic energy and functional activities appropriate to the limb affected.

Chronic injuries

The important aspects of the management of chronic injuries are:

1. To identify the cause of the repeated trauma to which the ligament is subjected.
2. To treat the ligament.
3. To prevent recurrence.

Identifying the cause demands careful, logical analysis of the patient's life-style. It is important to include positions that may cause long-term stress, e.g. sitting with the feet held in inversion stretches the lateral ligament of the ankle joint; always running clockwise round an athletics track stretches the right lateral and left medial ankle ligaments with shortening of the opposite ligaments. Poor posture tends to put long-term stress on ligaments. Changing the grip of a racquet or golf club can stress the ligaments of the hand and wrist. The patient can often trace the onset of pain in a ligament back to a change in technique or equipment at work or at play but may have to be prompted by the physiotherapist to remember this.

Treatment is directed at achieving the following aims:

1. To mobilize the ligament from underlying structures.
2. To restore flexibility to the ligament.
3. To strengthen the muscles related to the ligament.
4. To re-educate proprioception.
5. To re-educate function and the patient's confidence.

Mobility of the joint is regained by soft-tissue manipulation to reduce swelling and to restore mobility to all soft tissues within their fascial planes.

Active exercises are essential. Mobilizations are usually required and are generally essential to restore accessory movements especially where there is a complexity of joints involved, e.g. tarsal, carpal, elbow, intervertebral joints. Where pain is a restricting factor, pulsed electromagnetic energy, or interferential treatment may be used.

Flexibility of the ligament can be regained by using transverse frictions, passive stretching, ultrasound and active exercise.

Strengthening of the muscles is achieved by active exercise resisted manually or mechanically.

Proprioception can be re-educated by propriocep-tive neuromuscular facilitation techniques, weight-bearing activities, coordination exercises, and for lower limb injuries, balance (wobble) boards.

Prevention of recurrence

This starts by eliminating, where possible, the causative factors or repeated stress.

General fitness is important with an exercise programme designed to increase the flexibility of ligaments. Before activity, which may be high-level competitive sport or the occasional weekend gardening, warm-up is essential. This includes stretching and jogging for anything from 5 to 20 minutes beforehand depending on the intended activity.

Clothing needs to provide warmth and protection together with freedom of movement. Equipment must be reliable and appropriate to the activity as well as to the individual.

Complete rupture

As with acute injuries, early management is vital to enable good long-term outcome.

The two principal methods are:

1. Surgical repair followed by immobilization.
2. Immobilization in a shortened position.

In both instances, the joint is fixed so that the ligament is in a shortened position.

During the period of fixation the main aims are:

1. To encourage healing.
2. To minimize adhesion formation.
3. To maintain the strength of the muscles related to the ligament.
4. To maintain function.

The main themes are therefore active exercises, functional use of the limb and specific exercises to work the muscles isometrically over the fixed joints.

After the fixation is removed the principles of treatment are similar to those for chronic ligament injuries.

Principles applied – Ankle ligaments

The ligaments of the ankle are injured when the plantar-flexed foot is forced suddenly into inversion (lateral ligament) or eversion (medial ligament). Injury of the lateral ligament is the most common.

Acute sprain – lateral ligament

Aetiology

This injury is common in sports activities such as pole vaulting, cross country running and hiking. It is also quite common in general terms when a person slips off a pavement or walks on uneven surfaces. The mechanism is for the foot to be forced into inversion and plantar flexion. The site of the injury is generally between the centre and the distal attachments of the middle and anterior bands of the ligament.

Clinical features

History – The patient describes 'going over' at the ankle.

Pain – There is sharp pain just below and anterior to the lateral malleolus at the time of the injury. Passive stretching and weight bearing increase the pain.

Swelling – This is present from the lateral border of the tendo Achillis, over the lateral malleolus along the dorsum of the foot. In severe injuries, the swelling may spread to the dorsum of the toes and up the leg.

Bruising – This appears under the lateral malleolus and over the dorsum of the foot.

Loss of function – All weight bearing is painful so the patient cannot run and has a gait with a very short stance phase on the affected foot.

Treatment

Immediate

Application of cold – The foot and leg may be immersed in ice-cold water to mid-calf level for 20 minutes. Alternatively, the leg may be placed in elevation and a towel, wrung out in icy water, wrapped round the foot and ankle for 20 minutes.

Compression and support – A minor sprain may be treated with a crêpe or elastic bandage (Figure 6.1(a)), which may have reinforcing zinc oxide strips (Figure 6.1(b)). A more severe injury requires a pressure bandage. Walking can be permitted in a minor injury but running, jumping and such activities must be avoided for a few days. In severe injuries, the patient is advised to rest with the limb in elevation and to use crutches for getting about. The foot should be moved up and down five times every hour when the limb is elevated.

Subsequent treatment

After 2–3 days the treatment may be as follows.

Ultrasound applied over the site of the injury helps to limit adhesion formation by moving inflammatory exudate. It also stimulates repair of collagen. Generally the dosage would start at 3 MHz, pulsed 0.25 W cm^{-2} for 5 minutes. As healing takes place, this may be altered to an intensity of 0.5–0.8 W cm^{-2} and a time up to 10 minutes to accelerate the rate of recovery.

Massage may be applied in the form of kneading and effleurage to soften and clear the oedema. This must be done as early as possible to prevent consolidation of the fluid resulting in chronic oedema and permanent impairment of function.

Exercises

Free active exercises practised every hour may be: lying (legs elevated):

1. Feet pushing down and pulling up.
2. Feet turning out and holding.
3. Feet turning out and upwards.
4. Feet turning out and downwards.

Notes

1. Performing the exercises with both feet provides a comparison for the patient for full range between affected and non-affected foot.
2. Each movement is repeated 5–10 times.

The same exercises may be repeated with the patient in half-lying and then in cross-legged sitting.

Manual resistance is then added by the physiotherapist. The patient may then be taught auto-resistance using the other foot or the hand.

As the pain subsides – within 7 days – active inversion must be started. The patient is instructed to turn the foot in at both forefoot and heel, hold at the point of stretch and release. The movement should be eased into new range and plantar flexion added.

About 6 days after a minor strain and 2 weeks after a more severe injury the ligament is treated by passive stretching. If this is virtually pain free, weight-bearing exercises may be started, such as:

1. Sitting:
   (a) Marking time, raising heels and toes alternately.
   (b) Turning feet and heels in and out.
2. Standing (holding onto chair or wall) – exercises as above.

Repeat these exercises standing without support.

In all these exercises it is important that the movements are restricted to the foot and ankle, so the patient must keep the legs still.

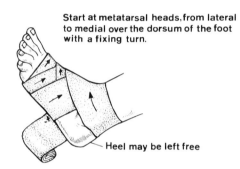

Start at metatarsal heads, from lateral to medial over the dorsum of the foot with a fixing turn.

Heel may be left free

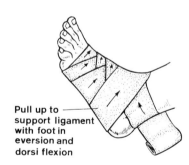

Pull up to support ligament with foot in eversion and dorsi flexion

(a)

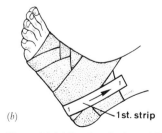

(b)   1st. strip

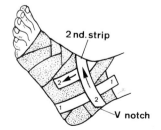

2nd. strip

V notch

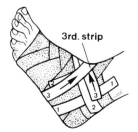

3rd. strip

Figure 6.1 (*a*) Bandage for lateral ligament of the ankle. (*b*) Zinc oxide reinforcement

Balance must be practised

1. Standing on affected leg – holding steady:
   (a) Eyes closed, hold steady.
   (b) Moving arms in different directions.
   (c) Throwing and catching a ball.
2. Standing on a balance board (wobble board):
   (a) Hold board level and steady.
   (b) Stand on affected leg only. Hold. Progress as above.
3. Propulsion activities:
   (a) Spring start position: alternately bend one leg up and thrust other leg back.
   (b) Standing:
       Bob jumps, increasing height.
       Sideways jumping either side of a line.
       Star jumps.
   (c) Skipping.
   (d) Hopping.

Activities are then tailored to the patient's individual needs (see Appendix I).

Walking re-education

Concurrent with the exercise programme it is important to progress walking. In minor injuries a walking aid is not usually necessary. In more severe injuries, the patient should be able to walk with one stick in the opposite hand by 2 weeks and discard this support in 3–4 weeks. The pain initially reduces the stance phase, and so even pacing and timing must be taught. The push-off also needs practice as the plantar flexion pulls on the anterior band of the ligament. Final re-education involves walking over uneven surfaces.

Other treatments

Interferential therapy or pulsed electromagnetic energy may be used to relieve pain and reduce swelling.

Transverse frictions are usually necessary to soften adhesions and restore pliability to the ligament.

Passive stretching may also be used to restore pliability – the patient should be taught to stretch by plantar flexing and inverting the foot then pulling the heel inwards. It is essential to repeat this until there is no discomfort so that the ligament is mobile and less prone to further injury.

Mobilizations are essential to restore accessory gliding of the ankle, subtalar and intertarsal joints. In addition physiological movements to regain inversion are often useful.

Support

As swelling is reduced, the pressure bandage is replaced by a crêpe elastic bandage or elastic strapping. A support which can be removed for electrical treatment and soft-tissue manipulation is sensible, but if the patient cannot attend for physiotherapy an elastic adhesive strapping should be used. Tubigrip (elasticated tubular bandage) may be used for weight bearing activities up to 3 weeks after severe injury, or 4–6 weeks after a severe injury. Protective strapping may be necessary for another 4 weeks for stressful sporting activities.

Chronic sprain – lateral ligament

Identifying the cause

Causes may be:

1. Poor reflex coordination of peronei to prevent twisting during walking over uneven ground.
2. Poor support from footwear – worn heels or old shoes which have become too large.
3. Prolonged sitting with feet turned in (causes lengthening).
4. Poor foot posture with feet everted (causes shortening).

Clinical features

Pain – Dull ache over ligament which may become more sharp during prolonged walking or running.

Swelling – Thickened swelling is often present under the lateral malleolus and along the tendo Achillis.

Loss of movement – Plantar flexion with inversion is limited and feels tight.

Instability – Balancing on the affected leg is more difficult than on the other leg even though muscle power may not be remarkably diminished. This tends to lead to the ankle 'going over' especially on uneven surfaces.

Treatment

Transverse frictions

These are necessary to restore pliability to the anterior and middle bands of the ligament.

Passive stretching

This is appropriate where the ligament is shortened and the patient should be taught how to pull the calcaneum medially to stretch the middle band.

Mobilizations

As accessory and physiological movements these are usually required to restore mobility to one or more of the intertarsal, the ankle and possibly inferior tibio-fibular joints. Meticulous examination is required of the accessory movements of the intertarsal joints with the foot at the limits of plantar/dorsiflexion and inversion or eversion as sometimes the stiffness causing the problem is quite subtle.

Ultrasound

Given with the ligament on a stretch this can help to mobilize adhesions or reduce any chronic swelling, e.g. $0.8\,W\,cm^{-2}$ $3\,MHz$ continuous: 5 minutes, to start with and if greater effect is required, increase to $1\,W\,cm^{-2}$.

Interferential therapy and pulsed electromagnetic energy

These may be used to reduce swelling and relieve pain.

Resisted exercises

Where peroneal muscle incompetence or weakness is a feature PNF slow reversals, or resistance in pattern with holds in eversion are invaluable. The commonest pattern used is dorsiflexion, eversion with knee extension and medial rotation at the hip. Spring resistance may be applied with a sling round the foot and the spring fixed medially.

Free active exercises

Mobility of the joints is gained and retained if the patient practises in half-lying and cross-leg sitting:

1. Foot circling with emphasis on keeping leg steady and making a big circle.
2. Foot pulling up and in, then pushing down and out.
3. Foot pulling up and out then pushing down and in.

Balance boards

After correct foot posture awareness has been grasped by the patient, balance board practice should be given as in recovery from acute sprain. Balancing practice at home may be carried out with the affected foot on the bottom step of the staircase and the other leg swinging backwards and forwards.

Support

Support is generally indicated if the patient intends to walk or run for some distance so that swelling is controlled and the danger of going over causing further trauma is minimized. Double-layer Tubigrip may be sufficient, for support. To control swelling a C-shaped pad of adhesive felt is placed under the lateral malleolus and along the lateral side of the

tendo Achillis. On top of this, a crêpe or elasticated bandage is applied as for acute sprains.

Walking re-education

The most common fault is lack of correct push-off. The patient must be taught how to push with ankle plantar flexion, push-off from the big toe and propulsion in a straightforward direction. This component of gait should be practised as an exercise (Figure 6.2).

Complete rupture – lateral ligament

This is caused by a violent force which produces plantar flexion, inversion and adduction of the foot – often the patient falls with the foot twisted under the body weight.

Clinical features

Pain – Severe pain over the ligament area.

Swelling – Immediate swelling denoting severe injury occurs on the lateral side of the ankle and over the dorsum of the foot.

Instability – There is excessive range of inversion and adduction.

Loss of function – The patient is unable to walk or to take any weight at all on the foot.

Radiograph – Abnormal sideways tilt of the talus demonstrated on X-ray.

Treatment

The ligament is usually surgically repaired and immobilized for 6–8 weeks in a below-knee plaster cast. Immobilization alone may be used for 6–8 weeks. Within 2–3 days, a rocker is applied to the plaster so that the patient can walk with crutches or sticks. Walking pattern should be as normal as possible.

While the plaster is on the patient follows an exercise regimen to maintain muscle power and promote healing, whilst retaining function. When the plaster is removed treatment follows a similar pattern to the programme for an acute sprain. Hydrotherapy for retraining gait and using hydrostatic pressure to reduce swelling is indicated at this stage.

Non-weight-bearing exercises are used at first and progressed to resisted weight-bearing exercises. Support is usually required for 2–3 weeks in the form of double layer Tubigrip with the top layer extending from metatarsal heads to the knee and the underneath layer extending half-way up the calf. The patient may use a stick for 2–3 weeks depending on age. Full rehabilitation should be expected in a young person 4–8 weeks after removal of plaster but in an older person there may have to be a review programme for up to 8 months.

Principles applied – Knee ligaments

The ligaments at the knee joint commonly damaged are:

1. The medial collateral.
2. The lateral collateral.
3. The anterior and posterior cruciates.

The medial collateral ligament

Anatomy

Attachments are the medial femoral condyle and the medial tibial condyle. The deep fibres are attached to the medial meniscus. It stabilizes the knee against valgus strain.

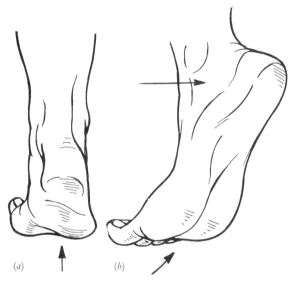

(a)   (b)

Acute sprain

Aetiology

The site of the injury may be at the level of the joint line where it is attached to the capsule and medial meniscus, or at the femoral attachment.

The cause is usually an abduction force where the foot and tibia are fixed and the femur is forced medially. A rotation force of the femur on the fixed tibia will also injure the ligament. A combination of these two forces produces a severe injury often affecting the medial meniscus, and, if severe enough, the anterior cruciate ligament. It is common in sports activities such as football, high jumping and skiing. It sometimes happens in swimming during an excessively forceful kick in breast stroke.

Clinical features

History – The patient describes the injury.

Pain – There is sharp, sudden pain over the medial side of the knee. In minor strain the pain is momentary but in more severe injuries the pain stops movement.

Swelling – This does not usually occur with minor injuries but if there is severe injury then there is swelling visible over the medial side of the joint. There may also be effusion in the medial compartment of the tibio-femoral joint.

Loss of function – The joint may feel unstable and walking is impaired because the joint will not extend to bear weight during the stance phase.

Palpation – The ligament is tender especially over the joint line.

Tests – Valgus stress (pushing the tibia laterally) produces pain over the ligament site and the end feel

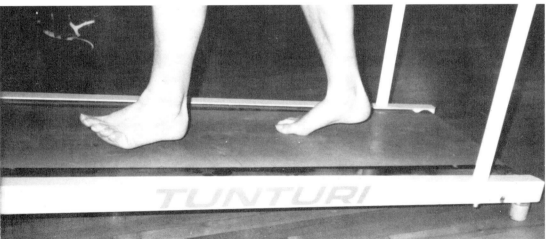

Figure 6.2 (*a*) Correct push-off. (*b*) Incorrect push-off stress on the lateral ligament. (*c*) Travelator in use for re-education of walking
(*c*)

is soft rather than firm. This test is performed with the knee flexed to 30 degrees so that the cruciate ligaments are relaxed. If the test is repeated with the knee in full extension and there is joint opening, then there is likely to be anterior cruciate ligament damage as well.

X-ray – Joint opening can be seen if the above tests are performed.

Arthrography – If the dye remains within the knee, the ligament is intact; if it is disrupted, the dye will escape into neighbouring tissues.

Treatment

Immediate

This follows the principles of ice towel, compression bandage and rest which should be in lying with the leg elevated. If the patient has to get about, then crutches and non-weight-bearing walking are necessary.

Subsequent treatment

For minor injury, the compression bandage will be retained for a week (Figure 6.3).

For more severe injuries, the support may be back splint and bandage for 2 weeks or, for very severe injury, 6–8 weeks in a plaster cylinder.

During fixation

Exercises – Static quadriceps exercises must be practised: five contractions every waking hour. Depending on severity, partial weight-bearing, walking with one stick in the opposite hand, or two sticks or perhaps elbow crutches, should be practised every day.

Rest and elevation – Whenever the patient is sitting it is essential to have the whole leg fully supported, preferably in elevation. In bed, the bedclothes may need to be raised so that there is no pressure on the knee and the foot is clear so that there is no twisting force on the lower leg.

After fixation

Pain relief is obtained by ice or interferential therapy or by pulsed electromagnetic energy. Also as mobility is restored there is less tension in the tissues and therefore pain is reduced.

Swelling is reduced by the pain-relieving massage modalities of kneading and effleurage. If the patient's lifestyle involves a large amount of standing or walking, a crêpe bandage or Tubigrip should be used to control swelling. If there is a lot of sitting in the lifestyle then the patient should straighten the knee or stand up and sit down every 20–30 minutes.

Mobility

Transverse frictions are usually necessary to restore mobility and pliability to the ligament and to the part of the capsule between the upper border of the patella and the femur.

Non-weight-bearing free active flexion and extension of the knee has to be practised, five movements every hour.

Mobilizations are generally necessary to restore caudad/cephalad movement of the patella and antero-posterior movement of the tibia on the femur. In the final stages of rehabilitation, flexion and medial rotation mobilizations may be necessary.

Weight-bearing mobility exercises (squats, star jumps, stepping on and off a form) should begin when flexion is 90°, extension is 0° and there is no effusion.

Strength

Quadriceps and hamstrings must be progressively strengthened and monitored against the strength of the other leg so that a muscle imbalance is not created. Monitoring may be by testing the 1 or 10 repetition maximum or by measuring muscle bulk with a tape measure but is more accurate with a repeatable method such as a Cybex.

Weight-bearing mobility exercises (squats, star jumps, stepping on and off a form) should begin when flexion is 90°, extension is 0° and there is no effusion.

Walking re-education

When there is full knee extension, walking aids should be discarded. It is important to ensure that the calf muscle strength is maintained so that there is power for push-off in walking, running, jumping and landing. The patient may reduce the stance phase on the affected leg which can be corrected by walking to a metronome or counting, or by practising balancing on the affected leg whilst moving the other leg forwards, backwards or sideways. A useful exercise is: standing on the affected leg, pushing a bean-bag or ball round the foot with the other foot. During push-off it is important that the patient does not exaggerate the natural valgus stress at the knee as this will lead to chronic strain of the ligament.

Final rehabilitation

This varies according to the needs of the individual. If the patient participates regularly in sport, then training and return to the sport may take place when strength is 75% of the other leg. For the 'holiday only' sport patient it is important to teach a pre-activity exercise regimen and to encourage general fitness which helps to minimize recurrence.

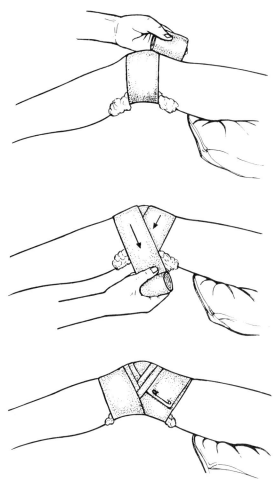

Figure 6.3 Knee supported with a crêpe bandage

It is also important for the patient with a relatively sedentary lifestyle to have full confidence in running, stopping, starting, going up and down stairs without trying to protect the injured knee. Otherwise, the uneven stresses so caused lead to musculoskeletal strain in other parts of the body.

Chronic sprain

Identifying the cause

This is associated with repeated minor injury by, for example, a habit of sitting with the knee twisted, or by walking with a valgus stress on the knee. Often the problem is related to poor foot and hip posture. It is also present in patients who did not have full pliability or mobility restored after an acute injury, fail to warm up and stretch before activities, or have excessive valgus stress during push-off in walking.

Clinical features

Pain – Niggling, sharp, stabbing, intermittent pain over the ligament which is generally absent at rest.

Swelling – Not common although there may be a small chronic effusion.

Loss of movement – Full extension of the knee is sometimes limited.

Function – This is not usually seriously impaired but the patient becomes aware of a pain which becomes more persistent with activity or time.

Sometimes the knee gives way on going down a step.

Treatment

Transverse frictions – Applied to the superficial vertical fibres with the knee in extension or to the deeper posterior fibres in flexion will restore pliability. Pain-free range of movement should increase immediately if the technique is accurate. Sometimes frictions can clear the problem completely.

Ultrasound may be appropriate to mobilize scar tissue and may be used prior to frictions.

Exercises – Progressive strengthening of the quadriceps muscle is usually appropriate and is achieved by weight resistance. If on examination the vastus medialis is especially weak, proprioceptive neuromuscular facilitation techniques may be used, e.g. knee extension within the flexion/adduction/lateral rotation pattern of the leg, with holds in extension.

Balance boards – Balancing practice is necessary because the ligament is the main structure that stabilizes the knee against valgus stress. Foot posture correction plus balancing are, therefore, essential to increase stability and reduce giving-way episodes.

Support – If a patient has to perform a particular activity, e.g. a tennis or golf match, or work demands stress on the knee, then strapping applied to the knee effectively reinforcing the ligament will help between treatments until the problem is clear.

Prevention of recurrence – The patient must avoid postural stress. This may involve ensuring that shoes are adequate to support the medial longitudinal arch of the foot.

Exercises

Daily practice is important to maintain mobility of the knee and strength of the quadriceps. Examples:

1. Lying: bending alternate knees and hips.
2. Prone lying: bending alternate knees.
3. Prone lying: one leg – point toes, tighten quadriceps, lift leg. Repeat with other leg. (This exercise works the extensor thrust muscles together.)

4. Standing with one foot on low block (or first step of stairs): straighten and bend the knee and hip. Progress by increasing number of repetitions (up to 20) and by holding weights in hands or strapping weights round the other ankle.
5. Standing (at work or in queues): tighten quadriceps – hold count 10. Repeat × 10.
6. Sitting: knees, hips and ankles at right angle; turn toes to touch, then turn heels to touch – produces rotation at the knees.

General warm-up exercises are also necessary before activity, which may range from regular sport to the occasional football or cricket with the children or grandchildren.

Complete rupture of the medial ligament is usually associated with severe trauma and requires surgery. Postoperative management is considered later.

The lateral collateral ligament

Anatomy

Attachments are the lateral femoral condyle and the head of the fibula. It has no connection to the lateral meniscus. It stabilizes the knee against varus strain.

Acute sprain

Aetiology

This injury is much less common than in the medial ligament and is caused by a varus stress. It may happen when there is a sideways fall, for example, off a motor-cycle or bicycle when the vehicle lands on the lower leg. Severe twisting may tear this ligament and is likely to affect the medial ligament as well.

Clinical features

These are similar to the features for the medial ligament but related to the lateral side of the joint.

Treatment

This follows the principles as for the medial ligament and full recovery is expected because of the other stabilizing structures on the lateral side of the knee – the iliotibial tract, biceps femoris and, supporting the lateral compartment on the posterior aspect, the popliteus tendon and the arcuate ligament.

Chronic sprain

This is more common in the lateral ligament than acute strain.

Cause

This is usually overuse and occurs particularly in long-distance – especially cross-country – runners and in long-distance skiing.

Clinical features

Pain – Comes on gradually. At first it is a slight ache, which goes with rest but gradually the intensity of pain increases, it comes on earlier in the activity and takes a longer time to settle. It is over the lateral side of the knee towards the head of the fibula.

Tenderness – It is sore over the ligament just above the head of the fibula.

Function – Often the pain is not present unless the causative activity is being performed.

Treatment

Identifying the cause is a vital part of treatment. This may involve analysing the effects of the causative activity and whether technique needs to be improved. Athletic shoes or ski equipment need to be examined in case faulty equipment is causing a varus stress on the knee.

Examination is required in detail because there may be a tight iliotibial band or an imbalance with hamstrings so that the biceps femoris is weak, throwing stress on the ligament.

Often, there is a stiff superior tibiofibular joint and sometimes there is tightness of the lateral ligament of the ankle joint.

Treatment must, therefore, be directed at treating the abnormality found on examination.

Ice – An ice cube moved over the area of the ligament by the patient will relieve the pain immediately after activity.

Rest – The patient should be persuaded to avoid the aggravating activity until any mechanical abnormality is cleared.

Transverse frictions – These may be appropriate; the commonest site treated is just above the fibular attachment.

Mobilizations – Antero-posterior passive movements to the superior tibiofibular joint are frequently required to relieve the pain described, especially in cross-country runners. The movement at this joint is small but important during knee movements.

Other treatments

Stretching of the iliotibial band may be appropriate together with ultrasound.

Strengthening of the biceps femoris may be necessary, for example by PNF slow reversals with knee flexion in the extension/adduction/lateral rotation pattern of the leg.

Anterior cruciate ligament (ACL)

Anatomy

Attachments are the medial surface of the lateral femoral condyle and the tibial plateau between the tibial spines – making its direction postero-superior to antero-inferior. It stabilizes the knee, preventing anterior displacement of the tibia on the femur. It also controls hyperextension and internal (medial) rotation of the tibia.

Aetiology

The causative force is often hyperextension with internal rotation stress on the tibia with the foot fixed. The ligament is also injured in a severe valgus stress with the joint in flexion and the tibia rotated externally where the medial ligament and medial meniscus have already been injured. Basket ball, skiing and hockey can produce injuries of the ACL alone.

Clinical features

History – This is related to the causative forces described above and the patient often feels 'something go' inside the knee.

Swelling – At the time of injury there is a haemarthrosis: a jelly-like swelling which makes walking impossible although not necessarily painful.

The injury at this stage may settle with ice, rest and quadriceps exercises and the patient can have full functional recovery.

With time, however, the patient presents with repeated episodes of the knee giving way. After each episode, there is swelling and some pain which clears up. The patient, however, gradually becomes more uncertain of the knee and stops sport – at least at a competitive level.

The classical test is to draw the tibia forward on the femur with the patient in crook lying. If the anterior cruciate is weak, the range of movement is greater than in the other knee and the end-feel of the movement is 'empty' or 'spongy' feeling instead of the firm elasticity of an intact ligament. If the tibia is rotated medially and this range is increased, then ACL tear is the most likely lesion.

Treatment

A complete rupture requires surgical repair. Sometimes this involves opening the knee and sometimes the approach is through an arthroscope. Partial tear, or chronic laxity, may be treated surgically by procedures to obtain anterior stability of the tibia on the femur. The iliotibial tract may be detached and moved forward on the lateral tibial condyle or the tendons of sartorius, gracilis and semitendinosus may be moved forwards on the medial tibial condyle. The operation depends on the state of the medial collateral ligament and the medial meniscus. It also depends on the surgeon's experience and the patient's age and requirements.

Physiotherapy

Following operation, the knee is usually immobilized in plaster for 2–3 weeks. Then for the next 4–6 weeks, the plaster is bi-valved and removed for physiotherapy. The two halves may be replaced and held by elastic bandage or only the posterior half used as a back splint.

If there is no surgery, the periods of complete and partial immobilization may be as above. During the complete immobilization period, foot and toe muscle exercises are performed by the patient for 5 minutes every hour. Walking with hip updrawing is taught to maintain a swing-through pattern. Walking aids may be sticks or elbow crutches.

When the plaster is removed the ideal treatment is hydrotherapy. Buoyancy assisted extension of the knee can regain the movement and help realign the healing collagen without a strong anterior force being exerted by the quadriceps on the tibia. Buoyancy resisted flexion can strengthen the hamstrings and gain movement by the patient performing repeated contractions (hold – move – hold – move) against buoyancy. Exercises to maintain strength of the hip, ankle and foot muscles can be performed either with buoyancy counterbalanced or resisting.

Coordination exercises in water can be started early in the programme with the patient standing on the affected leg and moving the other leg in different directions, or moving bats through the water with the hands.

The criteria for gym work to be started are:

1. Good co-contraction of quadriceps and hamstrings.
2. Free, nearly full-range extension and flexion.
3. Minimal swelling.

A programme of progressive strengthening for quadriceps and hamstrings is then followed. Finally, a circuit including, e.g. stopping, starting, jumping, running, walking whilst carrying objects and general fitness exercises is devised for the individual's requirements. A Cybex is very useful for monitoring the progress of hamstrings and quadriceps together with the corresponding muscles on the other side. It is essential in these patients to ensure a balance of muscle power so as to avoid torsional or uneven stresses.

In general

Ligamentous injuries of the lower limb need a period of rest and immobilization to enable healing but the big disadvantage is the atrophy of both muscle and ligamentous (normal ligaments) tissue which occurs. Early controlled mobilization and surgical repair, therefore, constitute the optimum management.

Elbow ligaments

The ligaments of the elbow are:

1. Medial collateral.
2. Lateral collateral.
3. Capsule.

The medial collateral ligament

This is the most commonly injured ligament of the elbow, when the force is insufficient to produce a fracture.

Aetiology

The site of injury is central and may be the anterior component if the elbow is extended and the posterior component if the elbow is flexed.

The cause is usually a fall on the outstretched arm with a valgus strain on the forearm. The common flexor tendon is usually injured at the same time.

Clinical features

History – The patient relates to an injury (e.g. a fall in skiing).

Pain – This is usually localized to the medial side of the elbow.

Treatment

Ice applied for 10 minutes twice a day for 2–3 days reduces pain.

Exercises should start as soon as possible. Examples:

1. Free active full-range flexion and extension of the elbow.
2. Free active full-range pronation and supination of the radio-ulnar joints.
3. Squeezing a ball or sponge in the hand with the elbow in extension is important to maintain mobility of the flexor tendon.
4. Throwing and catching a ball above the head.

Weight-bearing exercises should start in 7 days, e.g. modified press-ups on a table or wall.

Complete tears are usually associated with joint dislocation or fractures (see Chapter 4).

Ligaments of the fingers and wrist

The principles of treatment are the same as those for the injuries already described. Ice treatment should not last longer than 2–3 days to reduce swelling and pain. Free active full-range exercises must start as soon as possible to facilitate collagen alignment. It is important to remember to exercise the whole limb and to include weight-bearing activities.

Knee meniscal lesions

The two menisci in the knee joint are composed mostly of collagen fibres with some elastic tissue. The fibres run longitudinally from anterior to posterior and there are reinforcing bands running in an in-to-out direction (Figure 6.4).

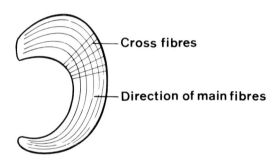

Figure 6.4 Medial meniscus, direction of fibres

The menisci are dependent on synovial diffusion for nutrition except at either horn and the outer margin where there are blood vessels. Nerve endings are present in the horns and the periphery.

The functions of the menisci are:

1. Shock absorption.
2. Deepening of articular surfaces of the tibial condyles.
3. Facilitation of rotation of the knee:
   (a) Lateral rotation of tibia on femur giving 'screw home' at limit of extension (close-packed position of joint).
   (b) Medial rotation of tibia on femur to unlock during flexion.

The medial meniscus is torn three times more often than the lateral partly because it is firmly attached to the medial collateral ligament. The lateral meniscus is separate from the lateral collateral ligament. Types of tear are illustrated in Figure 6.5.

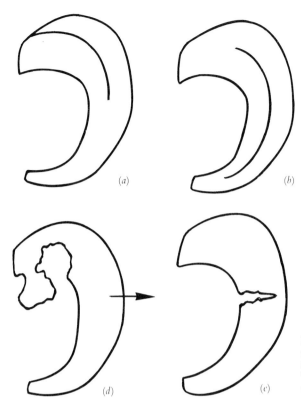

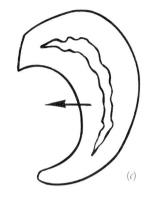

Figure 6.5 Meniscal injuries. a = Slit in posterior horn undisplaced. b = Split along line of longitudinal fibres. c = Split increases and the free margin goes into the joint. d = The middle portion displaces away from the joint. e = A transverse tear

Aetiology

Age – Commonly 18–45.

Sex – Mostly males but the incidence in females is increasing.

Occupation – Professional sport, miners and labourers.

Sport – Football, rugger, golf, tennis.

Cause

Sudden rotation of the knee in partial flexion, during weight bearing causes the meniscus to be trapped between the joint surfaces, e.g. catching the foot in a rabbit hole during brisk walking or running causes the femur to rotate on the tibia. An abduction stress (tibia forced laterally) tears the medial ligament and the medial meniscus with it.

Clinical features

History – The patient can describe a twisting injury.

Pain – There is acute pain in the knee joint often round the medial margin and 'deep' in the joint.

Effusion – Excess synovial fluid forms and collects in the suprapatellar bursa as well as between the joint surfaces.

After rest – The knee may return to normal.

Later – There may be another episode of twisting or the patient may feel the knee give way or lock. Locking is due to the free margin moving into the joint (Figure 6.5(c)). 'Catching' is due to tears such as Figure 6.5(d) and (e).

Range of movement – Thickened effused fluid may prevent full extension because the joint surfaces cannot 'screw home' into the close-packed position.

Muscle power – Quadriceps atrophies rapidly, especially vastus medialis.

McMurray's test

1. *Medial meniscus* – The knee is flexed fully, then extended with the tibia laterally rotated and abducted. If a 'click' is felt the test is positive.
2. *Lateral meniscus* – The test is the same except for the tibia being adducted and medially rotated. This test can be false positive or false negative.

Arthrography

This is very useful in clarifying that the patient's problems are due to a torn cartilage and not to cysts or ligament injury.

Arthroscopy

Tears can be seen during this procedure although posterior horn damage can be missed.

Management

The initial acute episode is treated conservatively following the principles described for a ligament injury.

Persistent pain, locking, giving way or effusion requires removal of the meniscus.

Surgery

Arthroscopy: the cartilage may be removed by the surgeon using an arthroscope.

Open operation: when the posterior horn is affected an anteromedial or anterolateral incision is used and the whole meniscus removed.

Sometimes the peripheral part is left. A pseudo-meniscus, which is much more fibrous than normal, forms during the weeks after surgery.

Physiotherapy in relation to open surgery

Surgeons vary in their beliefs as to how patients should be rehabilitated. The factors that vary are:

1. When flexion should be started.
2. When the patient should go home.
3. Use of walking aids and splints.

The aims of physiotherapy are common to all operations and these are to:

1. Prevent effusion and haemarthrosis.
2. Prevent muscle atrophy of the quadriceps and hamstrings.
3. Enable tissues to heal.
4. Teach the patient use of walking aids.
5. Progressively regain mobility of the knee.
6. Strengthen muscles.
7. Restore confidence and return to function.

Effusion and haemarthrosis

This is prevented by pressure bandaging, possibly by the use of a splint (plaster back slab) and instruction to the patient NOT to bend the knee until the sutures are out. No weight bearing for 10 days post-operatively is also an important theme. The foot end of the bed can be raised so that even at home there is elevation of the limb.

Prevention of muscle atrophy

Within 24 hours of the operation, quadriceps contractions must be practised – five times every hour to a count of five is usually within the patient's capabilities (pre-operative training helps). Straight leg raising starts just after 24 hours and it is essential that the physiotherapist palpates to check that all components of the quadriceps are contracted *before* the leg is raised. If this is not meticulously carried out, the leg can be raised by the hip flexors and the knee is kept straight by the pressure bandage. The patient must be taught to palpate the muscles to make sure they are working. It is at this stage that a quadriceps leg may develop and is disastrous for the future wellbeing of the joint. If necessary, faradism may be applied if the muscle is not working within 48 hours.

Healing

Rest and the above exercises ensure that circulation is maintained, collagen is laid down in the correct lines and healing takes place.

Walking aids

Elbow or axillary crutches are necessary if non-weight-bearing is to be taught, and hip hitching is essential so that the knee is not held in flexion. During the swing phase of partial weight-bearing there must again be hip hitching and the patient must feel the knee is straight before weight is taken (usually 10–20% weight on knee and 90–80% on the arms at first). Within 4–5 days the percentage of weight bearing can progress to 50–50. Some surgeons apply a plaster cylinder and the merit of this is that the patient cannot 'forget' and bend the knee.

Mobility

After 10–14 days from the operation, provided plaster and sutures are removed and there is a good full quadriceps contraction, knee flexion can start. At first this is non-weight-bearing. The patient is encouraged to bend the knee to the point of 'tightness' – then straighten, 10–15 times every hour. No forcing should be allowed. The scar may need mobilizing with kneading and picking up. Mobilizations (antero-posterior-tibia on femur) may be applied and passive patella movements are useful.

Mobility, strength, confidence and function

These are regained by a progressive programme similar to that for ligament repair. The main difference is that progress can be quicker.

Weight-bearing activities must not start in the presence of effusion and there must be 90° flexion available. At 6–12 weeks after the operation the knee should be fit for a gym programme of light training depending on the individual patient's life style and previous history.

Hydrotherapy is indicated at the stage where sutures and plaster are removed. The walking pattern can be re-educated. Buoyancy counter-balanced (side-lying) positions can be used to regain flexion. Bicycling action in float lying is also useful. Knee and hip extensors can be strengthened, e.g. standing (flipper on foot) knee and hip bending and straightening. The leg kick in breast stroke should not be used until the later stages of rehabilitation as it is a stressful exercise for the knee.

Physiotherapy following cartilage removal by arthroscopy follows similar principles to those of open surgery. The big difference is the reduction in time scale. The rehabilitation programme may be condensed into 3 weeks. A professional sportsman may return to full activity 3–4 weeks after operation.

Tendon injuries

Tendons are strong structures which connect muscles to bones. The epimysium blends with the tendon at the teno-muscular junction and the tendon blends with the periosteum at the teno-periosteal junction. Some tendons are enclosed in a synovial sheath (e.g. the flexor digitorum and superficialis). Tendons that do not have a synovial sheath slide smoothly within a compartment of deep fascia.

Types of injury

1. Strain or partial rupture.
2. Complete rupture.
3. Tenosynovitis.

Causes of injury

These may be traumatic or spontaneous.

Traumatic

1. Direct cuts: window glass, road traffic accident, knife accidents (e.g. in a butcher's business or a kitchen). Complete rupture is most likely.

2. A sudden stretch when the muscle is contracting:
   (a) Sometimes the tendon gives, sometimes the muscle gives.
   (b) The injury may be partial or complete.

Spontaneous

Degenerative changes may weaken a tendon which then ruptures without apparent trauma. For example: long head of biceps brachii; supraspinatus; extensor pollicis longus (particularly after a Colles' fracture has healed and the radius is roughened, producing friction on the tendon).

Tendons commonly affected

1. Tendo calcaneus (tendo-Achillis).
2. Ligamentum patellae.
3. Hamstrings.
4. Rotator cuff, especially supraspinatus.
5. Long head of biceps brachii.
6. Common extensor tendon (tennis elbow).
7. Common flexor tendon (golfer's elbow).
8. Extensor pollicis longus.
9. Abductor pollicis longus and extensor pollicis brevis.
10. Finger flexor or extensor tendons.

Sprain (partial rupture)

Pathology

1. Some of the tendon fibres tear and others are intact.
2. Tendon is a poorly vascularized tissue, and only a small amount of blood may be released from damaged blood vessels.
3. Low-grade inflammatory changes take place.
4. Granulation tissue forms at the site of injury.
5. Tendon cells invade the area and tendon fibres are laid down, so that healing takes place.
6. If there is extensive damage then fibrous (non-tendon type) scar tissue may form as well and this can bind the tendon to surrounding tissues.
7. Repair can take from 3 to 6 weeks depending on the degree of injury.

Clinical features

1. *History* – A sharp, stabbing pain and tearing may be heard or felt.
2. *Loss of function* – The patient is unable to produce the action of the muscle.
3. Swelling and bruising may appear 2–3 days after injury.

Management

This comprises fixation to allow healing, and rehabilitation out of fixation.

Fixation

1. This may be by plaster of Paris where the injury is severe.
2. Strapping is used for less severe injuries.
3. Rest or working splints may be used made from a firm, washable material.
4. The main principles of fixation are to hold the tendon in a shortened position, prevent movement at the injury site and therefore allow healing. It is also important to enable the patient to use the limb as normally as possible.

Physiotherapy during fixation

The main aims are to:

1. Maintain circulation through the muscle to promote healing.
2. Minimize adhesion formation.
3. Maintain muscle strength.
4. Encourage functional use of the affected limb.

Methods used

1. Free active exercises for the joints and muscles out of fixation.
2. Functional activities – the patient is encouraged to try out activities to identify those that are possible and those that must be avoided. For example, for a lower limb walking may have to be with the aid of a walking stick; writing, cutting food or combing hair may be difficult with an upper limb involved.
3. Isometric work for the muscle to which the injured tendon is attached may start 7–21 days after the injury, according to severity. Overflow is useful – i.e. resistance applied to neighbouring muscles will produce contraction of the affected muscle by overflow or irradiation. For example, resistance on the ankle dorsiflexors will produce quadriceps contraction where the quadriceps tendon has been partially ruptured. Resistance to the left shoulder muscles will produce a contraction in the right shoulder muscles. Isometric contraction helps compress the joint surfaces of the immobilized joints, maintaining synovial sweep and fluid flow which reduces adhesion formation.

Rehabiliation out of fixation

Physiotherapy

The main aims are to:

1. Regain mobility of the affected tendon and the strength of the muscle.
2. Regain mobility of joints.
3. Restore general muscle strength.
4. Regain the patient's confidence in the tendon.
5. Regain full functional use.
6. Prevent recurrence.

Methods used

Physiotherapy starts the day fixation is removed.

Soft-tissue techniques

Finger kneading, picking up and effleurage are used to mobilize the soft tissues in the vicinity of the tendon and to clear oedema. Frictions may be required after a few days to mobilize the tendon or the adjacent muscle fibres. Lanolin or oil may be necessary at first if the limb has been fixed in plaster of Paris.

Exercises

Hold–relax, repeated contractions may be used to regain the length of the muscle. Free active exercise, encouraging full range without forcing should be practised regularly by the patient. The movement which stretches the tendon and muscle should be performed to the point of 'tightness', held for a few seconds, and released. Careful controlled practice of this will regain range without endangering the tendon. Hydrotherapy is particularly useful at this stage for lower limb and shoulder injuries. Strengthening techniques using weights, springs or malleable substances can start as soon as the patient can work the muscle without pain in the middle to inner range. PNF slow reversals technique is particularly useful to work the muscle in pattern through the available range. Once the patient can confidently move the muscle freely through full range, an appropriate functional activity programme should be devised, i.e. appropriate to the patient's requirements, hobbies, work and to the affected muscle.

Complete rupture

Pathology

Spasm of the muscle causes retraction of the free end of the tendon so that a gap forms. Haematoma fills the gap. Granulation tissue forms in the haematoma. Tendon cells may lay down tendon fibres but generally fibrous tissue fills the gap. This renders the tendon virtually useless because the fibrous tissue stretches. Suturing is therefore essential to enable tendon fibres to reunite the tendon.

Where the rupture is spontaneous, the poor blood supply and frayed ends of the tendon make spontaneous healing impossible and suturing is difficult. Repair may require a graft.

Clinical features

1. History:
   (a) Knife injury (fingers).
   (b) Hand going through window (wrist).
   (c) Sudden snap on sudden activity (tendo Achilles).
   (d) Sudden stretch with muscle contracting (quadriceps tendon).
2. Immediate loss of function.
3. The gap may be palpable.
4. Pain and nausea may be present at the time of injury. A nagging ache and local tenderness are often present with a spontaneous rupture.

Management

Surgical repair is essential:

1. The two ends may be sutured or wired together.
2. It may be necessary to use another tendon (e.g. palmaris longus or plantaris) to provide a graft to bridge the gap.
3. Tendon transplant may be used, e.g. extensor indices may be transposed to replace extensor pollicis longus.

Following surgery there is fixation which keeps the muscle and tendon in a shortened position. Plaster of Paris is usually used for lower limb tendons and a polythene type of material is used for the upper limb.

Time in fixation varies from 3 to 9 weeks. During this time adjustments may be made so that fixation is reapplied with the muscle in a longer position.

Physiotherapy

During fixation

The principles are essentially the same as for partial rupture fixation but the surgeon may wish activities to be curtailed to ensure that the tendon has every chance to heal. The physiotherapist must explain the balance to the patient between activity to maintain circulation and muscle power with the control required to avoid stress on the suture.

After fixation

Again, this follows the pattern for rehabilitation after partial rupture.

Lanolin or arachis oil may be incorporated into the treatment for the first 2–3 days to help improve the skin.

A Faradic type of current may help to re-educate a contraction in the muscle, e.g. quadriceps or supraspinatus.

The rehabilitation period is much longer and requires perseverance and patience on the part of both patient and physiotherapist.

At the beginning, mobility of the tendon, muscle, scar and neighbouring tissues is vital and is obtained by skilled soft-tissue techniques. Mobilizations – accessory movements particularly – help to regain movement in joints that have been fixed, without stressing the injured site. The exercise programme follows that of the partial rupture.

Patient, surgeon and physiotherapist have to discuss return to function. This may be totally possible for some patients but sadly may mean that a talented individual may be handicapped in his or her self-esteem (e.g. in sport or musical instrument playing). It is important to note that hypertrophy of muscles in top-class sport training programmes can generate such force in a muscle that the tendon is too weak to cope with it, and this predisposes individuals to injury.

Tendo-calcaneus (Achilles)
Principles applied to particular tendons

(complete rupture) (*Figure 6.6*)

History

1. The patient feels a sharp pain as if a blow has been imparted to the calf muscle (e.g. from a tennis ball).
2. A test for complete rupture, with the patient in prone lying: if the calf muscles are squeezed in the lower third, the ankle normally slightly plantarflexes. If it does not, the tendon is ruptured.
3. Walking is impossible immediately.

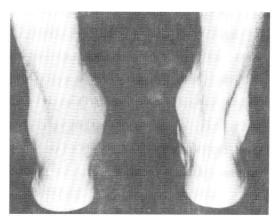

Figure 6.6 Rupture of the left tendo calcaneus (Achilles) (From Muckle, 1982, p. 29, with permission).

Management

The tendon must be sutured as soon as possible. Immobilization is usually in plaster of Paris for up to 9 weeks. The plaster is changed twice to enable stitches to be removed and to alter the angle at the ankle joint which starts in slight plantarflexion and is altered to 90° dorsiflexion.

Physiotherapy

During fixation

Non-weight-bearing and later partial weight-bearing walking must be taught.

Functional activities with crutches must also be taught, i.e. opening, shutting doors, coping with transport, stairs, toilet.

An exercise programme is taught to maintain mobility of toes, knee (if out of plaster), hip and to maintain muscle power.

After fixation

Inner and middle range, non-weight-bearing exercises are started immediately.

Mobilizing techniques for all the foot joints, and tibiofibular joints are given. The scar may be mobilized with finger kneading and the thickened swelling around the ankle must be dispersed with kneading and effleurage.

Spring resistance to strengthen the calf muscles is useful. Weight-bearing exercises begin when there is pain-free dorsiflexion to just beyond a right angle.

Stabilizations standing on the affected leg are important for giving the patient confidence. Walking may at first be with a stick in the opposite hand and a pad under the heel. The particular gait problems are lack of ankle dorsiflexion during heel strike and lack of push-off.

For the first problem, the patient should practise ankle dorsiflexion: 2–3 times to point of stretch every hour. For the second problem the patient should practise:

1. Sitting, heel raising with manual resistance applied to the thigh.
2. Standing (hand on wall or chair), heels raising.

Balance board practice is important. The mini-trampoline is useful.

Final rehabilitation, depending on age and lifestyle of the patient, should include hopping, skipping, jumping from various heights, running, stopping and starting. Even for an elderly patient some of this should be included, because jumping and running may be necessary in an emergency.

Ligamentum patellae

History

This tendon is ruptured when the foot is fixed and the knee is forcibly flexed with the quadriceps contracting strongly.

Walking is severely impaired.

Management

The tendon is sutured – often with wire.

Immobilization is in a plaster cylinder for 6–10 weeks, with the knee in slight flexion.

Physiotherapy

During fixation

Non-weight-bearing walking may be taught at first and it is important to teach the patient to 'hip hitch' to hold the affected leg up. This avoids excessive use of the rectus femoris as a hip flexor which occurs if the patient holds the leg forwards.

Partial weight-bearing walking may be started with a heel pad in the shoe at 4–6 weeks.

Quadriceps contractions – checked by palpation of the muscle just above the plaster – are started when the surgeon allows (4–5 days).

After fixation

Mobility of the tendon is regained by passive side-to-side movement. Swelling is reduced by kneading and effleurage. Curapulse or ultrasound may be used to help soften indurated swelling around the knee. Skin mobility must be regained by finger kneading and picking up.

Passive patellar movements are essential.

Mobilizations – accessory at first and then physiological movements – are used to mobilize the knee.

Free active exercises regain knee movements and when there is full extension and flexion is 90°, weight-bearing exercises may begin.

The Cybex is useful to regain power balance between hamstring and quadriceps muscles.

The gait problems are:

1. Lack of heel strike due to loss of knee extension.
2. Short stance phase on affected leg due to a feeling of insecurity.

Knee mobilizing takes care of the first problem. The second problem is overcome by balance-board practice, stabilizations standing on the affected leg, walking practice using a travelator and then a balance form.

Final rehabilitation should incorporate jumping, crouching, running and activities involving the lower limbs which enable the patient to forget the injury.

Hamstring tendons

History

Hamstring tendons are usually torn when the patient sprints suddenly from cold, unprepared or fatigued. It may occur in an athlete who has had a previous injury or has congenitally short hamstrings or a 'non-athlete' who runs for a bus or plays unaccustomed sport, e.g. cricket.

Pain

This is usually sudden, stabbing pain in the back of the thigh, but there may be a gradual onset of twinges which develop into constant pain. For example, a sprinter with a bad technique may develop chronic strain.

Site

The ischial attachment is often injured. Less often the distal tendons may be injured. Complete rupture of a tendon is rare because the muscle tissue usually tears first.

Management

Following an acute injury, a bandage may be applied to the thigh and the limb is rested.

Physiotherapy

This follows the principles applied in the case of muscle tissue injury.

Chronic strain is treated with ultrasound, frictions (deep and accurate), stretching – firstly passive, then auto stretches. Hold–relax may be used to lengthen the muscle component.

The cause (poor technique or posture) must be identified to prevent further stress.

Rotator cuff tendons

The muscles are:

1. Supraspinatus.
2. Infraspinatus.
3. Teres minor.
4. Subscapularis.

The tendons blend with the capsule of the glenohumeral joint and are often implicated in capsulitis.

Anatomy

The tendons attach to the greater tuberosity from anterior to superior to posterior. Whenever the arm is moved from the side, these muscles steady the head of the humerus and hold it down in a force couple action enabling deltoid muscle (in particular) to raise the arm. Without these muscles, the deltoid would jam the upper end of the humerus against the acromion process. At about 60° abduction, the tendons lie between the humerus and acromion (separated from the latter by the subacromial bursa) (Figure 6.7). By about 120° abduction the tuberosity has moved medially and the head of the humerus

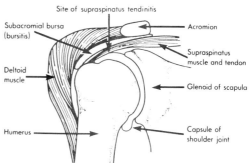

Figure 6.7 Supraspinatus tendon and subacromial bursa (From Hickling and Golding 1984, with permission.)

rotated laterally so that the tendons no longer lie directly between the two bones.

Elevation from 0° to 180° is in a ratio of 60° ($\frac{1}{3}$) to 120° ($\frac{2}{3}$) – scapula (glenoid cavity) to humerus.

Types of lesion

1. Tendinitis.
2. Partial rupture.
3. Complete rupture.

The muscle most commonly injured is the supraspinatus.

Supraspinatus tendinitis

History

This may occur as a result of one accident (e.g. a fall on the shoulder), over-exercise (e.g. aerobics) or a series of minor stresses (e.g. long periods of writing).

Pain

A toothache-type pain is often present – possibly most of the time – radiating from the acromion process to the deltoid insertion.

Painful arc: abduction to 60° is pain free, 60–120° is painful, 120–180° is pain free. This is a classical picture of the inflamed tendon being compressed between the acromion and humerus (see Anatomy, above).

Movement

1. Shoulder/arm movements are full (but have a painful arc).
2. Resisted abduction in outer range is often painful.
3. Often lowering the arm from elevation is very painful. If this movement is resisted, the pain is less. This is a test used to determine whether it is bursitis or tendinitis. Bursitis remains painful on resisted lowering of the arm.

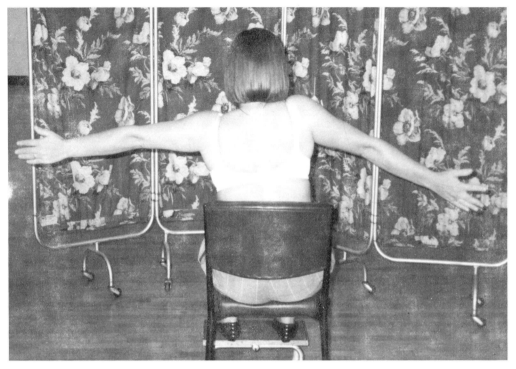

Figure 6.8 Reversed glenohumeral rhythm of the right shoulder

4. There is reversed glenohumeral rhythm – the scapula moving more than the humerous (Figure 6.8).

Function

This can be severely limited in a patient who has to carry (e.g. dresses on coat hangers).

Management

A hydrocortisone injection is often very effective in reducing the inflammation.

Non-steroidal anti-inflammatory drugs are also very effective.

Physiotherapy

Rest in an arm sling is appropriate for severe pain especially following a traumatic episode. Two days should be sufficient.

Ultrasound can be helpful in removing inflammatory exudate – but must be applied to the tendon, i.e. with the shoulder in extension and medial rotation.

Ice applied either in a towel to the superior aspect of the shoulder or as a cube, stroked over the tendon, can relieve pain and reduce swelling. The patient may benefit from treatment at home with ice – especially 10–20 minutes before bed if there is a problem with night pain.

Exercise

Auto-assisted elevation through flexion and adduction should be practised once every hour to prevent adhesion formation between the capsule, tendon and bursa. Re-education of glenohumeral rhythm is usually necessary. This may be achieved by:

1. PNF slow reversals.
2. Gravity counterbalanced (patient lying), carry the arm sideways until the scapula elevates, stop, correct the position, teach correct feeling, give stabilizations.
3. Patient sits with elbow resting on a table (30–40° abduction), palpates acromion and greater tubercle of humerus, lifts elbow, feel depression which forms between the bones; if scapula rises, stop, rest elbow on table, try again. It may help to palpate the correct movement on the opposite side.
4. Sitting with arm by the side, practise pushing the arm down (fingers to floor) (this keeps the head of the humerus sliding down in the glenoid cavity – an essential accessory movement for all shoulder movements).

5. Sitting with hand on shoulder, practise pushing elbow down and out – do this with both arms and look in a mirror to compare movements.

Mobilizations

If the glenohumeral joint is stiff, longitudinal movement (humeral head moving down on the glenoid) should be given – either by applying a force to the lower end of the humerus or to the greater tuberosity.

Frictions

Transverse frictions may be applied to the tendon with the shoulder in extension, medial rotation and adduction. This technique should not be applied in the presence of acute pain but is very appropriate 7–10 days after injury or in the case of repeated minor stress. The tendon is mobilized, adhesions are softened and stretched and pain-free movement can be restored very quickly. This is the first technique of choice if examination findings indicate that a chronic tendinitis has led to thickening and adhesions of the tendon.

Prevention

The cause should be identified if possible and new techniques of lifting or advice on rest may help to prevent recurrence of tendinitis. Often protraction and depression of the shoulder girdles need to be practised because poor posture has predisposed to stress on the tendon. The pectoralis major may be tight, preventing lateral rotation of the humerus during elevation – this stresses the rotator cuff muscles.

Calcified deposits in the supraspinatus tendon

This can cause a painful arc. Sometimes it clears spontaneously. Surgery is usually the only successful treatment. Physiotherapy has little to offer, but is essential to restore movement after surgery.

Partial rupture of the supraspinatus

History

A fall on the shoulder or carrying a heavy weight often precipitates a partial rupture.

Pain

1. Sharp pain in the shoulder.
2. Referred pain down to the elbow.
3. Tenderness is present on palpation of the tendon.
4. A painful arc is present.
5. Resisted abduction is painful.

Movement

Passive elevation is pain free. There is reversed glenohumeral rhythm.

Management and physiotherapy

1. These follow the principles for tendinitis.
2. Pulsed electromagnetic energy is very beneficial to increase the circulation to promote healing.
3. Progress is slower than with tendinitis and more exercises may be required to strengthen the shoulder muscles.

Complete rupture of the supraspinatus

History

A fall on the point of the shoulder with the arm adducted can cause a complete rupture.

There may be a history of aching in the shoulder and painful arc, then suddenly there is a sharp pain and an inability to initiate abduction. This is a spontaneous rupture due to degenerative changes.

Pain

There is general aching round the shoulder which gets worse at night.

Movement

1. Abduction cannot be initiated.
2. Passive movements are full range.
3. The arm can be elevated actively if it is first passively moved to 20–30°.

Management

Spontaneous rupture usually occurs in an elderly person and surgery is unrealistic. Treatment is similar to that for tendinitis. The patient has to be taught how to cope with functional activities.

Surgery is indicated for a younger patient. The tendon is sutured and the arm is fixed in a plaster or steel and polythene splint at 90° abduction and 45° lateral rotation.

Fixation lasts for 4–6 weeks.

Physiotherapy

During fixation

The patient is taught to exercise the hand and elbow joints and muscles. Isometric contractions for deltoid – which will include the supraspinatus – start in 2–5 days. It is important to prevent adhesions between tendon, subacromial bursa and capsule, by working the muscles in inner range as soon as possible.

After fixation

After fixation is removed rehabilitation involves re-education of glenohumeral rhythm.

Slow reversal technique is particularly useful for retraining coordination and strength.

Finger kneading is necessary to mobilize the scar and tendon. General kneading and picking up are used to mobilize the soft tissues round the shoulder region.

Free active abduction starts with the patient in lying and the hand on the shoulder (short lever) so that gravity is counterbalanced. This is progressed by straightening the arm. A further progression is to have the patient (hand on shoulder) in sitting and assistance is applied for the first 30°. Alternatively the patient may side-flex to the affected side so that the arm falls into abduction and then the movement is continued actively. It is important to remember that when the patient is in side-lying with a weight in the hand and raises the arm, this is advanced work for the abductors in outer range. Weight-bearing activities, for example in prone kneeling, should be included. For an athletic patient activities with medicine and gymnastic balls are useful. Swimming should also be encouraged. `

Hydrotherapy is of particular benefit 2–3 days after fixation is removed because buoyancy assists abduction when the patient is sitting. Activities with bats and floats, or holding the bar and swinging the trunk, can be graduated to strengthen and mobilize the muscles.

Other rotator cuff tendons

Infraspinatus

This muscle and tendon are subject to trauma resulting in inflammation, more often chronic than acute.

There is a painful arc and resisted lateral rotation is painful.

On palpation the tendon is thickened and the muscle fibres are tight.

Teres minor

This is similar to the infraspinatus.

Physiotherapy

1. Friction is the most effective technique and should clear the problem in 3–4 treatments.
2. Ultrasound may be beneficial.
3. Hold–relax to gain medial rotation is very helpful, especially if the scapula is fixed.
4. Passive stretching – i.e. the arm is moved into flexion, medial rotation with the scapula held – is also very useful.
5. Spring resistance for both arms like a 'chest expander' strengthens the lateral rotators.

Subscapularis

This is similar to the two above except that resisted medial rotation is painful.

Bicipital tendinitis

This tends to occur where the tendon of the long head lies in the bicipital groove.

Pain is provoked by resisted supination of the forearm and flexion of the elbow.

Frictions and ultrasound are the treatments of choice.

Biceps – long head tendon

Complete rupture can occur and the muscle contracts, forming a bulge in the lower third of the upper arm (Figure 6.9). It is usually spontaneous and is due to degenerative wear and tear.

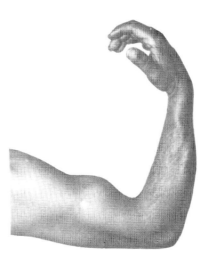

Figure 6.9 Ruptured biceps long head (From Muckle, 1982, p. 119, with permission.)

There may be no treatment at all if the patient is elderly and can manage with the short head being intact.

Surgery may be appropriate – in which case the distal end of the tendon is sutured to the short head. It is not possible to suture the two free ends because the proximal part is loose inside the joint.

Tennis elbow

Definition

This is a condition characterized by pain and acute tenderness on the lateral side of the elbow usually related to the common extensor tendon.

Aetiology

Age – 30–60 years.
    Sex – Equal distribution according to activities.

Cause

Excessive use of wrist extensors. For example:

1. Carrying a heavy case.
2. Wrong technique at sport (e.g. tennis, golf, badminton, fencing).
3. Unaccustomed gardening or carpentry.

Pathology

A tear occurs at the teno-muscular junction, in the tendon or at the teno-periosteal junction (Figure 6.10). The resulting inflammation produces exudate in which fibrin forms to heal the torn tissue. If

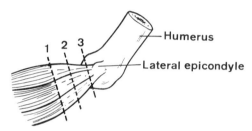

1 = Teno-muscular junction
2 = Tendon
3 = Teno-periosteal junction

Figure 6.10 Sites of lesion in tennis elbow

excessive fibrin is formed fibrous tissue will result in adhesions between the tendon and the neighbouring tissues. This causes pain on being stretched and impairs function. This may occur in one episode but is more commonly a long-term low-grade process. A subperiosteal haematoma may form.
    Repeated use and minor injury to the tendon prevent healing and excessive scar tissue can form.

Clinical features

Pain – Gradual onset present after activity, disappears with rest. With time it takes longer to go, is more easily aggravated and may be more intense.
    Referred pain – Aching or sharp pain over the wrist extensors from elbow to wrist.
    Movements – Elbow, radio-ulnar, wrist and hand joints have full active range. Resisted wrist extension is painful; passive movement is pain free.
    Muscle power – This is normal at first but becomes diminished as the patient stops using the arm.
    Palpation – Tenderness is present over the tendon and is more acute at the site of the lesion. There may be thickening of the tendon and loss of mobility.

Long term – Accessory movements of the elbow and superior radio-ulnar joints may be reduced in a long-term problem.

Physiotherapy

This has to relate to whether the condition is acute or chronic.

Acute

Ice applied after a game or activity helps to reduce inflammation. It is usually applied in a towel for 15–20 minutes.
    Rest is also appropriate. A splint which holds the wrist in extension may be used for 2 or 3 weeks, until resisted extension is pain free.
    Strapping may be used in the form of adhesive elastic tape applied to the forearm to restrict the movement of the tendon and ensure that healing occurs without lengthening.
    Once healing has occurred, the cause of the injury should be analysed, e.g. the thickness of the racket grip.
    If there is residual thickening or immobility of the tendon, this responds well to deep transverse frictions.

Chronic

This is the more common form of the condition because the patient at first thinks the pain will go away and seeks help only when it becomes constant or functionally restricting.
    Examination must be meticulous to enable identification of the lesion.

Modalities used

Deep transverse frictions applied for 5–10 minutes for 3–4 days can restore mobility and stretch adhesions. Progress is tested by resisted wrist extension which will become pain free if the lesion has been correctly treated.
    Ultrasound is often successful – given at dosages of, for example, $1\,\mathrm{W\,cm^{-2}}$, continuous beam for up to 10 minutes before frictions.
    Pulsed electromagnetic energy or ice may be applied after the frictions to ease the tenderness. (It is not sensible to use more than two modalities in one treatment session.)
    Strapping – zinc oxide 2–3 cm wide, applied completely round the forearm just below the teno-muscular junction – helps to reduce stretch on the tendon during everyday activities. This should be kept in position on days between treatment sessions. Where the history is that the pain clears completely but returns following sport, the patient may find it helpful to apply this type of strapping to protect the tendon during sport.

Laser therapy may be dramatically effective if applied to the exact site of a lesion.

It is important to differentiate a lesion in the tendon from other causes of pain on the lateral side of the elbow. These may be:

1. Strain of the lateral ligament.
2. Synovial fringe entrapment between head of radius and capitulum.
3. Arthritis of the radiohumeral or superior radio-ulnar joint.
4. Strain of the teno-periosteal attachment of extensor carpi radialis longus.
5. Radial nerve (or a branch) entrapment possibly within the brachioradialis or supinator.
6. Nerve root pressure in the neck – C5/C6.

Guidelines for physiotherapy in relation to other causes of pain on the lateral side of the elbow

Strain – lateral ligament

Findings

Pain is reproduced by an adduction force applied to the forearm with the elbow in extension and the radio-ulnar joints in supination.

Modalities used

Ultrasound or interferential may obtain pain relief.

Mobilizations – longitudinal movements of the radius or adduction movements of the forearm – help to stretch adhesions in or around the ligament.

Synovial fringe entrapment

Findings

Compression of the radio-humeral joint is painful. Anteroposterior accessory movement may be limited between head of radius and capitulum.

Modalities used

Mobilizations as for the lateral ligament may be useful. Anteroposterior movements of the head of radius may also be successful.

Electromagnetic energy pulsed or continuous given after the mobilizations is helpful in relieving treatment soreness.

Arthritis – of the radio-humeral and radio-ulnar joints

Findings

Active and passive elbow movements are painful – especially where there is a load in the hand (e.g. ironing) or prolonged use of the arm in one position (e.g. holding the telephone for long).

Accessory movements of the joints are limited.

Modalities used

Continuous electromagnetic energy given to obtain heat, followed by mobilization (accessory and longitudinal) to restore synovial sweep across the joint cartilage.

Muscle strengthening is usually required – slow reversals technique is very useful.

Weight lifting may be given to the wrist extensors (patient in sitting) or elbow extensors (patient prone lying with elbow flexed over edge of table). Later – holding weight in hand – bend elbow, stretch arm up and lower.

Strain of teno-periosteal attachment of extensor carpi radialis longus

Findings

Palpation identifies tenderness on the lateral supra-condylar ridge.

Modalities used

Transverse frictions usually clears this lesion.

Nerve entrapment (radial nerve or branches)

Findings

The pain is quite stabbing and sharp and the brachioradialis muscle may be sore. There may be weakness of the wrist extensors so that the patient feels the hand function is impaired.

Modalities used

Deep, wide sweeping kneading to all the soft tissues through which the neve passes on the lateral side of the elbow may help.

Stretching of the radial nerve may be achieved by holding the fingers and wrist in flexion, the radio-ulnar joints in pronation, the elbow in extension and the glenohumeral joint in abduction and lateral rotation. If an adduction stress is added to the forearm, adhesions round the nerve may be released.

Nerve root pressure

Findings

Pain in the neck may or may not be present.

Neck movements are usually restricted – this may be at one segment only and requires close observation to be detected. Side-flexion with overpressure to the side of the painful elbow may reproduce the pain.

Palpation over C4, 5, 6 especially on the side of the painful elbow may reproduce the pain and/or be particularly tender, and there may be spasm of the scalenii.

Modalities used

Cervical traction can have dramatic effects on relieving the pain. If this is the correct treatment, pain should diminish in 2–3 sessions. Mobilizations, e.g. lateral flexion away from the painful side may release tethered nerve roots.

Other treatments

1. Local steroid injection can be very effective when the lesion is identified and the drug reduces the inflammation.
2. Tenotomy to release a fibrosed tendon can be effective.
3. Radial nerve decompression may be carried out for long standing, disabling pain.
4. Excision of a synovial fringe can be very successful.

Golfer's elbow

Definition

This is a condition characterized by pain and acute tenderness on the medial side of the elbow. It affects the common flexor origin.

The principles of treatment are the same as for tennis elbow.

Wrist and hand tendons

Some of the problems arising with these tendons are:

1. Knife wounds – often one tendon only is severed, e.g. extensor pollicis longus.
2. Injuries with glass – a hand or fist through a window can result in cuts of several of the flexor tendons – grasping a sharp surface can cut the finger flexors level with the proximal phalanges.
3. Road, rail or air accidents can cause rupture of any number of tendons.
4. Sudden forced flexion of a finger tip can avulse the extensor digitorum tendon from the distal phalanx (Mallet finger).
5. Sudden forced flexion of the proximal interphalangeal joint avulses extensor digitorum tendon from the middle phalanx resulting in a boutonnière type deformity (Figure 6.10).
6. Spontaneous rupture of the extensor tendons occurs in rheumatoid arthritis.
7. Spontaneous rupture of extensor pollicis longus following a Colles' fracture.

Pathology

Cut tendons

The two ends separate because the part attached to the muscle is retracted owing to elastic recoil or contraction of the muscle fibres. Healing will not take place without good management. Sutured tendons are healed by collagen, scar tissue which starts to form 2–3 days after injury and consolidates over 3 weeks.

Avulsed tendons

If immobilized, scar tissue reattaches the tendon to the periosteum over 3–6 weeks.

Management

1. *Avulsed tendons* – the finger must be immobilized in a splint which fixes the joint or joints so that the tendon is in a shortened position.
2. *Ruptured tendons*
   (a) Suturing of the two ends is performed as soon as possible.
   (b) For spontaneous rupture, a graft may be necessary. The Palmaris longus tendon or one of the extensor digitorum brevis tendons from the foot may be used to provide the graft.

Immobilization may be from 3 to 6 weeks.

Physiotherapy

Mallet finger

A splint is slipped over the finger to hold the distal interphalangeal joint in hyperextension. Physiotherapy is important after the splint is removed (5–6 weeks). The finger joints are mobilized with accessory movements. Finger kneading may be given to mobilize the tendon and effleurage added to reduce swelling. Carefully controlled passive stretching is applied to regain flexion. The patient is taught to hold the middle phalanx initially in extension and practise flexion – 5 bends to the limit of stretch, rest, 5 bends, should be performed every hour because this gradually lengthens the adhesions. Progress can be made by increasing flexion of the proximal interphalangeal joint. A splint may need to be worn for manual activities until full control is regained. This is an irritating injury because it is caused by a trivial force, the joint may become fixed in extension and 'gets in the way'.

Boutonnière deformity (see Figure 9.6, page 135)

A splint must be applied to keep the proximal interphalangeal (PIP) joint in extension and to avoid hyperextension at the distal interphalangeal (DIP) joint. Immobilization is 3–6 weeks. Incorrect splinting can lead to a permanent flexion deformity of the PIP joint which is painful and irritating. Following fixation, mobilizations (postero-anterior accessory movements), kneading and passive stretching are needed to mobilize the joint and soft tissues. If a deformity has developed, passive stretching and thumb kneading must be applied to the tight PIP flexors. Longitudinal stretching to the whole finger helps. Postero-anterior pressure over the posterior aspect of the PIP joint should be applied and taught to the patient to do at home. Auto-resisted finger extension and lumbrical action must also be practised.

Finger flexor or extensor tendons

Following surgical repair, a splint is applied which holds the tendon or tendons in a shortened position for up to 3 weeks, depending on the surgeon's directions. The splint used may be fixed or 'lively'. The latter incorporates a spring or rubber band which pulls the finger into the movement which shortens the tendon. The advantage of this is that the antagonist muscles can work actively and the joint mobility can be maintained. During fixation, the patient must be taught to exercise the free joints. During the second week, resisted exercises for the whole arm should be applied and taught for the patient to practise so that hand muscles are worked isometrically by overflow. Every hour the hand should be placed behind the neck, behind the back, on the opposite shoulder and above the head. It is essential that the hand is not 'carried about like a parcel'.

When the splint is removed, daily physiotherapy is important. Massage, e.g. finger kneading, modified picking up, should be applied to mobilize the scar. Also similar techniques are used to mobilize the tendons especially within sheaths. Carefully controlled passive stretching is applied. Resistance is applied to the antagonist movement and assistance to the movement performed by the tendon.

The patient has to be taught to practise active exercises. A goal is helpful, e.g. for finger flexors, a pole is placed on the palm and the patient has to touch it then hold the fingers on it. Progression is to a thinner object, e.g. a pencil, a ruler, then to the skin of the palm. Squeezing a cotton-wool ball from large to small regains grip, then a hard ball (tennis or squash) should be used to harden the skin and practise the grip.

A night splint should be applied to protect the fingers and tendons until almost full range is regained.

Hard work and determination is required on the part of both patient and physiotherapist to obtain a good functional result. If stiffness, pain and muscle weakness persist, physiotherapy follows the principles for crushed hand.

Tenosynovitis

Definition

This is inflammation of the synovial sheath of a tendon. (Tendinitis is inflammation of a tendon which does not have a sheath.)

Cause

The commonest cause is over-use, but pressure may also cause the condition.

Pathology

Inflammatory changes occur within the tissues of the sheath resulting in excess synovium production and inflammatory exudate. Over 1–2 weeks fibrin forms and can consolidate into adhesions which can impair tendon movement. With correct treatment, the inflammation subsides, the excess fluid is absorbed and the tendon plus sheath return to normal within 2–3 weeks. Over-use and abuse can cause chronic inflammation.

Clinical features

1. *Pain* – Sharp pain is felt at the site of the inflammation and spreads in line with the tendon both distally and proximally.
2. *Redness* – This appears over the line of the tendon.
3. *Swelling* – There is swelling, sometimes sausage shaped, along the length of the sheath.
4. *Crepitus* – 'Grating' can be felt over the sheath as the tendon moves within it.
5. *Loss of function* – This is a disabling condition, the patient being unable to perform any of the movements involving the tendon.

Common sites

1. *Wrist tendons* – caused by over-use, e.g. at a keyboard, prolonged knitting or writing, change of grip (technique or 'handle') in sport.
2. *Extensor pollicis longus* – caused for example by using scissors excessively.
3. *Tibialis anterior* – caused for example by sudden extra-fast walking.
4. *Extensor tendons (toes)* – caused for example by pressure from an ill-fitting shoe or extra walking in tight shoes.

Physiotherapy

Rest is essential for 2–3 weeks. This may be applied by splint (polythene or plaster) and, in the case of the lower limb, crutches.

Splintage may continue if necessary, e.g. a working splint in a light, washable material to enable the patient to work without stressing the tendon further.

Strapping – This may be more effective in supporting the tendon e.g. for finger or thumb tendons.

Ice – An ice bath for up to 10 minutes twice a day will help to reduce inflammation.

Isometric work – After 2–3 days rest, the appropriate muscle is exercised: 5 contractions 2–3 times per day keeps the tendon moving a little and reduces adhesion formation.

Ultrasound – Low dosage (0.25 W cm^{-2}, pulsed) may be applied along the length of the tendon to decrease swelling and relieve pain, 3–7 days after onset.

Frictions – This may be appropriate 2–3 weeks after onset to mobilize the sheath on the tendon and if appropriate, the sheath and tendon or underlying structures.

Prevention of cause – This is essential because the condition may become chronic. A rest–activity ratio is established. For example:

1. At a keyboard, stop every 10 minutes, bend and stretch fingers, wrists, stretch arms upwards, put hands behind head. If possible do not type for longer than 1 hour without a break – try to find another job to do for 5 minutes.
2. Cut then tear material rather than use scissors.
3. Check grip technique or thickness of racquet/bat handle if sport is involved.
4. Change shoes that produce pressure on the foot tendons or use padding to protect them.
5. Correction of gait may be required.

Other techniques

Laser may be used because it can be localized to the tendon to promote absorption of inflammatory exudate.

PEME may also be used to reduce oedema. Where the condition arises in connection with sport, the patient can have access to good management by doctor and physiotherapist. Unfortunately, in some patients the condition becomes advanced or chronic before help becomes available. The appropriate physiotherapy is then:

1. *Ultrasound* – Higher doses (1 W cm^{-2}, continuous).
2. *Frictions* – Given for up to 10 minutes daily.
3. *Analysis of cause* – Apart from the causes mentioned above, the physiotherapist must examine thoroughly by passive movements all the joints over which the tendon passes. This is because the tendon may be subjected to stress by working on a stiff joint.
4. *Cortisone injections* may be used if inflammation does not resolve after 2–3 weeks rest.
5. *Surgery* – Splitting of the tendon sheath may be necessary in which case physiotherapy comprises gradually progressed active exercises.

Muscle injuries

Types of injury are:

1. Strain.
2. Rupture.
3. Contusion.

Strain ('pulled' muscle)

A few fibres are torn. Healing takes place by fibrous union.

Rupture

There is complete loss of continuity of muscle fibres. Both strain and rupture are caused by a sudden stretching force applied whilst the muscle is contracting.

Contusion

This is bruising without loss of continuity of fibres. It is caused by a blow to the muscle.

Pathology

1. Haemorrhage occurs from the damaged capillaries.
2. Inflammatory changes occur.
3. Swelling results from the exuded blood and inflammatory exudate.
4. Synovial fluid may escape into the muscle if there is accompanying damage to a tendon and its sheath.
5. The capillaries are closed by fibrin which consolidates over 2–3 days.
6. The blood clots and fibrin forms within the area resulting in organization. Consolidation of fibrin results in fibrous scar tissue uniting the damaged muscle fibres. This takes 7 days to 3 weeks depending on the degree of damage.

Strain and rupture

Clinical features

History – This is usually clear. The patient can identify the episode that results in the injury.

Pain – Sudden and sickening pain occurs which stops the patient's activity albeit temporarily, e.g. the athlete who tears a hamstring during a race has to stop and limp off the track.

Loss of function – This can be severe, e.g. with quadriceps, or slightly disabling.

Swelling – Appears at site of injury. On palpation there may be a palpable gap in the muscle and tenderness.

Physiotherapy

Strain

Immediate treatment is ice, compression, elevation and rest – as for all soft-tissue injuries. Ice is applied for 20–30 minutes.

Compression is applied by crêpe bandaging with cotton wool. To prevent oedema collecting distal to the bandaging it should start distally and progress proximally with decreasing pressure. Blood flow should be checked – by pressure on a finger- or toe-nail distal to the bandage. Blood should flow back as soon as pressure is released.

Rest may mean lying – on a settee or in bed. Crutches are necessary to avoid weight bearing on a lower limb.

Elevation is important to facilitate drainage of exudate. This regimen is followed for 48 hours to allow the capillaries to heal, then isometric contractions of the muscle should be performed, e.g. five times every hour. This vital to ensure that the scar tissue is laid down in the stress lines of the muscle. A scar with matted fibres running in different directions makes the muscle very vulnerable to further injury. Also adhesions binding the muscle to neighbouring tissues also predispose to further tearing of the tethered muscle.

Over 7–21 days after injury, exercises are gradually progressed from non-weight bearing, inner range to middle to outer range work. Then weight-bearing exercises are added, together with weight or spring resistance as appropriate.

Activities involving full stretching of the muscle as well as everyday functions are then incorporated.

Criteria for progressing are pain and swelling. As these diminish so the vigour of exercise can be increased.

Final rehabilitation must include the following:

1. Full-range movement of joints moved by the muscle.
2. Full power as demanded by the patient's lifestyle.
3. Full pain-free passive stretching.
4. The muscle working as an agonist, fixator and synergist, as well as paying out as an antagonist.
5. Coordination, stopping, starting activities to give the patient complete confidence.
6. A warm-up programme or patient education to minimize future injury.

Complete rupture

This must be sutured as soon as possible and immobilized. The surgeon will dictate when isomet-

ric work can start and non-weight-bearing crutch walking has to be taught for a lower limb muscle.

For example, quadriceps (immobilized in a plaster-of-Paris cylinder): 'isometric' contractions may be started 5–7 days after operation, with foot movements and non-weight-bearing walking. Partial weight bearing is allowed 2 weeks after operation and the plaster cylinder is removed 6 weeks after operation.

Rehabilitation follows the principles as for a strain but is obviously much slower.

Contusion (haematoma)

Clinical features

History – A direct blow to the area can be described by the patient.

Pain – A dull ache is present which can be sharp when the muscle is worked.

Swelling – At the site of the injury. This is tense and very tender on palpation.

Bruising – This may remain localized where it is intra-muscular but may track down fascial planes to quite a distance away from the original injury.

Physiotherapy

A contusion is treated similarly to a strain. In addition to exercises, other modalities may be used. These are:

1. Pulsed electromagnetic energy (PEME).
2. Laser.
3. Ultrasound.
4. Interferential.
5. Faradic type of current.
6. Strapping: splinting.
7. Soft-tissue manipulation.
8. Passive stretching.
9. Auto-stretching.
10. Mobilizations.
11. Hydrotherapy.

Times given relate to contusion or minor strain but could be considered for complete rupture after the stitches are out.

PEME

This may be used 48 hours after the injury, to reduce swelling and promote collagen synthesis. Relief of swelling reduces pain.

Laser

Laser may be used 48 hours after the injury to reduce the inflammatory reaction, therefore reducing exudate formation. Pain is reduced possibly by release of endogenous endorphins or perhaps by inhibition of prostaglandin release. Pain relief is most effective with a wavelength of 910 nm. Acceleration of healing may be obtained with a wavelength of 632.8 nm.

Ultrasound

Ultrasound may be used 48 hours after the injury to increase local arterial circulation and to increase the activity of phagocytes in removing damaged tissue components. This facilitates the growth of capillary buds which bring oxygen and amino acids to the area and accelerate the healing process.

Interferential therapy

This may be of value in relief of residual pain after healing. Useful frequencies are 90–130 Hz. Frequencies of 0–10 Hz may be used to produce a contraction of muscle fibres which is of value when reflex inhibition makes it impossible for the patient to contract the muscle voluntarily. The pumping effect of muscle contraction may be used to reduce oedema. Electrical equilibrium of cell membranes may be restored and this can accelerate healing.

Faradic type of current

This is used for the same purpose as low-frequency interferential. It is often the modality of choice because the length and frequency of contraction can be varied. This makes it possible to simulate the muscle's normal rate of activity. The muscle most commonly requiring this treatment is the quadriceps, but the method should be considered for any muscle with sluggish or no contraction, provided the nerve supply is intact.

Strapping and splinting

Adhesive elastic strapping is used to protect an injured muscle by providing support or limiting stretch, e.g. for a calf muscle (Figure 6.11). It is used for a patient who has to remain active while the injury is healing. Also it is applied for protection when the patient returns to full activity, especially if this includes sport. Generally, strapping should not be left on for longer than a week maximum; 3–4 days is average because there is a danger of the skin breaking down.

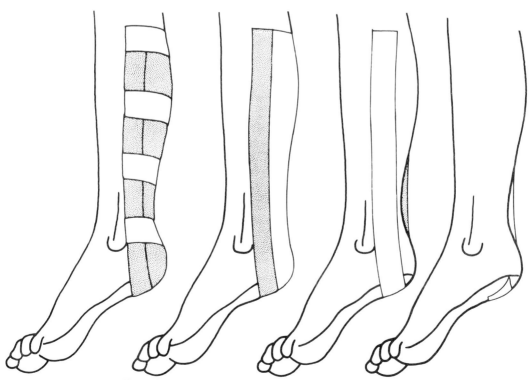

Figure 6.11 Strapping for calf muscle

Principles

1. Always think of the effect to be achieved when applying strapping.
2. Avoid heavy strapping over recent swelling because if oedema continues to form, it will compress blood vessels.
3. Avoid gaps between layers, wrinkles, excessive traction or creasing of the skin.
4. Avoid too much strapping and judge the tension by aiming for effect.
5. The patient should feel comfortable, not longing to have it removed.
6. Splinting may be appropriate for an injured forearm muscle, e.g. a polythene working splint.
7. Shoulder muscles are best rested in a sling.
8. A pad under the heel is a support for the calf muscles.

Tubigrip may be used to provide support when a plaster comes off. It should be in two layers, the underneath one stops short of the top one. The fold of the two layers is at the metatarsal heads or metacarpal heads. One layer is not very supportive but may keep the part warm.

Soft-tissue manipulation

Mobility of muscle tissue and removal of exudate is achieved by effleurage, kneading, picking up, wringing and cross-frictions. This starts after 48 hours and may be applied around the site of injury at first. The techniques encroach on the site around 4–7 days after injury, depending on severity. Frictions are not usually indicated before 14 days. It is essential at first to avoid stressing the tissues in such a way as to increase bleeding, and equally essential later to prevent consolidation of exudate which would cause intra- and extra-muscular adhesions.

Passive stretching

This is essential to maintain extensibility of the muscle and to avoid over-contraction of the new collagen. It should start around 2½–3 weeks after injury. The technique involves taking the limb to the position of maximum available stretch, holding for 10–15 seconds, easing a little further, then releasing. Repeat 5–10 times. As soon as the patient understands the principle, auto-stretching (see Appendix 1) should be started. This should be continued daily (2–3 stretches) for up to a year depending on severity. If the patient plays a sport or is an occasional gardener or decorator, a warm-up programme including stretching should be followed.

Mobilizations

In a neglected injury or low-grade chronic injury, the neighbouring joints may become stiff. Generally accessory movements clear this stiffness.

Hydrotherapy

This is particularly useful for treating a moderate to severe injury of a lower limb. Walking can be practised before it is possible on land because buoyancy relieves some of the body weight. Joint mobility is regained by free active exercises, buoyancy neutralized. Hold–relax repeated contractions may be used to regain muscle extensibility. Strengthening can progress from buoyancy neutralized to resisting. Swelling in the lower limb is reduced because water pressure is greatest at the ankle and foot and decreases proximally when the patient is standing.

Complications of muscle injury

1. Myositis ossificans.
2. Infection.
3. Cyst formation.
4. Acute becoming chronic.

Myositis ossificans (Figure 6.12)

An injury that tears the periosteum may release osteoblasts which ossify the haematoma. The bone tissue forms 4–6 weeks after injury and may consolidate into mature bone by 3–6 months.

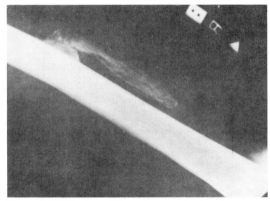

Figure 6.12 Myositis ossificans (arrowed). Anterior aspect of the thigh (From Muckle, 1982, p. 34, with permission.)

Prognosis

With early recognition of onset and good management the bone may be reabsorbed. If not, the bone tissue matures and may cause problems by pressing on blood vessels, nerves and muscle tissue.

Clinical features

1. Loss of range of movement.
2. Pain on muscle activity.
3. Firmness of tissue on palpation.
4. On X-ray there is a faint outline of bone tissue.
5. The commonest sites are:
   (a) Thigh – quadriceps.
   (b) Biceps brachii.
   (c) Supraspinatus.
   (d) Anterior tibialis.

Management

Early diagnosis is vital – and this is usually by the physiotherapist who recognizes the significance of diminishing range or poorer quality of muscle contraction. Physiotherapy must stop immediately.

Rest is so important that the limb is completely immobilized (e.g. in a plaster cylinder for quadriceps) for 3–4 weeks.

After the pain has subsided and the X-ray indicates reabsorption of the bone tissue, rehabilitation may be restarted. This follows a protracted programme similar to the one following an acute injury.

Sometimes surgical removal is necessary.

Infection

This is not common in an intramuscular haematoma but may occur in a subcutaneous area, e.g. anterior aspect of the tibia.

It is treated with rest and antibiotics until clear and then rehabilitation is as for an acute injury.

Cyst formation

A serous filled cavity forms owing to partial but not complete absorption of the haematoma.

Treatment is by incision to remove the fluid. A firm pressure bandage is applied for 2–3 days. Then rehabilitation follows the acute injury programme.

Acute becoming chronic

Poor technique or lack of full mobility following an acute injury can cause repeated minor trauma which causes low-grade chronic inflammation. This leads to excess scar tissue formation, and the muscle function is impaired.

The implications to the patient may range from an irritating twinge occasionally, to loss of a place in the team for a top-class athlete. The hamstring muscles are commonly affected by chronic recurrent strain especially in people with shortened hamstrings.

Physiotherapy

The first important step is to identify the site of the lesion by palpation and by resisting the various movements in which the muscle performs (e.g. for biceps femoris resist hip extension, knee flexion and lateral rotation and test stability of the knee with the patient standing on the affected leg with the knee in semi-flexion).

Once the site of the lesion is identified, ultrasound (e.g. continuous mode, intensity $1\,\mathrm{W\,cm^{-2}}$), deep frictions and passive stretching are usually effective. Muscle power should be developed – preferably monitored by Cybex to ensure that there is a proper balance between quadriceps and hamstrings. Warm-up, auto-stretching and a circuit of exercises appropriate to the patient's requirements must then be worked out. Sometimes strapping may be applied to protect the muscle for a big event, e.g. olympics, tennis final at Wimbledon or the FA cup final.

Fascia

This tends to be a forgotten tissue but it must be considered as the structure at fault in certain situations. These are:

1. Iliotibial tract syndrome.
2. Shin soreness; shin splints; anterior tibial compartment syndrome.
3. Interscapular pain.

Iliotibial tract syndrome

Anatomy

The iliotibial tract is a thickened band of fascia on the lateral aspect of the thigh. Proximally, the gluteus maximus and tensor fasciae latae are inserted into it. Distally it is attached to the lateral condyle of the tibia.

Pathology

The tract can become thickened and tight. The deep surface can become inflamed.

Cause

Excessive use in patients who participate in long-distance sport (running, walking) gives rise to this syndrome. It can also occur in people who habitually stand on one leg more than the other, e.g. a person who favours the left leg has a lengthened left tract and a tightened right tract.

Clinical features

Pain – Usually comes on gradually, over the lateral side of the thigh. It increases in intensity and comes on more readily until the patient decides to seek help.

Tenderness – The tract is tender on palpation, especially in the lower third.

Movements – Hip adduction is slightly limited.

Physiotherapy

1. Rest from the aggravating activity is necessary until the condition clears.
2. Ultrasound applied over the tender or thickened area reduces pain and inflammation.
3. Passive stretching can be applied in the following ways:
   (a) *Stride standing* – trunk and pelvis bend sideways away from tight side.
   (b) *Lying* – Carry both legs to the left, bend trunk to left sliding left hand down left thigh (stretches right iliotibial tract).
   (c) *Lying on right side* – Trunk supported on right hand, place left foot with knee bent behind right leg. Lift right leg off floor – active adduction which lengthens right tract.
   (d) *Lying* – Both legs held up, hips flexed to right angle, knees straight; lower both legs to left (stretch right iliotibial tract).
4. *Mobilizing* – May be required for hip, knee, ankle and foot. The tight tract can cause joint stiffness and vice versa.
5. *Posture* – The patient may require education on posture of the pelvis, legs and feet.

Shin soreness

This is related to a tight fascial compartment in which the anterior tibial muscles are contained. Exercise – especially long-distance walking or unaccustomed running or walking – brings on the pain over the anterior aspect of the shin. As the muscle exercises, fluid collects and the tightness of the fascia causes compression which causes the pain.

Physiotherapy

This is directed at ensuring the ankle and foot movements are full range, and at analysing gait. Any faults detected are then treated. Advice may be as follows:

1. Stop exercising when the pain comes on.

2. Lie with the legs in elevation and an ice towel applied over the painful area for 10–15 minutes. This reduces the swelling.
3. If the pain persists – an orthopaedic surgeon can operate and slit the tight fascia.

Interscapular pain

Longstanding tension in the interscapular muscles is associated with tethering of the fascia. This is a component in a vicious circle: tension in muscle → accumulation of fluid → discomfort → more tension → pressure within fascial compartments → stretching of fascia → reaction of thickening → tethering → more pain → more tension.

Physiotherapy

1. Deep kneading and finger kneading can stretch and loosen tight fascia.
2. 'Springing' – i.e. flat-handed oscillations over the thoracic spine – is essential to mobilize the structures of the vertebral column.
3. Passive, full-range stretching movements of the scapulae restore mobility.

After these techniques have been applied the patient must be taught:

1. Relaxation.
2. Active exercises – particularly shoulder girdle circling with emphasis on retraction.
3. Also, bilateral PNF arm patterns should be practised daily.

Fascial tightness can occur anywhere and must be treated if maximum pain relief and restoration of function are to be obtained.

Bursitis

Definition

Bursitis is inflammation of a bursa. A bursa is a membranous sac lined with endothelial cells. It may or may not communicate with the synovial membranes of joints. The function of a bursa is to prevent friction between two structures (e.g. tendon and bone or tendon and muscle) or to protect bony points.

Common sites

1. Prepatellar bursitis ('housemaid's knee').
2. Suprapatellar bursitis.
3. Subdeltoid bursitis.
4. Miner's or student's elbow (olecranon bursitis).
5. Achillodynia (inflammation of one of the bursae around the tendo achillis).

Causes

1. Trauma – one episode, or, more often, repeated minor episodes.
2. Associated disease, e.g. rheumatoid arthritis, gout.

Pathology

Acute inflammatory changes occur. Chronic inflammation may arise with repeated minor trauma.

Clinical features

Pain – Over the bursa especially on compression.
Swelling – A large fluctuating swelling may be present.

Treatment

Aspiration – Where the bursa is a problem, the fluid may be aspirated. A cortisone injection may be appropriate to reduce inflammation.
Physiotherapy is not generally appropriate, but may be for suprapatellar and subdeltoid bursitis especially if the condition has become chronic.

Suprapatellar bursitis

In the acute stage, ice and a support bandage may be applied, until the swelling goes down. The quadriceps may require progressive strengthening.

In the chronic stage, the principal clinical features are:

1. Dull pain over the knee.
2. Limited knee flexion – particularly weight-bearing crouching.
3. Thickened palpable swelling with adhesions above the patella.

Physiotherapy

1. Ultrasound to the suprapatellar bursa with the knee in flexion (to just short of the limit) – usually 0.8 or 1 W cm^{-2} continuous is applied.
2. Frictions and finger kneading are applied to soften the thickened swelling.
3. Mobilizations (knee in flexion): longitudinal oscillations applied to the patella – directed distally – will stretch the adhesions in the bursa.
4. Later oscillatory flexion is applied at the limit of flexion to regain the last few degrees of movement.
5. Progressive quadriceps strengthening is then required.

Subdeltoid bursitis (subacromial bursitis)

This condition is characterized by a painful arc on shoulder abduction. It is present between 60° and 120° on both active and passive movements when the bursa is passing underneath the acromion process together with supraspinatus tendon, the long head of biceps and the capsule of the glenohumeral joints.

PEME is effective in relieving pain. Mobilizations can also be effective. Longitudinal oscillations or distraction of the glenohumeral joint mobilize adhesions and restore pain-free movement.

Capsulitis of the glenohumeral joint

Pain at the shoulder joint area can arise from:

1. Rotator cuff lesions.
2. Subdeltoid (subacromial) bursitis.
3. Bicipital tendinitis.
4. Osteoarthritis.
5. Rheumatoid arthritis.
6. Osteosarcoma of the humerus (often secondary to breast cancer).

Referred pain may arise from:

1. Pressure on C4, 5 or 6 nerve roots.
2. Acromio-clavicular or sterno-clavicular joints.
3. Cervical rib.
4. Spasm of the scalenii.
5. Diaphragmatic irritation.
6. Gall-bladder problems (right shoulder).
7. Heart problems (left shoulder).

It is evident, therefore, that meticulous examination is required to ensure that the pathology giving rise to shoulder pain is identified.

Capsulitis is generally a reasonable diagnosis when all shoulder movements are limited, the pain is eased by rest or analgesics, and general health is good.

Definition

Inflammation of the capsule and synovial membrane leading to adhesion formation.

Aetiology

1. *Age* – 40 plus.
2. *Sex* – Females tend to be affected between 45 and 55 years and males between 50 and 60 years.
3. *Cause*. This is often not identifiable but may be:
   (a) Trauma: (i) 'wrench' or fall on to the shoulder; (ii) dislocation; (iii) fracture (surgical neck humerus).

(b) Secondary to: (i) cervical spondylosis; (ii) cerebrovascular accident (hemiplegia); (iii) coronary thrombosis.

Pathology

1. Inflammatory changes take place in the capsule and synovial membrane.
2. Exudate accumulates within the capsule especially the dependent part.
3. Adhesions form within this exudate.
4. The inflammatory changes may spread to other periarticular structures.

Clinical features

Pain

1. A dull ache comes on which becomes more intense and constant over a few weeks or months.
2. Sharp pain is produced at the limit of all active or passive movement.
3. The pain is over the acromioclavicular joint and deltoid at first, then gradually spreads down to the elbow and up to the neck.
4. Often the pain is worse at night especially if the patient lies flat.

Movements

All glenohumeral movements are limited by pain at first and 'fibrous stiffness' later.

Muscle spasm

Usually this is present in pectoralis major and latissimus dorsi.

Muscle atrophy

This may occur in deltoid, pectoralis major and the rotator cuff muscles.

Functional loss

The patient is incapacitated because of being unable to reach to high shelves and to put the hand behind the back. Sudden movements and any activity reaching forwards, sideways or backwards are painful.

Posture

Often pectoralis major, pectoralis minor and serratus anterior are tight, with corresponding lengthening of the middle and lower fibres of trapezius. The upper fibres of trapezius are often tight with the shoulder girdle held in elevation. There is, there-fore, a muscle imbalance which impairs glenohumeral rhythm. Often, the head is held with the chin thrust forwards (Figure 6.13).

Anxiety/personality

Often there is an underlying anxiety which must be alleviated before full recovery can be expected.

Management

Capsulitis is one of the most difficult conditions to clear. There are many reported instances of patients who have pain, then stiffness with less pain, then gradual recovery over 2 years, and based on this, several patients are told to take analgesics and 'live with it'.

Physiotherapy has a considerable help to offer provided that the treatment is based on the findings of thorough examination, and regular analysis of progress.

Possible treatments

Interferential therapy applied generally with suction electrodes is effective for relieving pain – especially night pain. Higher frequencies are used for recent-onset high-intensity pain (e.g. 100–140 Hz) and for more chronic lower intensity aching 50–100 Hz may be helpful.

Pulsed electromagnetic energy (PEME) is effective in reducing pain where there is a history of identifiable trauma.

Ultrasound may also be effective if there is a history of injury or repeated minor trauma, by facilitating removal of inflammatory exudate.

Ice therapy is effective in relieving pain in some patients. It may help if the patient is taught to apply an ice towel 10–20 minutes before going to bed so that night pain is reduced. This treatment should not generally be continued for more than 3 weeks.

Heat in the form of an electrical heat pad or rubber hot-water bottle helps to relax muscle spasm and can relieve pain provided that the patient can relax with the arm well supported.

Mobilizations

Accessory movements to the glenohumeral joints are essential for restoring the gliding between joint surfaces necessary for every movement. Physiological movements applied at the limit of available range restore movement when fibrous resistance is the main limiting factor. Lateral and medial rotation must be regained if glenohumeral movements are to be restored. It is important, however, to avoid

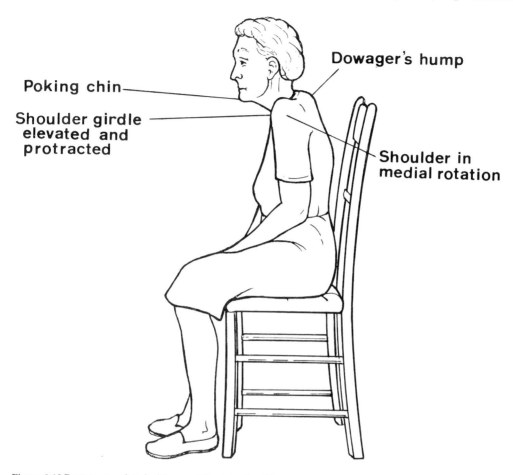

Poking chin

Shoulder girdle elevated and protracted

Dowager's hump

Shoulder in medial rotation

Figure 6.13 Posture associated with capsulitis of the shoulders

treatments aimed at regaining both rotations in the same treatment session because as one is gained the other is lost. Generally, longitudinal oscillations, anteroposterior and postero-anterior oscillations, lateral rotation, elevation and medial rotation (possibly combined with postero-anterior oscillation) form the basis for a mobilizations programme for capsulitis. The acromioclavicular and sternoclavicular joints may require mobilizations and sometimes it is necessary to apply mobilizations to the cervical or thoracic spine to clear the pain. Meticulous examination and regular re-examination is essential to ensure that all the components of spinal and shoulder movements are restored to as near normality as possible. For example, lateral vertebral pressure applied to C7 spinous process can clear shoulder pain even though there is an apparently obvious history of glenohumeral injury. Also, arm elevation through flexion can increase in range following mobilizations to the 9th thoracic spine.

Soft-tissue manipulation

Kneading, wringing and passive stretching are often necessary to relax and lengthen the upper fibres of trapezius. Kneading and finger kneading are used to soften thickenings in the inter-scapular muscles. Finger kneading may also be appropriate applied to the para-vertebral muscles and to the iliac attachment of latissimus dorsi. Passive scapular movements in every direction including oblique patterns may be used to ensure that the shoulder girdle can contribute the components of movement essential in all arm activities.

Frictions may be appropriate to restore movement to the supraspinatus tendon and to the infraspinatus and teres minor muscles.

Mobilizations and soft-tissue manipulation must be combined to regain full functional range. For example, elevation may be applied as an oscillatory end-of-range technique, but may be preceded by deep kneading or passive stretching to the pectorales minor and/or major or latissimus dorsi. The 'hand behind back' functional activity is regained by placing the arm in the position (just short of the comfortable limit) and applying one or two of the following: glenohumeral extension, adduction, medial rotation, postero-anterior movement, elbow flexion, scapular protraction or depression. With the arm in the same position, kneading and finger kneading may be applied to the tissues on the anterior aspect of the glenohumeral joint (at which site the patient feels pain when the arm is brought forward from the hand-behind-back position).

Posture/position sense

Capsulitis – especially of insidious onset – is often associated with poor posture. Shoulder girdle retraction and depression require practice, together with head retraction. Total spinal posture and pelvic symmetry may also require attention. For example, a right-handed patient who writes a lot and tends to sit more on the left buttock than the right can develop shortening of the right paravertebral structures with lengthening on the left. This over time can create unequal movement, and stress occurs at the glenohumeral joint because 'hand above shoulder' activities stretch the tight paravertebral structures.

Relaxation

Relaxation practice should go together with posture training. It is particularly important for the patient to learn to recognize the state of tension in the shoulder girdle elevators and protractors, during everyday activities. Shoudler girdle retraction and depression with a 'hold' then release should be practised regularly throughout the day. General physiological relaxation will also help the patient especially if it is put into practice before going to sleep (see spondylosis and relaxation in Obstetrics).

Movement

Various forms of active movement are appropriate. For example:

1. Proprioceptive neuromuscular facilitation (PNF).
2. Sling suspension.
3. Free active exercises.
4. Resisted active exercises.
5. Group work.
6. Hydrotherapy.

PNF

Stabilizations are appropriate at the stage of acute pain, to maintain muscle power, and fluid flow through the glenohumeral joint tissues. The patient should be taught:

1. Interlink hands together – push together – count 5.
2. Interlink hands together – pull apart (without separating hands) – count 5.
3. Place one fist on top of the other – push together – count 5.
4. Place other fist on top – push together – count 5.

If this pattern is repeated five times 2–3 times per day, all the shoulder muscles are worked without pain. There is less likelihood then of exudate collecting between the joint surfaces and in the dependent part of the capsule, and adhesion formation is minimized. Shoulder girdle retraction should be practised at the same time – also held for count of 5 and repeated five times. Otherwise an imbalance can occur between the pectoral muscles and the shoulder girdle retractors, together with the glenohumeral lateral rotators.

Hold–relax technique is nearly always appropriate to gain lengthening of the pectoralis major and latissimus dorsi.

Repeated contractions are also useful to gain elevation, lateral and medial rotation and to strengthen the muscles producing these movements.

Slow reversal technique applied to both arm patterns is especially useful in regaining coordination as well as strength and should be used in the later stages of treatment to maintain the range gained by mobilizations. Scapular patterns may also be appropriate, to strengthen the lower fibres of trapezius and serratus anterior. Both of these muscles have to act in coordination with the upper fibres of trapazius (force couple effect) to control the scapula and ensure that it provides a firm base for arm movements. The arm muscles as such can be quite strong but if the scapular muscles are weak or out of balance then the whole arm feels weak.

Sling suspension

Abduction or flexion can be practised in a pain-free range with gravity counterbalanced and this gives the patient confidence. If the arm is carried to the limit of, for example, abduction, held and pushed a little further, with the shoulder girdle (scapula) held in depression then the feeling of correct glenohumeral rhythm can be re-educated. This is useful when the active range of movement is poor and painful.

Free active exercises

'Pendular' exercises are very useful for regaining and maintaining range. It is important that the patient stands in walk standing then leans forwards from the hips, bending the front knee, keeping the back straight and placing the hand or forearm on a table. The affected arm should then hang free and a good arc of movement is obtained. A weight in the hand (0.5–1 kg) helps to apply traction to the humerus and increases momentum.

Standing 'walking the fingers up the wall' is a useful exercise for gaining elevation and can be used to monitor progress by having a weekly measurement taken of the distance up the wall.

Auto-assisted elevation – either by clasping one hand with the other or reciprocal pulley – is helpful for the stiff rather than painful shoulder. The patient must be carefully instructed not to bend sideways or backwards and also not to overforce the shoulder.

Towelling action is helpful for regaining hand-behind-back and hand-behind-neck activities. Exercises with a pole, small ball, or bean bag can all be made enjoyable and therapeutic for regaining function.

Some patients benefit by practising sitting (hands on shoulders), elbows raising sideways and watching the movement in a mirror. This helps to regain glenohumeral rhythm because the patient tries to perform the same movement with the affected arm as can be seen in the non-affected arm.

Resisted active exercises

Sitting (weight in hand), elbow bending, straightening (into elevation) and lowering helps to strengthen the elevator muscles.

Sitting (weight in hand) arm raising sideways strengthens the deltoid. This is not necessarily appropriate for every patient. A strengthening programme must be geared to individual patient's requirements.

Group work

Patients require education in posture, relaxation and active exercises which can be well covered in a group of 6–8. Exercises with small apparatus and to music can restore confidence and morale in patients (see Appendix 1).

Hydrotherapy

Where pain is a dominating feature, with muscle spasm also present, hydrotherapy is very beneficial. Relaxation in float lying, hold–relax and trunk movement with the arm fixed all help to reduce pain and regain movement. Exercises with bats and against turbulence help to regain strength, and swimming may help to regain confidence as well as general fitness.

Whiplash of the cervical spine

Definition

This is a set of clinical features which arise from the cervical spine and can be definitely related to an episode of injury.

Aetiology

Age – Any group can be affected, the range is between mid teens to late sixties. Most patients are aged between 20 and 50.

Sex distribution – Equal male and female.

Cause – The classic cause is a deceleration injury in a road traffic accident. If the patient is travelling forwards and comes to a sudden stop, inertia carries the head forward, then it is flicked back into hyperextension and forwards again. If the patient is stationary and a car hits from behind, there is neck extension followed by hyperflexion followed by extension.

Any sudden change in direction can cause injury to the neck, and therefore may be considered as producing 'neck strain'.

Pathology

During hyperflexion, there is stress and possibly rupture of the posterior neck muscles, ligamentum nuchae, interspinous ligaments, capsules of facet joints, posterior longitudinal ligament and possibly nerve roots. There is compression of the anterior structures.

During hyperextension, there is stress in the anterior part of the annulus of the intervertebral discs, the anterior longitudinal ligament and anterior neck muscles. The facet joints, nerve roots and spinous processes tend to be compressed.

If the neck is rotated or side-flexed at the time of the injury, the damage is more extensive.

Damage to the soft tissues of the neck may vary from slight to extensive.

Inflammatory changes take place with exudate and haematoma formation within the damaged tissues. These changes occur over 2–4 days which is why the patient may feel progressively worse after an accident. After 1–3 weeks exudate and haematoma absorption occur and fibrous collagen tissue is laid down. Contraction and remodelling of the collagen fibrils takes place as the patient recovers normal movements.

Clinical features

These again vary according to severity but may be a combination of the following:

1. Pain in the neck, aggravated by movement especially in the direction of the aggravating movement.
2. Referred pain which may radiate to the shoulders, scapula, one or both arms, thoracic spine or head.
3. The nature of the pain is sharp on movement, and for the first few days there may be a constant ache.
4. Paraesthesiae may be present, especially in the ulnar border of the hand.
5. Dizziness or unsteadiness may be present.
6. Spasm of the neck and shoulder girdle muscles.
7. Loss of neck movements – the patient is very protective of the neck and turns the trunk to look round rather than the head.
8. Less commonly, there may be:
   (a) Blurring of the vision.
   (b) Tinnitus (ringing in the ears).
   (c) Dysphagia (difficulty in swallowing – this may be due to retropharyngeal haematoma and the patient must be referred to a doctor immediately).
9. Chest pains and bruising may be present due to the force of a seat belt.

Management

This clearly varies with the intensity of the symptoms. The principles to be followed are:

1. Rest.
2. Mobilization.
3. Relief of pain.
4. Muscle strengthening.
5. Restoration of confidence.
6. Advice and reassurance.
7. Prevention or treatment of chronic problems.

Rest

This is necessary for all but the mildest of cases.

It may be achieved by bed rest in hospital where there is dyaphagia or marked dizziness.

The patient may rest in bed at home or 'rest' may be at home, up and about, off work. In bed, a soft collar or butterfly pillow supports the neck.

Up and about, a firm collar should be worn during the day and a soft one at night. When sitting, the patient should support the arms and neck with pillows in a high-back chair. Generally, the collar should be used as little as possible and discarded as early as possible.

A period of rest is essential to minimize further injury but 48 hours' complete rest is generally long enough.

Mobilization

Mobilizations and soft-tissue techniques

Two to three days after the injury, it is important to start movement so that the inflammatory exudate is absorbed and collagen scar tissue is laid down in the lines of movement. This is important because many patients are not treated at this stage and may attend for physiotherapy months later when fibrous stiffness plus continual, irritating pain are dominant features. Effleurage and kneading applied smoothly and rhythmically relieve muscle spasm and by moving fluid through the tissues, help to clear inflammatory exudate.

Mobilizations (postero-anterior to the spinous processes) grade I or II help to keep the facet joint surfaces moving (especially if the direction of force is applied parallel to the plane of the facet joints). The number of vertebrae treated may be three or four according to palpation examination findings. As the pain settles and physiological movements become easier, progress is by increasing the grade, the number of oscillations or changing to postero-anterior unilateral techniques (sometimes an antero-posterior approach is required, applied to the transverse processes of C3, 4, 5 or possibly 6). Postero-anterior flat-handed 'springing' to the thoracic spine and rib cage is often appropriate for these patients. Hold–relax technique must be used to relax muscle spasm which is still present 4–5 days after the injury so that free active neck exercises can begin around 6–7 days. These should be in lying (non-weight-bearing). Generally it is kind to start with rotation and side flexion and then to add in assisted flexion plus extension (pushing down into the pillow). Flexion and extension may be practised in side lying, performed slowly and within the limits of pain. When the patient is confident that there is no danger or pain in moving the neck, free active exercises may begin in sitting. The final progression should be oblique pattern movements and combined movements.

Relief of pain

Rest, mobilization and analgesics generally obtain pain relief. Residual pain in the neck and shoulders may be relieved by use of a heat pad for 10 minutes 2–3 times a day. Cervical traction may be appropriate to relieve nerve root pain or pins and needles. Generally it is not started until 3 or 4 days after injury and low force (3 kg, 7 lb) for a short time (10 minutes) should be used, on a daily basis. The choice of intermittent or continuous form depends on the degree of injury, i.e. the more severe the injury the more appropriate it may be to use intermittent traction.

Residual pain present at a level unacceptable to the patient 2½–3 weeks after injury may be relieved with pulsed electromagnetic energy.

Muscle strengthening

Isometric work against manual resistance should be applied to the neck muscles in mild to moderate cases 3–4 days after injury. This maintains muscle strength and also helps to clear inflammatory exudate. As mobility recovers, and pain diminishes, manual resistance should be applied throughout full range firstly by the physiotherapist, then by the patient.

Restoration of confidence

The patient may need to talk through the accident and any medico-legal circumstances surrounding it. The physiotherapist should listen but avoid offering advice related to the case. Relaxation techniques may be useful for the patient who is tense. Vertigo exercises are helpful for the patient who is recovering from dizziness and vision problems.

It is sometimes advisable for the patient to wear a collar when travelling, so that sudden unguarded movement will not cause further damage. The patient must not drive a car wearing a collar and it is wise not to drive until neck movements are full, controlled and can be performed quickly, or slowly.

Advice and reassurance

The nature of the injury should be explained to the patient and that recovery is possible just as a 'sprained ankle' recovers. Advice relates to the individual's requirements and must include the following:

1. *Collar* – When to wear and when not to wear.
2. *Sleep* – Position so that the neck and head are supported.
3. *Relaxation* – Practise in lying, sitting, standing, working, walking.
4. *Exercises* – Performed regularly and progressed as treatment progresses.
5. *Work* – Return depends on the nature of the work, e.g. concentrated reading or writing may give rise to headache and neck pain – therefore, part-time work may be better.
6. *Spare time* – Lighter sports, e.g. badminton and tennis, may start before games like rugby. Swimming is helpful only if performed with correct head movement and breathing.

Prevention or treatment of chronic problems

Many patients attending for physiotherapy to relieve neck pain can on close questioning relate the onset to an episode of trauma.

It is essential, therefore, to ensure that full mobility is regained as much as possible. This may mean grade III or IV mobilizations to ensure that each segment is moving followed by auto-mobilizations for the patient to practise at home. It is also important to stress that exercises through full range must be performed daily.

Chronic problems are treated according to examination findings. Deep kneading and passive stretching are often necessary to mobilize tight soft tissues together with mobilizations, posture training and active exercises.

Crush injuries

Crushed hand

Definition

Damage to the hand from a crushing injury may be severe enough to damage nerves, arteries, tendons and bones or it may be minor enough to cause only soft-tissue damage.

Aetiology

Crushed hand injury can occur at any age and to women and men equally. Injuries may be due to the hand being caught in machinery, gates or doors, under a heavy object or in road or rail accidents.

Pathology

1. Nerves may require suturing and will regenerate (see peripheral nerve injuries).
2. Fractures of metacarpals and phalanges may require immobilization for a minumum period (see fractures).
3. Blood vessels must be sutured within 6 hours so that tissues can be revitalized.
4. Skin which is lacerated must be sutured once infection is cleared. Healing of the skin takes place over 3 weeks. If skin is lost, grafting may be required (see Skin grafts).
5. Tendons may require immobilization or suturing (see tendon injuries).

Even without any of these above injuries, oedema formation takes place. This is very serious in the hand because, although the dorsum has loose skin which can accommodate excess fluid, the palm and fingers have tight fascial compartments. Fluid collects in muscles, tendon sheaths, ligaments and between joint surfaces. If allowed to remain, consolidation and fibrin formation takes place which seriously impairs tissue mobility, and hand function can be very limited.

Clinical features

Assuming there is soft-tisue injury only with the skin intact:

1. *Pain* – Present as a dull ache and sharp on movement.
2. *Movement* of the fingers may be limited to a few degrees of flexion. The fingers and thumb are held in slight flexion.
3. *Function* – Loss of function is severe if the whole hand is involved and is irritating if only one finger is affected.

Physiotherapy

The main aims of physiotherapy are to:

1. Reduce oedema.
2. Regain mobility of the joints and soft tissues.
3. Strengthen and regain coordination of muscles.
4. Toughen the skin.
5. Regain function and confidence.

Reduction of oedema

A pad of wool in the palm, cotton wool between the fingers and a pressure bandage should be applied for 24–48 hours after the injury. An arm sling is advisable to keep the hand elevated while the patient is moving about; when the patient is sitting or lying the hand must be elevated.

Two or three times in the day, the bandage should be taken off and the hand dipped in iced water for up to 10 minutes.

Exercises should start as soon as the patient can tolerate the discomfort.

Isometric work for the hand muscles is applied by manual resistance to the finger and thumb tips. PNF slow reversals and holds should be applied to the arm so that overflow causes isometric work for the hand muscles. The patient must practise this at home.

Contrast baths should be applied at home once or twice a day. After 3–4 days the bandage may be left off during the day but re-applied at night for protection whilst the patient is sleeping.

Pulsed electromagnetic energy applied daily helps to reduce the oedema.

Kneading and effleurage applied fairly firmly within the limits of minor discomfort will reduce oedema and mobilize soft tissues. Passive or assisted active movements should be taught for the patient to practise every hour so that joint surfaces are moved and tendons slide within sheaths. Also at home, the patient should practise squeezing a bandage 4–5 times hourly with the hand in elevation.

Mobility

Mobilizations applied as accessory movements at first and then physiological movements to the finger joints regain mobility and the patient is encouraged to practise mobilizing exercises immediately after mobilizations. Progression from gripping a tennis ball, to a golf ball, to a piece of dowelling, to a pencil helps restore gripping.

Strength and coordination

The gripping exercises and PNF help to regain strength at the same time as reducing oedema. Coordination is regained by various activities such as: throwing and catching beanbags, tennis or botton wool balls; precision exercises with marbles, cards, corks, newspaper, tying knots in ropes.

Toughening the skin

This involves weight bearing which may simply be leaning on a table or prone kneeling for some patients. For athletic patients rope climbing or bunny jumps are advanced weight-bearing hand exercises.

Function and confidence

An exercise programme must be devised which will include power, pinch, precision and hook grips. Steady weight bearing (as in gardening in prone kneeling) and protection as in falling should be practised (the latter can be practised in prone over a gymnastic ball with the patient balancing on one hand then the other). Lifting and carrying is important and should include different shapes – a cup of tea or a hand towel, a pane of glass for a glazier, a briefcase for a businessman and hot, heavy cooking utensils for a chef.

Residual stiffness

A patient may present for physiotherapy 5–6 weeks after injury, having not been given any instructions. Intensive daily mobilizing is then necessary. Mobilizations for the finger and thumb joints have to be given at grade III (Maitland, 1986). Intercarpal and metacarpal movements must be vigorously applied. Deep kneading must complement the mobilizations and then squeezing exercises in warm water should be practised. If the swelling becomes softer, it may appear to increase at first and a pressure bandage may be necessary especially at night for 2 or 3 days. Contrast baths should be taught for the patient to practise at home. Auto-resisted (manually or with an elastic band) exercises should be applied to each finger in turn. Bilateral exercises help such as:

1. Holding big ball, carry over head, out to one side, then the other.

2. Screwing lid off coffee jar – first with good hand, then affected hand.
3. Two-handed Indian-club swinging.
4. Holding pole in both hands, carry up over head, behind head, up and down.
5. Pass ball right hand over right shoulder to catch behind back with left hand and vice versa.
6. Ultrasound and PEME may help to mobilize the fluid prior to mobilizations.

Occupational therapy would be very helpful for this patient. In the ideal situation, the hand would be treated with mobilizations, kneading and passive movements and then the patient would have a functional hand programme in the occupational therapy department.

That this constitutes multiple treatments, preferably daily, reflects the vigour with which a stiff hand must be treated if permanent disability is to be avoided.

Sensory loss

Sometimes there is loss of sensation in the fingers even though the main nerves are intact, because the terminal branches become implicated in the oedema.

Stereognosis

Sensation should recover and can be re-educated by stereognosis.

A tray of different objects is presented to the patient. With the eyes open, the patient is asked to pick up one object, hold it and move it around in the hand, register how it feels, close the eyes, and go on feeling, then replace it for another one with the eyes open again. This process is repeated until the patient feels reasonably confident. The patient is then instructed by the physiotherapist to close the eyes and pick up a nominated object; the greater the number of objects the harder it is. If this is too difficult it may be necessary for the physiotherapist to start by placing an object in the patient's hand (eyes closed) and asking him to identify it by feel alone.

Examples of objects:

1. *Different textures* – Cotton thread reel, piece of India rubber, cotton wool, crêpe bandage, newspaper, felt.
2. *Different shapes* – Pencil, ball, polystyrene cup, box.
3. *Different sizes* – Jam jar, marbles, safety pin.
4. *Different weights* – Golf ball, table tennis ball, polystyrene cups with different amounts of sand.
5. *Different coins* – £1, 50p, 20p, 2p, 1p, 5p, 10p.
6. *Different everyday objects* – Pencil, ball of wool, piece of paper, washing-up cloth, soap dish, towel, buttons, buckets, door handles.

7. *Tasks (eyes closed):*
   (a) Put marbles into jam jar.
   (b) Put different shaped pegs into corresponding shapes in a board.
   (c) Write letters, numbers, draw pinmen.
8. Thermal sensation may be re-educated using tubes with hot and cold water.

Two-point discrimination may be re-educated by teaching the patient to feel two pins – far apart, then brought close together. Note that the index finger and thumb are more sensitive, therefore should register two points which are quite near and would feel like one on the dorsum of the hand.

Self-massage for oedema (kneading and effleurage) and auto-resisted exercises will also help to re-educate sensation.

Crushed foot

A foot crushed by a weight falling on it or someone standing on the foot (e.g. at a disco) can be as disabling as a crushed hand. If there are no bones broken, the principles of treatment are similar to those for crushed hand.

First 48 hours

The foot should be dipped into a bucket of water and ice (two-thirds ice: one-third water) in and out for up to 10 minutes. A crêpe bandage should then be applied from the metatarsal heads up to the lower third of the leg. This should provide enough compression but if it is felt that there is oedema accumulating on the dorsum, then an elastic pressure bandage may be applied. The foot should be rested in elevation whenever possible for 48 hours and one or two sticks used as necessary to relieve pain on weight bearing.

After 48 hours

Contrast baths should be used. Effleurage and kneading should be applied to reduce oedema. Exercises should be practised – if possible with the patient sitting on a bed or on the floor with the feet against a wall.

The exercises are:

1. Lumbrical action.
2. Toe spreading.
3. Toes pushing against wall – lifting and pushing.
4. 'Walk' foot up wall and down.

The bandage should be re-applied whenever the foot is to be weight-bearing.

Mobilizations – Intermetatarsal movements and intertarsal movements should be given to prevent oedema consolidating and forming intra-articular adhesions.

As pain subsides, intrinsic foot exercises, walking re-reduction, and progressive activities should follow a similar programme as for a sprained ankle ligament.

Spinal pain

Published statistics on spinal pain tend to relate to working days lost or GP/hospital attendances and probably do not give a true picture of the prevalence of the problem. There are people who seek treatment from sources other than so-called ortho-dox medicine, or who do not happen to be working and therefore do not feature in the 'working days lost' list or who self-treat by 'over-the-counter drugs'. Suffice it to say that in any population within most industrialized countries it would be difficult to find a person over the age of 40 who could claim to never having had pain in the spinal region. Physiotherapy has a well-recognized part to play in the management of people with pain of spinal origin especially where the cause is considered to be 'mechanical' or 'structural'.

Pain in the spine may arise from a number of diseases or disorders, classified as follows:

1. Structural and traumatic:
   (a) Fractures (see Chapter 4).
   (b) Sprains and strains of ligaments and muscles.
   (c) Postural or occupational stress.
   (d) Disc lesions (see Chapter 11).
   (e) Spondylolysis and spondylolisthesis (see Chapter 8).
   (f) Spondylosis (see Chapter 8).
   (g) Spinal stenosis.
   (h) Congenital deformity.
2. Inflammatory:
   (a) Ankylosing spondylitis (see Chapter 9).
   (b) Rheumatoid arthritis (see Chapter 9).
   (c) Sero-negative arthropathies (see Chapter 9).
   (d) Infections.
3. Neoplasms:
   (a) Primary tumours.
   (b) Secondary tumours from, for example, kidney, pelvic organs or breast.
4. Visceral referred:
   From abdominal organs, kidneys, heart, oesophagitis, bronchitis, pleurisy, aortic aneurysm or ear problems (cervical spine).
5. Bone diseases (see Chapter 7):
   (a) Paget's.
   (b) Osteoporosis.
6. Metabolic:
   Gout (see Chapter 10).

Given the right kind of management some patients become pain free while others learn to have a reasonable quality of life with the pain at a controllable level.

Physiotherapy for structural or mechanical disorders

The spinal ligaments and muscles like others in the limbs are subjected to acute and chronic sprain or strain. Acute injuries tend to settle and the patient may not seek professional medical help. Rest and 'over the counter' analgesics are often sufficient to satisfy the patient that all is well. Unfortunately, if there is a true injury (due for example, to a fall, a slip with one foot on ice, a sudden twist or stretch) the pain will settle but unless the patient performs specific exercises, the healing scar tissue will be laid down in an irregular matted fashion which predis-poses the spine to further injury; therefore patients often do not present until the pain or discomfort has been present for several months or there is a history of repeated episodes of disorder or dysfunction.

In this case, the physiotherapy should be con-ducted as follows:

1. Examination.
2. Assessment of findings.
3. Decision to treat.
4. Selection of technique and of test for determining effect of treatment.
5. Discussion with patient regarding prevention of recurrence or management of chronic pain.

Examination

Subjective

During this component of the examination the physiotherapist must try to formulate a working hypothesis for the objective component, identify indications for methods of treatment and rule out contraindications (see Appendix 2).

The patient's lifestyle must be discussed and this often identifies poor posture at work or leisure togehter with a dominance of flexion.

The onset may be insidious, which is associated with poor posture and degenerative changes, or there may be an identifiable sudden onset. This may be following an accustomed exercise, e.g. decorat-ing, gardening, building a garage, playing cricket with the grandchildren, or 'ever since my rugby playing days' or 'since my first pregnancy'.

Pain that is persistent, worse at night, does not ease with analgesics or by changing from movement, position or rest should be considered with great respect. It may indicate neoplasm, or inflammatory disease if associated with general malaise or a poor colour. Meningitis can start with a stiff neck, toxaemia can give rise to mild backache. Clearly, it is important that the physiotherapist has these possibilities in mind when examining a patient with spinal pain whether or not the patient has been referred from a doctor. It is also important to remember that evidence of a non-mechanical disorder may develop as the patient attends for treatment and the physiotherapist must then report the findings to the appropriate medical practitioner.

Objective examination begins as soon as the patient arrives in that the physiotherapist can learn a lot by watching how the patient walks, responds to the initial welcome and invitation to sit or lie down. Subjective examination continues whilst movement and palpation are being performed and it is important to interlink the two aspects. However, before observation, movement testing and palpation there should be a clear picture of the site and nature of pain-aggravating factors, easing factors and the effect of the pain on the patient's life-style. Clearly the patient who has pain that is easily stirred and takes a long time to settle will have much less testing than the one who has little pain, aggravated only by vigorous exercise and settling quickly. Symptoms such as pins and needles and feelings of numbness must also be noted so that they can be taken into account during the objective examination.

Aspects of objective examination

Observation, complemented by palpation with the patient in standing and sitting is essential to obtain a clear picture of bony alignment and position together with soft-tissue tension and mobility. Figure 6.14 shows bony points for guidance. Note must also be taken of leg positioning and of the state of the structures indicated. Leg abnormalities – e.g. unilateral tightness of hamstrings, tendency to stand on one leg, curved tendo Achillis (pronated foot) – has a direct bearing on pelvic symmetry and unilateral stress on the lumbar spine during walking and standing. Activity such as lifting and carrying or golfing based on asymmetry is almost bound to lead to pain at some time. Treatment must then be directed at the structure at fault, e.g. correcting foot posture or mobilizing stiff tibiofibular joints.

Movements of the spine as a whole should be examined for range, quality, and limiting factors. Again it is important to look beyond the area the patient immediately associates with the pain. Muscle power must be tested and attention paid to the quality of contraction as well as asymmetry of tone or tightness. As with movements, muscles must be tested which are not necessarily adjacent to the painful area. For example, the hip abductors must be tested because unilateral abnormalities can give rise to pelvic torsion which may result in stress with pain in the thoracic spine. Also, limited shoulder movement may result in pulling on the latissimus dorsi which in turn can distort the hip bone and cause sacroiliac strain. Palpation and passive physiological intervertebral movements performed with the patient in lying identify hypo- or hypermobility at individual segmental level and are essential for clarifying the abnormalities contributing to the patient's pain. There are many tests that may be appropriate before there is sufficient information to plan a treatment programme (see Further reading).

Assessment of findings

This is a vital step in the treatment of the patient. The physiotherapist must consider the findings and try to put them in an order of importance, then decide what the patient might start to do immediately as self-help and what has to be achieved by the skilful application of physiotherapy techniques.

For example, the patient may be encouraged to consider changing a habit, such as sitting on the floor in side sitting always on the right side. This causes shortening of the left trunk side flexors, amongst other problems.

At work there may be a situation where the patient is sitting with filing cabinets on the left so that throughout the day there is torsion to the left. The situation should be remedied by moving some files to the right or by establishing some compensating activity to the right. A patient may develop pain in the left side of the neck due to a habit of holding a telephone receiver between the left shoulder and the neck whilst writing with the right hand. This can be rectified by having a desktop loudspeaker.

A patient may participate regularly in a predominantly asymmetrical sport, for example rowing in pairs, fours or eights, which causes unequal development of trunk muscles.

Decision to treat

The physiotherapist has then to decide if the patient's problems can be treated by physiotherapy. This means that the findings indicate a musculoskeletal problem or problems that are likely to respond to physiotherapy skills. This is not always easy because it may involve sending the patient away without 'treatment', e.g. the patient who has neck pain but is anxious about an imminent driving test, who is advised on relaxation of the neck and shoulder muscles and asked to return when the test is over.

Selection of technique and test

The physiotherapist must then select a technique of treatment directed at achieving a goal, e.g. stretching a tight muscle, mobilizing a stiff segment, relaxing muscle spasm. The methods may be mobilizations for regaining vertebral movement or passive stretching to stretch a muscle. Clearly it is essential to tailor the treatment to individual findings based on a working hypothesis, and each patient is different. As the patient improves, techniques must be adjusted, e.g. postero-anterior

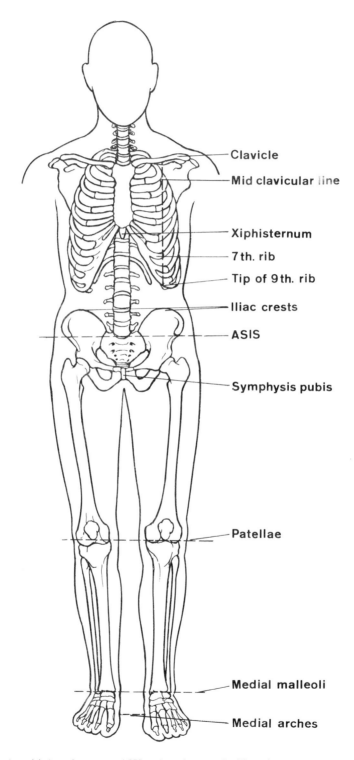

Figure 6.14 Bony points. (*a*) Anterior aspect. ASIS = Anterior superior iliac spines

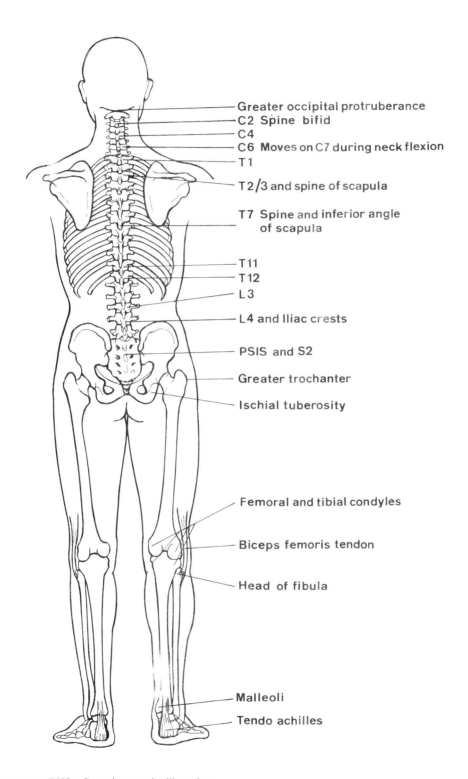

Greater occipital protruberance
C2 Spine bifid
C4
C6 Moves on C7 during neck flexion
T1

T2/3 and spine of scapula

T7 Spine and inferior angle
    of scapula

T11
T12
L3

L4 and Iliac crests

PSIS and S2

Greater trochanter

Ischial tuberosity

Femoral and tibial condyles

Biceps femoris tendon

Head of fibula

Malleoli
Tendo achilles

(*b*) Posterior aspect. PSIS = Posterior superior iliac spines

mobilizations may be directed cephalad to a spinous process with the spine in a position of total flexion to restore movement to a segment which does not contribute its component to flexion as a whole. Frictions to the supraspinous ligament or localized muscular thickenings should also be applied in a position of stretch.

Exercises must be equally logically selected. For example, for a lordosis, lumbar isometric flexion exercises (LIFEs) are indicated and inner range extension exercises are contraindicated. Conversely, LIFEs are contraindicated where there is flattening of the lumbar spine for which auto-passive extension in prone lying may be indicated (McKenzie, 1985). Sometimes exercises must be asymmetrical, e.g. prone kneeling right arm and leg stretching for shortening of the right side flexors.

A test may be a limited movement and improvement may be increase of range, same range but less pain or easier to perform. As the patient improves

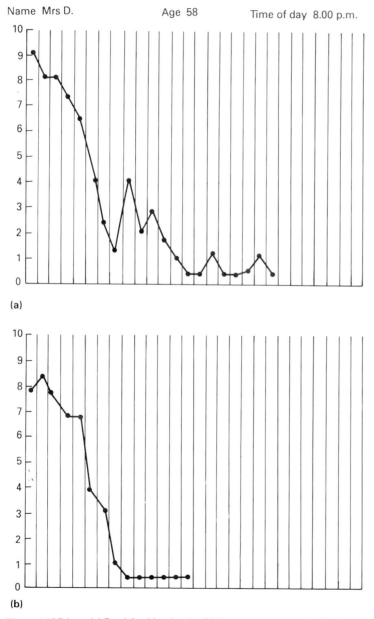

Figure 6.15 Diary. (*a*) P_1, right side of neck. (*b*) Test movement: neck side flex

the movement may have to be sustained or repeated quickly or combined with another movement. Sometimes the test may have to be time related, e.g. pain comes on later in the day, or is intermittent where it was constant.

To assist both the patient and the therapist in monitoring progress it is helpful if the patient keeps a diary (Figure 6.15).

Discussion of prevention of recurrence

Once the spine is moving smoothly and intersegmental movement is restored the patient should have a programme of exercises to perform every day. For example, if there is chronic supraspinous ligamentous strain due to prolonged flexion as a component of the patient's lifestyle then extension stretching should be performed every day. Stretching exercises for tight hamstrings, rectus femoris or calf muscles may be appropriate (see Appendix 1).

It is also helpful for the patient to continue the principle of the diary and to accept that 'level 2' is 'liveable with' whereas 'level 3' and rising means the exercises that may have been neglected have to be restarted. This is often sufficient to contain the problem. At 'level 6' the patient should have the facility to contact the physiotherapist for immediate help. Pain that is intractable may be managed with TNS, or group therapy which encourages the patient to participate in activities and create a lifestyle in which the pain (although at level 6–8) does not dominate.

Hydrotherapy is of particular value for the patient who has widespread spinal pain which is aggravated by weight bearing and eased in lying. The warmth and support of the water afford pain relief and relaxation of muscle spasm. Mobility and muscle power can be restored by large range exercises. Posture training is readily practised in sitting and standing with the support of the water. Swimming is an excellent exercise for the spinal muscles and general body fitness, particularly where the patient's lifestyle is dominated by flexion (sitting job, sitting hobbies, drives to work). It is important, however, to note that swimming is not the answer for all patients – two types in particular. One is the patient whose pain is aggravated by extension and the other is the patient who keeps the head up to breathe and as a result swims with the neck in hyperextension. Backstroke may, of course, be used instead of crawl or breaststroke. Once a patient has benefited from hydrotherapy, it is worth suggesting a swimming session twice a week as a prophylactic exercise and for general body fitness.

Patient recording of pain intensity and daily occurrence (Figure 6.15)

The patient is asked to consider the pain on a scale of 0 to 10, where 0 = no pain and 10 = the pain at its worst. At the same time every day the patient considers the last 24 hours and records the highest pain level experienced. Sometimes it is helpful to select the time of day when the pain is generally at its worst. If there are several pains then the worst should be chosen. For example, if the worst pain is in the neck and there are secondary pains in the shoulder or scapular area then it is the intensity of the neck pain which is recorded. 'T' can be put on the days of treatment as this can help to monitor effects of the treatment. Graph (a) represents a pain diary. Where the patient records a higher level than the previous day, it is helpful to note any activity, e.g. long journey, several hours' disco dancing, change of diet. This helps to identify possible aggravating factors. Graph (b) represents the record of a test movement. This monitors objective progress by the patient's assessment of pain produced by the movement (this could be more objectively tested if the patient has a method of measurement that is reasonably repeatable). It is useful to have both graphs because as can be seen by the sample the movement may improve but the pain lags behind. The patient, however, recognizes progress, is encouraged and feels better able to cope with life.

References

Evans, P. (1980) The healing process at cellular level. *Physiotherapy*, **66**, 256–259

Hickling, P. and Golding, J. (1984) *An outline of Rheumatology*, Wright, Bristol, p. 3

McKenzie (1985) *Treat Your Own Back*, 3rd edn. Spinal Publications, London, p. 60

Maitland, G. D. (1986) *Vertebral Manipulation*, 5th edn, Butterworths, London

Muckle, D. S. (1982) *Injuries in Sport*, 2nd edn, Wright, Bristol

Chapter 7

Diseases and disorders of bones and joints

Definition of deformity
Causes of disease and disorders
Principles of general management

Physiotherapy management
Specific conditions of lower extremity,
* spine and upper extremity*

Some diseases and disorders of bones and joints are discussed elsewhere in this book, as for example the Rheumatology section (Chapters 8–11). However, those conditions that are not encompassed under other headings, and are of significance to the physiotherapist, are grouped in this chapter. They may be those in which the physiotherapist is involved in the management or where the disease or disorder leads to the development of a secondary condition, as for example osteoarthritis, which requires physiotherapy. The majority of the conditions described in this chapter result in a temporary or permanent deformity.

Definition of deformity

An abnormal position of a bone or joint, or abnormal development as in achondroplasia (short limb), phocomelia (aplasia of proximal part and presence of distal part of limb – 'seal limb'), or absence of a limb or part of a limb.

Causes of diseases and disorders

These may be either congenital or acquired.

Congenital

These are faulty developments that occur *in utero* and are present at birth, although in some instances the problem may not be recognized until later.

There may be a genetic abnormality, for example mutation of whole chromosomes as occurs in mongolism, or part of a single gene as may occur in achondroplasia.

Congenital abnormalities may also be caused by environmental factors – radiation, rubella, drugs such as thalidomide, and anoxia. The abnormality depends on the time of incidence relative to the stage of development of the fetus.

Sometimes abnormalities may be due to a mixture of genetic and environmental factors.

Acquired

Trauma – Fractures, dislocations and subluxations have been covered in Chapter 4. Permanent deformities of the bone or joint can arise from these and may lead to further compensatory deformities as for example a short leg following a fractured femur may result in a postural scoliosis. Deformities of joints may arise as the result of damage to the cartilage, or soft tissues that may contract and hold a joint in an abnormal position.

Muscle imbalance – This may be a cause of deformity of a joint if there is a weakness or paralysis of muscles (flaccid or spastic) which develops as the result of another condition.

Endocrine disorders – For example, osteitis fibrosa from hyperparathyroidism, acromegaly from hyperpituitarism.

Metabolic disorders – For example, rickets.

Infection – Some of the infections such as osteomyelitis and tuberculosis are far less common since the advent of antibiotics.

Bone diseases – Carcinoma, Perthes'.

Diseases and degenerative disorders of joints – See Chapters 8–11.

Other diseases and disorders of unknown cause – For example, idiopathic scoliosis.

Acquired joint deformities

These fall into the various categories described below depending on the cause and the resultant changes taking place.

1. There are no structural changes and the position can be corrected by the patient. There may be weakness of some muscles giving an imbalance around the joint and so the patient has difficulty in retaining the correct position. Alternatively the person may develop a habit of holding the joint in an incorrect position which could lead to muscle weakness. In either instance the patient will lose 'position sense'.
2. Paralysis of muscle, whether flaccid or spastic, will give joint deformity. Initially it is not a fixed deformity and can be corrected by the physiotherapist but it cannot be held by the patient. If the abnormal state of the muscle persists this may lead to structural change.
3. There may be structural changes of soft tissues leading to contractures which will give a fixed deformity. There may be a slight change of bone structure and if correction cannot be obtained a secondary osteoarthritis will probably develop resulting in further deformity.
4. Severe structural abnormality affecting bone and consequent soft-tissue contracture around the joint will give a fixed deformity which cannot be corrected without surgical intervention.

Principles of general management

Medical or surgical

In some diseases or disorders a cure may be effected or the disease process halted and the development of deformity prevented provided that the diagnosis is established early. Endocrine and metabolic disturbances can be cured or halted in this way, and infections can be treated with antibiotics. Some disorders can be corrected by early positioning and immobilization as in congenital dislocation of the hip or talipes equinovarus but the result will depend on the severity of the abnormality and whether any structural changes have taken place.

Patients with acquired postural deformities may not require any medical or surgical treatment but may be referred to the physiotherapist for advice and/or treatment.

Deformities where there is contracture of soft-tissue structures and which may include some bone change may be treated by passive stretching and/or surgical release. In those deformities where there are severe bone changes and a fixed deformity the only possible treatment may be by surgical intervention. This can occasionally result in improved function and a better cosmetic appearance.

Physiotherapy management

This will vary according to the medical and/or surgical treatment and to the type of deformity present.

Deformities with no alteration in bone structure or contracture of soft tissues

The joints are usually mobile and the deformity can easily be corrected by positioning.

If physiotherapy is indicated following an assessment by the physiotherapist then the aims of treatment will include:

1. Relief of pain caused by stretching of soft-tissue structures.
2. Strengthening of any weak muscles.
3. Teaching the patient how to correct the position and re-educating an awareness of this position.

The specific aims of treatment must be considered in the context of the whole problem.

Postural deformities occur quite commonly in children and may or may not need treatment. For example, a child who grows quickly and is tall in comparison with other children in her age group may develop a stooping posture so that her height is not as obvious. Generally such deformities correct themselves as the other children grow and any difference is less marked. Posture is often a reflection of psychological reactions – shyness, depression, insecurity – and physical treatment will not cure these deformities unless the underlying psychological problem is dealt with. Other deformities in this group may be the result of muscle imbalance, in which case the weak muscles need to be strengthened.

This type of deformity can be secondary to another abnormality and the aim should be to prevent this occurring if possible. For example, a short leg due to a fractured femur tends to give a compensatory postural scoliosis and this can be prevented or the scoliosis minimized if the surgeon gives the patient a shoe raise. However, the patient may still need postural and gait re-education as well as advice from the physiotherapist. Other secondary deformities such as a scoliosis resulting from a prolapsed intervertebral disc will not change unless the primary problem is treated.

Deformities with contracture of the soft tissues

The physiotherapist may be concerned with passive stretching of the contracted soft tissues and positioning in a corrected or over-corrected position, particularly in conditions such as talipes equinovarus or torticollis. This must be accompanied by exercises to strengthen weak muscles and by postural re-education. In the case of babies the mother may be taught how to do the passive stretching and positioning, but it must be carefully monitored by the physiotherapist to ensure that the treatment is effective. The desired movements may be obtained by reflex activities and the use of toys.

Following the surgical release of tight structures and immobilization in the corrected position the physiotherapist can teach static contractions of the muscles which will hold the corrected position, and then active exercises and postural re-education after the removal of the fixation.

The important aim in the above cases, whether they are treated conservatively or by surgery, is for the physiotherapist to try to maintain corrected positions by muscular activity and re-education of position. There will be other aims and objectives which will depend on the particular condition and the assessment of the individual by the physiotherapist.

Severe deformities with bone changes and soft-tissue contractures

There is nothing the physiotherapist can do to decrease deformities of this type. However, help may be required in various ways, for example patients with severe thoracic scoliosis may develop chest infections which may need physiotherapy or the patient may need treatment for the relief of muscular pain. Active exercises may be required to maintain the mobility of other joints, to strengthen muscles and to maintain as good a position as possible.

When surgical intervention is necessary the physiotherapist will be one of the team concerned with the management of the patient. The aims will depend on the specific surgery and the correction achieved.

Specific conditions of lower extremity, spine and upper extremity

Lower extremity

Congenital dislocation of the hip

This condition may affect one or both hips and the dislocation may be partial or complete. Girls are more often affected than boys in the ratio of about six to one.

Cause

Generally the cause is genetic and the failure in development *in utero* may affect the bone or

ligaments, or both. There may be a defective development of the acetabulum which is often bilateral and predisposes to subluxation or dislocation. Ligamentous laxity may occur as the result of the release of the hormone relaxin by the fetal uterus in response to oestrone and progesterone in the fetal circulation. Breech delivery sometimes predisposes to a congenital dislocation or subluxation.

Pathology

Bones

The acetabulum is shallow and the upper part fails to form the horizontal roof. Sometimes it may appear normal at birth but then fails to develop further and fills up with fibrous tissue and fat. As a result of this the head of the femur rides up on the ilium and by exerting pressure may indent the bone forming a pseudo-socket which is rarely deep enough to make a firm support.

The femoral head is poorly developed and may become more deformed as a result of the displacement. It is usually displaced backwards and upwards although more rarely it can be displaced anteriorly to lie below the anterior superior spine.

The neck of the femur is usually anteverted.

Ligaments

There may be a developmental laxity of the ligaments or they may be stretched as the result of the displacement of the femoral head. The capsule is gradually elongated and the anterior portion is stretched across the acetabulum and may become adherent to the rim.

The ligamentum of the head may be missing or poorly developed. The glenoid labrum is often folded into the acetabulum and this may impede reduction.

Muscles

The changes are those that occur mainly as a result of the subluxation or dislocation, particularly when early treatment is not successful. These changes will make reduction more difficult to obtain. The long muscles passing from the pelvis to the femur, or to the tibia or fibula will tend to become shortened and these will offer resistance to reduction (hamstrings, sartorius, rectus femoris, the adductors).

The short muscles attached between the pelvis and the femur are altered in direction and this alters their function. Gluteus medius and gluteus minimus become more horizontal in direction and this makes their angle of pull largely ineffective, not only as abductors of the hip but in their important function of keeping the pelvis level during weight transference.

In posterior dislocations the tendon of psoas major is displaced so that it compresses the capsule of the hip joint producing an 'hour-glass' shape. It thus stretches between the origin and insertion like a sling, and the pelvis is supported on it, and on the capsule.

Clinical features

Early diagnosis is very important if a good result is to be achieved. The clinical features are not very obvious until the child begins to walk, but the observer should look for asymmetry in the buttock folds, a shortening of one leg and restricted abduction in flexion. If the condition is bilateral detection may be more difficult but there will be a wider perineum than normal and a lumbar lordosis may be noted quite early. Later features include the following:

1. *Trendelenburg's sign* – As described above, the patient cannot hold the pelvis level when standing on the affected side, because the abductors are at such a disadvantage that they cannot function effectively. This dropping of the pelvis towards the sound side when the patient stands on the affected side constitutes Trendelenburg's sign, and accounts for the peculiar gait.
2. *Gait* – In unilateral cases there is a very marked limp, the patient dropping the pelvis towards the sound side every time the weight is placed on the affected limb. In order to counteract this the trunk is jerked in the opposite direction (i.e. towards the affected side). In bilateral cases the gait is an exaggerated waddle, the pelvis being dropped alternately on either side, and the trunk jerked correspondingly from side to side.
3. *Lordosis* – This occurs in posterior dislocations because the pelvis is tilted forward and the back is hollowed to compensate for this. It disappears when the hip is flexed, as in the sitting position. It is much less marked in the unilateral cases than the bilateral.
4. *Scoliosis* develops in unilateral cases, the convexity of the curve being towards the sound limb, because the pelvis is dropped on this side.
5. *Apparent shortening* – There is apparent shortening of the leg (2.5–4 cm, 1–1½ in) because the head of the femur is displaced upwards. This can be demonstrated by placing the child in crook lying on the plinth, when the affected knee will be found to be lower than the other.
6. *Position of the great trochanter* – This lies above Nélaton's line (i.e. a line drawn from the anterior superior spine to the tuberosity of the ischium), instead of on the line. Since it protrudes above the upper border of the gluteus maximus it is prominent, though this is more noticeable in adults than in children.
7. *Buttocks* – In bilateral cases the buttocks are broad, flat, and somewhat triangular in shape, owing to the altered position of the gluteus maximus. Also, in bilateral cases, the perineum is wider than normal.
8. *Pain* – As a rule children do not suffer any pain, but as they grow older there is fatigue on exertion, especially in bilateral cases. Spasm of muscles may also cause considerable pain. The symptoms tend to become worse as the patient advances in age.

Management

Treatment of this condition has improved with better post-natal care and early diagnosis. The aim is to replace the femoral head in the acetabulum and maintain it in position until normal development of the acetabulum occurs.

Between birth and 6 months – If the hip is unstable after 3 weeks the baby is immobilized in moderate abduction for about 3 months.

6 months to 6 years – As a result of early diagnosis there are fewer presenting with this condition in this age group. Treatment is first attempted by closed reduction. Initially weight traction is applied through a frame or 'Gallows' traction and then the hips are gradually abducted until about 80° is reached. Usually this takes 3 or 4 weeks. Then the legs are immobilized in plaster of Paris with moderate medial rotation and moderate abduction for several months. This position has superceded the 'Frog' position that was previously used because of the possible danger to the blood supply.

Operative reduction – If the above conservative treatment is not successful then some form of surgery may be necessary. The actual procedure will depend on the particular problem. Anteversion of the neck of the femur may require an osteotomy using a fixed plate and screws. The patient is then immobilized in plaster for 6 weeks and then all splintage is removed. Other procedures may be used to correct the defective acetabulum. If osteoarthritis develops when the patient is older it may be necessary to perform a total hip replacement.

Physiotherapy management

Early conservative treatment as outlined above may not require any physiotherapy unless the child has any problems following removal of the fixation. Hydrotherapy is useful for encouraging general leg activity, and in particular abduction, and the child can be supported easily. It is very important to gain a good walking pattern when the child is ambulant in order to try to prevent further trauma to the hip.

Children who have had an open reduction may need a more active mobilizing programme after the removal of fixation, combined with strengthening exercises and walking re-education.

If the patient has not been treated successfully at an early age then she is likely to develop problems in adult life. Osteoarthritis is likely to develop with consequent pain and stiffness which may require surgical intervention. The management of osteoarthritis and total hip replacement is dealt with in Chapters 8–11.

Slipped femoral epiphysis

This occurs in young people before the bones have ossified. It affects boys more than girls in the ratio of 5:1 and, at approximately 14–16 years of age in boys and slightly younger in girls.

The femoral head slips in relation to its position on the femoral neck resulting in the head facing more posteriorly and the limb is laterally rotated.

Cause

It may happen following a twisting injury or sometimes there is a gradual slipping which is probably due to a less violent trauma.

Clinical features

In cases of a twisting injury the features are similar to a fracture with acute pain and an inability to move the leg. When the displacement is more gradual the child develops a limp and complains of pain which is often referred to the knee. The leg tends to lie in a laterally rotated position and medial rotation is limited.

Management

In the acute case the surgeon will reduce the displacement and then fix it with pins. When there is a gradual displacement reduction is not attempted as a rule because of the danger of damaging the arterial supply to the head of the femur with a resultant avascular necrosis. Usually the head is held in place with a pin and this may be followed by a subtrochanteric osteotomy at a later date.

Physiotherapy management

This is similar to the treatment for a fracture with emphasis on mobilizing the hip joint and strengthening the muscles, particularly the abductors. The leg should not be adducted across the midline of the body. Walking re-education is very important to try to prevent further trauma to the hip which could be caused by an incorrect gait pattern.

Perthés' disease (Legg–Calvé–Perthés' disease)

This is due to an obstruction of the blood supply to the femoral head giving an avascular necrosis which may result in the partial collapse of the subchondral ossification centre. In some patients it may occur in other epiphyses such as those of the vertebral bodies. Usually the sex and age incidence is that of boys between 6 and 8 years. This is a relatively uncommon condition, and the cause is unknown.

The necrosis may result in a flattening of the head of the femur and a short broad neck. The disease is self-limiting and the normal density of the head, as seen on radiographs, returns after about 18 months. Unfortunately any flattening of the head that has occurred during the acute stage of the disease will be permanent. This may lead to the development of osteoarthritis in adult life. However, the earlier the onset, the better the prognosis, and about 75% of the patients suffer very little permanent disability.

Clinical features

In the early stages the hip is painful and the child has a slight limp. There may be slight limitation of abduction and medial rotation. The necrotic changes and deformity of the femoral head will be seen on X-ray.

Management

Orthopaedic surgeons have varying opinions about the treatment of this condition. However, the main emphasis today seems to be to give no active treatment but to keep the child under observation. Sometimes it may be necessary to maintain a position of abduction and medial rotation for a period of time.

Physiotherapy management

Physiotherapy is rarely required unless a period of immobilization necessitates gentle mobilization of the hip and walking re-education after the fixation has been removed.

Coxa vara

The normal angle of the neck of the femur to the shaft is approximately 125°. A decrease of this angle is known as coxa vara and it may occur for a number of reasons. Some may be due to a congenital defect whereby part of the neck of the femur remains as unossified cartilage and gradually bends. Others can occur as the result of fractures in the trochanteric region or a slipped femoral epiphysis. Coxa vara may also occur when the bone is softened by disease as in rickets, osteomalacia or Paget's disease.

Clinical features

There is shortening of the leg and impaired efficiency of abduction, which results in a positive Trendelenburg sign.

Management

This depends on whether the underlying cause can be treated. If the patient is left with a mild abnormality no treatment may be necessary, but a severe deformity may require an osteotomy to correct the angle between the neck and the shaft.

Physiotherapy management

This would depend on the above treatment. If there is no surgical treatment then physiotherapy may not be necessary although sometimes it is advisable to strengthen muscles, particularly the abductors of the hip, and to re-educate gait. Following surgery the aims of treatment will be to mobilize the hip, strengthen the muscles around the joint and re-educate walking.

Genu valgum (knock-knee)

There is abduction of the tibia on the femur so that in standing the knees come close together and there is a gap between the feet. This condition may be the result of a developmental abnormality or disease which affects the structure of the knee joint.

Management

When the condition occurs in young children it often corrects itself and generally no treatment is required. Because of the position of the legs it is usually associated with postural flat feet.

When the condition is the result of a disease process, for example rheumatoid arthritis, then treatment may be necessary. If the deformity is due to changes in the soft-tissue structures, lengthening of the medial ligament and weakness of muscles, correction may be achieved by splinting. However, if bone changes have occurred surgery may be required. In some cases a wedge osteotomy may be indicated whereas in others, particularly when there is constant pain, a knee replacement may be considered.

Physiotherapy management

Treatment is not usually required for children with postural defects unless the postural flat feet persist, when the management will be as described in the section on flat feet (see page 94).

Patients treated by splinting may be helped by some form of treatment to relieve pain, strengthening exercises for the muscles, and re-education of gait possibly with the help of crutches or a frame.

Patients who have had surgery will require pre- and post-operative treatment as described in Chapters 8–11.

Genu varum (bow legs)

In this condition there may be adduction of the tibia on the femur, or there may be a bowing of the whole leg with the femur and tibia both being curved. The causes may be similar to those for genu valgus although the postural form in children is less common.

Management

This will depend on the cause and the type of deformity. It may not be possible to correct a deformity involving a bowing of the femur and the tibia unless a complicated osteotomy is performed. The principles of treatment for an adduction of the tibia on the femur will be similar to that for genu valgum.

Physiotherapy management

This will depend on the surgical management and will be similar to that described for genu valgum.

Disorders of the feet

Talipes equinovarus (Figure 7.1)

This is the commonest of the deformities occurring at the region of the ankle, subtaloid and mid-tarsal joints. The foot is plantar flexed at the ankle joint, adducted and inverted at the subtaloid and mid-tarsal joints. The condition may be unilateral or bilateral.

Causes

The usual cause appears to be a defect in fetal development. When talipes equinovarus is the only

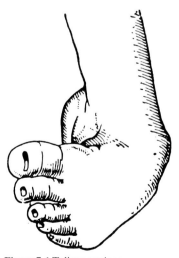

Figure 7.1 Talipes equinovarus

defect present there may be a family history of this condition indicating a hereditary factor. The deformity may be one of a complex series of deformities in children with cerebral palsy or spina bifida. The condition can be acquired as the result of disease or injury. However, the commonest causation is congenital and is the one that will be dealt with here.

Pathology

Initially there may be little bony abnormality although there is usually a subluxation at the talo-navicular joint, so that the navicular lies partly on the medial instead of the distal part of the talus. The soft tissues on the medial side of the foot are underdeveloped and shorter than usual. The calf and peroneal muscles are underdeveloped. With early diagnosis and treatment it may be possible to obtain a good result and good function. However, in some cases there may be further deterioration with the tarsal bones becoming misshapen and then the joint deformities will become fixed.

Management

When this condition is diagnosed early, treatment may be conservative with the aim of correcting the deformity and then holding the foot in the corrected or over-corrected position. Passive stretching is performed gradually, correcting the adduction and inversion deformity first with the foot being taken slowly into the neutral position and then if possible the foot is taken into the abducted and everted position (Figure 7.2(a)). This is followed by a correction of the equinus deformity (Figure 7.2(b)). The corrected or over-corrected position may be held in metal splints (Denis Browne splint) (Figure 7.3), or plaster which is extended to the upper part of the thigh with the knee flexed 90°, or adhesive strapping (Figure 7.4). If plaster is used it is retained for approximately 3 months – initially it is changed weekly and then every 2–3 weeks. The choice of the above methods will depend on the severity of the deformity, the age of the infant, and the orthopaedic surgeon responsible for the child. Some surgeons prefer not to use rigid splints as this inevitably restricts all foot movements and retards the development of muscles.

Physiotherapy management

Immediately after birth, when the condition is mild and the foot is relatively mobile, the physiotherapist may carry out the passive stretchings. It is important to fix the lower end of the tibia and keep the knee flexed to prevent damage to the lower tibial and fibular epiphyses and to the knee joint. The plantar flexion deformity must be corrected by pressure on the heel and not on the forefoot. Ideally the mother should be taught to do these movements several times a day, but the physiotherapist must check that the movements are being performed correctly and that the mother is doing them a sufficient number of times.

If adhesive strapping is used to hold a corrected position this may be applied by the physiotherapist and replaced once or twice a week. A physiotherapist must be experienced and skilled in the use

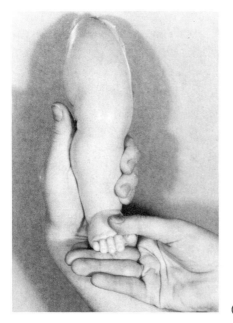

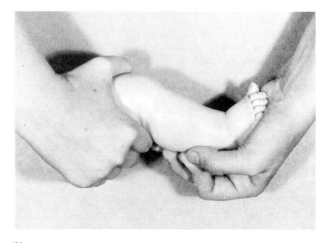

(b)   **Figure 7.2** Passive correction of talipes equinovarus

(a)

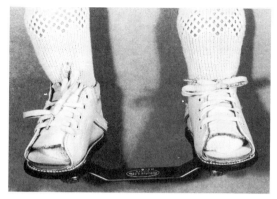

Figure 7.3 Splints to correct talipes equinovarus

of strapping as there are dangers involved in incorrect strapping – for example it could be too tight thus impeding the circulation, or cause pressure sores, or the pressure may be greater than the child can tolerate. The mother must be taught to watch for any problems with the strapping, or with other methods of fixation and report at once if there is a problem.

If the deformity cannot be corrected conservatively then surgery may be necessary. The extent of the surgery will depend on the severity of the deformity but the taut ligaments on the medial side of the foot are divided and similarly a tendon if it is too tight. The tarsal bones are manipulated into as correct a position as possible. Then the limb is placed in plaster of Paris for 2–3 months. If the child has already walked then this may be a walking plaster. Following the removal of the fixation the physiotherapist aims to maintain the correct position by passive movements and active exercises, with particular emphasis on the dorsiflexors and evertors. If the child has been ambulant then a correct walking pattern must be taught, but if not then the child should be observed as weight bearing starts. The child may require a surgical shoe, or if not, the physiotherapist should advise on suitable footwear. It is important in all the above methods of treatment that the child is seen at regular intervals by one of the members of the medical team after treatment has ceased, to see that the corrected position and function have been maintained.

Other ankle disorders

Other disorders occurring in the region of the ankle and foot are talipes calcaneum, talipes equinus, talipes varus and talipes valgus. These are not as common as talipes equinovarus and will not be described here. The treatment will depend on the cause and severity of the deformity.

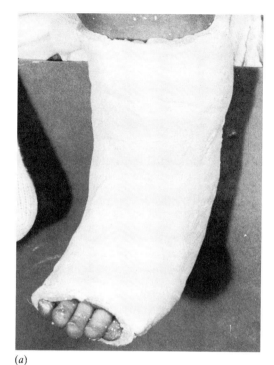

(a)

(b)

Figure 7.4. (a) Plaster to correct talipes equinovarus. (b) Strapping to correct talipes equinovarus

Flat feet (pes planus)

Normal function of the feet

The complexities of the walking pattern are described in Appendix 1. However, to aid understanding of the effect of disorders of the foot on walking the function and anatomy of the foot is described briefly here. This should serve to remind the reader of the basic principles, but a further study of anatomy and biomechanics is necessary to give a fuller understanding of the subject. The foot has two main functions: to support the weight of the body in standing or when moving, and to propel the body forward in walking or any other weight-bearing activity. To fulfil the first function the foot could be a flat plate but this would not allow the distribution of weight over the whole foot as occurs with an arched foot. Also there would not be the same control over postural shift, which is important in preparing to move. Thus an arched foot gives a better distribution of weight for a variety of activities. To fulfil the second function of propulsion the foot must be capable of forming a strong lever as well as supporting the body weight. Mechanically a segmented lever needs to be built in an arched form to work efficiently.

In standing the weight is distributed between the feet and so there is a larger base of support. In walking the weight of the body is taken on one foot in the stance phase and then carried forward over that foot and then through to the other foot as that comes into the stance phase. In running and jumping the weight distribution is more crucial as the weight comes onto the foot as it hits the ground; and even more importantly, only part of the foot is in contact, as the heel is kept off the ground by the strong propulsive thrust of the plantar flexors.

The bony structure of the foot, the ligaments and musculature all assist in fulfilling the above functions. The foot has three arches: two longitudinal, one medial and lateral, and one transverse. If the feet are placed together there is a second transverse arch, lying posterior to the other, formed by a transverse section of the two medial longitudinal arches. These arches differ in height in different individuals, at different ages, and in differing actions. The foot of a baby appears flat because of the amount of fatty connective tissue in the sole and because the muscles working on the arches have not been used in walking. The arches normally become apparent between the ages of 3 and 4. The lateral arch lying between the posterior part of the inferior aspect of the calcaneum and the heads of the 4th and 5th metatarsals is low compared with the medial arch. It is relatively immobile and is concerned with the transmission of weight and thrust to the ground. The medial arch lies between the posterior aspect of the calcaneum and the 1st, 2nd and 3rd metatarsal heads and is generally higher than the lateral. It is

mobile and varies considerably in shape according to whether the individual is standing, walking or running. During standing the arch is low with the muscles relaxed and the strain probably taken by the ligaments. During activity the intrinsic muscles of the foot contract giving stability to the segments of the lever and allowing the extrinsic muscles to exert a strong propelling force. During strike action in walking the heel hits the ground first followed by the lateral side of the foot and then it rolls across to take the weight over the foot and onto the metatarsal heads. Thus in the stance phase the foot is supinated. Then as the heel lifts off the ground the medial arch is raised and the foot pronated, and the main thrust occurs through the ball of the great toe.

There is still controversy about the part played by the various muscles in the various functional activities.

Flat feet

This condition is characterized by the diminution or disappearance of the longitudinal arches of the foot (Figure 7.5). As can be appreciated from the

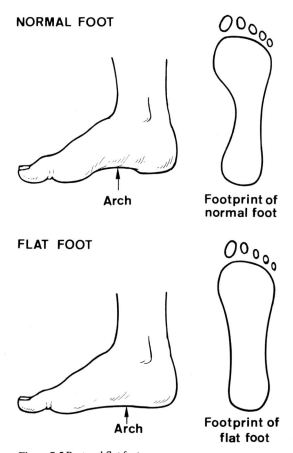

Figure 7.5 Postural flat feet

description of the normal function this will affect the propulsive force, given by the muscles acting on the segmented levers of the foot, to a varying degree depending on whether it is a postural or structural deformity.

Postural flat feet

In children under the age of 3 years the arches are normally flat, as described under normal function. Some children under 5 years of age have postural flat feet associated with a postural genu valgum. The condition is painless but it may cause concern to the parents. It is generally agreed that the majority of children do not require active treatment for the condition, but advice should be given to the parents on suitable footwear.

School children have regular medical examinations and so postural or structural abnormalities will be seen then, or may be reported by the parents. In some cases the foot is painless, the joints are mobile and the muscles are strong and these children probably do not require any treatment. However, in others the feet may be painful and the muscles weak. Initially the joints may be mobile but if the condition is not treated they may become stiff. Occasionally there is some slight structural abnormality of the bones.

Adults may develop a painful flat foot (or feet) for a number of reasons. Certain occupations, particularly when there is prolonged standing, may lead to the development of a painful flat foot. In standing the ligaments are stretched and if this is continued with very little muscular activity the foot may become painful. The muscles may be weak already or the pain may prevent the normal muscular activity and they will become weak. People who are overweight place a similar stress on the arches of the feet. Flat feet may result from disease, for example rheumatoid arthritis, and in these cases there may be structural abnormality. If there is an altered joint position of the hip or the knee due to disease or disorder this may result in a secondary postural flat foot. Poor footwear may be a contributory factor in deformities of the feet.

Pes planovalgus (Figure 7.6)

This is more common than a pes planus and occurs when the foot rolls in to lie in an everted position in standing. Usually there are no structural changes although there may be a slight tightness of the tendo calcaneus.

Peroneal spastic flat foot

This seems to be caused by an irritative focus in the tarsus giving peroneal muscular spasm and resulting in a painful flat foot. This is most commonly seen

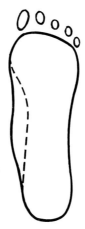

Figure 7.6 Pes planovalgus

when there is a congenital fusion between the calcaneum and the navicular (calcaneo-navicular bar), or more rarely it may be due to a low-grade osteitis. Usually it becomes evident during adolescence and affects boys more than girls.

Management

Cases of painless postural flat feet in children usually do not require any treatment, but advice should be given on suitable footwear. Painful flat feet are usually referred to the physiotherapist for advice and treatment if necessary. In adults the treatment will depend on the cause and whether there is any structural abnormality. Painful flat feet due to occupational stress may be helped by physiotherapy and advice. If this is not successful the patient may be advised to consider a change of occupation if this is possible. If the patient is overweight they will be given advice on diet and may be referred to a dietitian. Again these patients should be advised about suitable footwear and in some instances it may be helpful for them to have an arch support. If the patient regains sufficient muscle power and postural sense then the support can be discarded. Flat feet caused by disease can be treated similarly to postural flat feet if there are no structural changes. Treatment for patients with structural changes will depend on the severity of the deformity and the actual structures affected. If there is a fixed deformity surgical shoes or shoes with an arch support may help to give relief of pain and allow the patient to be ambulant. In some cases surgery may be necessary to relieve pain and if possible restore function.

Children with peroneal spastic flat foot may be treated by immobilization in plaster for a period of time. If this is not successful surgical intervention may be required to excise the calcaneo-navicular bar. In some cases it may be necessary to perform a triple arthrodesis with fusion of the subtalar, calcaneo-cuboid and talo-navicular joints.

Physiotherapy management – postural flat feet

Children

If the foot is mobile the emphasis should be on strengthening the muscles supporting the medial longitudinal arch, particularly the tibialis posterior, tibialis anterior, flexor digitorum longus and brevis. If the joints are stiff then mobilizing techniques must be used in conjunction with the strengthening exercises. The child must be taught to control the position of the whole body in standing and walking. In young children the parents should be shown the exercises so that they can continue the treatment at home. The child should be encouraged to take part in physical activity as general strengthening of all the muscles of the legs and trunk are important in conjunction with specific treatment for the feet. The parents must be advised about suitable footwear with the requirements mentioned below. If the treatment is to be effective the child and parents must appreciate the importance of regular exercise. If the child is normally active and participates in games and/or other activities then a fairly short period of treatment may suffice. However, the feet should be checked regularly to see that the correction has been maintained.

Adults

The treatment will depend on the cause, the severity of the condition and the functional needs of the patient. For example, physical treatment is not very likely to help obese patients unless they lose weight. Pain may be relieved by rest and if necessary some form of heat or contrast baths. Once the pain has decreased then active exercises for the muscles supporting the medial arch can be started. The muscles supporting the anterior arch are usually weak as well and so exercises for the intrinsic muscles should be included. It may be useful to use faradic foot baths to start with to help the patient regain the feeling of movement and to see which movements are possible. This may also assist in relieving pain as the active contraction and relaxation of the muscles will help the circulation and help to relieve any muscle spasm. Faradic foot baths must always be used in conjunction with exercises and should not be used as a substitute for exercises.

In assessing the patient it is important for the physiotherapist to look at the whole posture, and to assess the strength of the muscles and the mobility of the joints in the leg. Sometimes treatment can be too specific, and the effect of the condition on other parts of the body is not appreciated. The plan of treatment and its effectiveness will depend on a good assessment. Specific exercises for the muscles supporting the medial and transverse arches will form part of the treatment plan, but it must include posture correction, re-education of gait and advice on footwear. In formulating plans it is important to consider the cause of the condition and its severity, the age and ability of the patient, occupation and/or leisure activities.

Footwear

The shoes must be well fitting and comfortable. The inner side of the shoe should be straight and the upper edge of the shoe should fit closely, but not tightly, to the foot particularly round the heel. The toes should not be compressed from the front or from the sides. The shoe should be pliable both in the upper part and in the sole so that the normal movements are not restricted. The shoes may have a small heel but it should not be so high that it throws the weight of the body forward over the front of the foot. Attractive shoes can still measure up to these requirements.

Physiotherapy management – structural abnormalities

When there is a fixed deformity the physiotherapist may be able to give symptomatic relief of pain depending on the cause. If surgery is not indicated the patient may be given permanent supports and the physiotherapist will make an assessment to determine whether any active treatment is required apart from re-education of gait and advice on functional activities.

If the surgeon decides to operate, any post-operative treatment will depend on the nature and purpose of the procedure.

Metatarsalgia

This is a condition, as the name implies, where there is pain in the metatarsal region. It is usually felt under the metatarsal heads and is commonly found in the middle aged or elderly, and more often in women than men.

Causes

Metatarsalgia may be due to weak intrinsic muscles allowing the anterior arch to collapse. As the metatarsal bones splay out this stretches the transverse ligaments and causes pain. The initiating causes may be similar to those for postural flat feet in the adult as described previously. Also it can occur in relation to certain other foot deformities, as for example talipes equinus or pes cavus. Patients suffering from rheumatoid arthritis may develop metatarsalgia, or it may occur following fractures of the metatarsal bones. Unsuitable footwear may be a contributory factor, particularly if the heel is high enough to throw the weight of the body forward on to the metatarsal heads. A heel of this type also causes the metatarso-phalangeal joints to be passively extended.

Morton's disease – In this instance there is an enlargement of the plantar digital nerve, usually in the cleft between the 2nd and 3rd toes or the 3rd and 4th. The digital vessel may be affected and the lumen of the vessel obliterated.

Clinical features

The type of pain varies, it may be dull and aching in character or take the form of intermittent periods of excruciating pain. In the case of Morton's disease the pain is usually acute. The metatarsal heads are usually prominent on the sole of the foot with callosities forming over the heads. The interphalangeal joints are usually flexed, giving a clawing of the toes, and callosities may form over the dorsal aspects of the joints. The walking pattern will be affected, with the spring and resilience of the foot being lost.

Management

The feet should be rested as much as possible to relieve the pressure on the metatarsal heads and the patient should be advised not to stand for any long periods. The patient should be advised about suitable footwear, particularly if they have been wearing shoes with a high heel. A metatarsal pad may be used to relieve pressure on the metatarsal heads until the intrinsic muscles have been strengthened to support the arch. It is very important that this pad is placed correctly *behind* the metatarsal heads and it should follow the shape of the bones. This pad can be fixed to the foot with adhesive strapping or a wide band of elastic. If the pad needs to be permanent it may be incorporated into the shoe but it must fit correctly.

Morton's disease – Usually this requires surgical intervention to remove the neuroma.

Physiotherapy management

If there is any stiffness of the joints passive mobilization may be helpful in increasing the movements. Passive moulding of the arch helps to give the patient the feeling of the movement produced by the intrinsic muscles. The intrinsic muscles supporting the arch, namely the lumbricals and the interossei, must be strengthened. Initially faradic foot baths may be given to re-educate the pattern of movement. However, it is essential, as emphasized previously, that this is accompanied by active re-education of the intrinsics. Assessment of the whole limb and the general posture of the patient must be considered in planning the treatment programme. The programme will include re-education of walking and advice on general weight-bearing activities. The physiotherapist should advise the patient on correct footwear and apply a metatarsal pad if necessary. If a metatarsal pad has already been supplied the physiotherapist must check that it is being worn in the correct position. The patient must continue to practise the exercises at home, and follow the advice given, if the treatment is to be effective.

Morton's disease – The postoperative treatment will be similar to that described above with particular emphasis on re-education of the intrinsics and correction of gait.

Hallux valgus (Figure 7.7)

This is a common condition in which the deformity of the great toe consists of abnormal abduction of the 1st metatarsal and adduction of the phalanges.

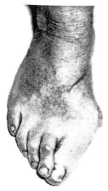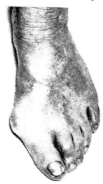

Figure 7.7 Hallux valgus

In severe cases the toe may lie under or over the 2nd toe. This condition seems to affect women more than men and can appear in adolescence or later life depending on the cause.

Causes

A hallux valgus may be due to an abnormality in development of the metatarsals with a varus position of the 1st metatarsal. This may not become apparent until adolescence and if the deformity is slight it may not cause any problems at this time. However, it may become more pronounced in adult life and require treatment. A hallux valgus developing in an adult may be the result of disease such as rheumatoid arthritis or gout. As with most foot deformities the problem can be exacerbated by unsuitable footwear, although this is not the primary cause.

Pathological changes

The joint space is increased medially and decreased laterally thus stretching the medial structures and producing an adaptive shortening of the soft-tissue structures on the lateral side. The lateral deviation of the base of the proximal phalanx results in a subluxation of the 1st metatarso-phalangeal joint and this increases the deformity. Degeneration of the articular cartilage occurs as a result of the altered joint mechanics. When rheumatoid arthritis is the causal factor there may be erosion of bone. New bone is laid down on the inner side of the metatarsal head, leading to the formation of bony outgrowths – exostoses. The prominence of the metatarsal head results in increased pressure and the formation of a callosity which is called a bunion. This inflames the underlying tissues and in some cases may suppurate.

Clinical features

Initially this condition may not cause any disability but as the deformity increases and a bunion develops there will be increasing discomfort and pain. It will be difficult to wear ordinary shoes because of the pain caused by the pressure of the shoe on the bunion. Walking will inevitably be affected because of the normal pattern of weight transference and thrust through the great toe.

Management

Adolescent – The majority do not require surgery but if it is necessary the contracted structures on the lateral side of the 1st metatarso-phalangeal joint are released, the adductor hallucis is divided and reattached to the metatarsal head to correct the varus of the metatarsal bone. Sometimes an osteotomy may be performed.

Adults – There are various surgical procedures that can be used and the method will depend on the individual problem and the particular surgeon. In a young adult the method of choice may be an osteotomy whereas with an older person the choice may be a Keller's excision arthroplasty. In the latter case the proximal half of the proximal phalanx is excised to give a false joint and the bunion is trimmed. Another operative procedure is to excise the metatarsal head (Mayo's operation).

In cases when surgery is not indicated it may be necessary to provide the patient with surgical shoes.

Physiotherapy management

In mild cases and in the younger patients, when surgery is not indicated, the patient may be helped by strengthening the intrinsic muscles, in particular the adductor hallucis. The patient must also be given advice on suitable footwear and a correct gait.

Following surgical procedures management would include strengthening the intrinsic muscles and walking re-education.

The spine

Normal structure

The spine is normally curved antero-posteriorly to give a concavity backwards in the cervical region, a convexity backwards in the thoracic region, a concavity backwards in the lumbar region and there is a fixed convexity backwards in the sacrum. The thoracic and pelvic curves develop *in utero* and are called primary curves, whereas the cervical and lumbar curves are secondary. The cervical curve begins to develop at the end of the intra-uterine period and increases as the baby begins to lift its head and then to sit up. The lumbar curve develops when the infant begins to crawl and stand upright. When the spine is viewed from the back or the front it appears to be fairly straight, although it is normal to develop a slight lateral curvature in the thoracic region which may be convex to the right in a right-handed person and conversely to the left for a left-handed person.

The curves of the spine brought about by the shape of the bodies and the intervertebral discs gives the spine some elasticity in absorbing shocks during movements and also assists the mechanics of movement.

The curves may be influenced from above by the position of the head and below by the position of the pelvis and the lower limbs. The normal antero-posterior tilt of the pelvis is approximately 30° when measured with a pelvic inclinometer with one arm placed over the symphysis pubis and the other over the posterior superior iliac spines.

Posture

Posture is a term used to denote the alignment of the body segments to each other and usually refers to the standing position. However, it may be equally important for the physiotherapist to consider the 'posture' in sitting and lying as these may also show up differences from the normal. In some instances an abnormal posture in standing may not be apparent in the sitting or lying position and this may indicate a postural rather than a structural deformity. A normal posture is difficult to describe as no two people measure the same in all dimensions of arms, legs and trunk. People of the same height may have variations in the lengths of legs and trunk. Also there will be variations between amounts of fat and its distribution, the bulk of muscles and their relative weight and the weight of bone. Apart from these anatomical variations each individual uses their body differently depending on their personality and reactions to the environment. Also it is interesting to notice the variations between different races, and even between people living in different parts of the same country. The posture of people living in mountainous country may be very different from people living in cities or plains.

To give a balanced posture the line of gravity must pass through the base. The weight of the body should be distributed evenly between either side of the base, and also between the front and the back. If this does not occur then the individual has to adjust to maintain a balance, with the consequent strain on soft tissues and muscles. The body is in equilibrium if the vertical line through the centre of gravity falls within the base, and the nearer to the centre of the base the less is the stress on the muscles and other soft tissues.

A good posture must be that from which all activities of the body can take place with the minimum of effort, and from which the systems of the body (respiratory, circulatory, digestive, etc.) can function normally.

There has been a tendency to give too much consideration to the posture in standing when in fact an individual is very rarely stationary for any length of time. There is a continual interchange of activity between various muscle groups to accord with changes of position in standing, sitting or even lying positions. Nevertheless, it is important for the physiotherapist to study posture in the standing position as deviations from the normal parameters will lead to stress on muscles and other soft-tissue structures. Postural deformities will lead to stress in working positions and inefficiency in work activities.

Students interested in further study of people in relation to their work, or other physical activities, should study some of the textbooks on ergonomics.

Maintenance of posture

There are many factors that interrelate to control the posture of the body. Muscle contractions to adjust a position are brought about in response to the sensory input by complex reflex mechanisms. The sensory receptors which relay changes in the position of the body are situated in a number of tissues within the body and are correlated to give the required response in normal postural activity:

1. Cutaneous receptors, particularly those of touch and pressure, respond to contact between the body and another surface. They are particularly important in the feet, responding to variations of pressure and surface textures on different parts of the feet.
2. Joint receptors react to changes in the position of the joint. The type 1 endings, which are slow adapting receptors in the capsular structures, seem to be important in static positional sense and therefore in control of posture.
3. Neuro-tendinous organs of Golgi respond to passive stretching of tendons.
4. Eyes – afferent stimuli from the eyes pass to the brain to integrate with information received from the other sources.

5. Labyrinths of the ears (semicircular canals) – afferent impulses relating to the position of the head are relayed to the brain.
6. Muscle spindles – previously the muscle spindle was thought to play a major role in postural control but it now seems likely that they are not involved in appreciation of limb position and are more concerned with monitoring the extent of muscle contraction.

At one time it was thought that there was no complete relaxation of all the motor units in a muscle and that there was always a rotational activity of a few motor units giving 'muscle tone'. However, it has now been shown by electromyographic studies that a muscle may be completely relaxed with no motor activity. Nevertheless a normal muscle has resistance to deformation given by its elastic and viscous properties and this may give the so-called 'tone' which is different to the texture of a flaccid muscle.

It is important to realize that a person may be deficient in one of the senses contributing to posture control and yet still be able to maintain a normal posture. This requires the adaptation of the other senses to compensate for this loss. The efficiency of this compensation varies from one individual to another.

Loss of one part of the body, for example an arm or leg, will require a change in posture to bring the line of gravity within the base.

Readers should study up-to-date physiology textbooks to gain further information on the neuromuscular control of posture.

Postural deformities (Figure 7.8)

Antero-posterior curves

A mobile spine can easily move into different positions and can just as easily be corrected. Many of these changes occur normally and do not require any treatment. However, changes that result in an altered sense of position being held habitually will lead and this may require treatment depending on the cause.

Amongst the factors likely to alter the antero-posterior curves is a variation in the tilt of the pelvis. The antero-posterior tilt is normally controlled by the activity of the hip and trunk musculature. Contraction of the abdominals and/or the hip extensors will decrease the angle of tilt and will flatten the lumbar spine, whereas contraction of the back extensors and/or the hip flexors will tilt the pelvis forward and increase the concavity of the lumbar spine posteriorly. There will be compensatory adjustments to the curves in the thoracic and cervical regions and possibly downwards to the knees and the ankles. The pelvic tilt may be changed

NORMAL   **LORDOSIS**   **KYPHOSIS**   **FLAT BACK**   **SWAY BACK**

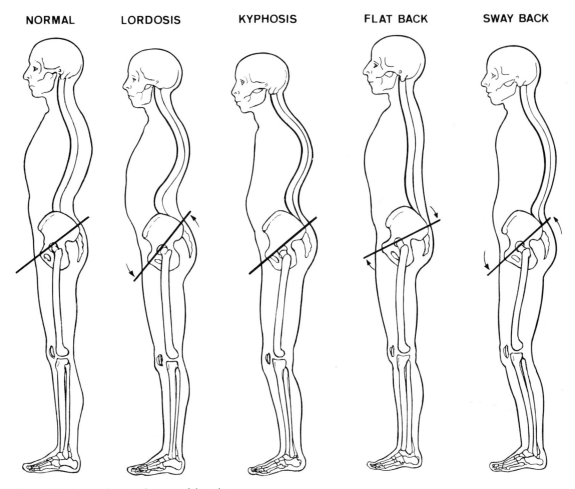

Figure 7.8 Abnormal postural curves of the spine

as the result of deformities occurring in the lower limbs, particularly flexion deformities of the hips or knees.

Lumbar spine

Lordosis – This is an increase in the posterior concavity.

Flat back – This is a decrease in the posterior concavity.

Sway back – The pelvis is tilted forward but instead of producing a lordosis the spine bends back at the lumbosacral angle and then there is a compensatory thoracolumbar kyphosis. This may be due to an existing thoracolumbar kyphosis rather than the other way round. To keep the centre of gravity over the base the legs are inclined forward slightly at the ankles, and the line of gravity falls behind the hips.

Thoracic spine

Kyphosis – This is an increase in the posterior convexity.

Cervical spine

The normal posterior concavity of the cervical spine can be increased or decreased.

Lateral curves

A lateral curve of the spine is called a scoliosis and is named according to the convexity. Thus a curve that is convex to the right in the thoracic region is termed a right thoracic scoliosis. The curve may be single or there may be two or more curves in different directions. For example, a double or 'S' curve could be left cervical and a right thoracic, or a right thoracic and left lumbar and so on. There can be triple or even quadruple curves although the latter are very rare, and these types are not usual as postural deformities. Postural scoliosis occurring in children is usually mild and is often a single curve. Normally those occurring in the thoracic region are not accompanied by vertebral rotation.

Causes

Lordosis, kyphosis, alterations in the cervical curves and scoliosis are fairly common postural deformities. They can be the result of any one of the following factors or sometimes a combination of factors:

1. Muscle imbalance with one group being weak in relation to the opposing group. There may be generally weak musculature leading to a slack posture, and this will be particularly evident if the antigravity muscles are affected.
2. Psychological factors can be an important cause of postural deformities particularly in children and adolescents. For example, a child lacking in confidence and feeling insecure may develop a postural deformity.
3. Poor physical health or tiredness.
4. Compensatory to another deformity or disorder. The other deformity could be postural as when one deformity develops another may be necessary to maintain the line of gravity over the base. Postural deformities can be secondary to structural deformities or other disorders. For example, a short leg will result in a compensatory scoliosis with the curve to the side of the shortened leg. Disorders or diseases of the spine such as a prolapsed intervertebral disc, a tumour, tuberculosis (now rare) or muscle paralysis can all lead to compensatory postural deformities.

Occasionally a postural curve will become structural depending on the initial cause and whether this could lead to contracture of soft-tissue structures and any abnormality of bone.

Management

The management will depend on the cause of the deformity and the age of the individual. In children and adolescents physiotherapy may be an important part of the management but it must be remembered that many of these deformities are linked with psychological factors and should therefore be considered in relation to the total management.

Compensatory deformities will depend on treatment of the primary cause. A short leg may require a shoe raise to prevent a compensatory scoliosis. A scoliosis caused by an intervertebral disc lesion will not change until the disc problem has been resolved.

Physiotherapy management

The physiotherapist makes an assessment of the whole child, adolescent or adult with regard to the physical, psychological and social factors before deciding on the aims and objectives of treatment, or indeed whether physiotherapy is the most effective way of dealing with the problem.

The physical assessment will include an examination of the whole posture in the standing, sitting and lying positions. Observations in the standing position will be made from the back, side and front of the patient as indicated in Figure 7.9. Postural deformities can be corrected and the physiotherapist should show the patient how to adjust to the correct position. Apart from these observations the range of joint movements and the strength of muscles will be tested. It is important to see whether the deformity has any effect on gait or other functional activities.

If physical treatment is considered appropriate then the aims will include re-education of postural sense and strengthening of muscles to control the corrected position. If there is any stiffness of joints these will be mobilized but it is likely in a postural deformity, particularly in children, that the spine is mobile. In treating children it is helpful to encourage general physical activity but this is only possible if the child is willing to participate. Very often children with postural deformities are lacking confidence in their own ability and feel insecure. If this is the case the physiotherapist should try to instil self-reliance and self-confidence in the child but care must be taken to see that the child does not become dependent on the physiotherapist.

Pain may be a feature, particularly when the patient is tense, and with prolonged stretching of the soft-tissue structures. The physiotherapist may help by teaching relaxation and by the use of modalities to relieve pain. Compensatory deformities should be prevented whenever possible and physiotherapists should consider this whenever treating patients with diseases or disorders which are likely to develop a secondary postural deformity.

Structural deformities

Antero-posterior curves

Lordosis – This is more often a postural than a structural abnormality. Sometimes when it is compensatory to another deformity such as bilateral congenital dislocation of the hip or the result of paralysis of the abdominal muscles there may be adaptive shortening of the soft-tissue structures.

Flat back – This may be linked with diseases affecting the spine, as for example ankylosing spondylitis.

Kyphosis – There are a number of diseases or disorders which contribute to a structural kyphosis. Scheuermann's disease affects adolescents, usually

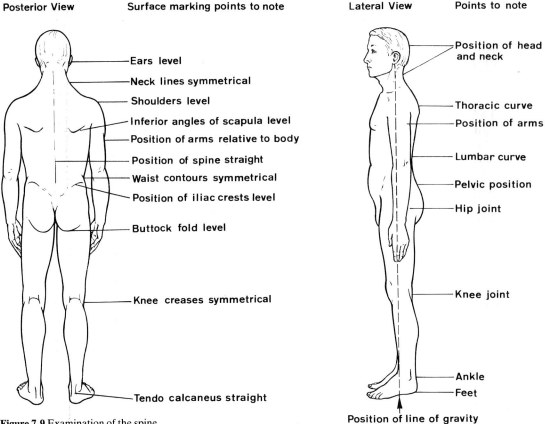

Posterior View **Surface marking points to note** **Lateral View** **Points to note**

- Ears level
- Neck lines symmetrical
- Shoulders level
- Inferior angles of scapula level
- Position of arms relative to body
- Position of spine straight
- Waist contours symmetrical
- Position of iliac crests level
- Buttock fold level
- Knee creases symmetrical
- Tendo calcaneus straight

- Position of head and neck
- Thoracic curve
- Position of arms
- Lumbar curve
- Pelvic position
- Hip joint
- Knee joint
- Ankle
- Feet

Position of line of gravity

Figure 7.9 Examination of the spine

boys, between the ages of 13 and 16. It is an uncommon condition and the cause is unknown. There is a disturbance of the normal development of the cartilage plates and the ring epiphyses, possibly because they are damaged by disc contents bursting through cartilage into adjacent vertebral body. Usually it affects several vertebrae in the thoracic region. The patient suffers pain, weakness of the back extensors and a kyphosis develops. A kyphosis may develop in elderly people, particularly women, as a result of senile osteoporosis which causes collapse of the vertebral bodies. A compression fracture of one or more vertebral bodies in the thoracic region may result in a kyphosis. Patients with ankylosing spondylitis may develop a kyphosis if care is not taken in maintaining a good posture. In the past tuberculosis affecting the vertebrae could cause a severe kyphosis, but fortunately this is rare today.

Cervical spine – Diseases and disorders can affect the cervical curve. The posterior concavity is decreased in ankylosing spondylitis and there may be a collapse of one or more vertebral bodies in patients with rheumatoid arthritis.

Lateral curves

Idiopathic scoliosis accounts for most of the cases of structural scoliosis other than those caused by disease or injury of bone. Occasionally there may be a failure in the development of the spine with a resultant hemivertebra when the body of the vertebra is wedge shaped. However, this is a rare cause of scoliosis.

Idiopathic scoliosis can occur either in childhood or adolescence and may affect any part of the thoraco-lumbar spine. Usually the primary curve is followed by a secondary postural curve either above or below depending on the position of the primary. The curve tends to increase until cessation of skeletal growth. Structural curves usually comprise rotation of the bodies of the vertebrae and in the case of the thoracic vertebrae this will include rotation of the rib cage. The prognosis depends on the age of onset and the site of the primary curve. Thoracic curves have the worst prognosis because of the rotation of the rib cage and the consequent effect on respiration and possibly on the cardio-vascular system (Figure 7.10).

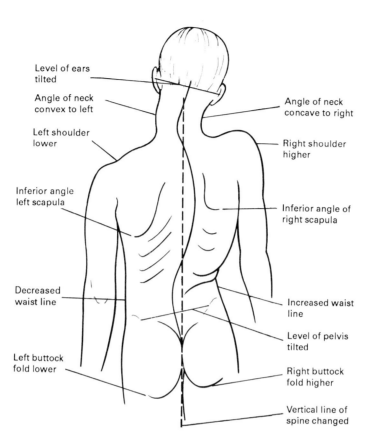

Level of ears
tilted

Angle of neck
convex to left

Left shoulder
lower

Inferior angle
left scapula

Decreased
waist line

Left buttock
fold lower

Angle of neck
concave to right

Right shoulder
higher

Inferior angle of
right scapula

Increased waist
line

Level of pelvis
tilted

Right buttock
fold higher

Vertical line of
spine changed

Figure 7.10 Scoliosis with rotation of the thoracic cage

Management

Antero-posterior curves

This will depend on the particular disease or
disorder. Changes due to ankylosing spondylitis or
rheumatoid arthritis are dealt with in Chapters 8–11.
There is little that can be done to halt a kyphosis
that is due to senile osteoporosis, although studies
are being carried out into the cause of osteoporosis
in the elderly and whether anything can be done to
prevent it.

Adolescent kyphosis due to Scheuermann's disease may be helped by postural correction and
strengthening exercises for the back extensors, if
wedging of the vertebrae has not occurred.

Lateral curves

Idiopathic scoliosis will be assessed by the orthopaedic surgeon to determine the degree of the curve
and the changes that have occurred. If the curve is
not severe and the prognosis is good the surgeon
may review the patient every 6 months to check that
there has been no deterioration. However, when the
curve is increasing and the prognosis is poor the
patient may require an appliance to try to prevent
further deterioration and to stretch the curve if
possible. In the past the stretching was done by a
hinged plaster jacket (Risser jacket), and then a
Milwaukee brace was used to hold the correction.
This was followed by a spinal fusion and then a
plaster jacket to maintain the corrected position.

Now some surgeons prefer to use Harrington's rods which are wedged between the vertebrae on the concave side. These are gradually elongated to open the curve and then this is followed by spinal fusion.

Physiotherapy management

Physical treatment cannot alter a structural curve when there is a change in bone structure. However in some cases it may be possible to prevent further deterioration by positioning and by strengthening muscles. The physiotherapist may be able to give symptomatic relief for patients who have pain and discomfort caused by the stretching of soft-tissue structures.

Antero-posterior curves

Patients with a kyphosis due to senile osteoporosis may suffer considerable discomfort and pain. They will tend to sit in a flexed position which will further stretch the soft tissues and increase the deformity. Treatment may be given using techniques for the relief of pain, and if tension is a problem this may be relieved by teaching relaxation. Advice should be given to the patient on posture and general positioning – sitting in a chair with the back straight and well supported, finding the best position for sleeping, suitable positions for housework or an occupation. Strengthening exercises for the back extensors may help to relieve the stretch on the tissues and enable the patient to maintain a better position.

As mentioned above adolescent kyphosis may be helped by posture correction and strengthening exercises. The physiotherapist must emphasize the importance of maintaining a good position, and of doing exercises to strengthen the back extensors. Hydrotherapy may be a useful modality as the warmth help to relieve pain and gain relaxation. Also mobilizing and strengthening exercises may be given in water.

Lateral curves

If the prognosis is good and the child is not to have surgical intervention it is important that the child is taught to hold a good position and to do active exercises to strengthen the muscles of the trunk. It may not be necessary for the child to have a long period of treatment as once the child can maintain a correct position and knows how to do the exercises these can be carried on at home. However, it is important that the physiotherapist monitors progress and any deterioration in the posture is reported at once to the surgeon.

When a child is to have surgery the management will include pre- and post-operative treatment, with particular emphasis on chest treatment. Later management will aim to teach the child to adjust to the new posture, and strengthen the appropriate muscles both to hold the position and to undertake normal function. Again hydrotherapy may be a useful modality once the child is mobilizing freely.

Torticollis

This is usually an acquired condition which arises after birth and is probably due to an interference with the blood supply of sternomastoid during birth. This results in fibrous tissue formation and a consequent shortening of the muscle which causes the cervical spine to be side-flexed on the affected side, and the head rotated to the opposite side. If this deformity is not corrected early an asymmetry of the face occurs.

Management

When diagnosed early these patients are usually referred to the physiotherapist. In cases where treatment is not successful or has not been carried out for some reason it may be necessary to have surgical intervention. This will entail dividing the sternal and clavicular heads of sterno-mastoid close to their origin and severing any contracted bands of fascia.

Physiotherapy management

The physiotherapist will carry out passive stretchings and position the baby to correct the deformity. The mother should be taught how to do the passive stretchings, how to hold the baby, and how to position the baby in the cot. The physiotherapist must continue to watch the mother doing the passive movements and positioning until she is satisfied that the treatment is being carried out properly. Some mothers are frightened of doing the treatment in which case it may be necessary for the physiotherapist to continue. The condition of the baby must be monitored at regular intervals until the physiotherapist and the surgeon are satisfied that no further treatment is required.

Spina bifida

This is a congenital abnormality in which there is a failure of the embryonic neural plate to fold over and form a closed neural tube, or of the mesodermal tissue to invest the neural tube fully. It may be only a defect in the vertebral canal but more severe abnormalities include defects in the spinal cord and meninges.

This will be dealt with in more detail in Chapter 22.

Upper extremity

Congenital abnormalities are found far less frequently in the upper than the lower extremity. A number of children were born with amoelia (absence of a limb) or phocomelia following the use of the drug thalidomide during pregnancy. In a few children these abnormalities occur for no known reason. There are a few other abnormalities such as Sprengel's shoulder and arthrogryposis multiplex congenita but they are very rare.

The physiotherapist may be involved in the management of children with the loss of an arm or the partial absence of a limb to aid and encourage the child in making use of an artificial arm or in making the best use of an underdeveloped arm.

Acquired deformities are not as common in the upper limb and the majority of those caused by diseases or disorders are covered in other chapters of this book.

Chapter 8

Degenerative arthropathies

Introduction

Rheumatic diseases constitute one of the commonest causes of pain, disability and economic loss in mankind. 'Rheumatism' in its broadest sense has been recognized since the fifth century BC. Today there is a wide range of treatments, some of which are very successful. The bewildering nature of 'rheumatism' is that people with apparently identical clinical features benefit from different treatment. Acupuncture, ultrasound, cortisone injections, manipulation – all have their devotees as constituting the cure for them. Physiotherapy for 'soft-tissue rheumatism' is closely related to soft-tissue injury and therefore features in Chapter 6. Chapters 8–11 cover physiotherapy for joint disorders or diseases.

Anatomy and physiology

Joints are fibrous, cartilaginous or synovial.

Synovial joints

1. Articular surfaces are covered in hyaline cartilage.
2. Joint capsule and ligaments unite the bones, provide stability and direct movement.
3. Synovial membrane lines the capsule and secretes synovial fluid.
4. Intra-articular structures are present in some joints such as menisci and cartilaginous discs.
5. Nerve supply is generally from the nerves supplying the muscles acting on the joints (Hilton's law).
6. Nerve endings in the capsule and ligaments are mechanoreceptors, which register movement, proprioceptors to register the position of the joint and nociceptors to register pain. There are also autonomic (sympathetic) nerve endings on blood vessels.

Joint lubrication and nutrition

All joint components are supplied with blood vessels except for the articular cartilage.

Synovial fluid provides both joint lubrication and nutrition for articular cartilage. Movement of joint surfaces over one another, compression and distraction are all important in the provision of synovial fluid sweep and therefore maintenance of healthy cartilage.

Cartilaginous joints of the vertebral column

Articular surfaces are superior and inferior surfaces of vertebral bodies, which are covered by cartilage end-plates. The intervertebral disc is between the two bodies.

Structure of the disc

Each disc has two basic components – a central nucleus pulposus and a surrounding annulus fibrosus.

The nucleus pulposus is a semifluid gel, containing cartilage cells and irregularly arranged collagen fibres. As it is fluid it cannot be compressed but transmits force as well as dissipating it all round.

The annulus fibrosus is a series of collagen layers with fibres running obliquely at right angles to each other. These layers control and direct movement at a vertebral level; all the fibres in one lamella are parallel with each other.

Functions of the disc

1. Allows movement between vertebrae.
2. Transmits load.
3. Provides height to the vertebral column.

Nutrition of the disc is dependent on fluid flow from blood vessels in neighbouring tissues and this occurs during spinal movement, especially flexion and extension.

Osteoarthritis (OA)

Definition

A chronic degenerative disease of joints with exacerbations of acute inflammation.
  Synonyms – Degenerative arthritis, degenerative joint disease, arthritis deformans.

Aetiology

Studies have shown that in the UK three and a half million people over the age of 65 suffer from the condition. Many working days are lost because of the effects of osteoarthritis.
  Both men and women are affected but the joint distribution pattern is different. In men, the order of affected joints is hip (most common), knee, spine, ankle, shoulder, fingers. In women the order is knee, finger, spine, hip, ankle and shoulders.

Classification

There are two types – primary and secondary. In primary OA there is no obvious cause. Secondary OA arises as a consequence of other conditions such as:

1. Trauma after severe injury, resulting in fractures of the joint surfaces.
2. Dislocation:
    (a) Repeated minor trauma.
    (b) Occupational, e.g. miners, knees are at risk; tailors, first carpometacarpal and metacarpophalangeal joints; pneumatic drillers, elbows and shoulders.
3. Infection:
    (a) Tracking into a joint from an open wound.
    (b) Tuberculosis of a joint.
4. Deformity.
5. Obesity.
6. Haemophilia.
7. Acromegaly.
8. Hyperthyroidism.
9. Tabes dorsalis, syringomyelia – Charcot's joints.

Cause

The cause is unknown but a number of predisposing factors may be considered:

1. Conditions already mentioned in relation to secondary arthritis.
2. Hereditary. There is a significantly higher incidence of the condition in families.
3. Poor posture.
4. The ageing process in joint cartilage.
5. Climate has not been shown to be related to the pathological changes but pain is greater in cold, damp climates.
6. Defective lubricating mechanism and uneven nutrition of the articular cartilage.
7. Crystals (calcium pyrophosphate and hydroxyapatite) have been associated with synovitis in osteoarthritic joints.

Pathology

This will be considered in relation to each joint structure as follows:

1. Articular cartilage.
2. Bone.
3. Synovial membrane.
4. Capsule.
5. Ligaments.
6. Muscles.

Articular cartilage

Erosion occurs, often central and frequently in the weight-bearing areas. Cartilage is usually the first structure to be affected. Fibrillation which causes softening, splitting and fragmentation of the cartilage occurs in both weight-bearing and non-weight-bearing areas.
  Collagen fibres split and there is disorganization of the proteoglycan – collagen relationship such that water is attracted into the cartilage which causes further softening and flaking. Flakes of cartilage break off and may be impacted between the joint surfaces causing locking and inflammation.
  Proliferation occurs at the periphery of the cartilage.

Bone

Eburnation – The bone surfaces become hard and polished as there is loss of protection from the cartilage.
  Cystic cavities form in the subchondral bone because eburnated bone is brittle and microfractures occur allowing the passage of synovial fluid into the bone tissue. There can also be venous congestion in the subchondral bone.

Osteophytes form at the margin of the articular surfaces where they may project into the joint or into the capsule and ligaments. Bone of the weight-bearing joints alters in shape – the femoral head becomes flat and mushroom shaped. The tibial condyles become flattened.

Synovial membrane

This undergoes hypertrophy and becomes oedematous. Later there is fibrous degeneration. Reduction of synovial fluid secretion results in loss of nutrition and lubrication of the articular cartilage.

Capsule

This undergoes fibrous degeneration and there are low-grade chronic inflammatory changes.

Ligaments

These undergo the same changes as the capsule and according to the aspect of the joint become contracted or elongated.

Muscles

These undergo atrophy which may be related to disuse because pain limits movement and function. Without adequate exercise the muscles may undergo fibrous atrophy.

Clinical features

1. Pain.
2. Muscle spasm.
3. Stiffness.
4. Loss of movement.
5. Muscle wasting and weakness.
6. Joint enlargement.
7. Deformity.
8. Crepitus.
9. Loss of function.

During active inflammation:

10. Heat.
11. Redness.
12. Swelling.
13. Pain.

Pain

The onset is of low intensity and can be described as three types:

1. Pain on weight bearing, severe aching, due to stress on the synovial membrane and later due to the bone surfaces, which are rich in nerve endings, coming into contact.

2. During and after exercise there is pain described as being around the joint.
3. At night especially after a very active day there is severe aching. This is thought to be due to venous congestion in the bone ends. It is worse in patients with varicose veins and can be reduced if the end of the bed is raised.

Nature of pain

1. Aching is dominant, at first fleeting and then becoming more constant.
2. Referred pain is described as passing down a limb distally from the affected joint.
3. Sharp stabbing pain is associated with a loose body becoming impacted in the joint.
4. Throbbing is related to an episode of inflammation and is worse at night.

Muscle spasm

This occurs over one aspect of the joint and is initially protective but where it remains beyond the acute episode it must be treated to prevent contractures.

Stiffness

This is present after rest and takes a little time to wear off with movement. It may be due to loss of joint lubrication, chronic oedema in the periarticular structures or swelling of the articular cartilage.

Loss of joint movement

This is different from stiffness because it does not wear off. It may be permanent where there is articular cartilage destruction but will respond to physiotherapy where it is due to muscle spasm or soft-tissue contracture.

Muscle wasting and weakness

Muscles become weak often on the aspect of the joint which is opposite to contracures (e.g. hip extensors).

Joint enlargement

Chronic oedema of the synovial membrane and capsule together with muscle wasting makes the joint appear large.

Deformity

Each joint tends to adopt a characteristic deformity.

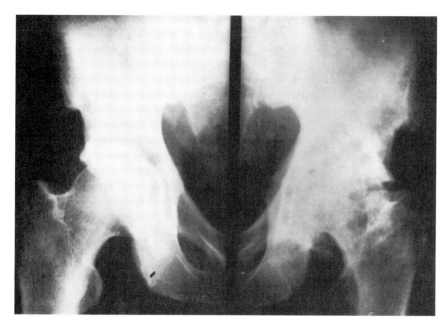

Figure 8.1 Radiograph of osteoarthritic hip joint. Note, in the left hip, subchondral cysts, loss of cartilage (i.e. loss of 'joint space'), osteophyte formation and sclerosis of bone. The right hip is normal

Crepitus

The flaked cartilage and eburnated bone ends grate with a characteristic sound on movement.

Loss of function

Pain, muscle weakness, giving way lead to inability to use the limb normally and can be severely disabling.

Radiograph

1. Loss of joint space.
2. Sclerosis.
3. Altered shape of bone ends.
4. Osteophytes (Figure 8.1).

Clinical features relating to specific joints

Hip

1. Pain is over the abductor aspect and is referred down the anterior aspect of the thigh to the knee.
2. Muscle spasm occurs in the adductor, flexor and lateral rotator muscles.
3. Deformity is flexion, adduction and lateral rotation.
4. Muscle weakness occurs in all muscles. The most functionally restricting is the weakness of the extensors and abductors.

5. Loss of function is difficulty in getting up from sitting and in walking far. The characteristic gait is Trendelenburg due to weakness of the abductor muscles. When the patient stands on the affected leg the pelvis drops to the non-weight-bearing side because the hip abductors are too weak to hold the pelvis horizontal. To balance and to maintain the line of gravity passing through the base, the trunk is side flexed over to the side of the affected leg. Therefore, during the stance phase of walking the patient's trunk is thrust sideways, and this is a characteristic of a Trendelenburg gait (Figure 8.2).

Knee

Pain is described as round and through the joint, and may be referred up the anterior aspect of the thigh or down to the ankle. Muscle spasm may be present in the hamstring muscles. Deformity from prolonged hamstring spasm is flexion and there is deformation of the tibia with valgus deformity. The joint is enlarged and there is quadriceps atrophy especially vastus medialis. There is a limp due to pain and a tendency for the joint to give way especially during stepping down.

Hands

Heberden's nodes are characteristic of OA. These are cartilaginous or bony outgrowths on the margins of the distal interphalangeal joints.

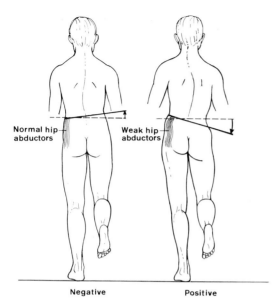

Normal hip abductors

Weak hip abductors

Negative   Positive

Figure 8.2 Trendelenburg's sign

Prognosis

There is not a cure but with good diet, exercise and common sense there can be good function. Function can be regained by surgery, including joint replacement.

Management

This involves the doctors, dietitian, pharmacist, occupational therapist, surgical appliance officer and physiotherapist.

Doctors

The general practitioner prescribes and monitors drugs. The rheumatologist may be consulted as the condition advances. The orthopaedic surgeon may perform an arthroplasty, arthrodesis or osteotomy.

Dietitian

Most patients need advice on weight reduction.

Pharmacists

There are many analgesics on the market and all have side-effects to varying degrees. A pharmacist can help the patient recognize side-effects and advise on the alternative drugs.

Occupational therapist

The patient will need aids for daily living if there is severe disability. This may include provision of aids, for example for dressing or adaptations to the house for mobility.

Surgical appliance officer

Sometimes the patient may benefit from a shoe raise, for example if there is a fixed flexion deformity of a knee or hip.

Physiotherapy

This may be hospital, health centre or community based. The advantage of having the patient attend a hospital department is that a wide range of treatment is available, including hydrotherapy.

The aims of physiotherapy are to:

1. Relieve pain.
2. Strengthen muscles.
3. Mobilize joints.
4. Teach maintenance of joint range and muscle power.
5. Improve coordination.
6. Minimize deformity.
7. Train position sense to reduce postural stress.
8. Advise rest/activity relationship.
9. Help maintain function.

Modalities used

These are selected, based on the assessment of the patient's needs. Necessarily, therefore, they are many and various. Appropriate procedures are as follows.

Pain relief

1. *Pulsed electromagnetic energy or inductothermy* is effective in some patients especially in reducing a dull ache. The localized increase in arterial blood flow may improve the nutrition to the joint cartilage. Some patients report an increase in aching and this could be due to venous congestion in the cysts in the subchondral bone, e.g. in the head of the femur.
2. *Wax therapy* is useful for hand pain.
3. *Superficial heat* – Infra-red radiation, heat pad or a hot pack can bring relief to patients especially where there is associated muscle spasm and the pain is exacerbated by cold. The hot pack is safer because the heat starts at a given temperature and gets cooler.

4. *Ice therapy* is useful if there is acute pain and swelling as can happen at the knee when a loose flake of cartilage becomes trapped between the joint surfaces. Often there are varicose veins near to an osteoarthritic knee and a fat pad on the medial side. In either case it is unwise to apply ice. Chronic thickened swelling does not respond to ice therapy.

5. *Ultrasound* – This is useful for treating chronic swelling as it softens fluid and loosens scar tissue so that subsequent exercises can be effective in reducing the swelling and gain pain relief, especially deep aching.

6. *Free active exercises* and mobilizations by restoring mobility and improving circulation can contribute to pain reief.

7. *Group therapy* can provide encouragement to lose weight, carry out home exercises, monitor muscle bulk and by providing moral support to enable the patient to cope with the pain.

Muscle strengthening

The general principle is to work the muscles at a high repetition rate and against low resistance. The main muscles requiring strengthening are generally as follows.

Quadriceps

At regular intervals throughout the day it is helpful to practise inner range contractions held to a count of 5. This can be in standing, sitting or lying and incorporated into everyday activities such as watching TV, waiting for a bus, before rising in the morning and on going to bed at night.

For weight lifting, the patient is in half crook lying, a weight is attached to the straight leg. Instructions are given to keep the knee straight and to lift the leg to the level of the other thigh. The sequence then is 10 lifts, rest, repeat three times. The principle underlying this method is that the muscle can be strengthened without the joint surfaces being moved under load (especially the patello-femoral joint). If there is a quadriceps lag, then the patient should be treated with PNF slow reversals, repeated contractions and inner range isometric work. A quadriceps lag is present if the knee has full passive extension and the muscle cannot keep the knee straight when the leg is lifted with the patient in lying.

The weight lifted should be in the order of 75% of the patient's 10-repetition maximum (RM). If there is no swelling and the diagnosis is 'early OA' the exercise may be changed to sitting (weight as before) one knee straightening and bending. If there is pain in the hip and the above exercise is contraindicated the patient should lie with firm pillows to support the thighs with the knees in flexion; alternate knee straightening is then performed. Weights may be added as before.

A general fitness programme may achieve an improvement in the quadriceps function without the use of direct weight resistance.

Hip abductors

The patient lies in side lying, with the underneath leg flexed for stability; a weight may be attached to the top leg just above the ankle. The knee is kept straight with the toes pointing forward and the leg lifted slowly 10 times every day. If weight lifting is not practical then the leg should be raised to the horizontal and bicycling action performed. This maintains flexion and extension of the hip at the same time as the abductors are working isometrically which is akin to their function in maintaining the lateral tilt of the pelvis.

Hip extensors

The patient lies prone. Each leg is lifted straight, alternately, slowly. This is an important position for the patient to practise as it stretches tight structures over the anterior aspect of the hips; weight resistance may be added. Slow reversals, repeated contractions are useful for strengthening muscles, because specific muscles can be worked maximally at different ranges or through range. Although these muscles often require particular strengthening, it is important to perform a daily programme of free active exercises to help maintain muscle balance.

Other muscle groups

Resisted exercises are important for the muscles of any joint in which there are osteoarthritic changes.

Appropriate proprioceptive neuromuscular facilitation (PNF) techniques are slow reversals (in pattern for the whole limb as well as modified to work at a specific joint level) repeated contractions, stabilizations. These techniques are particularly useful for working the muscles in the range appropriate to the patient's requirements.

Auto-manual resistance is useful for some muscles, e.g. sitting, one knee straightening against resistance of the other leg. Arm exercises can also be resisted by the other arm. Spring resistance is useful for certain muscle groups such as the elbow extensors, wrist extensors, latissimus dorsi muscles together with the shoulder girdle retractors. Rubber bands or balls are useful as resistance for hand exercises.

In the hydrotherapy pool, buoyancy-resisted exercises strengthen selected muscle groups. Patterns of movement against resistance to the water flow (Bad Ragaz) are particularly useful for hip, knee, shoulder and spinal joints.

Mobility of joints

Realistically, when the joint surfaces are destroyed, mobility will be restored only by joint surgery. Success with physiotherapy in restoring mobility depends on the limiting factors which may be:

1. Pain.
2. Chronic thickened swelling.
3. Muscle spasm.
4. Fibrous contracture.

Pain relief may be obtained by the methods already mentioned. This includes free active exercises which may release endogenous opiates and thus relieve pain.

Chronic thickened swelling can be softened and at least partly cleared by ultrasound. Whole hand and finger kneading together with effleurage can also help. Where appropriate, the patient may wear an elasticated support on, for example, the knee so that during walking the oedematous fluid is compressed and should pass into the lymphatic channels. Interferential therapy can also be effective.

Muscle spasm is best relaxed by hold–relax, repeated contractions and possibly by pulsed electromagnetic energy or radiant heat. If there is spasm in a lower limb muscle it is worth considering encouraging the patient to use a walking aid to reduce the weight taken during the stance phase of walking which in turn reduces the pain and diminishes the development of muscle spasm. Ice may be appropriate when there is acute pain and spasm.

The commonest muscles affected are: hip adductors and flexors and the spinal extensors. Techniques are hold relax, repeated contractions, heat, cold and relaxation.

Sling suspension is helpful for regaining hip, knee and shoulder movements in the presence of pain or spasm and also where there is fibrous tightness limiting movement (free swinging particularly).

Fibrous contracture tends to occur in the muscles which produce deformity. This may be successfully treated by ultrasound, friction or finger kneading and passive stretching applied as a slow sustained stretch.

Mobilizations as either accessory or physiological movements are invaluable at the earlier stages of the condition. Stretching the capsule and applying rhythmical movement facilitates synovial sweep across the cartilage and may help to diminish degeneration by improving nutrition. Compression and distraction are useful for the same reason. Mobilizations may be applied in the hydrotherapy pool with great success (pain relief and increased function) especially for the hip and lumbar spine. Grades I and II relieve pain and grade III reduces resistance – fibrous thickening and tightening.

Free active exercises

Non-weight-bearing exercises including pendular movements are of particular value in regaining range of movement. These should be performed daily in every direction for the affected joints.

Examples

1. Hip:
    (a) Standing, shadow walking (heels together – toes together) for hip rotation.
    (b) Standing, alternate knee raising with clasping the knee and flexing further up onto the chest.
    (c) Lying on a smooth surface:
        (i) Slide one leg sideways and back, repeat with the other leg.
        (ii) Roll legs in and out.
    (d) Crook lying – pelvic raising and lowering.
    (e) Stride sitting – trunk bending forward and stretching back.
    (f) Stride sitting – trunk bending side to side.
2. Knee:
    (a) Lying on a smooth surface – alternate knee and hip bending and stretching.
    (b) Sitting on a high surface – bend and stretch knees with a swing.
    (c) Sitting – turn heels to touch then turn toes to touch (hips as steady as possible to produce knee rotation).

Maintenance of joint range and muscle power

Every patient with OA should practise a programme of exercises designed to move the joints and muscles through full range at least once each day. Attendance at a group therapy session from time to time encourages the patient to practise (e.g. a knee school). Joint range, muscle power and bulk measurements can be taken regularly to identify any evidence of rapid regress.

Coordination

Frenkel's exercises can be used to work the joints and muscles through smooth coordinated purposeful movements. Stabilizations in standing help to gain co-contraction around the hip, knee and ankle joints. Balance-board work is also of value in re-educating proprioceptor function. Damage to these nerve endings in thickened fibrous tissue may possibly be a contributing factor to a feeling of instability at the lower limb joints. The patient may be taught to stand on one leg for 2–3 minutes at home with corrected leg posture. PNF slow reversals and correctly performed free active exercise also contribute to coordination.

Gait re-education may include teaching the patient to take slightly shorter steps so that there is a relatively shorter hip movement during stance phase. A walking stick may be necessary to relieve weight and pain, held in the hand opposite to the affected joint (where there is only one limb affected) so that gait pattern can be smooth. It is sometimes necessary to persuade the patient that this reduces stress on the joints and therefore reduces the rate of wear and tear.

Minimizing deformity

This is achieved by educating the patient in the mechanism of development of deformity and in the importance of exercise and good posture. Also the patient should avoid sitting for hours on end if the hips and knees are affected. It is helpful to 'stand up turn round, sit down' every 20–30 minutes.

Position sense

'A badly hung gate creaks', and the same can be said for joints. Poor posture leads to stress and muscle imbalance which predispose to the changes of OA. For example, a forward pelvic tilt tends to stretch the hip extensors and shorten the flexors. Rounded shoulders result in lengthening of the shoulder girdle retractors, shoulder extensors and lateral rotators with shortening of the opposing muscle groups especially the pectorals. A habit of standing with body weight more on one leg than the other causes shortening of the hip abductors of the favoured side and can be associated with tightening of the iliotibial tract. Instruction on a balanced posture in standing, sitting, relaxing positions and lying is essential.

Advice to patients

1. Walking is good for lubrication and nutrition – walk a little every day within limits of pain. Monitor pace and distance by recording effects. Use walking aids to relieve pain and stress and to help balance.
2. Rest 5–10 minutes every hour but avoid being in one position for longer than half an hour. If this is not possible, e.g. in a train or car, then practise isometric muscle contractions every so often.
3. Exercise daily. If bed rest is necessary, e.g. because of 'flu', once the acute fever stage is passed and the joints have stopped aching try to move each joint in every direction every half hour or so. Also, practise isometric contractions.
4. Weigh regularly – at least once a week. Try to keep weight under control. Perhaps go to weight-watchers.
5. Avoid sitting with the knees crossed to prevent deformity. Do not sit or lie with a pillow under the knees.
6. Avoid putting sudden strain on the joints, e.g. lifting heavy loads, long spells of gardening or decorating. Use a bag on wheels for shopping – try to do a little every day rather than one big exhausting 'shop' once or twice a month. Carry two small bags, one in each hand.
7. Do a little housework every day.
8. In cold weather, wrap up well; cold predisposes to muscle spasm. Do not exercise from cold, use a rubber hot water-bottle or electric heat pad to warm the muscles prior to exercise.
9. Buy a heat lamp if heat helps but a hot water-bottle is less dangerous and can mould to the part. A heat pad is more versatile.
10. Although there is no cure, the effects of OA can be minimized so that functional capacity can be maintained. Patients sometimes need to be reassured that OA is not crippling rheumatoid arthritis.

Maintenance of function

As already explained this is achieved by the patient following a programme of exercise, rest and diet.

Surgery

Replacement arthroplasty is very effective in relieving pain. Osteotomy may be performed (see below).

Spondylosis

Definition

Spondylosis is a condition in which there are degenerative changes in the intervertebral joints between the bodies and the discs.

OA results in degenerative changes in synovial joints and therefore can occur in the apophyseal joints of the spine. Clinically the two conditions often occur together.

Aetiology

The age range is 30 years onwards and is most common around 45. Women are more commonly affected than men. The type of person is often anxious and worrying by nature.

There are a number of predisposing factors which are:

1. Poor posture associated with anxiety, habit.

2. Occupational stress, e.g. typists at poorly positioned desks, coalminers, drivers, people whose work involves lifting, twisting and carrying.
3. Body type. Necks that are thickset with a 'Dowager's hump' and long backs are prone to spondylosis.

The sites commonly affected are:

Cervical – C4 to T1.
Lumbar – L2 to L4.
Thoracic – T4,5,6.

It is important to note that although these are the levels at which changes start there are effects in other parts of the spine where there are compensatory adjustments.

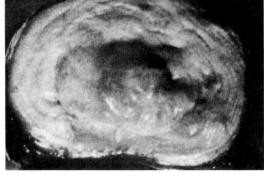

(a)

Pathology

The pathological changes that occur are the same regardless of site but the difference in anatomy gives rise to different signs and symptoms.

Intervertebral discs

1. The annulus fibrosis becomes coarser, the collagen fibres tend to separate and cracks appear at various sites.
2. The nucleus pulposus loses fluid and becomes more fibrous.
3. Thd disc overall loses height.
4. These changes occur as part of the ageing process of the discs and can be present without causing any signs or symptoms.

(b)

Vertebral bodies

'Lipping' of the vertebral bodies occurs. This is due to alteration of the disc mechanics producing traction of the periosteum by the attachments of the annulus fibrosis. There can be decalcification within the bodies which predisposes to crush fractures.

Ligaments

The intervertebral ligaments may become contracted and thickened especially at the sites where there are gross changes.

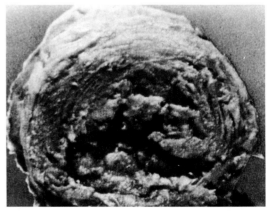

Meningeal sleeves

The dura mater of the spinal cord forms a sleeve round the nerve root and this undergoes inflammatory changes because as the disc space narrows there is diminihsed lumen of the intervertebral canal. The inflammation is low grade and chronic in nature resulting in adhesions round the nerve root.

(c)

Figure 8.3 Intervertebral discs. (*a*) A normal disc with translucent nucleus pulposus and collagen arrangement in the lamellae of outer annulus. As the disc becomes adult (*b*) the central nucleus area will be more fibrous and collagen fibres coarser. In the old disc (*c*) there are signs of degeneration

Apophyseal joints

These undergo the changes of OA. Osteophytes form at the margins of the articular surfaces and these together with the capsular thickening can cause pressure on the nerve root and reduce the lumen of the intervertebral foramen.

Prognosis

All tissues degenerate but at different rates in different people. It is important to note that not all people whose tissues are undergoing the ageing process develop pain that is intrusive enough to make a patient seek help. There is, therefore, always some precipitating factor (anxiety, poor posture, habitual poor movement) that aggravates the pain. Physiotherapy can be of great benefit in teaching pain management. Pain relief can be obtained and, given a clear explanation of the causative factors, the patient can learn to keep the pain at a level compatible with everyday comfortable living. This is important because too many of these patients are dismissed by some doctors as 'it's your age, put up with it'. The painkillers administered under this regimen are expensive (for the patient or, under the present system, for the NHS) and likely to play havoc with the patient's digestive system.

Clinical features

These vary according to the site and will be considered as cervical, lumbar and thoracic.

Cervical spine – clinical features

Onset

This may be precipitated by fatigue or worry and may be traced to an episode in the patient's life.

Pain

1. Headaches due to upper cervical pathology.
2. Neck-ache usually due to mid-cervical pathology.
3. Shoulder girdle, shoulder and arm pain due to pathology from C4 to T2.

Muscle weakness

Neck postural muscles are often weak, i.e. the upper cervical spine flexors, lower cervical spine extensors and the side-flexors. If there is pressure on a nerve root, there may be weakness in the muscles (myotome) supplied by that root.

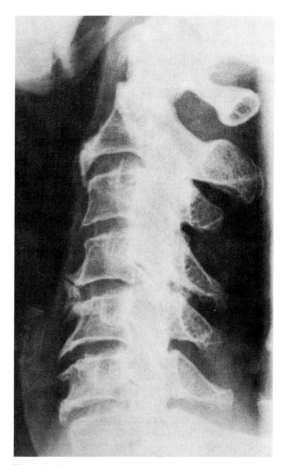

Figure 8.4 Lateral radiograph of cervical spine showing osteophytes, disc space narrowing and sclerosis of apophyseal joints, i.e. degenerative joint disease or cervical spondylosis

Radiograph

Lipping of the vertebral bodies, osteophytes at the margins of the apophyseal joints and diminished space between the vertebral bodies can be seen. It is important to remember that severity of signs and symptoms and X-ray findings do not very often correlate (Figures 8.4 and 8.5).

Treatment

Physiotherapy is directed at:

1. Relief of pain.
2. Restoration of movement.
3. Strengthening of muscles.
4. Education of posture.
5. Analysis of precipitating factors to reduce recurrence of the patient's problems.

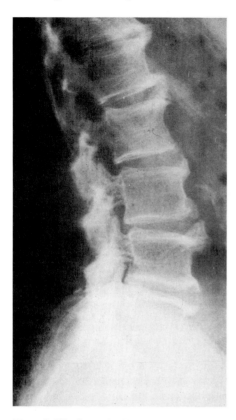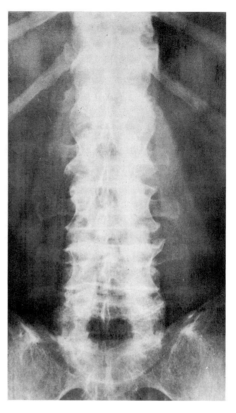

Figure 8.5 Radiograph of lumbar spine showing degenerative joint disease. Note osteophytes, loss of disc height and sclerosis of the posterior facet joints (apophyseal joints)

Examination – A scrupulous examination is essential to identify precipitating factors in the patient's lifestyle; for example:

1. Working conditions that demand concentration resulting in 'poking chin and round shoulders'.
2. Habit of holding the telephone on one shoulder.
3. Sitting or standing still for long times.
4. Driving for a long time, especially in traffic jams.
5. Sleeping in awkward positions.

Referred pain

1. There may be no pain perceived in the neck but there is pain in the arm.
2. Pain down to the elbow – could be C5.
3. Pain to thumb and index finger – could be C6.
4. Pain on middle three fingers and forearm – could be C7.
5. Pain on inside of forearm, little finger and possibly chest –could be C8/T1.
6. In addition pain may be referred down to the thoracic area, for example the medial border of the scapula.

Nature of the pain

The pain is described as dull aching superimposed by sharp stabbing pain and from time to time as cramp-type throbbing.

Paraesthesia

Pins and needles or altered sensation may be present in the area supplied by an impinged nerve root (dermatome).

Muscle spasm

There is always increased tone in the upper fibres of the trapezius which causes an imbalance as the middle and lower fibres become lengthened and relatively reduced in tone.

Spasm is often present in the scalene muscles usually more on one side than the other.

Limitation of movement

1. Neck movements are all limited often bilaterally but during an acute episode of pain one side is

more affected than the other. It is important to note that upper cervical spine flexion is often very limtied together with lower cervical spine extension.
2. Muscle spasm and muscle tightness.
3. Limitation of movements, including limiting factors and exact vertebral levels affected.
4. Loss of accessory intervertebral movements detected by palpation.
5. Loss of soft-tissue mobility also detected by palpation.

These findings are assessed together with the details of the pain picture and a logical treatment programme is planned. The following treatments may be used.

Heat

A heat pad applied with the patient in lying or half-lying so that the neck is supported can reduce muscle spasm and increase the circulation which brings nutrition to the neck structures and removes metabolites.

Other heat treatments may be from electromagnetic or electrostatic energy (pulsed or continuous), a hot water-bottle or moist heat from a heat pack.

If a patient's pain is relieved by warmth (aggravated by cold) then it is perfectly valid for that patient to use a heat pad or hot water-bottle for 10–20 minutes once or twice a day during an acute episode of pain. A 'heat lamp' is not so appropriate because the patient cannot adopt a position of support and relaxation for the neck.

Relaxation

Tension in the neck and shoulder girdle muscles is nearly always present in a patient who presents with pain from cervical spondylosis, and education in relaxation is therefore an essential component of the total management.

Physiological relaxation (Laura Mitchell method) is the best approach as it can be applied in various positions and at rest, work or play.

To encourage relaxed sleeping the patient and physiotherapist work out a position of comfort and support. Prone lying should be strongly discouraged. In side-lying there should be sufficient pillows to fill in the space between the shoulder and the head so that the neck is straight. A pillow between the legs or under the top knee plus another folded up and positioned to support the top arm are important so that the patient can truly relax in a position of support. The patient is instructed to push the legs down into the bed, feel the support and stop pushing. This is then repeated with the trunk, arms, and head until the whole body is fully supported and muscular tension is reduced to a minimum. The mouth is stretched open as in yawning and allowed to close gently. The eyes are closed and the eyebrows raised with a feeling of 'smoothing' the scalp back over the top of the head. The patient should then be encouraged to think of something pleasant, e.g. a piece of music, lying on a warm sunny beach, making a floral display, playing a sport. This promotes refreshing sleep making the patient feel better and breaking the cycle of pain, spasm, loss of sleep, anxiety, pain. If the patient sleeps supine one pillow under the head (not shoulders) is best and another pillow under the knees to flatten the lumbar spine is helpful. If a patient has a problem that precludes lying flat, the upper thoracic spine may be supported on pillows but there must be a pillow for the head alone – possibly 'butterflied' i.e. flattened in the middle so that the ends support the head on either side.

In sitting, relaxation can also be practised. The position depends on the activity being pursued. Where the patient is relaxing, e.g. watching television, the head, neck and shoulders should be supported by a high-backed chair with a small pillow in the lumbar spine, the feet supported and the arms resting either on the arms of the chair or on a pillow on the lap. The same principles are followed of pushing the parts of the body into the supporting surface registering the support and stopping pushing. The fingers should rest in extension, the elbows in slight flexion and the shoulders slightly abducted. This is opposite to the position of tension. The shoulder girdles are positioned by pushing them down and back, holding and then releasing. If the patient practises this and checks for relaxation every half hour the reduction in muscle tension is of great benefit. Sitting at work (e.g. reading papers, typing, driving a car) should also include components of relaxation, especially pushing the shoulders down and back and stretching the head up 'out of the neck' at regular intervals. The same principles are applied to walking with the shoulder girdles relaxed.

Posture education

This is closely associated with the teaching of relaxation. The classical postural abnormality is much the same as the position of tension. This in the extreme is:

1. Head thrust forwards (stressing the C5/6/7 level and resulting in shortening of the upper cervical spine extensors).
2. Shoulders held up and forwards (causing excess tension in the upper fibres of the trapezius muscles).
3. Thoracic spine flexed and rounded (causing, with the shoulder position, shortening of the pectorals and lengthening of the shoulder girdle retractors).

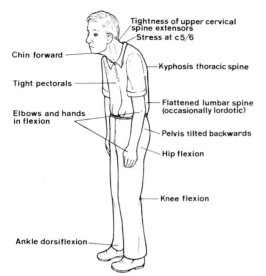

Tightness of upper cervical spine extensors
Stress at c5/6
Chin forward
Tight pectorals
Elbows and hands in flexion
Kyphosis thoracic spine
Flattened lumbar spine (occasionally lordotic)
Pelvis tilted backwards
Hip flexion
Knee flexion
Ankle dorsiflexion

Figure 8.6 Poor posture in spondylosis

4. Lumbar spine flexed, pelvis tilted backwards, hips flexed, knees flexed, ankles dorsiflexed, feet pronated (Figure 8.6). Correction of only one component will not succeed which is why it is essential to examine the posture of a patient from top to toe, identify abnormalities and teach alignment in total.

It is very important to impress upon the patient that it is perfectly possible to reduce the pain and discomfort associated with spondylosis by paying attention to posture.

Position sense needs to be developed so that the patient can think of correction during daily activities.

Collar

During a phase of acute pain, a firm collar will help to steady the neck and relieve pain especially during travelling or work. It is important to remind the patient that it is very unwise to drive or operate intricate machinery whilst wearing a collar because the altered input from the nerve receptors in the facet joint capsules results in impairment of coordination of upper limb activities. When the pain has subsided the collar should be taken off when the patient is resting (sitting in a high-backed chair). The periods without the collar should be gradually extended. Generally it is wise to keep the collar on for travelling until there is no pain at rest and neck movements are painfree for at least a third of full range. A soft collar is often helpful at night to prevent awkward positions of the neck during sleep. If the patient cannot tolerate a collar in bed then it is useful to put a rolled-up thick towel round the back of the neck crossed over in front and if necessary

tied with a pin. A 'butterfly' pillow may be used for the patient who likes sleeping supine. The pillow may be tied in the middle and this part supports the neck whilst the sides prevent the head and neck from rolling over.

Manipulative therapy

Mobilizations

These are undoubtedly essential in the treatment of patients suffering from pain related to spondylosis. Restoration of intersegmental mobility by accessory pressure and physiological techniques enables the patient to regain full functional pain-free movement. No other modality can achieve this. Scrupulous palpation is required to identify stiff segments. When there is acute pain and muscle spasm at C4, 5 there is often stiffness at C7, T1. These segments are not contributing the percentage they should to total spinal movement and therefore stress occurs above (C4, 5). Grade I and II techniques will settle the pain and spasm of C4, 5 and grade III techniques will mobilize C7, T1. The ribs often need mobilizing, especially 1–6. This is effectively and comfortably achieved by alternate flat hand pressure on the thoracic cage.

Soft-tissue techniques

Kneading to mobilize tethered fascia is required especially around the 'dowager's hump' C7–T2. Also, kneading helps to release tightness in the upper fibres of the trapezius. Finger kneading helps to mobilize the occipital attachment of the trapezius and the scalene muscles on the transverse processes of the vertebrae. Picking up, wringing and skin rolling achieve similar effects.

Finger kneading or frictions are often necessary to stretch interspinous ligaments (C7–T1 and T1–T2) or localized thickenings in the paravertebral muscles. The benefit of these soft-tissue techniques is underrated but can be objectively demonstrated in terms of increased pain-free range of movement in the neck, thoracic spine and shoulder girdle immediately after treatment.

Traction

Oscillatory traction is considered to be mobilizing, therefore is appropriate where the neck is generally stiff. Continuous traction is used to relieve nerve root pressure but if the target segment is stiff then it must be mobilized first otherwise the traction force is distributed between the other mobile segments. Also it is essential to ensure that the paravertebral muscles are relaxed and lengthened (e.g. by heat, hold–relax, passive stretching) prior to the application of traction.

Hydrotherapy

Total relaxation in float support lying, together with the warmth of the water gains relief of muscle spasm. Head, neck and trunk side-flexion (legs fixed) performed slowly through full range gains mobility and ensures that the muscles lengthen and shorten fully. To stretch tight paravertebral muscles the patient practises tucking the chin in and pushing the C4, 5 level into the neck float. Float support lying pushing one hand then the other towards the feet helps to relax the upper fibres of trapezius. Sitting, holding floats down with both hands works the lower fibres of trapezius and serratus anterior and trains the neck and shoulder joint receptors and muscles to hold a good position. Swimming is not advisable – except possibly for backstroke or if the patient is a very accomplished swimmer. Breast-stroke with the head held out of the water is the worst possible thing for the well-being of the cervical spine.

Movement

Hold–relax technique is necessary to lengthen the muscles especially the side-flexors and upper cervical spine extensors. Lengthening the shoulder girdle elevators is achieved by the physiotherapist holding the head steady and applying hold–relax to gain shoulder girdle depression. Lengthening the upper cervical extensors is achieved by deep longitudinal stroking and by teaching the patient to lift the head out of the shoulders pushing the back of the head backwards and upwards. Generally these techniques are applied with the patient in lying but half-lying or sitting can be used. Stabilizations are helpful to retrain correct muscle balance so that the upper cervical spine flexors and lower cervical extensors work to counteract the hypertonia in their antagonists. Free active exercises should be practised every day particularly oblique patterns (flexion, side-flexion rotation right to extension, side-flexion rotation left and repeat opposite way).

Advice

The patient who sleeps supine should have one or two (at the most) pillows under the head. In side-lying, two pillows should fill the gap between the neck and shoulder. A pillow to support the top arm and another to support the top knee helps to prevent the trunk rolling forward and twisting the neck.

During the day, every half hour or so, the neck should be stretched and moved through full range – especially in sitting, reading, writing, car driving and similar activities. If the neck starts to feel stiff it is advisable to see a physiotherapist soon so that movement can be restored before a severe acute episode of pain ensues.

Lumbar spine – clinical features

Onset

Usually the pain starts as a niggle and does not become a problem until a few months have passed when it becomes constant. Acute pain may be precipitated by unaccustomed activity, e.g. a weekend of gardening.

Pain

A common site for pain is across the sacrum between the sacroiliac joints. It may radiate down one or both buttocks and to the lateral aspects of one or both hips. Central pain can occur at L4, 5 S1 level.

Referred pain

1. Pain may radiate into a leg because of nerve root irritation. It tends to be dermatomal.
2. Groin –L1.
3. Anterior aspect thigh – L2.
4. Lower third anterior aspect thigh and knee – L3.
5. Medial aspect leg to the big toe – L4.
6. Lateral aspect leg to the middle three toes – L5.
7. Little toe, lateral border foot lateral side posterior aspect whole leg – S1.
8. Heel, medial side posterior aspect whole leg – S2.

Nature of the pain

Dull or severe ache superimposed from time to time by sharp stabbing pain.

Paraesthesia

This can follow dermatomal distribution and may be pins and needles, a sensation of 'creeping ants' or feeling of numbness.

Muscle spasm

There is usually increased tone in erector spinae and in one or both quadratus lumboram muscles. There is often unequal tone between the hip abductors and also between the adductors. Sometimes one hamstring muscle is tighter than the other. (Careful examination to detect these abnormalities is essential so that the patient's problems can be treated logically.)

Limitation of movement

All lumbar spine movements tend to be limited – on attempted flexion there is often no movement between S1 and L1. Hip movements are often limited asymmetrically. Limiting factors are generally soft-tissue tightness more than spasm or pain (except during an episode of acute pain).

Muscle weakness

The abdominal muscles have poor tone and may be weak. The gluteal muscles are often on one side. The muscles of the leg with referred pain are usually weaker than the other. Pressure on a nerve root can result in weakness of the muscles supplied by that root (myotome).

Radiograph

There is usually narrowing of the disc spaces and some lipping of the vertebral bodies. There is often little correlation between X-ray findings and the disability of the patient.

Treatment

Physiotherapy is directed at:

1. Relief of pain.
2. Restoration of movement.
3. Strengthening of muscles.
4. Education of posture.
5. Analysis of precipitating factors to reduce recurrence.

Examination

This, as in cervical spondylosis, identifies:

1. The pain picture.
2. Precipitating factors at work or leisure.
3. Posture abnormalities.
4. Muscle spasm and tightness.
5. Limitation of movements and the limiting factors.
6. Loss of accessory movement and soft-tissue mobility by palpation.

A logical treatment programme can be planned only after these findings are assessed.

The following treatments may be used.

Heat

A heat pad can help to relieve the aching which comes from prolonged muscle spasm. The best position is lying with one pillow under the head and two or three under the knees. Sometimes it is helpful to warm tight muscles in a stretched position. For the lumbar spine extensors pulsed or continuous electromagnetic energy can be applied to the patient, supported in side-lying with the knees, hips and lumbar spine flexed. If the patient's pain is relieved by warmth it is sensible to discuss wearing a vest or woollen body belt, especially during the winter. Often, there is a gap between shirt and trousers which chills the very muscles that are working, e.g. during gardening or DIY in the house. Chilling of the lumbar spine area is particularly common in the 'tee shirt and jeans brigade'.

Ultrasound

This is very useful for treating the thickenings in the periosteal attachments of erector spinae, quadratus lumborum and for thickened ligaments (sacrotuberous and sacroiliac).

Corsets

Generally corsets are not indicated in these patients because mobility and good postural muscle tone are the important themes. Short-term elasticated strapping may be helpful during an episode of acute pain.

Relaxation

This follows the same principles as described for cervical spondylosis.

Posture education

As in all postural deformities this includes training the patient in total body alignment. Foot and leg positions affect pelvic balance and can often be the underlying problem even when the patient insists that the pain is in the back and there is nothing wrong with the legs. (See Intervertebral disc lesions and postural deformities.)

For example, a habit of standing with the right knee slightly bent causes shortening of the hamstrings which pull on the ischial tuberosity attachments tending to cause backward rotation of the right hip bone which pulls on the quadratus lumborum and these muscles start to ache. Standing habitually on the right leg with the knee straight causes shortening of the right hip abductors and the left trunk side-flexors. Aching can then start in both these muscle groups. Breaking these 'habits of a liftime' may not be possible but the patient can certainly be trained in the habit of regular stretching in the opposite direction. Mobility of joints and soft tissues must be gained before posture training is possible. At first correct alignment feels squint to the patient but it is essential to persevere until good alignment feels normal.

Manipulative therapy

Mobilizations

Applied to stiff segments of the lumbar spine, sacroiliac and hip joints these techniques gain mobility at a target level which is not possible by exercise. It is important to remember that all of these joints must contribute movement to lumbar pelvic rhythm. Stiffness of one component throws stress on the others.

Soft-tissue techniques

Passive stretching of tight structures is also essential, e.g. the iliotibial tract is stretched by crossing the affected leg over the other together with side-flexion of the trunk.

Tight side-flexors are stretched with the patient in side lying over a firm roll and the legs lowered over the edge of the bed or table. The posterior sacroiliac ligament is stretched with the patient prone and the knee on the affected side flexed. The sacrum is fixed by the physiotherapist and the patient's leg carried outwards (medial rotation of the hip).

Kneading, finger kneading and frictions are all important in restoring mobility to supraspinous ligaments, quadratus lumborum, erector spinae (especially the sacral attachments), and glutei at their femoral attachment.

Traction

This is applied under the same principles as for the cervical spine.

Hydrotherapy

Provided the patient is happy in water, hydrotherapy is very beneficial. It is not sensible to have a patient in the pool who holds the head out of the water in float lying because the back pain is aggravated. Relaxation in float lying followed by the physiotherapist moving the patient through the water and gradually moving the trunk increasingly from side to side gains mobility. This is especially useful for the patient who is afraid to move the spine after an episode of severe pain. The patient joins in the exercise and eventually should be able to swing the legs from side to side adding in trunk extension or flexion. Trunk rotation in sitting gains range in a relatively weight-free position. Exercise against buoyancy – pushing both legs into the water in float lying strengthens the lumbar extensors. Swimming is generally beneficial. The freedom of the movement in the water gains mobility and strength more quickly than on land. Mobilizations given beforehand or in the water complement the benefits of the pool.

Movement

Hold–relax can be applied to gain flexion. At first the patient is in lying with the knees flexed and crossed. The physiotherapist applies the technique by pushing on the knees. Later, provided there is no danger of disc prolapse, the technique can be applied in long sitting. The side-flexors can be lengthened by hold–relax applied to alternate hip updrawing. Active exercise comprises teaching the patient pelvic tilting forwards, backwards and sideways in crook lying, prone kneeling, sitting and standing. Then smooth pelvic movement needs to be re-educated i.e. backwards to allow forward flexion, forwards to allow extension and sideways to allow side-flexion. Oblique movements should be taught for daily practice after discharge, i.e. standing hands clasped, feet astride – touch left foot, stretch up and back to the right, repeat to the opposite side. Also combined movements can be appropriate for some patients – especially younger age groups. These are standing – bend forwards then side to side in the flexed position, repeat in extension, bend sideways then bend forwards and backwards maintaining side-flexed position, repeat to opposite side.

Together with mobility, the patient should practise strengthening exercises for all the lumbar and hip muscles.

Advice

Sleeping on a firm mattress generally helps the patient whose problem is backache on waking, especially when the ache is aggravated by prolonged flexion. If the ache is aggravated by extension (where lordosis is the problem) a hard mattress can be quite wrong. If the patient sleeps in side-lying rather than supine the mattress should be soft enough to accommodate the body contour. Also the patient should try supporting the waist with a roll and the top arm and leg with pillows. During the treatment programme the physiotherapist and the patient should work out the precipitating factors, e.g. car seat, desk height, shape size and weight of objects handled at work, sitting position (including side-sitting always one way). Also the patient should understand the importance of general fitness in the prevention of recurrence.

Spondylolysis

Definition

A condition in which there is a defect in the pars interarticularis of a lumbar vertebra. The pars interarticularis is the spur of bone joining the inferior articular process and lamina to the superior articular process and pedicle.

Aetiology

Fatigue fracture or congenital abnormality results in fibrous tissue replacing the narrow part of the pars interarticularis.

Clinical features

1. Often there are none attributable to the defect directly.
2. The condition can be seen on radiographs and may be discovered by chance.
3. Commonest site affected is L4/5 and L5/S1.

Prognosis

1. The condition may not give rise to any symptoms.
2. The part of the vertebra above the defect may slip forwards and the condition is then known as spondylolisthesis.

Spondylolisthesis

Definition

This means that the body of a vertebra slips on the one below. Generally the direction of the slip is forwards; occasionally there is a backward slip (retrolysthesis).

Aetiology

Common sites are L5/S1 and L4/L5. The stability of the L4/5/S1 part of the lumbar spine depends on the pedicle, pars interarticularis and inferior articular facet locking over the superior facet of the vertebra below (Figure 8.7(a)). When the pars interarticularis 'gives', the vertebra slips forwards (Figure 8.7(b)).

Causes (after Newman, 1974)

1. Spondylolysis leads to separation of the pars interarticularis (Figure 8.7(b)).
2. Degenerative changes (Figure 8.7(c)) leads to subluxation of the facet joints.
3. Congenital underdevelopment of the superior articular facets can enable L5 to slip forwards on the sacrum (Figure 8.7(d)).
4. Fracture due to trauma.
5. Pathological weakening of bone (malignant or osteoporotic).

(4) and (5) are very rare.

Clinical features

These vary according to the cause:

1. Younger age groups are affected. Pain is in the back.

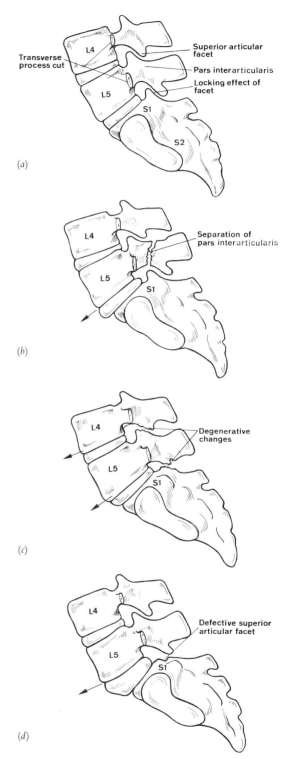

(a)

(b)

(c)

(d)

Figure 8.7 (*a*) Normal pars interarticularis and facet joints. (*b*) Separation of pars interarticularis. (*c*) Degenerative changes of facet joints. (*d*) Defective articular facet

2. Females are much more commonly affected than males:
   (a) Age group is 40 plus.
   (b) Backache is characteristic with muscle spasm a dominant feature.
   (c) Sometimes it feels as if the lumbar spine is locked in extension and the patient has a lordosis at L4/5/S1.
   (d) Pain is relieved on lying and aggravated by prolonged standing. Sitting may at first relieve but later aggravates.
   (e) Referred root pain in the legs can occur.

Treatment

Cause 2

1. Pain can be relieved by warmth. A lumbo-sacral support also helps to relieve pain.
2. Active exercises are essential when acute pain has subsided to strengthen abdominal and back extensor muscles.
3. Advice on posture, back care and lifting is essential.
4. Loss of weight is usually appropriate.
5. Mobilizations and soft-tissue techniques may be appropriate to restore movement to levels of the lumbar spine above the level of the lesion.
6. If root pain is severe or neurological deficit develops, spinal fusion may be appropriate.

Causes 1 and 3

These may need to be treated by decompression and fusion.

Joint surgery

1. Replacement.
2. Arthrodesis.
3. Osteotomy.

Replacement arthroplasty

The joints that are replaced most commonly are hips and knees. Shoulders, elbows, metacarpophalangeal joints and ankles are also replaced with varying degrees of success. The diseases that lead to joint replacement are rheumatoid arthritis, osteoarthritis, psoriatic arthritis, ankylosing spondylitis (hips) and juvenile arthritis.

The indications for surgery are:

1. Severe disabling pain.
2. Loss of range of movement causing severe impairment of function.

Elbow replacements

These are performed to relieve pain and enable the patient to use the arm. Physiotherapy is directed at encouraging the patient to believe in the new joint. Gravity counterbalanced or assisted active exercises are given daily – 2 or 3 movements only for the first few days. Thereafter the important theme is functional activity incorporating elbow movement, e.g. placing hand on head, neck, shoulder, opposite shoulder, above head; putting on/off jacket, cardigan, vest.

Shoulder replacements

Again the aim is to relieve pain and regain good function but full anatomical range is not possible. Re-education of glenohumeral rhythm is important and the scapula often needs mobilizing on the thoracic wall.

Metacarpophalangeal joints

These are replaced when there is subluxation and ulnar deviation. This improves the alignment of the flexor and extensor tendons and improves function.

Ankle joints

Re-surfacing of this joint is sometimes carried out. Arthrodesis is very successful for pain and instability of the ankle, therefore arthroplasty is less common.

Hip joints

Total hip replacement (THR) means that both the acetabulum and the head of femur are replaced (Figure 8.8). It is performed on patients aged 30–40 years for ankylosing spondylitis, rheumatoid arthritis or osteoarthritis due to congenital dislocation of the hip. It is also commonly performed on older patients with osteoarthritis, rheumatoid arthritis or fractured neck of femur. The materials used at present tend to last for 10–15 years and therefore ways of making revision easier are constantly under consideration.

Two methods are used: cemented and uncemented.

Cemented

This is good, but if the parts become loose, removing the old cement may be difficult, especially if the bone is poor. If revision is not possible a girdlestone operation may be required.

Uncemented

This method is becoming increasingly common because it is easier to revise and lasts longer. It is

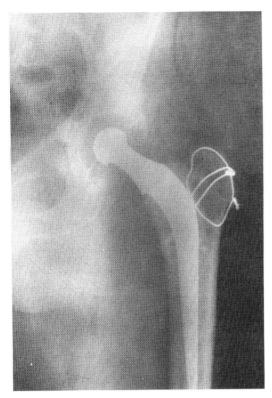

Figure 8.8 Charnley total hip replacement

therefore done in younger patients. The prosthesis has a greater surface area so that bone tissue grows around it thus making a natural fixation.

Materials used

Generally the femoral component is made of stainless steel alloy and the acetabulum is polyethylene. For fractured neck of femur there may be a THR or the femoral head alone may be replaced.

Physiotherapy

This is essential following a THR to enable the patient to regain a confident gait and mobility.

Preoperative

Prior to the operation, it is helpful for the physiotherapist to explain the postoperative programme to the patient.

Postoperative exercises are taught and the patient's respiratory function is tested. Expansion breathing exercises for the basal lung areas are taught. Walking aids can be assessed e.g. gutter crutches or frame for RA, elbow crutches for OA.

Postoperative

Management varies according to the following factors:

1. Cemented or uncemented.
2. State of the patient.
3. Approach used and surgeon's beliefs.
   The main aims are to:
   (a) Re-educate gait.
   (b) Regain the patient's confidence.
   (c) Advise the patient on how much to expect and any precautions necessary.
   (d) Regain movement and muscle strength.

Outline of progressive programme for a THR (cemented)

Day 1

1. Bed rest.
2. Assisted abduction and adduction to neutral.
3. Assisted hip and knee flexion and extension.
4. Isometric work for the hip abductors, hip extensors and quadriceps.
5. Active toe and foot exercises.
6. Prone lying, assisted hip extension should be tried, particularly if there has been a flexion deformity.

Precautions:

1. A sliding board helps the foot to move so that flexion and extension is easy.
2. A posterolateral approach – avoid flexion beyond 90°, medial rotation and adduction (a pillow must be placed between the legs, for both lying and side lying).
3. An anterolateral approach (this tends to be technically more difficult but it is more stable). Avoid lateral rotation.

Day 2

1. As above.
2. Practise getting to standing from sitting.
3. Sit on high chair and have bed high for sitting on the edge to get up.
4. Sit for meals – go back to bed for exercises.
5. Walking starts with elbow crutches or gutter crutches/frame as appropriate:
   (a) The patient should feel the weight is distributed comfortably between crutches and feet.
   (b) Shoes must be supportive.
   (c) The patient should be in trousers and top rather than nightwear.
   (d) Confidence is built up with the physiotherapist observing and instructing the patient, over a progressively greater distance.
   (e) Foot action is important (heel–toe push-off).

(f) The pelvis should face forwards (the patient may keep the pelvis on the affected side back).
(g) Even pacing and equal length steps are important.

Day 3–10/12

1. Physiotherapy continues as above until the stitches are out (10–12 days).
2. Going up and down stairs should be practised within 10 days.
3. Progression to sticks should be possible.
4. Independence must be developed so that the patient can get up, walk about and go back to bed at will.
5. Dressing, bathing, toileting, eating, cooking, should be practised with the occupational therapist.
6. Walking must be in shoes, preferably with a heel (not high or stiletto).

Discharge home

1. The patient is instructed to continue with exercises and walking practice and not to cross the legs when sitting or lying.
2. Community physiotherapy may be arranged so that activities at home are supervised every one or two weeks.
3. Going into and out of a car should be practised because the legs should be kept together. Driving is not allowed for 6 weeks because there is a loss of proprioceptive input to the hip joint.

Postoperative check (4–6 weeks from discharge home)

If the patient has stiffness and residual pain or a gait problem, then outpatient physiotherapy is arranged – hydrotherapy is particularly beneficial. Three months postoperatively, the patient should be walking easily and happily with pain-free function. Certainly by 6 months the patient should be following an active life of walking plus swimming or dancing if appropriate.

Differences with uncemented approach

1. Gait pattern is non-weight-bearing for 6 weeks then partial-weight bearing for 6 weeks. Walking aids (two sticks) are used for at least 3 months.
2. Discharge home is at 2 weeks when the patient is confident with crutches.
3. Thigh pain can be present for a month or two when the bone is growing into the prostheses.

These are successful operations, giving the patient independence, mobility, dignity and relief of pain.

Knee joints

Knee operations may be:

1. Uni compartmental.
2. Total knee replacement (TKR)
   (a) Unconstrained.
   (b) Constrained.

Uni-compartmental

Patients with a history of meniscus problems can develop arthritis in the lateral or, more commonly, the medial compartment of the knee. Both surfaces (femoral and tibial condyles) are replaced. The biomechanical advantage is that the joint is level (Figure 8.9).

BEFORE OPERATION

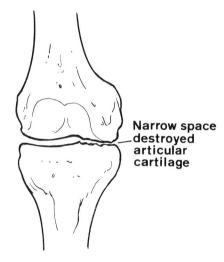

Narrow space
destroyed
articular
cartilage

AFTER OPERATION

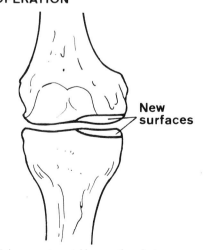

New
surfaces

Figure 8.9 Uni-compartmental knee arthroplasty

Physiotherapy

Following this operation, the physiotherapy is much the same as for TKR, but recovery is faster.

Total knee replacement

In unconstrained knee replacement both femoral condyles and both tibial condyles are resurfaced and a patella button is attached to the posterior surface of the patella. Insall Burstein replacement has a metal femoral component and a metal plus polyethylene tibial component. This allows 100° (at least) of flexion and some rotation. The cruciates are often sacrificed and soft-tissue tension in the other knee structures is essential for stability. Patients with this replacement may have a longer recovery period but revision is easier.

The constrained knee replacement (e.g. Stanmore) has long stems going into the tibia and femur. The components are linked and hinged. The patella is usually retained to maintain quadriceps function. Flexion is limited to between 90° and 95° and there is no rotation. This is the more usual replacement for patients with rheumatoid arthritis.

The approach to the knee is nearly always anterior central and longitudinal. The incision is 8 in (20 cm approx) long. The wound may take longer to heal in the presence of rheumatoid arthritis, especially if the patient is taking steroids.

Physiotherapy in total knee replacement

First 2 days

1. Toe and ankle active exercises are encouraged 2–3 times a day.
2. Quadriceps contractions are important – 5–10 contractions every hour.
3. Gluteal contractions are also important – 4–5 times every hour.
4. A radiograph may be taken to ascertain that all is well but generally the patient is up in the afternoon of the second day to sit with the knee supported in extension.
5. Drains are removed at the end of the second afternoon.

Days 3–10

1. Walking with crutches is practised – the amount of weight taken on the affected leg is as adjudged comfortable by the patient. As with the hip programme, the distance walked is progressed.
2. Stitches are out 10–14 days.
3. Flexion begins 2–5 days postoperatively, assisted manually by the physiotherapist and with the heel sliding on a re-education board.
4. As with the hip, shoes and day clothes should be worn as soon as possible.

Discharge home

The patient must know the exercises to practise and be able to go up and down stairs, stand up, sit down and any other appropriate function.

Some patients attend for out-patient physiotherapy and others are checked by the community physiotherapist. Treatment must continue until there is the optimum amount of flexion and full extension. Techniques used are free active exercises, free swinging in sling suspension, hold–relax and slow reversals. Hydrotherapy is very helpful at this stage. Some younger patients may join a group for exercises but the activity programme is geared to the individual patient taking into account the lifestyle and other joint problems. The scar often needs to be mobilized with skin rolling, picking up and wringing. Gait re-education progresses from crutches to sticks, and after 3 months no walking aid should be necessary for a patient who is fit and had only one joint affected. The commonest fault in gait is poor heel strike with the knee in flexion during stance phase. Heel strike with knee extension therefore requires practice.

Continuous passive movement machine (CPM)

The leg may be placed on a machine that provides steady, continuous flexion and extension. This starts immediately postoperatively. The range starts at 0°–40° and is gradually increased 5°–10° each day, 5° ahead of active movement, until active range of flexion is 90°. It may be used during the day (6 hours) only or on for 24 hours. The speed and range of movement is reduced during the night. If the wound starts seeping CPM is stopped. Accurate measurements are recorded by using a goniometer. There is some indication that CPM hastens recovery, but trials are still continuing.

Arthrodesis

This comprises nailing and/or bone grafting so that two joint surfaces are united. The hip, knee, ankle, wrist and sometimes glenohumeral joint may be treated this way. The operation usually produces a pain-free, stable joint. Function is not as restricted as may be imagined – but this is dependent on a good range of movement in neighbouring joints.

Physiotherapy is directed at regaining function and practising everyday activities.

Osteototomy

This comprises cutting through a bone and realigning the two ends so that there is altered distribution of stress through the bone. It is used for deformed osteoarthritic knee joints where the upper end of the tibia is realigned. Osteoarthritis of the hip may be treated by realignment of the shaft of the femur just below the lesser trochanter. There is usually considerable pain relief. Physiotherapy follows the principles outlined for fractures of these bones.

Excision arthroplasty

This comprises removal of the bony component of a joint, e.g. head and neck of femur, head of radius, head of ulna and proximal part of proximal phalanx of the big toe.

The resultant space fills with fibrous tissue, creating a false but pain-free joint. Physiotherapy is in the form of active exercise instituted as soon as possible to improve power and control over the joint. Following a femoral excision arthroplasty, the leg may be in skeletal traction for 2–6 weeks. Full weight bearing should be delayed for 6–10 weeks to reduce the shortening effect on the leg.

Reference

Newman, P. (1974) Spondylolisthesis. *Physiotherapy*, **60**, 14–16.

Chapter 9

Inflammatory arthropathies

Ankylosing spondylitis (AS)
Rheumatoid arthritis (RA)
Juvenile chronic arthritis

Reiter's disease
Psoriatic arthritis

Ankylosing spondylitis (AS)

Definition

This is a seronegative, progressive inflammatory disease presenting with pain and stiffness of the spine leading to bony ankylosis of the sacroiliac and spinal joints.

Aetiology

Age – Onset is commonest between 15 and 40 years although it can occur at any age.

Sex – It is commoner in men than in women, by a ratio of 3:1 but the ratio is changing as more women are diagnosed as having a form of AS.

Incidence – 0.6% of adult males are affected.

Heredity – The disease occurs 30 times more commonly in relatives of patients than in the general population.

Tissue type – 95% of patients with AS are HLA–B27 positive.

Associated conditions – Sacro-iliitis occurs in association with ulcerative colitis, Crohn's disease, or Reiter's syndrome.

Pathology

Changes start at the sacroiliac joints with synovitis. There is also cellular infiltration of periosteum to ligament or muscle junctions. These sites of attachment are termed entheses and enthesopathy is the name given to formation of new bone at these areas. As the disease continues the chronic inflammation leads to fibrosis which gradually becomes calcified and ossified. These changes occur in the structures of the spinal synovial and fibrocartilaginous joints with progression up the spine as the disease process continues. Bony ridges form at the periphery of the intervertebral joints owing to ossification of the annulus fibrosis and neighbouring tissues. (These are seen on radiographs and termed syndesmophytes.) The disease can progress to bony ankylosis of the sacroiliac joints, symphysis pubis, joints of the lumbar thoracic and cervical spines, costovertebral joints, and manubriosternal junction. Sometimes the shoulders and knees become affected. The changes undergo exacerbations and remissions.

Clinical features

Onset

This is often insidious with mild pain and stiffness in the lower lumbar spine. Sometimes the onset is acute with severe pain over the sacroiliac joints and lumbar spine.

Morning stiffness

This is common in the early stages.

Fatigue

This is also common.

Spinal features

There is pain and stiffness in the lumbar spine, pain radiating down the back of the leg (sciatica), muscle spasm of the lumbar paravertebral muscles and flattening of the lumbar spine. All movements are lost in the spine and straight leg raising is limited bilaterally. As the disease progresses, these features are present in the thoracic and then cervical regions.

Thoracic features

Diminished costovertebral and manubriosternal movements result in the loss of thoracic expansion. The patient becomes dependent on the diaphragm for respiration and there is a reduction in vital capacity.

Deformity

Without instruction and exercises the patient can become fixed in spinal flexion which is very disabling. This is because the weight of the head compresses the vertebral bodies and forward flexion takes place. In order to restore the line of vision the upper cervical spine is hyperextended.

Peripheral joints

Pain and stiffness may develop in the shoulders, hips and knees.

Iritis

Painful inflammation around the iris occurs in 10–30% of patients.

Cardiac

Aortic incompetence.

Constitutional

Weakness, general wasting and lassitude.

Radiograph

Sacroiliac joints – There is erosion and sclerosis of the bone near to the articular surfaces with ankylosis later.

Spine – Erosions occur at the apophyseal joints. There is squaring of the vertebral bodies with ossification of disc margins and longitudinal ligaments. Syndesmophytes are seen passing vertically from neighbouring vertebral bodies. There is bamboo spine due to calcification of the longitudinal ligaments and the syndesmophytes (Figure 9.1).

Skin

Associated psoriasis.

Colon

Ulcerative colitis.

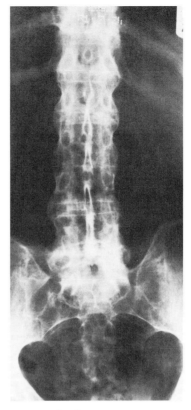

Figure 9.1 Radiograph showing bamboo spine

Neurological disease

The spinal cord is at risk when there is a fracture of the spine.

Prognosis

The disease is with the patient for life but does not shorten it. The course of the disease is variable but whereas some patients become very stiff, the majority, whilst having some limitation of function, can lead a full active life provided that contact sports are avoided. There are exacerbations of acute pain and muscle spasm and long periods of apparent quiescence.

Treatment

Non-steroidal anti-inflammatory drugs such as indomethacin or phenylbutazone reduce stiffness.

Analgesics are appropriate if pain is acute but are not generally needed in the long term.

Physiotherapy

Regular physiotherapy is essential in the management of a patient with AS.

Fibrous tissue is being continuously laid down as a result of the mild inflammation and regular physiotherapy with a monitored exercise programme moulds this fibrous tissue along lines of stress which do not restrict the patient's movements.

During an exacerbation

The aims are to:

1. Relieve pain.
2. Mobilize joints affected.
3. Minimize deformity.
4. Regain fitness.

Relief of pain and muscle spasm may be obtained by heat from hot packs which can be applied locally to the specific joints and muscles affected.

Muscle spasm that persists after the acute inflammation has died down is treated best by hold–relax technique.

Relief of pain and muscle spasm together with restoration of mobility is readily obtained by hydrotherapy.

Examples of procedures

1. *Float lying* – Relaxation practice.
2. *Float lying* – Arms and legs pushing down into the water and resting.
3. *Lying on half-stretcher* – Deep breathing exercises.
4. *Lying on half-stretcher* – Legs pushing down.
5. *Lying on half-stretcher* – Legs pushing down and out.
6. *Float lying* – Arms stretching sideways and upwards.
7. *Sitting* – Trunk turning side to side. Progress by holding arms forwards and grasping a bat.
8. *Prone lying grasping rail* – Breast stroke action of legs.
9. *Swimming* – Progress to underwater swimming.

A programme of hydrotherapy and gymnasium work three times a week for 3–4 weeks is very beneficial for the patient to regain mobility, strength and fitness before returning to a home exercise regimen with class once a week and swimming once to twice a week.

Suitable exercises for the gym work are as follows.

Lying

1. Physiological relaxation.
2. Practise feeling a position of a straight extended spine.

3. Push arms and legs into the floor (static contractions for quadriceps, gluteii and back extensors).

Lying with knees bent (crook lying)

1. Knees rolling from side to side.
2. Raise right arm upwards and outwards, turn head to watch hand. Repeat to left.
3. Deep breathing exercises with hands over upper abdomen – feel air fill under the hands and then sigh out feeling the hands sink down to encourage full use of the diaphragm.
4. Pelvic tilting forwards and backwards. (The range of movement is greater if the pelvis is on a small block, for example a book wrapped in a towel.)

Prone lying

1. Alternate straight leg raising and lowering.
2. Both legs raising and lowering.
3. Hands clasped behind back, thrust hands towards feet with head and shoulders raising and relaxing.
4. Place hands on floor, raise head and shoulders – walk hands to right and then to left (side flexion in extension), arms stretch above head (holding medicine ball), raise arms and ball plus head, shoulders and legs and lowering.

Sitting

1. Stretch head and neck upwards – posture correction.
2. Hands on shoulders – trunk turning from side to side.
3. Hands clasp – bend and twist to touch right foot, stretch upwards and backwards to the left, watching hands. Repeat to opposite side.
4. Head and neck turning from side to side.

Standing

1. Hands on shoulders – trunk turning from side to side.
2. Deep breathing.
3. Trunk bending from side to side.

Activities to be encouraged

1. Swimming.
2. Basketball.

After an exacerbation

The aims following recovery from an exacerbation are to:

1. Maintain mobility of the spine and peripheral joints.

2. Train the patient in postural awareness.
3. Improve and maintain fitness.
4. Provide motivation and encouragement.
5. Maintain mobility of the costovertebral joints and the vital capacity.

Programme to achieve these aims

A daily exercise regimen is essential for the patient. The exercises have to be simple and few so that it is realistic for the patient to carry them out at home and are selected from those already given. The principle to emphasize is that it is possible to maintain very acceptable functional ability by exercise. Daily, the spine must be moved full range in every direction, and the spinal extensor muscles must be worked in inner range. Swimming or a fitness activity should be undertaken three times a week.

Group therapy

Where it is possible, the patient should attend a class once a week. The class will include the exercises as listed previously. Other exercises may be:

1. Prone lying (over form) throw ball to partner.
2. Prone lying (over gymnastic ball supported on hands) stretch legs upwards and backwards.
3. Stride standing, pass ball to partner with trunk turning.

The advantages of group therapy are:

1. Patients offer mutual support.
2. Competition provides enjoyment at the same time as promoting physical fitness.
3. A forum is available for education for example lectures on research, diet and cardiovascular fitness.

Advice

The National Ankylosing Spondylitis Society provides information on research and problem solving.

The patient should avoid contact sports and must exercise every day. If the patient is ill it is still important that some attention is paid to exercise. Otherwise it is important for the lifestyle to suit the individual.

If leisure activities include sitting – for example reading, watching television, or driving – then spinal extension must be performed at intervals such as every quarter to half hour.

Monitoring

A spondylometer may be used. This is a framework which supports pegs. The patient stands on a

MEASUREMENT OF DEFORMITY IN ANKYLOSING SPONDYLITIS WITH SPONDYLOMETER

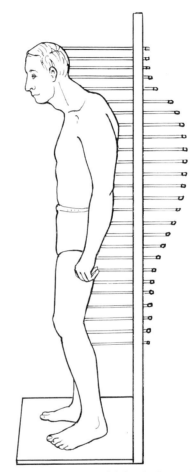

Figure 9.2 Measurement of deformity in ankylosing spondylitis with a spondylometer

platform with his back to the pegs which are then pushed through to touch each vertebra, and an outline of the spine is obtained (Figure 9.2).

A tape-measure or ruler may be used as follows:

1. Measurement can be made between the tragus of the ear and the wall behind. This gives a guide to the development of a flexion deformity of the spine and how upright the head can be held.
2. Measurement of forward spinal flexion may be obtained by placing the tape-measure or ruler vertically between the middle finger and the floor.
3. Chest expansion and vital capacity may be measured as in Chapter 12.
4. A spinal goniometer may be adapted for use to measure cervical spine side flexion.

It is very important that the patient has a simple method of measuring at least one movement at home and that a chart is kept. Should there be rapid loss of range he must seek help from a physiotherapist or doctor. Follow-up sessions are usually arranged at 6-month intervals.

Rheumatoid arthritis (RA)

This is a non-suppurative, systemic inflammatory disease of unknown cause characterized by a symmetrical polyarthritis affecting peripheral joints and extra-articular structures. The course of the disease is variable but tends to be chronic and characterized by exacerbations and remissions.

Aetiology

There are around 1.5 million people affected in the United Kingdom. Women are affected more than men in the proportion of 3:1. The age of onset may be as young as 16 years but is generally in the 20–55-year age group. Tissue type is an underlying factor, in that people with HLA DR4 are seven times more likely to develop RA than the average population. The cause is unknown but is related to a disturbance of the auto-immune system. The rheumatoid factor (RF) (an immunoglobulin IgM) is found in the serum and synovial fluid of 80% of patients with RA and the disease is known as a seropositive arthropathy.

There are a number of hypotheses relating to the cause. These are:

1. *Initiating factor therapy* – An initiating factor causes joint inflammation and does not switch off after the acute episode.
2. *Infectious theory* – Infections from diphtheroids and mycoplasms or from the viruses of rubella, herpes zoster, or Epstein–Barr may be implicated.
3. *Genetic predisposition* – relatives of people with RA are more prone to develop the disease than the rest of the population.

Pathology

RA is a generalized disorder of the connective tissue affecting articular and extra-articular structures.

Articular changes

The first joint structure affected is the synovial membrane which becomes inflamed and congested with blood. T lymphocytes, plasma cells and fibrin are present in the inflammatory fluid which histologically is granulation tissue. The membrane prolifer-ates and forms folds which are known as villi. There are sometimes focal areas of necrosis. The synovial membrane grows along the joint margins forming what is termed a pannus from which proteolytic enzymes are produced. These, plus lysosomal enzymes, erode the joint cartilage at the joint margins and non-weight bearing areas at first (Figure 9.3(b) and (c)) then the changes spread to the rest of the cartilage and articular surfaces of the bone. The erosion of the subchondral bone (Figure 9.3(d)) leads to joint subluxation and deformity. There is excess synovial fluid which is at first thin and watery (effusion) then as the disease progresses it contains fibrin which contributes to the stiffness of the joint and if it becomes consolidated will result in fibrous ankylosis. Locally secreted prostaglandins and increased activity of osteoclasts result in bones becoming osteoporotic especially in the areas near to the joints and also in the vertebrae and pelvis. Muscle tissue atrophies in the muscles which move the affected joints.

Non-articular changes

These may be nodule formation, vascular and reticuloendothelial. Nodules consist of a central necrotic core (with destroyed fibrin, collagen and cell fragments) surrounded by mononuclear cells, plasma cells and lymphocytes. They develop in areas of pressure and may be subcutaneous or intracutaneous. They may also be present in organs such as the heart and lungs.

Vascular changes constitute inflammation of the tunica intima of the arteries of all sizes. The lumen of small vessels can become obliterated.

Persistent overstimulation of the reticuloendothelial system occasionally leads to enlargement of the spleen.

Clinical features

Onset and progression of the disease is variable and may be:

1. *Symmetrical* – Peripheral polyarthritis starting distally and progressing proximally with acute episodes and remissions.
2. *Explosive* – Occurs in older age groups. The patient is alright one day and unable to move the next.
3. *Systemic* – Common in middle-aged men. The main features are non-articular, fever, anaemia, fatigue and weight loss. Joint disease may or may not be evident.
4. *Palindromic* – Irregular attacks of pain and swelling in one or two joints (usually hands, knees and shoulders). The pain may last a few days and then disappear. Nodules also may be

133

NORMAL JOINT

SYNOVIAL MEMBRANE INFLAMED AND THICKENED

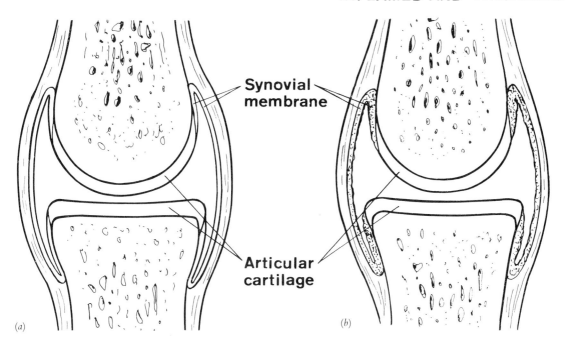

Synovial membrane

Articular cartilage

(a)

(b)

PANNUS ERODING ARTICULAR CARTILAGE

BONE EROSION AND OSTEOPOROSIS

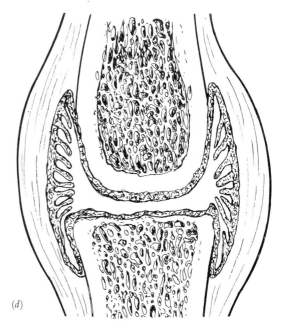

(c)

(d)

Figure 9.3 Pathological changes in rheumatoid arthritis

present and then disappear; 50% of these patients progress to RA changes.

5. *Polymyalgic* – There is diffuse joint pain and stiffness, but no synovitis. Joint disease and positive serum RF follow.

6. *Mono and oligoarticular* – There is pain and swelling in both knees. This occurs in young women and usually dies out after a couple of years with no long-term consequences.

Articular features

There is generally a symmetrical peripheral polyarthritis with early involvement of the small joints of the hands and wrists. The cervical spine, elbows, knees, ankles and metatarsophalangeal joints are often affected. Hip and DIP joints are often spared although in some forms of the disease any synovial joint may become affected (Figure 9.4). The main

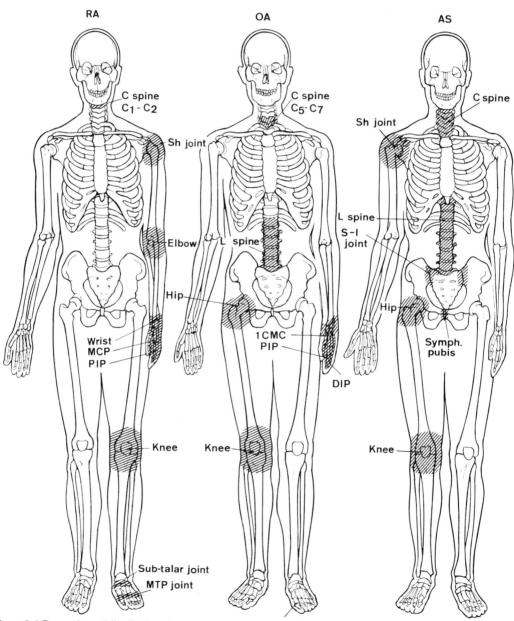

Figure 9.4 Comparison of distribution of rheumatoid arthritis (RA), osteoarthritis (OA) and ankylosing spondylitis (AS)

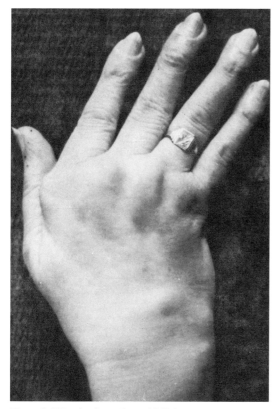

Figure 9.5 Hands of a patient with RA

features are pain, tenderness, swelling, warmth over the joints, loss of movement, muscle atrophy and deformity.

Pain – This is present at rest and readily exaggerated by movement. It can be a dull ache with sharp overtones.

Tenderness – This is present over the affected joints and can be aggravated by pressure of clothes or bedclothes.

Swelling – There is both effusion (intra-articular swelling) and periarticular swelling in the soft tissues. During an acute phase, the swelling is fluid but as the disease progresses the synovial membrane and other soft tissues become thickened so that the joints appear enlarged.

Warmth over the joints – The skin over the affected joints is warm during an exacerbation in association with the inflammation of the synovial membrane.

Loss of movement – This is initially due to pain but can become permanent as the swelling becomes fibrosed and the erosion of the joint surfaces leads to ankylosis.

Muscle atrophy – Occurs rapidly round the inflamed joints both as part of the disease process and because of disuse.

Deformity – During an acute exacerbation, the joints tend to be held in a position of comfort. As the disease progresses and irreversible joint changes occur, the deformity becomes permanent. Individual joint deformities are as follows.

SWAN NECK DEFORMITY

BOUTONNIERE DEFORMITY

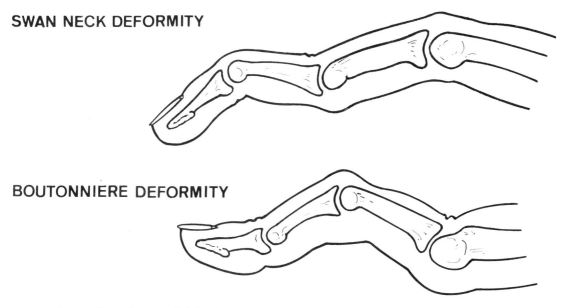

Figure 9.6 Boutonnière and swan-neck deformity

Hands (Figure 9.5):

1. Flexion and ulnar deviation at the metacarpophalangeal joints.
2. Boutonnière (buttonhole) – flexion at the proximal interphalangeal joints, extension at the distal interphalangeal joints (Figure 9.6).

3. Swan neck – flexion at the metacarpophalangeal joints, hyperextension at the proximal interphalangeal joints and flexion at the distal phalangeal joints (Figure 9.6).

Wrist – Flexion and subluxation of the head of the ulna plus ulnar deviation.

Knees – Flexion and/or valgus deformity (i.e. proximal end of the tibia is moved medially).

Feet – There is lateral deviation of the toes especially the big toe and the metatarsal heads are very prominent on the plantar aspect.

Cervical spine – There can be subluxation of the atlanto-axial joints and/or or C2/3, 3/4, 4/5 (Figure 9.7).

Elbows – There is flexion.

Other joints – Shoulders, hips and temporomandibular joints may become affected depending on the form of the disease. Shoulders and hips tend to develop flexion, adduction deformities.

Non-articular features

Systemic – Fatigue, weight loss, malaise, lassitude and sometimes low-grade pyrexia.

Skin – This becomes thin, papery and shiny.

Nodules – These form commonly over the elbows but can occur anywhere. They are round and firm but are not generally functionally disabling unless they interfere with tendon movement.

Vasculitis – Inflammation of blood vessels which can be fatal if large arteries become occluded.

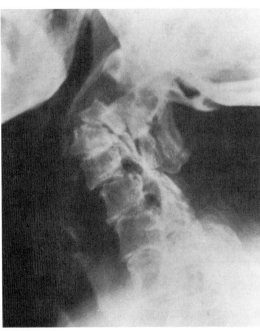

(a)

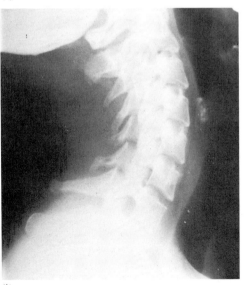

(b)

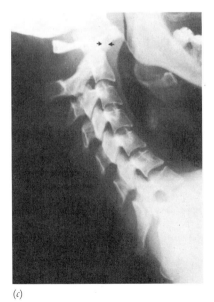

(c)

Figure 9.7 (*a*) Gross rheumatoid cervical spine disease showing subluxation resulting in acute quadriplegia. (*b*) and (*c*) Less severe changes showing subluxation of the atlanto-axial articulation on flexion of the neck (arrows show the gap between the body of the atlas and the odontoid peg. This normally does not exceed 3 mm.)

Cardiac involvement – Pericarditis is a feature in some patients.

Respiratory features – Pleurisy, pleural effusion and pulmonary fibrosis can all occur.

Sjögren's syndrome – Dry eyes and mouth may occur in some patients.

Ocular features – Inflammation and atrophy of the lacrimal ducts leads to scleritis and conjunctivitis.

Felty's syndrome – Enlarged spleen (splenomegaly) and leucopenia (raised white blood cell count).

Neurological features

There may be entrapment neuropathies, cervical myelopathy associated with subluxation, and peripheral neuropathies producing sensory changes in a glove or stocking distribution.

Complications

1. Septic arthritis – this is potentially fatal. It may be suspected when one or two joints are disproportionately inflamed, red, hot and painful especially if the patient is generally unwell.
2. Amyloidosis – extracellular deposition of fibrillar material in the kidney, spleen, liver, adrenal glands and bowel.
3. Osteoporosis.
4. Atlanto-occipital subluxation.

Investigations

Blood counts may show anaemia, leucopenia, plasma viscosity and raised erythrocyte sedimentation rate (ESR). Presence of rheumatoid factor (RF) in the blood is an indication of a poor prognosis. Latex fixation and sheep cell agglutination tests (SCAT) are positive in a high percentage of patients. In the latter test the patient's serum is added to globulin-coated sheep cells. If the serum contains the RF, the particles clump together and the test is positive. In latex fixation latex beads are used instead of sheep cells. Serum phosphatase activity may be high and serum albumin concentration may be low.

X-rays show loss of bone substance especially in the areas just below the articular surfaces. These can be used to detect early RA because there are detectable changes in the metatarsal heads before there are joint signs.

Diagnosis

The following criteria are used for diagnosing RA:

1. Morning stiffness.
2. Pain on movement or tenderness in at least one joint (observed by a physician).
3. Swelling in at least one joint.
4. Swelling of another joint within 3 months.
5. Symmetrical joint swelling.
6. Subcutaneous nodules.
7. Typical X-ray changes.
8. Positive SCAT, latex fixation:
   classical RA has seven criteria present;
   definite has five criteria present;
   probable has three criteria present (from the American Rheumatism Association).

Course and prognosis

The course of the disease is variable and unpredictable. Prognosis in terms of function is reasonably good:

25% remain fit for all-round activity.
40% have moderate impairment of function.
25% are quite badly disabled.
10% are wheelchair bound.

Prognosis is poor if RF is high, erosions of joint surfaces appear early, there are nodules, systemic manifestations and tissue-type is DR3/DR4.

The disease is characterized by exacerbations and remissions. In 50% of patients there are long periods of remission with little or no deformity.

Management

There is as yet no cure for the disease, and management is directed at alleviating the clinical features and achieving maximum functional capacity. Treatment depends on the stage and severity of the disease and is based on examination findings. Each patient requires regular assessment and individual management which demands a team approach.

The principles followed are:

1. Patient education is important related to the nature of the disease, the reasons for the tests, the treatment, diet and rest.
2. Drugs for pain relief, control of inflammation and reduction of the disease process.
3. Treatment of acute exacerbations and management of the chronic stage.
4. Orthopaedic surgery – joint replacement or reconstructive surgery is necessary in some patients to restore mobility and function.
5. Disability or immobility management has to be arranged according to the needs of the patient. Social workers, occupational therapists, home helps, relatives and neighbours have an essential part to play in keeping the very disabled patient mobile or at least comfortable.

Drugs for RA

Analgesics to relieve pain, e.g. aspirin, paracetamol and codeine.

Non-steroidal anti-inflammatory drugs (NSAIDS), e.g. indomethacin (relieves early morning stiffness), phenylbutazone.

Gold and chloroquine to suppress the disease process are used when NSAIDS have been unsuccessful.

Corticosteroids are used to reduce inflammation and pain and to limit deformity, e.g. prednisolone.

Local injections of corticosteroids are used to reduce the inflammation in, for example, knees, hips, elbows.

Immunosuppressive drugs, used when gold has not worked, for the effect of reducing the disease process: azathioprine, chlorambucil, cyclophosphamide.

Management of acute exacerbations

This includes local steroid injections, analgesics and NSAIDs, joint aspiration, physiotherapy and rest.

Physiotherapy

In-patient treatment

The patient may be admitted to hospital because of an acute exacerbation or because the drug programme needs to be changed and monitored.

The aims of physiotherapy are:

1. To relieve pain and muscle spasm.
2. To prevent deformity.
3. To maintain range of movement at unaffected joints.
4. To promote rest in the affected joints.
5. To maintain muscle strength.
6. To prevent circulatory or repiratory complications.
7. Later: to regain mobility of the affected joints; to re-educate function.

Methods

Rest, splinting, exercises and advice. Then during recovery ice towels or packs, heat (wax, shortwave diathermy, hot packs and hydrotherapy).

Rest

This is essential for actively inflamed joints because it allows the body's defences to overcome the irritant agent and relieves pain. Since RA is a generalized condition in many cases complete bed rest in hospital is essential. Where, however, only one or two joints are involved resting the affected joints in splints may be sufficient. During bed rest the position of the patient is carefully corrected on a firm mattress, with appropriate support during the day, i.e. a bed rest or carefully arranged pillows to maintain the head, shoulders and spine in a correct position. During the night there should be only one pillow under the head so that the patient lies flat. The feet should be supported in dorsiflexion with a cradle over them. The possibility of hip and knee flexion deformities must not be overlooked, and if the patient can lie flat for an hour during the day the risk of contractures is diminished. Whenever the patient is in supine lying or sitting up it is important that pillows are never placed transversely under the knees as this is conducive to the development of a flexion deformity. Constant posture correction is necessary and should be reinforced by nurses and therapists. The period of bed rest is from 1 to 3 weeks depending on the severity and extent of the inflammation.

Splintage

This is used for the neck, hands, wrist, knees and ankles to prevent deformity and encourage relaxation. The splint should be used for support and rest and not to over-correct a deformity. A variety of lightweight materials such as Plastozote, Polythene and Orthoplast are available but plaster of Paris is also effective. Rest splints must be worn during the acute phase of the disease for all night and all or most of the day. The joints are supported in a position of function.

Exercises

During the bed-rest stage, exercises are important to maintain muscle strength and function. All the main muscles of the affected joints should be worked isometrically every day as soon as there is evidence of the inflammation subsiding (e.g. ESR lower). Three to four contractions twice a day is generally enough. Muscles which work in the opposite direction to the deformity should be worked more than the others. (Gluteal muscles, quadriceps, ankle plantar flexors, shoulder extensors, elbow extensors, wrist extensors and abductors, finger flexors.) Where possible, the unaffected joints may be actively moved through full range with the physiotherapist guiding and supporting.

Exercises are progressed by increasing the number of repetitions, changing to free active exercises, increasing the range of movement and adding manual resistance.

Breathing exercises are important to keep the bases of the lungs ventilated and maintain venous return.

When the patient is allowed up, the physiotherapist gives stabilizations in high sitting, ensuring that the patient does not feel giddy. Balancing in stride standing and walk standing is then practised, followed by sitting down and standing up, from a high chair. An assessment is made for a walking aid and the appropriate one supplied. This will vary from a stick in the early stages to elbow crutches, gutter crutches or a frame where there is permanent disability. A splint may be necessary to support a knee in extension.

Hydrotherapy is indicated at this stage because there is pain reduction with weight relief. Buoyancy assisted movements are as follows:

1. Sitting, standing up (assisted extension), sitting down.
2. Sitting, shoulder abduction.
3. Prone lying (on half-stretcher), hip extension.

Progression is made by the patient exercising with buoyancy counterbalanced and then, if appropriate, against buoyancy. Walking re-education is very beneficial in a pool because correct pattern can be achieved with only 10–15% of the body weight being taken by the patient's feet.

During recovery

Cold therapy, applied as crushed ice in a towel, may be used to reduce swelling and relieve pain in a joint – particularly the knee.

Wax may be applied to relieve pain in the hands especially prior to exercise.

Heat – Where there is residual pain, especially if it is aggravated by activity, shortwave diathermy or a moist hot pack may be helpful.

Before the patient is discharged there should be a home visit. Ideally the physiotherapist and the occupational therapist should take the patient home for a review of the facilities and check that any necessary adaptations or alterations are put in hand. This important aspect of patient management may be attended to by the community physiotherapist or occupational therapist where this is more appropriate.

When the patient is ready for discharge it is important to emphasize a daily exercise programme and to provide advice. The exercise programme should move each joint through full available range and work each main muscle group isometrically if not isotonically five times daily. The patient must be encouraged to believe that during a quiescent phase daily exercise will maintain nutrition to joints and muscles as well as remove metabolic waste products which contribute to pain.

A ratio of rest to activity must be worked out for the individual needs and depends on the degree of joint destruction and disability. The points to consider are as follows:

1. Activities are important for general fitness.
2. The cardiovascular system benefits from regular exercise.

3. Breathing exercises improve the ventilation of the lungs making more oxygen available to all the organs including the brain and digestive system. This is important in maintaining a general feeling of well-being.
4. Rest does not mean simply sitting down but practising relaxation.
5. Many people with RA lead a very active and fulfilling life.

Management of chronic RA

The principles are:

1. Relief of pain by drugs, heat, splinting, exercise and relaxation.
2. Control of the disease with regular monitoring by a rheumatologist and drugs.
3. Prevention of deformity by exercise, rest, splints and advice.
4. Correction of deformity, possibly by serial splinting – this may be used for the correction of a flexion deformity of a knee or for gaining extension at a wrist. For a flexion deformity at the knee, a plaster-of-Paris cylinder is applied from just above the malleoli to the upper third of the thigh. The joint is held in as full extension as possible and the plaster left on for 1–2 weeks. A felt strip (1 cm thick) is placed on the outside of the leg under the plaster so that when the plaster scissors are applied to cut off the plaster they follow the line of the felt and the patient's delicate skin is protected. Felt is also placed over the malleoli. This procedure may be repeated at 2-week intervals until no more range is gained. Intensive quadriceps exercise must follow to maintain the range. Alternatively the plaster may be bivalved after 3–7 days and the patient attend the physiotherapy department for quadriceps strengthening. The procedure adopted depends on how easily the patient can attend for physiotherapy. This technique places a sustained stretch on fibrous tissue which gradually lengthens and is used in the chronic but quiescent stage. The patient has to be sure that if there is any discomfort that may lead to a pressure sore, immediate return to the physiotherapy department is essential.
5. Maintain joint range and muscle power by exercise.
6. Maintain functional independence by providing working splints, which are made of waterproof, light but durable material and hold the joint or joints in a position of function. They provide support so that the patient can perform everyday functional activities with minimum discomfort and maximum stability. It is important that these are easily applied with simple fastenings so that the patient can apply them himself.

7. Also supplied are aids for personal hygiene, dressing, eating, cooking, mobility (walking aids or a wheelchair).
8. Maintain quality of life by encouraging activities and hobbies compatible with disability. Possibly membership of a horticultural, bridge, disabled club or arthritis association may help.

Out-patient physiotherapy

In some instances a patient may attend for regular (1–2 per year) reviews of the home exercise programme and possibly treatment (6–8 sessions).

Appropriate procedures may then be as follows.

Muscle power

Manually resisted work for the trunk muscles with the patient supported on a high mat. Slow reversals and repeated contractions in pattern for the legs and arms. Resisted walking (resistance on the pelvis) in parallel bars. If these procedures are painful, stabilizations are used to apply isometric muscle work to the main muscle groups.

Joint range

Active assisted movements may be necessary to encourage movement but as soon as possible the patient should perform free active exercises. The principle is to encourage movement in one direction then to hold, try to go a little further then release. This approach is indicated when the limiting factor is fibrous tissue tightness and must not be used in the presence of muscle spasm. For this the appropriate method is hold–relax.

Hydrotherapy

Hydrotherapy is an ideal maintenance treatment as the warmth of the water relieves pain and patients benefit from the freedom of movement in a gravity reduced medium. The increased movement produces synovial sweep across the joint surfaces with consequent increased nutrition, and the quality of muscle work is improved because the muscles are warm. A course of 5–6 sessions every 6 months helps to keep patients mobile as well as boosting morale.

Group therapy

Patients derive mutual support from group meetings.

An out-patient class is useful for reinforcing education, and for checking home exercises. It also provides a forum for ensuring that the patient can seek advice should there be a problem arising from the arthritis. Patient association membership can be developed and social activities may be arranged that help to keep these people active and less dependent on the health service.

Community care

The community physiotherapist has an important part to play in the monitoring of patients with RA. It is often difficult for a patient to get to an out-patient department and it is essential that the community physiotherapist visits such a patient 2–3 times following discharge from hospital. Thereafter, regular checks on the home exercise programme are carried out, splints and aids are checked for wear and arrangements made for replacements.

Surgery

This is necessary in a small percentage of patients. The operations are:

1. *Synovectomy* – Removal of the synovial membrane, which relieves pain and swelling and may arrest the disease.
2. *Osteotomy* – Division of bone near to a joint to realign the bone and consequently alter the weight distribution used on the bones of the feet in RA.
3. *Arthroplasty* – Replacement of joints or joint surfaces.
4. *Tendon repair* – May be necessary where the extensor tendons of the fingers have ruptured.
5. *Arthrodesis* – Fixing of a joint permanently for the relief of pain and for improving function.

The joints operated on for RA are:

1. *Knee* – Replacement arthroplasty, synovectomy.
2. *Hip* – Replacement arthroplasty.
3. *Feet* – Excision of the metatarsal heads (Fowler's operation).
4. *Elbow* – Excision of the radial head and synovectomy, replacement arthroplasty.
5. *Shoulder* – Replacement of the head of the humerus.
6. *Hand* – Silastic replacement arthroplasty for the metacarpophalangeal joints.
7. *Cervical spine* – Arthrodesis of unstable segments.

For physiotherapy related to surgery in RA see joint surgery.

Juvenile chronic arthritis

Definition

Seronegative or seropositive chronic inflammatory arthritis starting before the age of 16 and of more than 3 months duration.

Classification

The arthritis can be classified according to the mode of onset.

Systemic (Still's) disease

The disease affects children aged under 8 who are often acutely ill with systemic symptoms – a spiky temperature, enlarged lymph glands, liver and spleen, pericarditis, pleurisy and unequal limb and finger development. In addition there is a maculo-papular pink rash which comes and goes and increases with external heat or a rise in temperature.

The patients are seronegative for the rheumatoid factor and the symptoms remit during the teens.

Polyarthritis

In some children (8–10 years old) the disease begins with polyarthritis instead of systemic features and is seronegative. The many joints involved swell and become destroyed with resultant bony ankylosis. The inflammatory process continues for longer than in the systemic type.

Pauciarticular

These children have less than four joints affected initially but more joints become affected in subsequent months. Some children have a positive antinuclear antigen (ANA) and often develop chronic iridocyclitis (eye inflammation) which may cause blindness. As the onset of eye symptoms is insidious all children likely to develop iridocyclitis should have regular ophthalmological tests.

Prognosis

The younger the age at onset the poorer the final outcome.

Systemic onset – These children generally do less well.

Polyarticular onset – Better prognosis but a proportion of children have abnormalities of limb growth and receding jaw.

Management

The overall management of the disease requires a team approach involving therapists, doctors, orthotists, social workers, school medical authorities and parents. There must be good communication among the team members both with the child and each other. The child should be encouraged to lead as normal a life as possible.

Drugs

These are prescribed to control the inflammatory process and reduce the severity of the acute episodes.

Soluble aspirin reduces pain, joint stiffness and fever if present and is the drug of choice. Indomethacin can be given. Where there is severe joint inflammation, systemic symptoms or iridocyclitis, corticosteroids are indicated.

Physiotherapy

Aims

1. To relieve pain.
2. To prevent deformities.
3. To increase joint mobility and muscle power.
4. To rehabilitate the child to be independent and educate the parents in the management of the condition.

Method: positioning and exercises

Each joint should be actively moved daily through full range (assisted by the physiotherapist if necessary). During acute episodes this should be performed twice daily.

Flexion deformities tend to occur in the hips, knees, spine, elbows and wrists; therefore, it is essential to strengthen the extensor muscles in prone and supine positions. Shoulder elevation in lying will stretch out tight structures and breathing exercises will keep the costovertebral joints mobile.

Strengthening the extensor muscles is achieved by isometric exercises progressed by increasing the repetitions but not adding weights. In the chronic stage, small weights of a few pounds may be used.

To prevent flexion deformities in the hips and spine, prone lying on a firm surface for at least 1 hour per day is necessary.

Splinting

Splints are used to rest inflamed joints, prevent deformities and aid mobility. Back slabs for the legs, working splints during the day, resting splints at night for the hands and insoles for the feet are all used. Serial plasters may be used, particularly for the knee to correct knee flexion deformities. Hip joints in the acute stage will benefit from skin traction to reduce intra-articular friction and thereby relieve pain.

Hydrotherapy

Children feel much better in the pool. All joints should be actively exercised through full range twice daily if possible. Due to buoyancy providing weight relief, re-education of walking can be given earlier than on land to improve the gait pattern. Swimming costumes with buoyancy floats incorporated around the middle, all or none of which inflate, can be used to support the child.

Passive stretching of tight structures is less painful in the pool. Although fixation is difficult, stretches into abduction and extension of the hip especially after soft-tissue release gain hip mobility.

Swimming (without buoyancy aids if possible) is encouraged to improve stamina and general muscle strengthening.

General exercises can be done in groups with individual treatment for the more painful joints. Parents can be encouraged to assist with treatment in the pool and taught suitable exercises to be done in the bath at home.

Games and activities can encourage younger children to move stiff joints without their realizing it. If any activity includes submerging the head, goggles must be worn to protect eyes from chlorinated water because they are frequently affected by the disease.

After pool treatment, exercises on land are encouraged, particularly for back and hip extensors.

Heat or cold

Hot packs may be applied locally to relieve pain and muscle spasm in the spine or large joints. For the hands or feet, wax is preferable. If swelling is the principal joint feature ice, either by towels or in a bath, is beneficial.

Heat or cold can be given prior to exercises or the application of splints. The choice of modality depends on whichever gives better relief of symptoms.

Gait re-education

Walking is started in the pool where pain relief and increased joint mobility allows improvement in the gait pattern. Hip and knee extension is encouraged during the stance phase together with the push-off and heel-strike at the beginning and end of the swing phase. A walking aid may be necessary if the child is limping.

Education

Since manual work is impossible for most patients with the disease, a good education is important. Nowadays this is likely to be integrated with the able-bodied and should be interrupted as little as possible. Good communication between the teachers and the rehabilitation team will help in better understanding and care of the child. Encouragement should be given to continue with an exercise programme but to avoid contact sports.

Reiter's disease

This is a seronegative polyarticular arthropathy.

Aetiology

The cause is unknown. Men are affected much more often than women. The age group commonly affected is 30–40.

Pathology

Inflammatory changes take place in the structures of the knees, ankles and foot joints. Also affected are the tendo Achillis, sheaths of the tendons round the ankle joint and plantar fascia.

Clinical features

Acute

Pain, swelling and loss of function occur in the foot, ankle and knee joints.

Chronic

Recurrent attacks may occur, and the clinical features can resemble ankylosing spondylitis.

Other features

1. Urethritis.
2. HLA-B27 is present.
3. Skin rash or lesions commonly occurs.
4. Oral ulcers may be present.
5. Conjunctivitis.
6. True Reiter's disease is usually sexually acquired.

Prognosis

The disease can be severe and progress rapidly although sometimes it is self-limiting.

Management

Non-steroidal anti-inflammatory drugs, antibiotics and analgesics are used. Corticosteroids may be used to control the disease and reduce tissue destruction.

Physiotherapy

During an acute episode

Aims of treatment are to:

1. Allow for inflammation to subside and relieve pain.
2. Mobilize joints.
3. Strengthen muscles.
4. Re-educate function.

Method

Ice applied in a towel wrapped round each joint may be helpful in relieving pain and inflammation. Rest with splintage to support the affected joints may be used but kept to a minimum. As soon as the acute inflammation is subsiding free active or assisted active movements for each joint must be started. Static and dynamic muscle work is then essential.

Walking should be encouraged with elbow crutches (four-point walking is progressed to two point).

Ultrasound may benefit tendonitis (tendo Achillis) or plantar fasciitis.

During the chronic stage

The physiotherapy approach is similar to that for ankylosing spondylitis.

Psoriatic arthritis

Psoriasis is associated with arthropathy which may resemble ankylosing spondylitis or Reiter's disease.

In some patients, however, there are features that appear to be more psoriatic related.

Clinical features

1. Inflammation and deformity of the distal interphalangeal joints of the fingers.
2. Psoriatic skin lesions may be mild affecting only a small area or widespread and severe.
3. Dry raised, red, skin over the extensor aspects of knees and elbows is characteristic.

Prognosis

Most patients with psoriatic arthritis can make a good recovery. The skin appearance is often the major worry for the patient.

Management

Gold therapy or non-steroidal anti-inflammatory drugs may be used.

Physiotherapy

This follows the treatment of infective arthritis, RA or ankylosing spondylitis according to the predominating features. It is important to remember that psoriasis is with a patient for life and that cervical or lumbar spondylosis may give pain and stiffness in later life. These should be treated exactly as outlined in Chapter 10.

Chapter 10

Metabolic arthropathies

Crystal arthritis
Connective tissue diseases

Infective arthritis
Haemophilic arthritis

Crystal arthritis

There is a group of arthropathies associated with the abnormal presence of crystals in synovial fluid or articular cartilage. In gout there are sodium urate crystals in joint structures. Pseudo-gout is associated with calcium pyrophosphate, and hydroxyapatite crystals have been identified in the cartilage of joints. These crystals have been identified in the cartilage of osteoarthritic joints in which synovitis is a feature.

Gout

This disease is characterized by arthritis in specific joints and the deposition in the tissues of sodium urate crystals.

Aetiology

Acute

Age group – 30–50 years is commonest.
   Sex – Men are much more commonly affected than women.
There is a familial tendency.
Diet, including alcohol, has an influence on blood uric acid values.

Pathology

The high concentration of uric acid in the blood results in deposition of urate crystals in the tissues – synovial membranes and sheaths, articular cartilage and subcutaneous tissues. These crystals are termed tophi and cause irritation leading to the changes of inflammation in these tissues. In joint structures there is increased synovial fluid production causing synovitis.

Clinical features

History – Recurrent synovitis with intervening periods of remission.
   Joints affected – Metatarsophalangeal joints of big toes, ankles, knees, wrists and hands.

Acute episode

The MTP joint of the big toe is hot, swollen, red and excruciatingly tender.
   After 3–5 days the inflammation subsides (Figure 10.1). The skin over the joints is dry and flakes off.

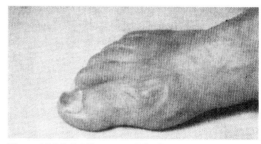

Figure 10.1 Subsiding gout of the first metatarsophalangeal joint

Chronic gout

This results after several acute episodes and causes thickened swelling with deformity of the hands or feet.

Management

1. Rest is essential with the limbs in elevation.
2. Non-steroidal anti-inflammatory drugs reduce the inflammation.

3. Colchicine, phenylbutazone and indomethacin are frequently used.
4. Long-term colchicine may be used prophylactically.
5. Diet should be considered both in terms of moderation of high-purine foods and alcohol as well as in weight reduction.
6. Monitoring and treatment of renal complications is important.

Physiotherapy

Currently, physiotherapy does not play a prominent part but advice on moderate regular exercise is important. The physiotherapist in a health clinic may well be involved in planning and teaching a programme of activities for individual patients.

Connective tissue diseases

This is a group of conditions which affect muscles and structures composed principally of fibrous tissue (collagen).

The effects of these conditions are far reaching as any alteration in the normal structures of support tissue of organs reduces the functional capacity of these organs. Joint structures are also affected and therefore there is impairment of the functions of the musculo-skeletal system.

Polyarteritis nodosum

This is a multi-system disease. Blood vessels are inflamed thus diminishing the lumen and denying blood supply with the loss of function of the affected organs and tissues.

Treatment is by corticosteroid therapy.

Scleroderma (progressive systemic sclerosis)

This disease is characterized by tethering of the skin to underlying structures. It affects the fingers first and progresses proximally. The facial skin is affected with tightness round the nose and eyes. The skin tightening becomes very disabling.

Physiotherapy

This is directed at stretching and mobilizing the skin and fascia by passive movements, passive stretching, skin rolling, kneading and active exercise where possible.

Polymyalgia rheumatica

This condition starts insidiously after the age of 60. The main features are:

1. Pain and early morning stiffness.
2. Poor health.
3. Poor limb function.
4. Synovitis in the hands and knees.
5. Raised ESR.

Treatment

Corticosteroids are very effective but may have to continue for several years with all the risks of side-effects. There can be spontaneous remission after 2 years but not everyone is so lucky.

Systemic lupus erythematosus

This is a disease that is becoming more common. It affects several of the organs and systems of the body.

Aetiology

Age of onset – Child-bearing years.
Sex – Ratio of 9:1 female to male.

Clinical features

1. Rash – especially 'butterfly' on the face.
2. General malaise – in the active stage.
3. Necrosis of the arteries.
4. Renal disease, cardiovascular disease, pulmonary problems, gastrointestinal system disorders, central nervous system disorders.
5. Arthritis resembling non-erosive rheumatoid arthritis. Deformities of the fingers.
6. Blood tests – raised ESR. Presence of antibodies ANA (anti-nuclear antibody) and anti-DNA (deoxyribonucleic acid).

Prognosis

This is improving to the extent that patients with good drug management and sensible lifestyle can live for a normal life span.

Physiotherapy

During an active exacerbation of arthritis the affected joints should be treated as for rheumatoid arthritis. Between exacerbations, a programme of active exercise should be devised for the patient to follow daily. It is important that the patient recognizes the symptoms of fatigue and tries to avoid prolonged anxiety or excess physical exercise. Patients with systemic lupus erythematosus are sensitive to ultra-violet rays. They are advised to use barrier creams and to avoid exposure to the sun.

Dermatomyositis

This is a condition in which there is inflammation in skin and muscle. There are exacerbations and remissions which follow an unpredictable course. The muscles affected most commonly are those of the pelvis and shoulder girdles followed by progression to the lower limb muscles. It occurs in both a childhood and an adult form.

Childhood form

In the childhood form joint inflammation occurs more than in the adult form. As the disease progresses, muscle tissue is replaced by fibrous tissue.

Physiotherapy

During an exacerbation, positioning of the patient with splints and pillows on bed rest is essential. As the acute inflammation subsides, free active exercises are started to improve muscle power and prevent contractures – particularly of the hips, knees and ankles. The physiotherapy programme has to be directed at maintaining maximum function, taking into account the fact that as the disease progresses there is involvement of cardiovascular, respiratory, gastrointestinal and reticulo-endothelial systems. Calcinosis (calcium deposits in muscle and skin) can cause fixed contractures of muscles.

Adult form

The disease is particularly characterized by inflammation of muscle producing considerable weakness. There may be acute exacerbations with swelling and tenderness of the muscles.

The pattern of affected muscles is the same as in the childhood form. There may be progressive disease of neck flexors, speech and swallowing muscles. When added to this the respiratory muscles are affected there is a great risk of pneumonia. Joint pains occur less often than with children but there is a skin rash. Some patients have a history of malignancy prior to the onset of the disease. In others only the muscles are affected, and the disease is then termed polymyositis.

Treatment

Steroid therapy and possibly immunosuppressive drugs are used.

Physiotherapy

This follows principles similar to those in children.

Infective arthritis

Arthritis in the true sense is inflammation of joint structures. Infective arthritis results from invasion of the joint or joints by an organism.

Bacterial infections

Bacteria may enter a joint through a puncture wound, through tissue from an infected wound (pressure sore, boil or traumatic) or from the blood (septicaemia). The causative organisms may be *Staphylococcus aureus*, Haemolytic Streptococci, and Pseudomonas.

Main local clinical features

These are:

1. Severe pain at rest making movement impossible.
2. Tenderness.
3. Redness of the skin around the joint.
4. Hot peri-articular structures.
5. Swelling.

The commonest joints affected are the knees.

Management

The principles of management are:

1. Rest with splintage.
2. Antibiotics.
3. Aspiration of effusion fluid.
4. Surgical drainage if necessary.

Physiotherapy

1. Splintage is applied during the rest period.
2. When the inflammation is resolving there is isometric work for the muscles round the affected joint.
3. Non-weight-bearing free active exercises are performed to move all the affected joints through full range.
4. Gait re-education is essential with crutches at first for partial weight bearing and progression to sticks as soon as pain has diminished.
5. Finally a fitness programme in the gymnasium is worked out for the individual patient.
6. Early mobilization is essential to prevent muscle atrophy and joint stiffness regardless of which joint is affected because loss of function can be very severe.

Other infections

These are related to: Gonococcus or syphilis, Meningococcus, brucellosis, tuberculosis, Salmonella, leprosy, viruses and fungi.

Unremitting pain that does not respond to pain-relieving modalities, e.g. ice, presence of a skin rash and general symptoms of malaise are the main features to recognize. It can be difficult to diagnose infective arthritis and it may be the physiotherapist who alerts the consultant or GP to the possibility of infection as the source of 'capsulitis', 'traumatic synovitis', 'bursitis', or metatarsalgia especially where there is no obvious swelling or heat. The patient can be labelled a hypochondriac if there are no obvious general signs and only one joint is affected (e.g. syphilis mimicking shoulder capsulitis and TB abscess mimicking osteoarthritis of the hip).

Treatment is essentially with antibiotics and rest with graded activity as the infection clears.

Haemophilic arthritis

This is an arthropathy associated with haemophilia in which factor VIII is deficient. Bleeding occurs into the joints (haemophilia).

Clinical features

Haemophilia is a disease of males. The genetic deficiency is transmitted by females. Pain, swelling and loss of movement occur locally in each affected joint (commonly knees, elbows and ankles). General symptoms of pyrexia and malaise may occur.

Treatment

Transfusion of blood or plasma with factor VIII is vital. The arthritis is treated with:

1. Rest and splintage.
2. Analgesics.
3. Aspiration of the blood.
4. Joint replacement surgery.

Physiotherapy

Movement starts when danger of bleeding is past. Mobilizing and strengthening exercises are progressed slowly. Hydrotherapy is of particular value following joint replacement. Buoyancy resisted exercises, walking re-education and swimming can be carried out quite vigorously. The water provides a medium for exercise with minimal risk of further damage to blood vessels.

Chapter 11

Neuropathies

Intervertebral disc lesions (PIVD)	*Thoracic outlet syndrome*
Entrapment neuropathies	*Bell's palsy (facial nerve palsy)*

Intervertebral disc lesions (PIVD)

There are various lesions that can occur in an intervertebral disc. The most common are protrusion and extrusion.

Aetiology

Intervertebral discs undergo the ageing process as described under spondylosis. The loss of fluidity of the nucleus makes true extrusion less likely to occur in older age groups.

Age – 20–55 (commonest). Can be older.

Sex – Males are more commonly affected than females. This is because disc damage is related to heavy, repeated work more commonly undertaken by males than females.

Sites – Most commonly affected sites are L5–S1 and L4–5, but all lumbar discs are prone to prolapse. C5–6 and C6–7 are vulnerable sites in the cervical spine. These are the levels at which there is a change from mobility to stability in the spine.

Pathology

Extrusion (Figure 11.1)

A split occurs in the annulus fibrosus, and since the nucleus is under tension fluid moves into the split.

Direction of movement of nuclear fluid

1. The nucleus may extrude upwards into the vertebral body above, through holes in the cartilage end-plate covering the inferior surface. This causes Schmorl's nodes and can be seen on a radiograph. This tends to occur in 15–18 year olds but is often symptomless until later when degenerative changes cause problems.
2. The nucleus may extrude centrally backwards but tends to be limited by the posterior longitudinal ligament. This ligament is narrowest over L4–5, L5–S1 and so the nucleus may extrude backwards at these sites.
3. The nucleus extrudes posterolaterally into the spinal canal. If the spine is forcefully flexed, the nuclear fluid can burst through the annulus with resultant damage to nerve roots (Figure 11.2), dura mater and possibly ligaments (posterior longitudinal and ligamentum flavum).

Healing

Fibrous tissue can close the split in the annulus and thus repair takes place although there is a weakness which can predispose to further lesions unless the patient follows a strict programme of spinal care. The extruded nuclear fluid is replaced by fibrous tissue which shrinks. This can cause adhesions between the ligaments, nerve root, dura mater and periosteum, and results in persistent pain if no attempt is made to restore mobility of these tissues.

Protrusion (see Figure 11.1)

The annulus may become weakened, the nuclear fluid then bulges into the annulus posterolaterally or laterally (occasionally anteriorly) and causes a bulge. This alters the mechanics of the segment (two vertebrae plus disc between). Two consequences of this may be:

1. A sudden burst in the annulus so that the nucleus extrudes.
2. Formation of osteophytes at the margins of the vertebral bodies. The annulus pulls on the

DISC EXTRUSION

Posterior

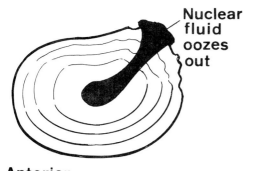

Anterior

Figure 11.1 Disc extrusion and disc protrusion

DISC PROTRUSION

Posterior

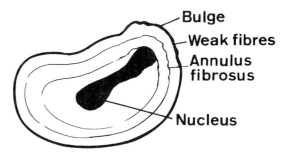

Anterior

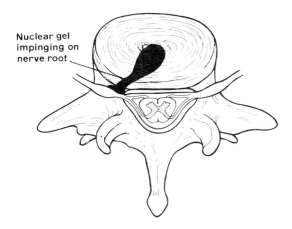

Figure 11.2 Disc extrusion with neurological involvement

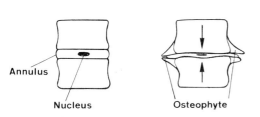

Figure 11.3 Osteophyte formation

periosteal attachment round the vertebral body margin and osteoblasts lay down bone at the traction sites (Figure 11.3).

Prognosis

Good management and sensible lifestyles can lead to full pain-free function. In some patients there is a vulnerability of the disc or vertebral segment and persistent episodic pain. Where this pain is an overriding feature of the patient's everyday existence, surgical intervention is justified.

Clinical features of lumbar disc lesions

History

Pain

The pain pattern varies greatly. Sharp pain in the back can arise suddenly as a result of a bending, twisting and lifting stress. Classically, the patient is unable to straighten up and is 'stuck' – often having heard or felt 'something go'.

Sometimes it appears gradually after several minor episodes of exercise or unaccustomed activity. In this case it starts as a niggle until gradually the patient becomes very aware of increasingly constant pain. A long journey (e.g. transcontinental air flight) can result in central backache, and the patient cannot straighten up.

The site of the pain may be:

1. Central in the back.
2. Diffuse over the lumbo-sacral area.
3. Referred down one or both legs.

Referred pain

This is of two main types:

1. Dull, poorly defined ache over the back, sacroiliac joint, buttock and thigh. This is thought to be due to pressure or stress on ligaments, muscles and fascia.
2. Searing, sharp, stabbing pain shooting down the leg, thought to be due to irritation of a nerve root (Figure 11.4). Generally the pain is aggravated by movements, especially flexion/extension, and eased by lying down.

Paraesthesia or numbness

Pins and needles may be felt in a nerve root distribution (dermatome) and numbness may be detected when tested by touch, pin-prick or temperature test tubes. There may be feelings of weakness. These are considered to be due to nerve root compression or irritation (Figure 11.4).

Muscle weakness

Compression of a nerve root that interrupts impulse transmission results in weakness of the muscles supplied by that nerve (Figure 11.5).

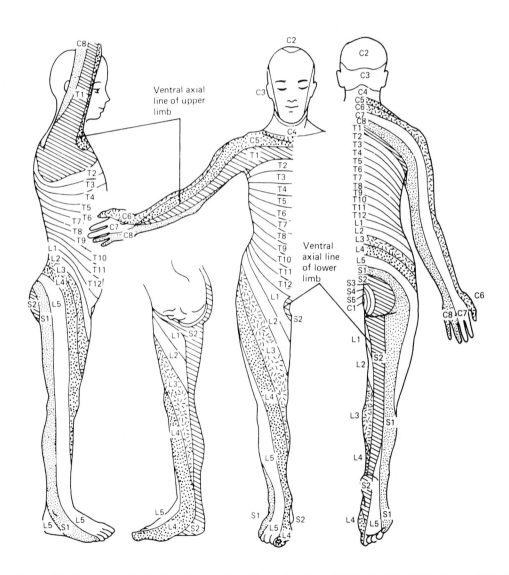

Figure 11.4 Dermatome distribution of paraesthesia (Reproduced from Maitland, G. D., 1985, *Vertebral Manipulation,* 5th edn, p. 46, by permission.)

Side-flexion is generally free to one side with some discomfort, and restricted to the opposite side.

Extension is not possible, beyond straightening of the lumbar spine, especially where there is a protrusion that cannot be compressed.

Standing posture

The spine is held rigid and in a scoliosis (Figure 11.6). This is termed an antalgic posture because straightening or correcting the position aggravates the pain in the leg. Eighty to ninety per cent of the body weight is taken on the non-painful leg.

Sitting

The patient does not like to sit and on trying to do so takes the weight of the trunk by pushing up on the

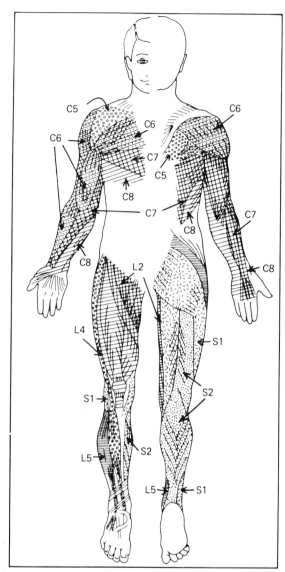

Figure 11.5 Myotome distribution of muscle weakness (Reproduced from Maitland, G. D., 1985, *Vertebral Manipulation*, 5th edn., p. 49, by permission.)

Tendon reflex changes

The quadriceps (L3/L4) and tendo-calcaneal (L5/S1) reflexes are diminished when there is pressure in the corresponding nerve roots.

Spinal movements

Flexion is very limited, erector spinae stands out in spasm and the movement that can occur usually deviates to one side.

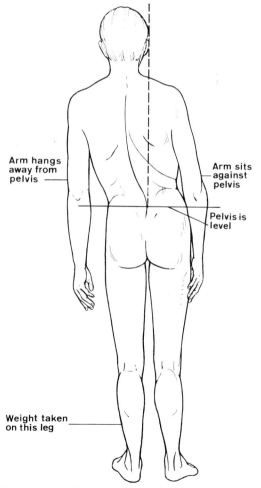

Figure 11.6 Sciatic scoliosis

fists. Standing up from sitting takes time and the patient 'walks the hands up the thighs'.

Lying

The patient likes to lie flat and the spine straightens out. A firm mattress usually affords the best relief.

Sleep

This is reasonably uninterrupted but the patient is stiff on waking and has to struggle to get moving.

Walking

There is a limp because the patient cannot take a normal stance phase on the affected leg. The pace is slow with no normal arm swing.

Sciatic nerve stretch (straight leg raising with foot dorsiflexion)

This is often slightly reduced on the unaffected leg and very limited on the affected leg.

Passive neck flexion (patient in lying)

This may aggravate the back pain and may aggravate the leg pain as well.

Coughing and sneezing

Back pain and leg pain are provoked by both coughing and sneezing. The latter is more painful because it is involuntary whereas the patient can often prepare for a cough. The pain is related to the raised abdominal pressure moving the affected segment and tending to force the nucleus backwards.

Tenderness

Palpation over the lumbar spine provokes tenderness and when pressure is applied can increase spasm. The skin may be slightly warmer and moist over the site of the lesion. In patients with repeated back problems, the skin may be thickened and tethered.

Conservative management

Physiotherapy

The main principles must be:

1. To allow healing.
2. To restore mobility.
3. To restore posture and strength.
4. Prevention.

Healing

Movements, especially rotation and flexion, are likely to cause more disc damage; therefore, resting in a firm bed to allow fibrin to form is helpful. The period of rest may have to be 7–10 days in severe cases but in others may be only 1–2 days. Although it is important to avoid prolonged rest, it is equally essential to persuade the patient that allowing healing will shorten the period of disablement and reduce the likelihood of recurrence.

Where bed rest is impractical, a corset to provide support and remind the patient to avoid flexion is essential, and if there is severe leg pain crutches are necessary.

If the pain and disability are minor then elastic, adhesive strapping applied over the back reminds the patient to avoid flexion and to maintain a lordosis (Figure 11.7). It should be used for up to 10 days and usually needs replacing 2–3 times during that period. Throughout all forms of management, it is essential to obtain a lordosis and for the patient to understand how vital it is to retain it. Within 10 days, fibrin should have been laid down and will start to shrink. If it does this with the disc in the position of lordosis, there is every likelihood that the posterior aspect of the annulus will heal in a shortened position and the nucleus will be retained centrally. Bending must be avoided and, if possible, the patient should support the loin–lumbar spine area with both hands before coughing or sneezing.

If the patient presents at a clinic unable to straighten up, it is worth lying the patient prone with 2–3 pillows (cushions) under the lumbar spine. After 1 hour, if the pain is less one pillow may be removed, then the others are removed until the patient is flat. Then the trunk is propped up – either by lifting the end of a plinth or placing pillows under the thorax. This relieves pain and gains a lordosis. A good working explanation related to this is that the gel-like nucleus is slowly shifted forwards. Then strapping is put on and the patient sent home with clear instructions to avoid bending and maintain the lordosis.

Mobility

During the period of rest, whether or not it is assumed the patient has an extrusion or protrusion, it is essential to keep the nerve roots mobile. If there is extruded disc material it is vital that the patient performs exercises such as alternate foot pulling up and down, alternate knee and hip bending and stretching, and alternate leg carrying sideways. As pain diminishes, passive straight leg raising should be given or crook lying, alternate knee straightening. A progression of this is to add foot dorsiflexion and circumduction to the knee straightening.

Gradually back mobility exercises are added, such as lying, alternate hip updrawing, crook lying, knees

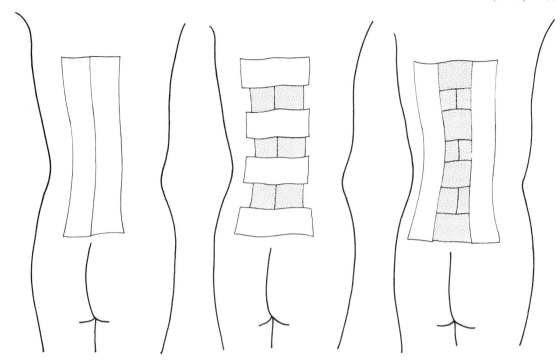

Figure 11.7 Strapping to maintain a lordosis

rolling side to side. Maintaining a lordosis remains important, and the patient must sit with a rolled towel or small cushion supporting the lumbar spine. Getting to upright from lying and vice versa must be correct, i.e. roll on to side, swing legs and trunk to upright in one piece – stand up; or sit on edge of bed, lie on to side and roll back. The objective is that the patient should not use the abdominal muscles to raise the trunk so that intra-abdominal pressure is raised and a force from anterior to posterior (direction of extrusion) is exerted on the discs. Mobility is increased by exercises such as:

1. Side lying (on a slippery floor), pelvis and legs on a blanket – bend and stretch lumbar spine by swinging pelvis and legs forwards and backwards.
2. Standing, pelvic tilting backwards and forwards.
3. Prone kneeling, spine humping and hollowing.

After 3 weeks from the onset it should be possible to start side-flexion and extension in standing. Also it is important to begin regaining flexion. To start with the patient may stand with the hands on a plinth and bend the trunk by bending the elbows. This is progressed by the patient putting both hands on a stool or chair seat and bending the trunk to touch the seat with the head. These are helpful exercises because the patient is confident enough to bend with the weight of the trunk on the arms.

As pain ceases and confidence returns, the patient should be taught to move the trunk in all directions.

For example:

1. Standing – feet apart – touch each foot with hands clasped together and stretch backwards and upwards to opposite sides.
2. Standing – feet apart – bend forwards and bend from side to side in the flexed position.
3. Standing – feet apart – bend to the side, then bend forwards and backwards.
4. Standing with a wall behind – keep feet steady, turn to touch the wall with both hands – repeat both ways.

The importance of exercises such as these is that the tissues of the lumbar spine, the joint cartilages and nerve roots are moved through full range. This prevents adhesions, helps fluid flow and, therefore, nutrition to all these structures. Also, collagen in the healed disc should follow the stress lines required for normal function.

Posture and strength

Strength of the lumbar spine muscles is important in supporting the spine. The extensors should be exercised in inner range (prone lying – head and shoulders raising) and then middle to inner range (prone lying over end of plinth – feet fixed – head and shoulders raising).

The abdominal muscles should be strengthened with graduated sit-ups so that intra-abdominal pressure is raised. This ensures a balanced support for the spine. The patient must be taught abdominal contractions prior to abdominal work. It is also essential that these exercises do not begin before healing of the disc has had time to occur (2–3 weeks from onset).

Posture training is essential so that the patient understands how vital it is to keep a lordosis, ensuring that the discs are compressed posteriorly. Posture work involves teaching the patient the corrected position in sitting, standing and lying and then basing activity on these positions. Balance board work is excellent for training the postural components of the lumbar spine muscles. The patient may stand or sit on the board. Gymnastic ball sitting balance practice is also helpful.

If the patient is shunted as in Figure 11.6 and the painful leg is the right, it is helpful to consider the following:

1. The disc protrusion may be above the nerve root – right lateral shift of the pelvis is painful. Lateral pelvic shifting to the left can relieve the pain.
2. The disc protrusion may be below the nerve root (Figure 11.8) – left lateral shift of the trunk is painful. Right lateral shift of the pelvis can relieve the pain.

If the patient understands this then lateral pelvic shifting can be practised to correct posture, starting with a little movement at first and increasing the shift until aligment is correct. On the other hand, if the pain is severe the patient can shift the pelvis away from the bulge and there is merit in doing this from time to time to reduce the irritation on the nerve root and reduce the danger of severe damage.

Prevention of recurrence

The predisposing factors in the patient's lifestyle should be identified. If prolonged sitting is necessary, then a 'lumbar roll' should be used to maintain the lordosis. Also, every 20–30 minutes, the lumbar spine should be extended. For example, standing (hands on back above pelvis) – bend back (Figure 11.9); or prone lying – push up on hands keeping pelvis and legs steady. Every day, the spine should be moved through full range in every direction. Two other important exercises are:

1. *Sitting on floor* – Stretch trunk forwards to touch toes with fingers.
2. *Star lying* – Carry right leg up and over so that right foot touches left hand. Repeat with left leg.

These exercises keep the nerve roots and dura mobile.

Lifting techniques must be corrected and common sense applied to make sure the patient knows how much lifting to attempt and when to seek help.

Concave on side of lesion

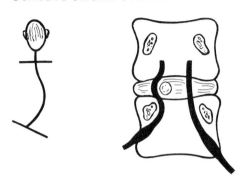

Convex on side of lesion

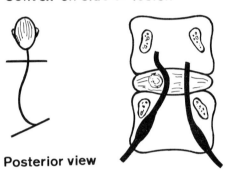

Posterior view

Figure 11.8 Disc protrusion impinging on nerve root, producing a spinal scoliosis. The spine is viewed from the posterior aspect

General fitness is important; bicycling and swimming are suitable activities. Excess weight causes excessive stress especially on the discs of L5–S1 and L4–5; therefore diet control is important. Protection with a broad belt during demanding physical activities is helpful. The back must be kept warm – wearing a vest in winter or a woollen band covering T12–S2 is sensible in outdoor activities in cold weather.

Manipulative therapy for PIVD

Where there is stiffness of a lumbar segment, mobilizations should be used to regain local mobility. This is an essential adjunct to mobilizing exercises that will work the mobile segments and not move the stiff segments. There may be a time, therefore, when it is appropriate to give mobilizations and to instruct the patient not to exercise between treatment sessions.

Soft-tissue techniques of kneading and skin rolling are often indicated to release tight paravertebral muscles, supraspinous ligaments and fascia.

If nerve root tethering is suspected, passive straight leg raising (SLR) is appropriate. If the

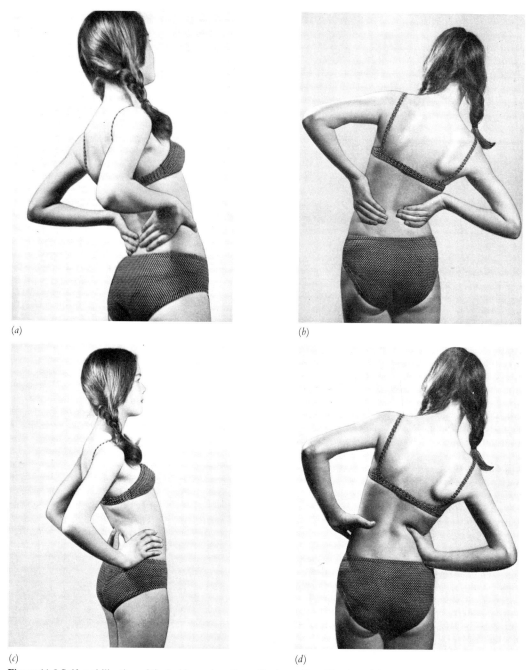

Figure 11.9 Self-mobilization of the lumbar spine, the patient standing. Fixation of the upper vertebra of the treated segment from above, with the hands: (*a*) back bending; (*b*) side-bending. Fixation with the hands from below: (*c*) back bending; (*d*) side-bending (Reproduced from Lewit, K., 1985, *Manipulative Therapy in Rehabilitation of the Motor System,* p. 247, by permission.)

problem is long-standing, hold–relax techniques may be added to SLR to lengthen tight paravertebral muscles.

Rotation mobilizations may be used for a patient whose clinical findings point to a small protrusion. The theory is that the oscillatory nature of the technique reduces the bulge and the nuclear material becomes central again.

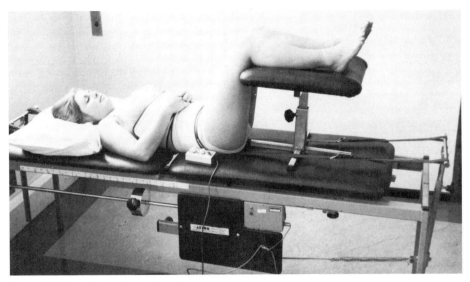

Figure 11.10 Traction to the lumbar spine

Traction (Figure 11.10)

The force exerted by traction tends to separate vertebrae; therefore, nerve root pressure can be relieved. Also, in exerting a longitudinal stretch on the annulus fibrosus plus anterior and posterior longitudinal ligaments, there is a centripetal force tending to move the nucleus centrally. Given for half an hour daily for 3–4 days, traction is very useful. The force applied should reduce the pain about 50% (no more, otherwise the pain comes back more severely when the traction is taken off). A respectable working theory is that blood and lymph flow are increased by reduction in nerve root compression, bringing nutrition and removing inflammatory waste products. Therefore, the leg pain is diminished at first and cleared by three or four treatments. The patient must get off the traction bed with the lumbar spine in lordosis and thereafter maintain it. It may be wise to put strapping or a corset on to remind the patient of this, otherwise the weight of the upper trunk will compress the disc and the protrusion will gradually recur.

Electrotherapy

Spasm in the paravertebral muscles is at first protective but later becomes a limiting factor to movement. Heat from a heat pad can relax this spasm and it is important to apply this for 10–15 minutes prior to exercise. Some patients report pain relief from pulsed electromagnetic energy (PEME) applied to the back and leg with a dual circuplode technique.

Medication

Analgesics are necessary for pain relief. The dose must be reduced and taken only as necessary as soon as possible. They can cause constipation which is unfortunate because straining for a bowel movement raises the intra-abdominal pressure. This then tends to make a protrusion worse because there is a strong anterior to posterior force on the disc.

Surgery

Indications for surgery are:

1. Severe pain which is causing disability such as to destroy the patient's lifestyle for several months.
2. Developing neurological signs, i.e. root signs or cord signs.

   Root signs are: loss of muscle tone and power, loss of tendon reflex and objective loss of sensation in dermatome distribution.

   Cord signs are: hypertonia of muscles, exaggerated tendon reflexes and altered sensation not in a dermatomal distribution.

   A physiotherapist must recognize these signs and refer the patient to a doctor.
3. Bladder or bowel disturbance which may be treated as a surgical emergency.

Surgery for PIVD

Operations that may be performed are: laminectomy and discectomy.

Laminectomy

This involves removing laminae to allow disc material to be removed – often a thick bundle of fibrous tissue is found compressing the nerve. The disc is removed at the same time.

Discectomy

An interlaminar approach can be used to remove the disc and is known as a discectomy or fenestration. This is much less traumatic for the spine than a laminectomy.

Postoperative management

This varies according to the surgeon's beliefs but physiotherapy follows essentially the same principles. These are:

1. Enable healing collagen to be laid down in functional lines and layers. (This is important because a pseudo-disc re-forms in the disc space and must allow movement without danger of tearing.)
2. Maintain nerve root mobility.
3. Restore mobility, posture and strength as for conservative management.
4. Teach back care.
5. Re-educate movements lost owing to nerve compression.

Healing collagen alignment

This is ensured by early mobility – free active mobilizing exercises for the spine and hips. Also isometric contractions for the lumbar spine extensors, abdominal muscles, hip and knee muscles must be practised 2–3 times every hour.

Gait must be re-educated as soon as the surgeon allows, with a normal arm swing, so that the patient's confidence is rapidly restored.

Maintaining nerve root mobility

This is achieved by straight leg raising. The leg on the affected side should be moved to full range (80–90° hip flexion) as soon as possible. At first the movement may be totally passive, then the patient may join in actively. The other leg should be flexed to protect the lumbar spine from hyperextension or increased intra-abdominal pressure.

In 7–10 days when surgeon, physiotherapist and patient agree, standing, touching toes with knees straight should start. Some patients find it easier to touch the toes with the knees bent, then to keep the fingers on the floor and gradually straighten the knees. If the patient has 'never been able to touch toes' then clearly the range to be used is the normal one for that patient.

Restoring mobility, posture and teaching back care

This follows the principles as for conservative management, particularly in regaining general fitness when the patient has had protracted disabling pain.

Re-education of movement

It may be necessary to re-educate the action and function of muscles, e.g. ankle dorsiflexors. Methods used are faradism, Rood and PNF (proprioceptive neuromuscular facilitation) techniques. This may necessitate prolonged out-patient physiotherapy. It is very important to remember that perseverance to obtain full function is both cost effective and humane since the patient will in the end be independent of orthotic appliances or walking aids.

In the author's experience, two patients had weakness of the ankle and toe dorsiflexors (grade 2, Oxford classification) persisting 2 years after an episode of PIVD. Grade 4 function was regained within 6 weeks of the patient's performing daily exercise to mobilize the lumbar spine and the nerve roots (L4, L5) as indicated in the conservative management of PIVD. Localized rotation mobilization combined with sciatic nerve stretch were also given for five treatments. The referring consultant and patients were delighted that surgery was unnecessary.

Cervical disc lesions

The diagnosis of disc lesions in the cervical spine is highly speculative. One theory is that a flake of annulus becomes dislodged and impinges on the anterior part of the dura mater (which has a nerve supply) or the nerve root. The second theory is that a postero-lateral protrusion of the disc occurs and causes pressure on the same structures.

Aetiology

In the flake theory, typically, the patient turns the head suddenly and becomes locked – often early in the morning. A second theory which explains the same clinical features is that a fringe of synovial membrane is nipped between the surfaces of an apophyseal joint so that movements (extension, side flexion and rotation to the affected side) are very painful.

In the protrusion theory there is a history of the patient having slept awkwardly or read in bed with the neck in prolonged flexion.

Age – Any age group can be affected but the most commonly affected are aged 18–45.

Flake theory

Clinical features

Pain is in the neck and aggravated by certain movements. It can be only a dull ache at rest and is more on one side than the other.

Posture – The head and neck are held to one side in slight flexion, side flexion and rotation to the opposite side (acute torticollis). This is a typical deformity. The shoulder girdle is elevated on the affected side.

Neck movements – Flexion is possible with persuasion. Rotation and side flexion are possible to the side of the deformity but not to the opposite side.

Management

These lesions usually settle without anything more than rest in 5–10 days. There is, however, often a residual movement limitation in the cervical spine and increased tone in the upper fibres of trapezius which predispose to further injury. Often the upper thoracic spine is stiff and this contributes to recurrence. Unfortunately, patients tend not to be referred immediately and therefore have long-standing problems by the time they attend a physiotherapy department.

Physiotherapy

In the acute phase, low force traction in the line of the deformity relieves pain. The patient usually cannot lie flat because of the pain; therefore half lying with full support is the position of choice. The force applied should be such as to ease the weight of the head off the painful joints (2–3 kg). After 15–20 min a collar should be applied and the patient advised to rest with the head supported. Next day, it may be appropriate to repeat the traction but if the muscle spasm has relaxed and the patient can lie flat, manual traction can be applied. When the patient is relaxed and painfree either mobilizations or manipulation can be performed. Generally, rotation to the least restricted side is successful in regaining pain-free movement. Alternatively, or as an adjunct, side flexion towards the least restricted side can be successful. A manipulative thrust in side flexion or rotation can clear the movements completely. The collar should be discarded. The patient should be reviewed in 2–3 days when a thorough palpation examination can be performed. Any immobile segments in the cervical or thoracic spines should be treated with mobilizations for the joints and frictions or kneading for the soft tissues. Thereafter, the patient should be taught to move cervical and thoracic spines through every range of movement once a day.

Protrusion theory

Clinical features

Pain –This radiates down an arm, and the medial border of the scapula as well as the neck. The patient looks grey and drawn because the pain interrupts sleep and is resistant to analgesics.

Movements – These are all restricted in the neck and affected arm.

Management

Rest is enforced because the pain is too severe for work. Driving a car is also impossible. A soft collar may help but does not relieve the arm pain.

Physiotherapy

The kindest approach to this patient is to apply traction in half lying. The force should reduce the pain by 50%. Pillows must be placed behind the head, the affected arm, across the thighs to support the forearms and under the knees. The pillow behind the head should be flattened in the centre so that the sides support the sides of the head ('butterfly' pillow). The traction may be left on for 20 min. Then the patient relaxes in the same position and may go off to sleep for the first time in days. The traction may be repeated another two times on the same day – and extended to 30 min duration. The patient goes home with a clear understanding of the relaxation position and often sleeps well that night. This regimen, repeated for two more days, usually reduces the pain by 80–90%. Relieving the last 10% of pain is brought about by restoring neck and thoracic spine movements. Mobilizations – postero-anterior unilaterals at C3, 4, 5 levels may regain side flexion and transverse vertebral pressure to C7, T1 regains the last few degrees of neck rotation. Hold–relax technique and passive stretching are often necessary to lengthen the upper fibres of trapezius muscle.

Thereafter the possible cause should be identified – e.g. prolonged flexion, poor posture at work or leisure. The patient is usually very keen to follow advice on maintaining movement and ensuring good posture because the pain is so excruciating.

Disc lesions in the thoracic spine

This is a rare diagnosis. The difference is that the thoracic spine is much less mobile and the discs are designed to fit the natural kyphosis, being wedge-shaped – i.e. narrow anteriorly and deep posteriorly. Rarely, a cyst can form which causes the disc and spinal cord to become adherent. As this progresses, the patient has pins and needles in the one or both legs together with a feeling of weakness. Lying on one side, the patient is pain free but lying on the other side causes local pain in the thoracic spine. It is easy to label the patient as a hypochondriac. The only treatment is surgical excision of the cyst.

Entrapment neuropathies

It is important to remember during examination that pain may be perceived in a limb (or intercostal space) as a result of compression anywhere along the course of a nerve. Commonly, nerve roots are compressed in the intervertebral foramen (by disc material, thickening of an apophyseal joint capsule, osteophytes or thickening of the surrounding loose connective tissue/fascia).

Nerve trunks, however, may be compressed in bony canals by muscle spasm or thickening of fascial bands and ligaments.

Sites

Radial nerve

1. Radial nerve, under triceps in the radial groove.
2. Deep terminal branch of radial nerve (posterior interosseous) in supinator muscle.
3. Superficial terminal branch of radial nerve where it is attached to the deep surface of brachioradialis.

These lesions can give rise to pain on the lateral side of the elbow and forearm – mimicking C6 dermatome and tennis elbow.

Median nerve

Median nerve between the heads of pronator teres and in the carpal tunnel.

These lesions give rise to pain, pins and needles and some muscle weakness in the thumb, index and middle fingers (C6, C7 dermatome).

Carpal tunnel syndrome – see Chapter 6.

Ulnar nerve

In the groove behind the medial epicondyle of the humerus, between the two heads of flexor carpi ulnaris and on the lateral side of a stiff pisiform bone.

These lesions give rise to pins and needles in the ring and little fingers. Weakness of the intrinsic muscles of the hand makes fine finger movements awkward (C7, C8 dermatome).

Thoracic nerves

Thoracic nerves in the intercostal spaces may be compressed by thickenings in the intercostal muscles. This causes pain radiating round the chest wall, aggravated by coughing and deep breathing.

Femoral nerve

The femoral nerve in the psoas and iliacus (these muscles are shortened in early osteoarthritis of the hip) may be affected. This causes quadriceps weakness and pain radiating down the anterior aspect of the thigh and through the saphenous nerve to the medial aspect of the leg and foot (L3, L4 dermatome).

Cutaneous nerve

Entrapment of the lateral cutaneous nerve of the thigh between the sartorius muscle, the inguinal ligament and the anterior superior iliac spine causes pins and needles, sharp shooting pain and numbness over the lateral aspect of the thigh – known as meralgia paraesthetica (L2, L3 dermatome).

Sciatic nerve

Sciatic nerve entrapment in front of the sacroiliac joint, under the piriformis, over the quadratus femoris, under the gluteus maximus, or between the hamstring muscles causes pain in the leg (L4, L5, S1, S2 dermatome).

Peroneal nerve

Entrapment of the common peroneal nerve as it passes along the medial border of biceps femoris and round the neck of the fibula causes pain on the lateral side of the leg and dorsum of the foot (L5 dermatome) and weakness of the peronei and anterior tibial muscles.

Tibial nerve

The tibial nerve may be entrapped in the popliteal fossa – as in sitting awkwardly. This causes the leg and foot to 'go to sleep'.

Sural nerve

Entrapment of the sural nerve between the gastrocnemius and soleus and behind the lateral malleolus. This causes pain on the lateral side of the ankle and foot (S1 dermatome).

Plantar nerves

Medial and lateral plantar nerves may be entrapped under the flexor retinaculum between the medial malleolus and calcaneum. This is often associated with poor foot posture – flattening of the medial arch and pronation of the foot. Pain is on the plantar aspect of the foot and may be burning in nature and worse at night.

Physiotherapy

Once the lesion has been identified or a logical working hypothesis has been derived, there are various methods that may help.

Electrotherapy

Ultrasound can penetrate to loosen adhesions deeply set (e.g. sciatic nerve at the hip joint).

Laser treatment can increase the circulation locally to reduce muscle spasm.

Pulsed electromagnetic energy helps to relieve muscle spasm.

Manipulative therapy

Passive stretching of soft tissues (muscles and fibrous structures), e.g. piriformis stretch for the sciatic nerve, carpal flexor retinaculum stretch for the median nerve.

Mobilizations to move neighbouring stiff joints, e.g. pisiform-triquetral for the ulnar nerve, tarsal bones for the medial and lateral plantar nerves, radio-humeral joint for the radial nerve.

Connective tissue massage can release tight or thickened tissues along the course of a nerve.

Frictions, e.g. to supinator muscle for the deep terminal branch of the radial nerve, or intercostal muscles for the thoracic nerves.

Deep kneading for any of the muscles or fibrous structures, e.g. sartorius for lateral cutaneous nerve of the thigh.

Movement

Hold–relax technique to lengthen muscles, e.g. psoas major for the femoral nerve.

Free active exercises to stretch gastrocnemius for the tibial nerve, or biceps femoris for the common peroneal nerve.

The physiotherapist has to consider the anatomy of the nerve course and distribution to apply an effective treatment. The patient has also to work out if there is a habit in the lifestyle, e.g. prolonged sitting – tight iliopsoas, which must be counteracted to avoid nerve entrapment.

Thoracic outlet syndrome

This results from pressure on the lower trunk or medial cord of the brachial plexus (C8 and T1 roots) and/or the subclavian artery. These structures are closely related to the first rib and lie between the scalenus anterior and scalenus medius (Figure 11.11). Pressure may be due to the following:

1. A stiff, elevated first rib.
2. Spasm or contracture of the scaleni.
3. A cervical rib.
4. A fascial band between the scaleni.

Clinical features

Pressure on the lower trunk or medial cord – The features are:

1. Pain – toothache type or dull but intense ache in the C8 T1 distribution, ring plus little finger and medial side of the upper limb.
2. Paraesthesias in the same distribution.
3. Weakness of intrinsic muscles of the hand (perceived often as stiffness or clumsiness of the hand).

Pressure on the subclavian artery – The features are coldness and discoloration of the hand.

The pain and paraesthesias of both sources are often worse at night. They are not reproduced by neck movements. On examination, the patient often has:

1. A depressed shoulder girdle on the affected side.
2. Loss of neck side flexion to the pain-free side.
3. Loss of neck side flexion, and rotation to the pain-free side especially if combined with extension.
4. On palpation, the first rib can be felt to be in elevation and stiff.

Management

It is clearly essential to ascertain the cause. Physiotherapy can help as follows.

Stiff, elevated first rib

The treatment of choice for this is mobilization applied to the superior surface of the rib in a caudad direction. Restoration of movement can be ascertained by palpating both first ribs at the same time with the patient in prone and asking the patient to turn the head from side to side. The ribs should rise (elevate) as the head turns away.

Loss of neck movements

Rhythmical passive side flexion of the neck away from the affected side with the shoulder girdle on the affected side fixed to stretch the scaleni.

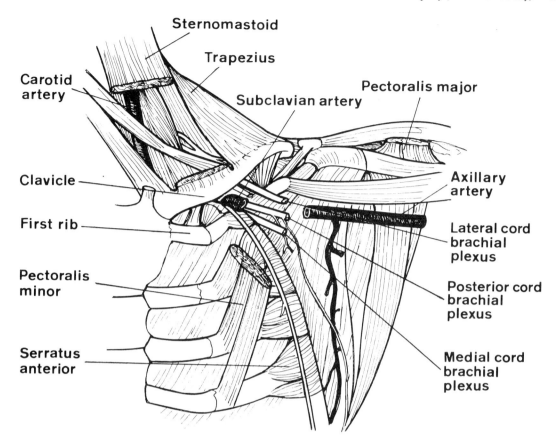

Figure 11.11 The structures around the brachial plexus

Hold–relax and repeated contraction techniques to lengthen the scaleni.

Posture training to keep shoulder girdles level and in correct retraction. Stretching of the pectoralis minor may be necessary to enable the posture to be corrected. The patient should be encouraged to turn the arms out (gleno-humeral lateral rotation) and pull the shoulders back (scapular retraction) 2–3 times every hour and 4–5 times after prolonged writing or reading.

It is important to avoid treating such a patient with cervical traction on the basis of the clinical features being of nerve root origin. Neck side-flexion with rotation to the affected side plus extension – even with compression – does not reproduce the pain or paraesthesia of thoracic outlet syndrome. If these symptoms are from root compression then this test would reproduce them, and traction is a treatment worth trying.

Bell's palsy (Facial Nerve Palsy)

This is a condition in which there is a lesion of the facial nerve and resultant paralysis in the muscles that it supplies. The main muscles affected are:

1. *Occipitofrontalis* – Raises eyebrow.
2. *Orbicularis oculi* – Closes eye.
3. *Corrugator and procerus* – Wrinkle skin between eyebrows and frowns.
4. *Zygomaticus major and minor, levator anguli oris, levator labii superioris* – Raise the corner of the mouth and upper lip.
5. *Buccinator* – Keeps the cheek against the teeth during mastication or sucking. Without it, food is trapped between the cheek and teeth which is functionally highly restricting.
6. *Orbicularis oris* – Closes the mouth.
7. *Risorius* – Pulls the angle of the mouth back, as in grinning.

8. *Depressor anguli oris and depressor labii in-ferioris* – Pull down the angle of the mouth and the lower lip.
9. *Mentalis* – Wrinkles the chin and is very important in drinking because it holds the lower lip on the cup and prevents dribbling.

The nerve also supplies taste sensation to the palate and anterior two-thirds of the tongue and the parasympathetic supply to the secretomotor salivary glands.

Aetiology

The cause is unknown. It can occur at any age and is not gender specific.

Onset

This is often sudden. The patient may have a history of earache or of having been in a draught. Often the patient wakes up with the paralysis, having been perfectly normal the night before.

Pathology

The facial nerve becomes swollen and hyperaemic within the facial canal, in which there is limited space. The nerve rapidly becomes compressed and conductivity is lost.

Prognosis

Fifty per cent recover within 3 months.

Clinical features – on the side of the lesion

1. Loss of facial expression.
2. Drooping of the face – lower eyelid, eyebrow and corner of the mouth sag.
3. Closing the eye is difficult.
4. Eating is difficult because food collects in the side of the cheek and fluids seep out of the corner of the mouth.
5. Speaking, whistling and drinking are impaired.
6. Non-verbal communication is lost as the patient cannot register pleasure, laughter, surprise, interest or worry.
7. The patient tends to sit with the hand over the side of the face.

Treatment

Oral steroids may be given to reduce inflammation. Surgery may be used in longstanding cases to improve appearance. The eyelids may be stitched together to protect the eye.

Physiotherapy

During paralysis

1. Ultrasound given over the nerve trunk just in front of the tragus of the ear may reduce the inflammation.
2. Massage may be taught to the patient:
   (a) Stroking in an upward, outward direction.
   (b) Slow finger kneading applied over the paralysed muscles maintains skin suppleness and muscle elasticity.
   (c) These techniques applied for 5 min or so daily help to maintain lymphatic and blood flow and prevent contractures.
3. Advice:
   (a) The patient should lie down at intervals throughout the day to reduce the effects of gravity on the paralysed muscles.
   (b) The eye should be bathed regularly because the normal blinking reflex is lost and dust particles collect, producing conjunctivitis.

Recovery stage

Mild infra-red treatment may be applied to warm the muscles and improve function – the eye must be protected with wet cotton wool.

PNF techniques are used for re-education:

1. Quick stretch technique can be applied to regain raising of the eyebrow and the movements of the corner of the mouth.
2. The physiotherapist can produce the movement passively then ask the patient to hold, then try to produce the movement.
3. Icing, brushing, tapping or brisk stroking may be applied along the length of the muscles, e.g. the zygomatics.

Exercises

1. Look surprised then frown.
2. Squeeze eyes closed then open wide.
3. Smile, grin, say 'o'.
4. Say 'a, e, i, o, u'.
5. Hold straw in mouth – suck and blow.
6. Whistle.

These exercises are performed in lying at first, then sitting up. The patient may assist at first then progress to resisting. A mirror is useful to enable the patient to observe the muscle activity. Generally, patients should practise these exercises twice a day with about five repetitions at a time so as not to fatigue the muscles. It is not necessary for the patient to be seen by the physiotherapist very often, but monitoring visits should be arranged.

Failure to recover

There is a tendency amongst the medical professions to 'let nature take its course' because so many make a complete recovery. This attitude, however, does not help those whose paralysis persists beyond 3 months. It is a serious handicap within society, and some people become withdrawn and depressed. It is very difficult with facial paralysis to run a business or perform work that demands inter-personal communication, and it is devastating for people such as television presenters or stage and film actors. Some people have the great misfortune to have bilateral paralysis.

Trophic electrical stimulation is therefore of enormous value to these people. This is an electrical current of: pulse width 80 s; frequency 5–8 Hz; voltage 0–18 V. Programme: 2 s on/2 s off for 3–5 h daily in two sessions. This modality, together with active re-education techniques, has been shown to improve muscle function and facial symmetry in longstanding cases of facial paralysis or palsy (Farragher, 1987; Farragher, Kidd and Tallis, 1987).

References

Farragher, D. J. (1987) Trophic stimulation for human muscle in chronic traumatic facial paralysis. In *Proceedings of the Tenth International Congress of WCPT,* Vol. 1, pp. 361–370

Farragher, D. J., Kidd, G. and Tallis, R. (1987) Eutrophic electrical stimulation for Bell's palsy. *Clinical Rehabilitation,* **1**, 265–271

Chapter 12

Introduction to diseases of the respiratory system

Anatomy and physiology
Effects of disease
General clinical features of diseases and
*   disorders of the respiratory system*
Investigations of the respiratory system

Drugs used in respiratory disease
Outline of physiotherpay examination
Medical conditions: principles of
*   physiotherapy treatment*

Anatomy and physiology

Before considering the pathology and treatment of these diseases a brief resumé of the anatomy and physiology of the normal respiratory tract will be given.

Anatomy

The respiratory system consists of air passages and lung tissue and may be divided into an upper and a lower tract.

The upper respiratory tract comprises nasal passages, the pharynx, larynx and upper part of the trachea. The lower respiratory tract comprises the lower part of the trachea, the bronchial tree and alveoli (Figure 12.1).

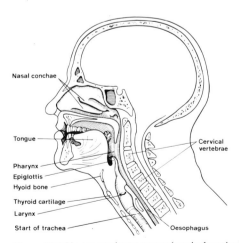

Figure 12.1 Upper respiratory tract (vertical section)

Nasal conchae

Tongue

Pharynx
Epiglottis
Hyoid bone
Thyroid cartilage
Larynx
Start of trachea

Cervical
vertebrae

Oesophagus

The nasal passages lie between the cribriform plate of the ethmoid bone above and the hard palate of the palatine bone below. The air sinuses in the maxillary, frontal, ethmoidal and sphenoid bones open into the nasal passages.

The pharynx extends from the nasal passages to the larynx and is a common pathway for air from the nose and food from the mouth.

The larynx is between the pharynx and trachea. It extends from the level of the 3rd cervical vertebra to the lower border of the 6th vertebra and is protected by the epiglottis which prevents food and liquid from entering the respiratory passages. The vocal cords lie below the epiglottis.

The trachea is between the larynx and the bifurcation of the two main bronchi (the carina). It extends from the level of the 6th cervical vertebra to the 5th thoracic vertebra. The upper end lies just below the skin and is the site of entry used for a tracheostomy. The tracheal walls are made up of C-shaped cartilages and smooth muscle. The cartilage keeps the airway open whilst the posterior muscular wall can allow for expansion of the oesophagus when the bolus of food is being transmitted.

The oesophagus lies behind the trachea (Figure 12.2).

The bronchial tree (Figure 12.3) starts at the bifurcation of the trachea. The right bronchus is more vertical, wider and shorter than the left. Each main bronchus divides into lobar bronchi which divide into segmental bronchi. A segmental bronchus together with the lung tissue it supplies is termed a bronchopulmonary segment (Figure 12.4).

Each bronchus continues to subdivide into branches of ever-decreasing lumen until terminal bronchioles are formed which do not have cartilage in the walls. Terminal bronchioles are followed by respira-

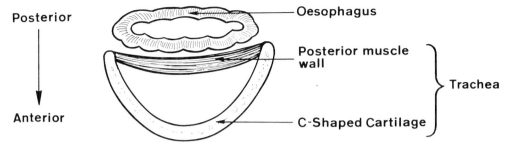

Figure 12.2 Horizontal section, trachea and oesophagus

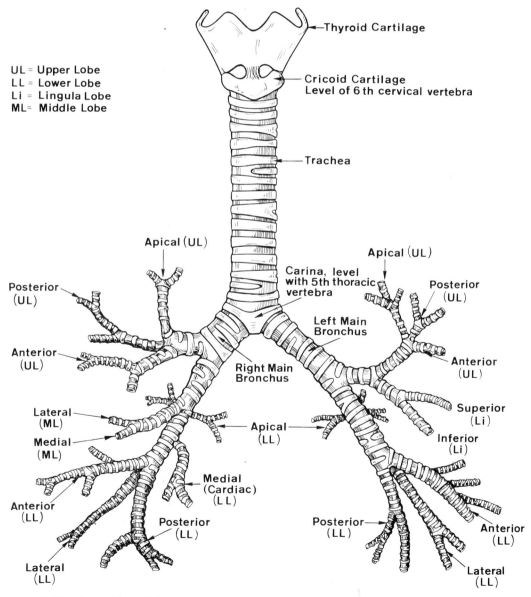

Figure 12.3 Trachea and bronchial tree

166

COSTAL ASPECT   RIGHT LUNG   MEDIAL ASPECT

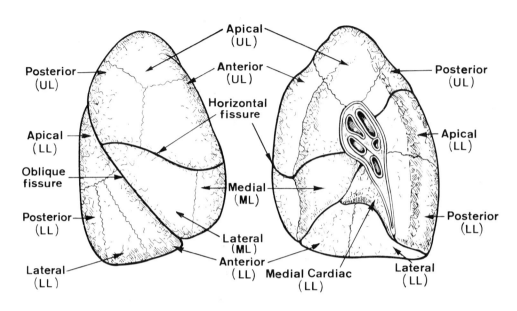

COSTAL ASPECT   LEFT LUNG   MEDIAL ASPECT

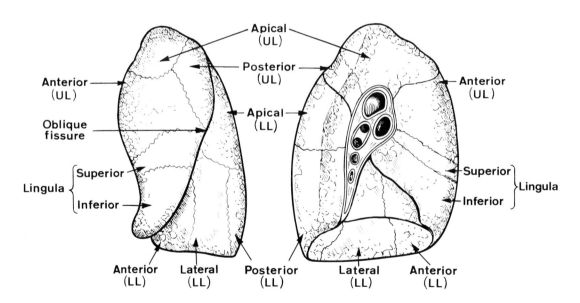

UL = Upper Lobe
L L = Lower Lobe
ML = Middle Lobe

Figure 12.4 Bronchopulmonary segments

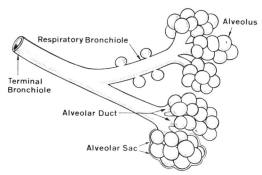

Figure 12.5 An acinus: bronchioles and alveoli

tory bronchioles which lead into the alveoli. An acinus is the respiratory bronchioles, alveolar ducts and alveoli from one terminal bronchiole (Figure 12.5).

Gaseous interchange takes place across the thin alveolar membrane immediately adjacent to which is a capillary network.

Alveolar membrane

The alveolar membrane consists of an epithelial lining, elastic and collagen fibres and blood capillaries. The epithelial lining is composed of a basement membrane together with pneumocytes (lung cells). The commonest cells are type I pneumocytes across which gas diffusion takes place. Type II pneumocytes produce pulmonary surfactant, which is a fluid (phospholipid) that reduces surface tension of the alveolar walls lowering the pressure (i.e. making it less negative) within deflated alveoli and therefore reducing the tendency of the alveoli to collapse. This reduced pressure also makes the work of expanding the lungs easier.

Compliance

This is a measure of the elasticity of the alveolar walls and is recorded as the change in volume produced by change in unit pressure, i.e. (volume change)/(pressure change).

Alveoli with high compliance expand more (i.e. volume change is greater) than those with low compliance for a given pressure. Lung tissue which is stiffened by disease has a low compliance and it is hard work for the patient to generate the force to expand the lungs therefore there is reduced ventilation.

Pores of Kohn

In the alveolar walls are openings known as pores of Kohn which allow collateral ventilation between neighbouring alveoli or segments. These help to prevent segmental collapse and allow air to pass into alveoli so that on forced expiration force from this air can be generated to dislodge secretions in bronchioles.

The surface marking of the lungs (Figure 12.6)

It is important for a physiotherapist to understand how the lungs and lobes relate to the surface of the thorax. The lung borders may be traced as follows.

Right lung

Anterior border – Start at the level of the apex 2–3 cm above the medial third of the clavicle, trace a line behind the right sternoclavicular joint vertically down behind the right side of the sternum to the 6th chondrosternal junction.

Inferior border – Trace from the 6th chondrosternal junction laterally on a line which crosses the 6th costal cartilage in midclavicular line and the 8th rib in mid-axillary line, then medially to the 10th rib in line with the inferior angle of the scapula to the 10th thoracic spine.

Posterior border – Trace from a point 2 cm right of 10th thoracic spine, vertically up the back to the level of the neck of the first rib, and thence to the apex.

Left lung

Anterior border – Same as right lung on the left side down to the 4th chondrosternal junction, then trace laterally along the lower border of the 4th costal cartilage for 3.5 cm turn down and curve slightly medially to the 6th costal cartilage 4 cm from midline of sternum (this curve is the cardiac notch).

Inferior and posterior borders are like those of the right lung.

Fissures

Oblique – This is traced from the posterior border of the right lung level with the spine of the 3rd thoracic vertebra to the 5th interspace in mid-axillary line and ends anteriorly near the 6th costochondral junction at the inferior border, 7.5 cm from the mid-line of the sternum. The oblique fissure of the left lung is equivalent on the left side.

Horizontal – This is traced from the oblique fissure of the right lung in mid-axillary line horizontally forwards and medially to the sternal end of the 4th costal cartilage. There is no horizontal fissure in the left lung.

Pleura

The right pleura starts 3 cm above the medial third of the clavicle, passes down behind the sternoclavicular joint and meets the left pleura at the sternal angle just left of mid-line. It passes vertically down

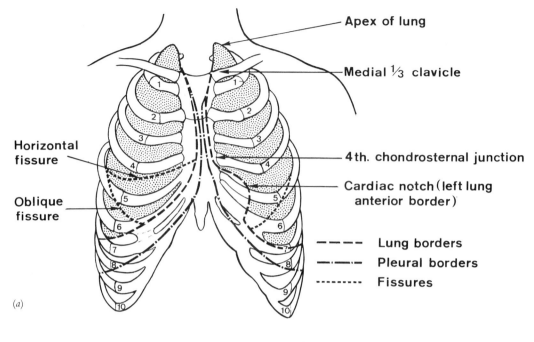

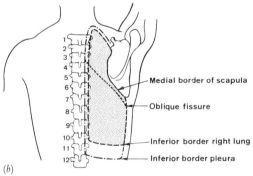

Figure 12.6 (*a*) Anterior aspect of thorax to show surface projection of lung. (*b*) Posterior aspect of thorax to show surface projection of right lung

to the level of the 4th chondrosternal junction and then obliquely to the 6th chondrosternal junction. It may then be traced laterally to the 8th costal cartilage in mid-clavicular line, the 10th rib in mid-axillary line, and the 11th rib in line with the inferior angle of the scapula to the level of the 12th thoracic spine, just lateral to midline.

The left pleura is traced in the same way as the right except that from the 4th chondrosternal junction it is traced obliquely laterally to the 8th costal cartilage in mid-clavicular line. Thereafter it is traced like the right pleura.

Mechanics of respiration

The principal effect of movements of the thorax is to alter the capacity of the thoracic cavity to enable air to be drawn in (inspiration) or expelled (expiration) and thus produce ventilation of the lungs. This capacity may be increased in three dimensions antero-posteriorly, laterally and vertically by the muscles of respiration which are the diaphragm and the intercostals. The amount of movement depends on the depth of respiration (ventilation).

Inspiration

The muscular fibres of the diaphragm contract and pull down the central tendon thus increasing the vertical dimension. The excursion of the tendon is limited by the abdominal organs and as the muscle fibres continue to contract the tendon becomes the fixed point and the lower ribs are pulled upwards and outwards. As inspiration continues the intercostal muscles also contract to produce these lower rib movements and in addition the upper ribs move forwards and upwards and then outwards. Thus the capacity of the thoracic cavity is increased in all three dimensions. Since the parietal pleura is attached to the upper surface of the diaphragm and inner surface of the thorax the negative intrapleural pressure is made more negative, thus stretching the elastic tissue of the lungs and increasing the volume of the air spaces. Air rushes in because the pressure inside the lungs is subatmospheric. The deeper the

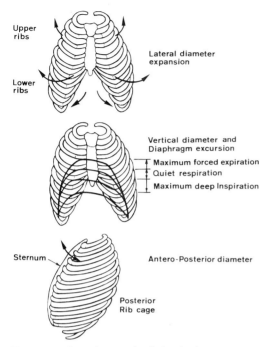

Figure 12.7 Thoracic excursion in inspiration

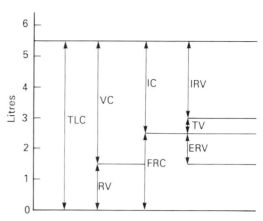

Figure 12.8 Lung volumes and capacities

inspiration the greater is the pressure difference and therefore the greater is the volume of air entering the lungs (Figure 12.7).

Expiration

This is a passive movement produced by the elastic recoil of the chest wall and the lung tissue which forces air out of the lungs. Momentarily, the pressure inside the lungs (alveolar pressure) is greater than atmospheric pressure, then when the two pressures are equal expiration stops. In forced expiration the abdominal muscles contract to aid expulsion of air by increasing intra-abdominal pressure.

Lung volumes and capacities (Figure 12.8)

The volume of air that passes in and out of the lungs and the total lung capacity varies according to age, sex and height. Deviations from the normal predicted values indicate a functional disorder.

Lung volumes

The total lung capacity can be divided into various volumes:

1. Tidal volume (TV) is the volume of air moved into or out of the lungs during quiet breathing at rest.

2. Inspiratory reserve volume (IRV) is the volume of air additional to TV that can be inspired during a maximum inspiration.
3. Expiratory reserve volume (ERV) is the volume of air additional to TV that can be expired during a maximum expiration.
4. Residual volume (RV) is the volume of air remaining in the lungs after a maximum expiration.

Lung capacities

1. Total lung capacity (TLC) is the total volume of air in the lungs after a maximum inspiration.
2. Vital capacity (VC) is the maximum volume of air that can be expired after a maximum inspiration.
3. Inspiratory capacity (IC) is the maximum volume of air that can be inspired from the end-point of quiet expiration at rest.
4. Functional residual capacity (FRC) is the volume of air remaining in the lungs at the end of quiet expiration at rest.

Tidal volume, inspiratory reserve volume, expiratory reserve volume, vital capacity and inspiratory capacity can be measured with a spirometer. Functional residual capacity can be measured indirectly using helium or nitrogen in a closed-circuit spirometer, a whole-body plethysmograph or radiographs. Residual volume and total lung capacity are calculated arithmetically from the measurements mentioned above.

Values for the average male adult:

TLC	5500 ml	RV	1500 ml
VC	4000 ml	IRV	2500 ml
IC	3000 ml	TV	500 ml
FRC	2500 ml	ERV	1000 ml

The values for the average female adult are 25% less.

In exercise the tidal volume gradually increases while both the inspiratory and expiratory reserve volumes decrease.

Respiratory rate – At rest a normal adult breathes in and out between 12 and 16 times per minute. During exercise this may increase to over 30 times per minute.

Respiratory minute volume = Tidal volume × respiratory rate, i.e. 500 ml × 14 = 7000 ml.

Anatomical dead space is the volume of air in the conducting airways from the nose and mouth to the alveoli and is 150 ml.

Forced vital capacity (FVC) is the maximum volume of air forcibly expired after a maximum inspiration.

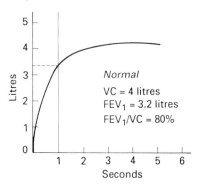

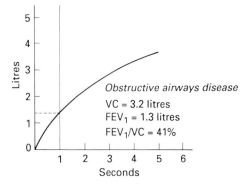

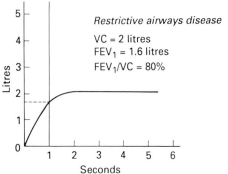

Figure 12.9 Graphs of lung measurements obtained with a vitalograph spirometer

Forced expiratory volume in one second (FEV$_1$) is the volume of air forcibly expired after a maximum inspiration in one second and this is usually 80% FVC.

Thus the ratio FEV$_1$/FVC in healthy people is 80%. Both FVC and FEV1 can be measured on a vitalograph as well as a spirometer.

Peak expiratory flow rate (PEFR) is the maximum flow rate of air from full inspiration during a forced expiration and is measured with a Wright peak flow meter. In the normal adult PEFR is over 400 litres min^{-1}.

These lung measurements are altered in respiratory diseases which have characteristic patterns (Figure 12.9).

In obstructive airways disease such as asthma, emphysema and chronic bronchitis there is a greater reduction in FEV$_1$ than FVC so that the ratio FEV$_1$/FVC may be as low as 30%. These diseases result in hyperinflation of the lungs and the TLC, FRC and RV are increased. PEFR can be reduced to less than 100 litres min^{-1}. In reversible airways obstruction the FEV$_1$/FVC and PEFR are improved after the administration of bronchodilators or corticosteroids and other measurements are nearer normal values.

In restrictive airways disease such as fibrosing alveolitis pneumonia, pleural and neuromuscular diseases and pulmonary collapse the FEV$_1$ and FVC are both reduced in the same proportion resulting in the FEV$_1$/FVC ratio remaining about 80%. The TLC, VC and RV are all decreased but PEFR is normal. Ankylosing spondylitis can produce results similar to restrictive airways disease.

Composition of air (Table 12.1)

Table 12.1 Composition of air (%)

	Inspired air	*Expired air*	*Alveolar air*
Oxygen	20.95	16.40	13.80
Carbon dioxide	0.04	4.00	5.50
Nitrogen	79.01	79.60	80.70

Alveolar air has the least amount of O_2 because it is from the alveoli that O_2 diffuses out into the blood. Similarly alveolar air has most CO_2 because CO_2 diffuses from the blood into the alveoli.

Expired air is a mixture of alveolar air and dead space air which has the composition of inspired air.

Blood gases

Oxygen:

Po_2 denotes the partial pressure of oxygen.

Pao_2 denotes partial pressure of oxygen in arterial blood.

Blood leaving the lungs, i.e. arterial blood, has a Po_2 of 13 kPa (97 mm Hg). Blood leaving the tissues has a Po_2 of 5.3 kPa (40 mm Hg).

Carbon dioxide:

Pco_2 denotes partial pressure of carbon dioxide. $Paco_2$ denotes partial pressure of CO_2 in arterial blood.

Blood leaving the tissues has a Pco_2 of 6.1 kPa (46 mm Hg).

Blood leaving the lungs has a Pco_2 of 5.3 kPa (40 mm Hg).

These values are affected by:

1. The efficiency of ventilation.
2. Ventilation – perfusion ratio (V/Q).
3. The oxygen carrying capacity of the blood.
4. The efficiency of the circulation.
5. The metabolic rate.
6. Acidity or alkalinity of the blood.

Efficiency of ventilation is dependent on normal inspiration and expiration. Inspiration is reduced by poor function of the respiratory muscles or lack of thoracic mobility. Expiration is impaired by loss of elastic recoil in the lungs or blockage or narrowing of the airways.

Ventilation–perfusion quotient (V/Q)
(Figure 12.10)

Ventilation is the movement of air into and out of the alveoli. Perfusion relates to the flow of blood through the pulmonary capillary network. Diffusion relates in respiratory terms to the transfer of O_2 and CO_2 between the alveoli and the blood in the capillary network. Ventilation (V) is normally 4.5 litres min^{-1} at rest. Perfusion (Q) is normally 5 litres min^{-1} at rest (i.e. cardiac output). The average V/Q is 0.9. Individual alveolar V/Q varies. Well-ventilated alveoli may have a poor blood supply so the V/Q rises. Po_2 of the blood is high, and Pco_2 could be low but may be high. This may occur with pulmonary embolism. Poorly ventilated alveoli may be well perfused and V/Q drops. Po_2 is low and Pco_2 is high. This may occur in pneumonia, asthma, chronic bronchitis, emphysema or pulmonary oedema.

Administration of oxygen can be helpful. The efficiency of the circulation, metabolic rate, acidity or alkalinity of the blood affect the level of blood gases which in turn affects the respiratory system. Generally low Po_2 and high Pco_2 increase the respiratory rate. Conditions causing abnormality of these factors may be blood, heart, blood vessel, metabolic or kidney disorders. Thus it is essential to ascertain the underlying cause of blood gas abnormality and not to assume that breathlessness, high Pco_2 or low Po_2 is due primarily to respiratory disease.

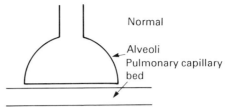

Normal ventilation of alveoli
Normal perfusion of capillaries
V/Q = 0.9

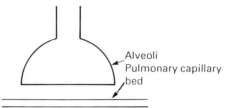

Normal ventilation of alveoli   V/Q higher than 0.9
Minimal perfusion of capillaries
Poor gaseous interchange but blood is oxygenated.
If many alveoli are involved CO_2 can accumulate in the blood

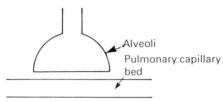

Very poor ventilation   V/Q may be 0
Adequate perfusion
Poor gaseous interchange, blood is not oxygenated therefore a venous type of blood returns to the heart

Figure 12.10 Ventilation perfusion quotient

Significance of ventilation perfusion quotient in different positions

When a person is lying on one side gravity tends to pull the pulmonary capillary blood to the underneath side. Ventilation is more efficient in the uppermost lung. There is therefore a mismatch of ventilation/perfusion. Normally there is some degree of compensation with capillaries opening on the upper side to shunt blood to the area of greater ventilation. In patients with respiratory disease, however, this compensation may not occur and it is undesirable for them to remain in side lying for any length of time. In the upright position there is greater perfusion in the lower lung areas whilst ventilation tends to be greater in the upper lung areas. There is much more efficient V/Q, therefore, if the basal areas of the lungs are used in respiration.

Oxygen therapy in relation to blood gases

Oxygen is indicated when the oxygen tension is low (P_{AO_2} below 6.6 kPa (50 mm Hg)) and the patient is hypoxic. These hypoxic patients often have CO_2 retention (hypercapnia) and a high P_{ACO_2} (above 9 kPa (70 mm Hg)). If there is a high P_{ACO_2} level patients lose their normal responsiveness to CO_2 and depend on O_2 to maintain the drive to breathe. Treatment with high concentrations of O_2 relieves the hypoxaemia but removes the O_2 drive depressing the ventilation and increasing the CO_2 retention. Oxygen therapy should be controlled by giving continuous O_2 at 24% concentration.

Effects of disease

Any part of the respiratory tract may become infected or diseased and the consequences may have far-reaching results. As in any other part of the body, the response to infection is an inflammatory reaction. The immediate result is hyperaemia and swelling of the mucous lining which gives rise to difficulty in respiration and a degree of hypoventilation. If the condition becomes chronic, fibrosis occurs. In the respiratory tract, particularly in the lung tissue itself, this means a loss of elasticity, with possible permanent decrease in ventilation. The oxygen uptake is impaired and carbon dioxide accumulates. The tissues become devitalized and the general health is impaired. The patient is easily fatigued, posture is poor and ultimately the heart begins to fail.

In addition to normal inflammatory reaction, there is increased mucus secretion, and the result is blocking of the airways with collapse of the lung tissue distal to the block. It is essential to regain expansion of the area as soon as possible because the collapsed tissue becomes fibrosed and necrotic with permanent reduction of the ventilation capacity of the lungs. If suppuration occurs large areas of lung tissue can be destroyed as a consequence.

General clinical features of diseases and disorders of the respiratory system

Dyspnoea

This is a state of disordered breathing, in which the patient has an unpleasant awareness of difficulty in breathing. The degree of distress varies considerably according to the stage of disease.

Orthopnoea is the name given to breathlessness that is aggravated when the patient lies flat and is relieved when the patient sits up.

Cough

Coughing is a protective reflex and is the commonest feature of all respiratory disorders. There is a brief inspiration, closure of the glottis, contraction of the expiratory muscles (principally the abdominals) resulting in a rise in intra-abdominal and intrathoracic pressures. This forces the epiglottis open and a rapid flow of expired air is produced, often carrying with it sputum and foreign particles. Cough may be dry or productive and the character varies according to the disorder or disease.

Sputum

Production of amounts of sputum in excess of 100 ml per 24 hours is abnormal (Flenley, 1981). Colour, nature and quantity of sputum varies according to the condition and stage of condition. Commonest variations are mucoid (clear or grey), purulent (yellow or green – infected) frothy (white and bubbly), red or black (due to blood or to atmospheric dust).

Haemoptysis

This is coughing up of blood. Differentiation must be made between this and haematemesis which is vomiting of blood.

Wheeze

This is a whistling sound normally heard on expiration caused by air flowing through airways, with a narrowed lumen, which may be due to mucosal oedema, tumour, bronchial muscle spasm or excessive mucous secretions. In severe asthma it is also heard on inspiration.

Stridor

This is a harsh vibrating sound heard on inspiration caused by obstruction of the larynx, trachea or main bronchi.

Cyanosis

This is the name given to the blue colour of the skin and mucous membranes. There are two types, peripheral and central. Peripheral cyanosis is due to reduced blood flow through the peripheries and is associated with cold extremities.

Central cyanosis is due to reduced oxygen saturation of arterial blood. It is noticed in the tongue, lips and ear lobes and is associated with warm extremities.

Chest pain

The parietal and diaphragmatic layers of the pleura are pain sensitive whilst the lung tissue and visceral layer of pleura have no pain nerve endings. Irritation of the pleura, therefore, causes a sharp stabbing pain especially during coughing and deep breathing. This pain may be referred to the posterior or lateral aspects of the chest wall, the abdomen or tip of the shoulder.

Retrosternal pain (felt behind the sternum) is a feature of tracheitis, but may be a symptom of heart disease (see Chapter 15). Deep aching chest pain may be caused by a tumour (carcinoma). Chest wall pain may also be due to rib fractures, strain of the intercostal muscles or tumours of the ribs.

Cor pulmonale

This is hypertrophy of the right ventricle resulting from disease affecting the function and/or structure of the lungs except when these pulmonary alterations are the result of diseases that primarily affect the left side of the heart or of congenital heart disease (World Health Organization, 1961). It is particularly associated with chronic lung diseases such as chronic bronchitis and bronchiectasis. This may lead to heart failure, and treatment must be directed to relief of the lung disease.

Reduced thoracic mobility

Loss of elasticity in the lung tissue results in the thorax being hyperinflated and in reduced thoracic movements.

Consolidation, collapse or fibrosis of one or more lobes is associated with localized or unilateral diminished movement.

Loss of elasticity of the costal cartilages as in old age and fixation of the costovertebral joints as in ankylosing spondylitis cause a general reduction of respiratory excursion.

Shape of the chest

There are several deformities of the chest that may arise:

Barrel chest – The thorax is held in inspiration with widened intercostal spaces which leads to widening of the antero-posterior and lateral dimensions.

Pigeon chest – This is raising of the sternum and is associated with childhood asthma.

Harrison's sulcus – A concave deformity of the lower ribs which is usually a result of chronic childhood asthma.

Kyphoscoliosis – A thoracic spinal deformity which is often associated with reduced vital capacity and breathlessness.

Postural changes

During respiratory distress the patient tends to hold the shoulder girdles elevated and protracted, and the chin is thrust forwards. In the long term this may become a permanent state.

Investigations of the respiratory system

Lung function tests (LFTs)

The following tests are associated with the examination of patients with respiratory disorders:

1. Ventilatory capacity tests.
2. Blood gas analysis.
3. Blood acid/alkaline reaction.
4. Exercises tolerance tests.

Ventilatory capacity tests

Vital capacity (VC), forced vital capacity (FVC) and forced expiratory volume in one second (FEV_1) are measured with a spirometer. Peak expiratory flow rate (PEFR) is measured with a peak flow meter. VC and FVC give an indication of the ventilatory capacity of the lungs. FEV_1 is useful in ascertaining the degree of reversibility in obstructive airways disease. These tests are used to assess the type of functional impairment (obstructive or restrictive), the effects of treatment and the severity or course of the disease.

Blood gas analysis

This is the measurement of the partial pressure of oxygen and carbon dioxide in arterial blood (P_{AO_2} and P_{ACO_2}). These tests provide an indication of the efficiency of the lungs in transferring oxygen and carbon dioxide between alveolar air and pulmonary capillary blood.

Blood acid/alkaline reaction

The normal pH of the blood is 7.4. A fall in blood pH is termed acidosis. Respiratory acidosis is caused by increased P_{ACO_2} which occurs in hypoventilation and chronic bronchitis. A rise in blood pH is termed alkalosis. Respiratory alkalosis is caused by decreased $P_{A}CO_2$ which occurs in hyperventilation, acute asthma and pneumonia.

Exercise tolerance tests

Exercise tests are of value in determining cardiorespiratory function using a step, treadmill or cycle ergometer. During these tests minute ventilation and oxygen consumption are measured. A useful test to assess pulmonary function involves the patient walking on a level surface at his/her own pace within a timed period of 12 minutes. Modifications of this test may utilize shorter periods of time, e.g. 6 minutes and 2 minutes (Butland *et al.*, 1981).

Bronchoscopy

A bronchoscope is a rigid metal or flexible fibreoptic tube which can be passed into the respiratory passages as far as the segmental bronchi. It enables direct inspection of the walls of the respiratory passages, a biopsy to be taken, or collection of bronchial secretions for testing.

Chest radiographs

Radiograph films are generally posteroanterior or lateral views taken at total lung capacity (i.e. at maximum inspiration).

Prior to reading a radiograph it is important to check the patient's name, whether it is postero-anterior or antero-posterior and to identify left from right.

The main features to identify on a postero-anterior film (Figure 12.11) are:

1. Clavicles – check level and position.
2. Scapulae – identify medial border which is well round the chest wall due to the protracted position of the shoulder girdles.
3. Trachea central and vertical.
4. Upper border of right hemi diaphragm is level with 10th rib at the back and 6th rib at the front. The left side is 1–3 cm lower.
5. The heart shadow – The width at its broadest part should not exceed 50% of the total width of the chest.
6. The right border of the heart shadow represents the border of the right atrium.
7. The left border of the heart shadow comprises from above down, the aorta, pulmonary artery and left ventricle.
8. Lung markings – Identify level of vascularity. This should decrease towards the periphery.

NB. Air shows as a dark area while bone and soft tissues which absorb X-rays appear light. Abnormal lesions that absorb X-rays show as grey/white areas and may be referred to as shadows or opacities.

Common abnormalities that may be detected on chest radiographs

Lobar collapse – Identify shift of trachea, raised hemi-diaphragm and fissures which may be obvious-

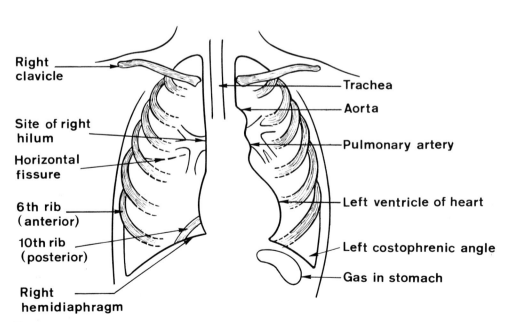

Figure 12.11 Main features on an antero-posterior chest radiograph

ly displaced. (A collapsed area looks like a homogenous opacity.)

Consolidation – Characterized by patchy opacity usually localized to a lobe or segment.

Pleural effusion – Always associated with loss of the costophrenic angles, and is seen as a dense opacity.

Coin lesion – Round dense areas anywhere in the lung fields may indicate carcinoma, tuberculosis or rheumatoid nodule.

Pneumothorax – No lung markings are seen, and the edge of the collapsed lung may be identified.

Lung abscess – Appears as a rounded opacity with concave meniscus at edges showing fluid level.

Other radiographic tests

Bronchograms – Radiographs are taken after a radio-opaque fluid has been introduced to the lung fields.

Tomography – Radiographs are taken with a specific area of the lung in focus and surrounding structures are blurred.

CAT scans – Computerized axial tomography provides views of horizontal 'slices' through the chest wall.

Auscultation

A stethoscope is used to determine the quality, character and intensity of breath sounds, vocal resonance and adventitious sounds.

Breath sounds

Normal breath sounds are of two types: (1) over the trachea, and (2) over lung tissue. Two tracheal sounds are heard: (1) on inspiration of low pitch, and (2) on expiration – at a higher pitch and for longer.

The two are separated by a pause, and are blowing in quality. The stethoscope diaphragm is placed near the root of the neck. Two lung tissue sounds are heard:

1. *On inspiration* – A 'wind through trees' sound heard throughout inspiration.
2. *On expiration* – A very short low pitched sound or no sound at all. There is no pause between the two and they are rustling in quality. They are often referred to as vesicular breath sounds. The stethoscope diaphragm is placed on various parts of the chest wall, covering each side equally (Figure 12.12).

Abnormal breath sounds

1. Tracheal breath sounds heard over lung tissue areas (often referred to as bronchial breathing).

This is due to transmission of these sounds by fluid or consolidation (e.g. in pneumonia). The sound is muffled by pleural effusion.

2. Absence of lung tissue sounds, occurs when transmission of sound is impeded (e.g. in pneumothorax, lung tissue collapse or pleural effusion). In severe asthma airflow obstruction may be so extensive as to prevent transmission of breath sounds and this is known as 'silent chest'.

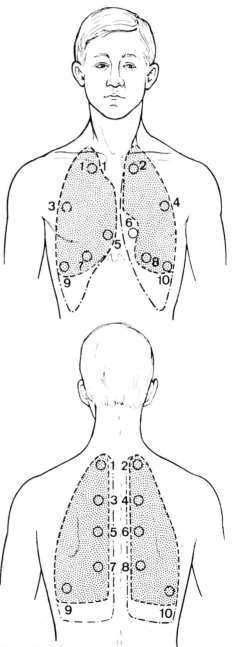

Figure 12.12 Stethoscope positions

Vocal resonance

These are the sounds heard through the stethoscope when the patient is asked to say 'Aaa' or '99'.

Normal

The sounds can be heard clearly over the trachea and are muffled and softer over lung tissue.

If the patient is asked to whisper, the sound can be heard over the trachea but not at all over lung tissue.

Abnormal

Increased sounds

Broncophony – The number '99' can be clearly heard over lung tissue.
Whispering pectoriloquy – The whispered '99' can be heard over lung tissue.

Both of these are due to consolidation.

Adventitious sounds

These are always a sign of abnormality. There are three types:

1. Rhonchi or wheezes.
2. Crepitations or crackles.
3. Pleural rub.

Rhonchi or wheezes indicate obstruction or narrowing of airways. They may be low pitched and sonorous or high pitched and whistling. The greater the narrowing, the higher the pitch of the sound.

Crepitations or crackles. These are short, interrupted sounds possibly due to the opening of previously closed airways. They are heard on inspiration and can help determine the site of abnormality as follows:

1. Start of inspiration – large airways.
2. Mid-inspiration – medium-smaller airways.
3. End of inspiration – small airways and lung tissue.

They may be coarse as in bronchiectasis or fine as in pulmonary oedema.

Pleural rub. This is a squeaky sound present on both inspiration and expiration. It is due to roughening of the pleural surfaces as in pleurisy.

Percussion

This is performed by placing one hand flat on the patient's chest and the middle phalanx of that hand is then tapped with the middle finger of the other hand. The resonance of the percussion note and resistance to percussion are identified. The note is affected by the nature of the underlying tissues being duller over the heart and liver and more resonant over air-filled lung tissue. Abnormal dullness may be caused by pleural effusion, lung collapse or consolidation or localized fibrosis. Increased resonance is indicative of pneumothorax or emphysema.

Drugs used in respiratory disease

Drugs required in the treatment of respiratory disease are mainly antibiotics, bronchodilators and corticosteroids.

Antibiotics

These are indicated for pneumonia, acute bronchitis, or bronchiectasis, asthmatic attacks with purulent sputum, lung abscess or empyema. Commonly used antibiotics are: penicillin, ampicillin, amoxycillin, cloxacillin, flucloxacillin, methicillin, carbenicillin, Septrin (trimethoprim and sulphamethoxazole), gentamicin, tobramycin, neomycin, and tetracycline.

Bronchodilators

These are indicated where relief of airways obstruction is required particularly in asthma and chronic bronchitis. Commonly used bronchodilators are: salbutamol (Ventolin), terbutaline (Bricanyl), aminophylline, and adrenaline.

Relief of airways obstruction is obtained mainly by relaxation of muscle spasm and by reduction of mucus secretion.

Corticosteroids

These are indicated in asthma or advanced chronic obstructive airways disease. Commonly used corticosteroids are: prednisone administered by mouth in tablet form, and beclomethasone (Becotide) administered by aerosol or nebulizer inhalation.

These drugs reduce bronchial hyperactivity by their anti-inflammatory effect which reduces oedema in the lining of the bronchial wall.

Steam inhalations

These are indicated in asthma and chronic bronchitis. Commonly used preparations are: benzoin tincture, and menthol and eucalyptus.

Hot water is added to these preparations and inhaling the hot moist air reduces the viscosity of the mucus secretions in the lungs.

Outline of physiotherapy examination

History

The patient must be warm and in a well-supported, relaxed position. It is important to ascertain the history of the illness, the patient's occupation and life-style, and how these are affected by the condition. The type and amount of sputum should be noted as should the nature and daily pattern of any cough. Smoking should be discouraged, therefore it is useful to record the number and type of cigarettes smoked.

Observation

General appearance, posture, colour, rate and depth of respiration, ease or distress when talking and presence of wheeze are noted. Shape of chest antero-posteriorly and laterally should be observed together with the pattern of breathing (e.g. upper chest or unilateral).

Palpation

The hands are placed over the various areas of the thorax to determine whether any area is not expanding.

Measurement of chest movements

Chest expansion can be measured with a measuring tape at the three levels of:

1. Upper lateral costal (4th costal cartilage) usually 2–3 cm.
2. Lower lateral costal (7th costal cartilage) usually 4–5 cm.
3. Diaphragmatic (9th costal cartilage) usually 7–8 cm.

The measurements are taken at full inspiration and at full expiration.

The measurement at expiration is subtracted from the measurement at inspiration to give the amount of expansion.

Percussion, auscultation, ventilatory capcity tests and exercise tolerance tests are performed as appropriate, and radiographs examined.

Following the examination, the physiotherapist must assess the findings to determine a logical treatment programme.

Medical conditions: principles of physiotherapy treatment

Aims

1. To mobilize secretions.
2. To teach effective coughing and remove secretions.
3. To teach relaxation.
4. To teach breathing patterns and control.
5. To teach postural awareness.
6. To mobilize thorax and shoulder girdle.
7. To advise on home management.

Methods of treatment

Loosening of secretions

Massage manipulations

Vibrations have a mechanical effect in moving secretions towards the main bronchi and may also be used to stimulate the cough reflex. They are performed throughout the expiratory phase of respiration.

Shaking has a more vigorous effect and is also performed during expiration.

Clapping has a loosening effect on secretions and can be applied during inspiration and expiration it should be performed over a blanket covering the patient's chest.

Breathing exercises

These may be general when the patient is encouraged to use the whole thorax, or localized where specific areas of the lung fields are to be expanded. Both have a mechanical effect on mobilizing secretions.

Postural drainage (Figure 12.13)

This comprises positioning the patient so that gravity helps drain a lobe or bronchopulmonary segment.

Positions used

1 *Right lung*:
   (a) *Upper (superior) lobe*:
       Apical segment – sitting upright.
       Posterior segment – one-quarter turn from prone right side up.
       Anterior segment – lying supine.
   (b) *Middle lobe* – one quarter turn to left from supine foot end of bed raised 30–35 cm.

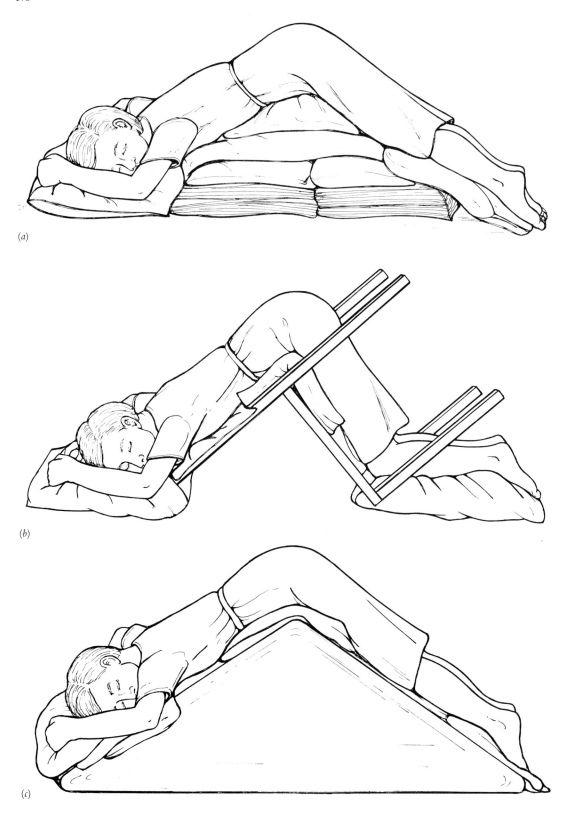

(a)

(b)

(c)

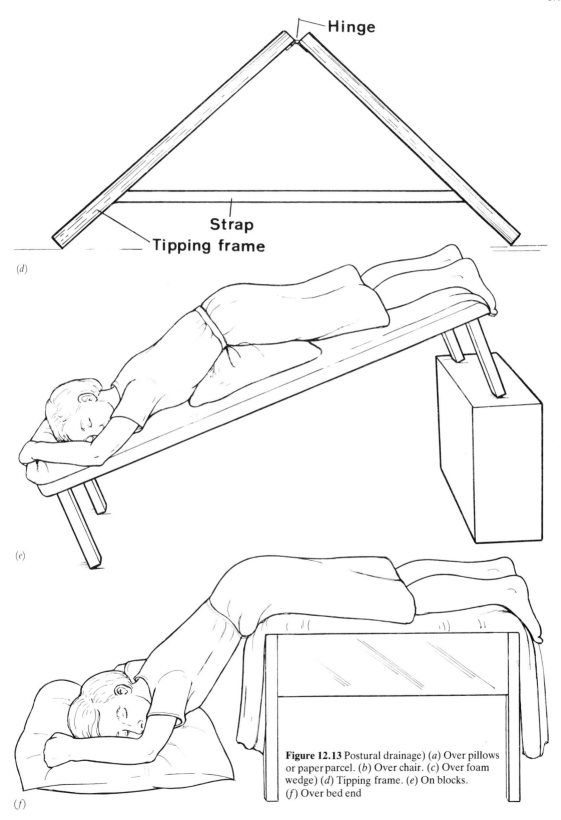

Hinge

Strap

Tipping frame

(d)

(e)

(f)

Figure 12.13 Postural drainage) (a) Over pillows or paper parcel. (b) Over chair. (c) Over foam wedge) (d) Tipping frame. (e) On blocks. (f) Over bed end

(c) *Lower (inferior) lobe*:
Apical segment – prone lying pillow under waist.
Anterior segment – supine lying. Foot of bed raised 45 cm.
Lateral segment – left side lying. Foot of bed raised 45 cm.
Posterior segment – prone lying two pillows under the hips. Foot of bed raised 45 cm.
Medial segment – right side lying. Foot of bed raised 45 cm.

2. *Left lung*:
   (a) *Upper (superior) lobe*:
   Apical and anterior segments – as for right lung.
   Posterior segment – one-quarter turn to right from prone. Left side up with head and trunk raised 30 cm.
   (b) *Lingula* – one-quarter turn from supine. Foot of bed raised 35 cm.
   (c) *Lower (inferior) lobe* – as right lung except that there is a medial segment and the lateral segment is drained in the position used for the medial segment, right lung.

The deep-tipped positions should be avoided in the following conditions:

1. Cardiac arrhythmias or cardiac insufficiency because the heart has to work harder to pump blood to the legs against gravity.
2. Severe hypertension because venous and lymphatic drainage from the legs is increased and puts extra stress on the heart.
3. Aortic aneurysms because the arterial walls are put under tension.
4. Pulmonary oedema because postural drainage is not the correct treatment and would cause severe dyspnoea.
5. Chronic obstructive airways disease with advanced emphysematous changes because the patient would become dyspnoeic.
6. Surgical emphysema because the air may track through the neck tissues to the face.
7. Severe haemoptysis. Should this occur during physiotherpay treatment must be stopped immediately.
8. Hiatus hernia because there is danger of regurgitation of gastric juices.
9. Oesophagectomy because postural drainage will cause strain on the anastomosis.
10. Head injuries or other conditions where it would be dangerous to increase intracranial pressure.
11. Facial oedema, for example following surgery or trauma to the face.
12. Eye surgery, because of the danger of increasing fluid pressure (intra-ocular pressure) behind the eye.

Home postural drainage

Postural drainage may be performed comparatively simply at home in a variety of ways:

1. Lying over a parcel of newspapers and pillows. The height of the parcel varies according to the area treated, e.g. 6–9 in (15–22 cm) for basal areas and less for lingual or middle lobe.
2. Lying over an upturned chair and pillows.
3. Using a wedge foam pillow.
4. Using a tipping frame.
5. Using blocks or a large trunk to put the feet of the bed on.
6. Lying over end of low bed.

Inhalation therapy

Mucolytic agents (which break up mucus) and bronchodilators (which produce relaxation in bronchial smooth muscle) may be administered by aerosol nebulizers, during intermittent positive pressure breathing (IPPB) or by steam inhalations.

Aerosols

These are hand-held devices which patients can use at home. Meticulous instruction in their use is essential. Rotahalers are often more beneficial for patients who cannot master the technique of use of aerosols.

Nebulizers

A nebulizer is a device in which the drug to be administered is broken down into fine particles to facilitate inhalation. It may be driven by compressed oxygen or air.

The patient using a nebulizer must be in a well-supported, relaxed position and encouraged to use the basal areas of the lungs. A face mask or mouthpiece may be used to deliver the nebulized drugs. The face mask is less efficient but may be necessary for young or disabled breathless patients, because the mouthpiece requires the patient to concentrate on holding the lips around it. The most useful pattern is relaxed breathing interspersed with one or two deep breaths during the 10–15 min it takes for the drug to be inhaled. This method helps to facilitate the penetration of the drug into the airways.

Humidification

The principle of humidification is that the patient breathes in air which is moistened by being passed through water vapour. There are several different types of humidifier but all are driven by air whether it be from a cylinder, piped or a compression unit (Webber, 1981). The moistened air is delivered to a free-breathing patient by a face mask, or a mouthpiece. Continuous moistening of the respiratory mucosa is normally obtained by the air passing through nose and pharynx. When this is inefficient, cilial action is impaired and secretions become viscid. Humidification may be used, therefore, to loosen secretions which are unusually viscid and thick.

Intermittent positive pressure breathing

This is a form of assisted inspiration in which air enters the bronchial tree under pressure provided by pressure-cycled ventilators (e.g. Bird or Bennett). It increases aeration of the alveoli and helps to mobilize secretions. Bronchodilator drugs may be administered by this technique and it is useful to reduce the energy expenditure in laboured breathing. These ventilators have a triggering device which can be set to provide the assisted air flow in time with the patient's breathing pattern.

Removal of secretions

Effective coughing

The patient is taught to take a deep breath in (high lung volume), tighten the abdominal muscles and cough. This ensures that the force of the expired air is sufficient to clear secretions from the trachea and main bronchi.

Huffing

The difference between coughing and huffing is that coughing starts as a forced expiration against a closed glottis whereas huffing is a forced expiration with the glottis open. The patient is instructed to take a medium-sized breath in (mid-lung volume), tighten the abdominal muscles, then give a hard 'huff' out through the mouth. The force behind the expired air is less than in coughing, but is none the less highly effective in moving secretions up from the lobar and segmental bronchi.

Forced expiration technique

This comprises teaching the patient to perform one or two huffs, followed by relaxed controlled breathing. The secretions thus mobilized are then cleared with one or two coughs. This technique ensures that the huffs which are performed from midlung volume to low lung volume move the secretions from the peripheral airways and that the coughs performed at high lung volume will clear the secretions from the central airways. The interspersed controlled breathing is essential to prevent or reduce bronchospasm (Pryor and Webber, 1979).

The effects can be enhanced with self-percussion or self-compression to loosen secretions.

Suction

This comprises passing a catheter through the nasopharynx or pharynx or, when appropriate, through an endotracheal or tracheostomy tube. The catheter is attached to a suction pump and therefore secretions that have accumulated in the main bronchi, trachea or pharynx are sucked out.

Relaxation (Figure 12.14)

The ability to relax is particularly important for patients with respiratory disorders especially during recovery from a frightening dyspnoeic attack. Conscious and physiological (Mitchell, 1977) methods are the most suitable. Neck and shoulder girdle relaxation should be practised every day. Upper chest relaxation together with controlled breathing needs practice in different positions.

The most commonly used positions are:

1. High side lying.
2. Forearm support (on table) forward lean sitting.
3. Forearm support (on thighs) forward lean sitting.
4. Back support (against wall) or relaxed standing.
5. Forearm support forward lean standing.

Breathing control

Patients suffering from chronic respiratory disease expend too much energy on breathing which in healthy people is virtually effortless. A patient should be supported in a relaxed position and taught breathing to establish a controlled pattern – counting 'one out – one in'. This is established at the patient's own rate which would slow down once control has been gained. To encourage the patient to use the basal areas of the lungs it is helpful to suggest 'tummy out with breathing in, tummy in with breathing out'. This counteracts the abdominal pattern which occurs in so many breathless patients when the abdomen is drawn in during inspiration and relaxes during expiration, with the result that the abdominal organs inhibit diaphragmatic excursion on inspiration.

Progression is made by altering the phasing to 'one, two out – one in' then 'one, two, three out – one, two in'. The patient's position is then altered to reduce support until he or she is able to stand, walk and go up or down stairs with breathing control. Such patients are encouraged to breathe out when bending down and to breathe in when straightening up during everyday activities (e.g. putting food in oven, tying shoe laces).

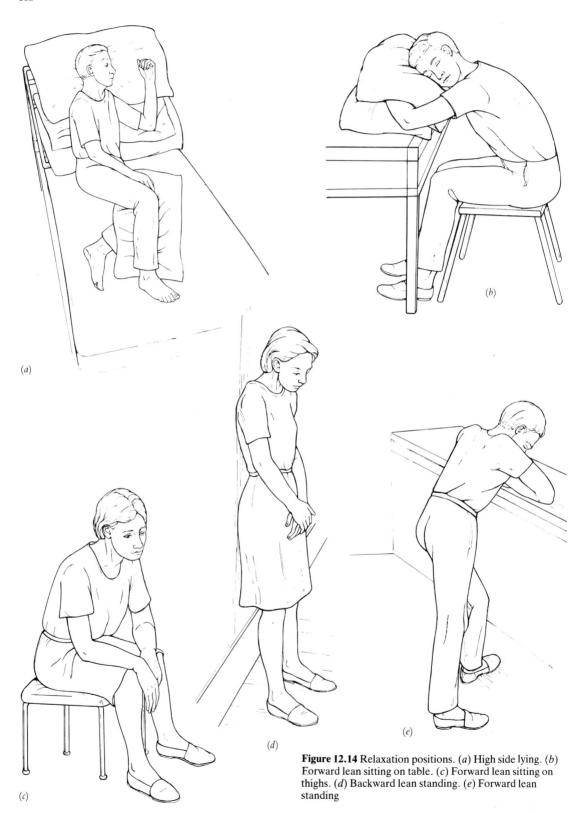

Figure 12.14 Relaxation positions. (*a*) High side lying. (*b*) Forward lean sitting on table. (*c*) Forward lean sitting on thighs. (*d*) Backward lean standing. (*e*) Forward lean standing

(*a*)

(*b*)

(*c*)

(*d*)

(*e*)

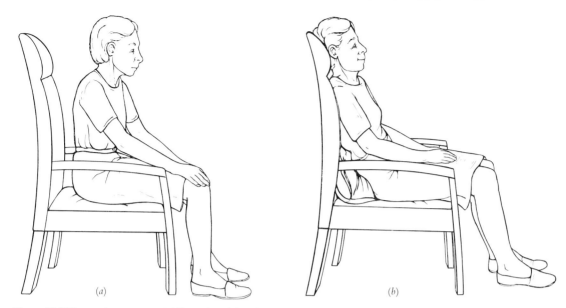

Figure 12.15 Postural awareness. (*a*) Tensed position. (*b*) Relaxed position

Postural awareness (Figure 12.15)

Rounded shoulders, thoracic kyphosis and head thrust forward are common postural abnormalities. The effect is to diminish thoracic spine mobility and chest expansion. Therefore it is essential to teach patients to relax the shoulder girdle, straighten the spine and keep the head erect. This must be applied in positions of work and when sitting resting, e.g. reading or watching television.

Mobilizing the thorax and shoulder girdle

Free active exercises are necessary for the patient to perform daily. Examples of exercises are:

1. Sitting; trunk turning with arms relaxed.
2. Sitting; trunk bending sideways.
3. Underbend sitting (fists on side of chest wall), trunk bending sideways.
4. Bend sitting; elbows circling backwards.
5. Crook lying; pelvic tilting forwards, backwards and sideways.
6. Crook lying; knee rolling side to side.
7. Lying; alternate hip updrawing.

5–7 are useful to help mobilize the lower part of the thorax and to encourage basal expansion.

8. Sitting; shoulder girdle circling backwards.
9. Sitting; trunk bending forwards with breathing out and trunk raising with breathing in.
10. Sitting; arms raising forwards and upwards, and lowering sideways.

11. Sitting trunk bending forwards and to the left and stretching upwards backwards and to the right – repeat to the other side.
12. As (11) add arm movements stretching in the same direction as the trunk.

Home management

The physiotherapist must discuss with each patient suffering chronic respiratory disease how treatment is to be carried out at home. This will include working out the feasibility of postural drainage positions, for example using a newspaper parcel to go under the hips rather than tipping the bed. Breathing exercises with a webbing belt helps the patient to practise basal expansion. Methods of disposing of sputum should be discussed. Self-percussion, drug administration and regular exercise have to be fitted in to the patient's daily lifestyle.

Overall management of the patient

Many disciplines are involved in the overall management apart from physiotherapists, including nurses, doctors, radiographers, occupational therapists, physiological measurement technicians and social workers. Management extends from intensive care for the acutely ill to the health centre, the patient's home and hospital or hospice for the terminally ill.

References

Butland, R. J. A., Pang, J. A., Gross, E. R., *et al.* (1982) 2, 6, and 12 minute walking tests in respiratory disease. *British Medical Journal,* **284**, 1607–1608

Flenley, D. G. (1981) *Respiratory Medicine,* Ballieré Tindall, London

Mitchell, L. (1977) *Simple Relaxation,* John Murray, London

Pryor, J. A. and Webber, B. A. (1979) An evaluation of the forced expiration technique as an adjunct to postural drainage. *Physiotherapy,* **65.10**, 304–307

Webber, B. A. (1981) The use and abuse of inhalation equipment. *Physiotherapy,* **67**, 5

World Health Organization (1961) Definition and description of pulmonary disease with special reference to chronic bronchitis and emphysema. *WHO Technical Report Series,* **213**, 15

Chapter 13

Chronic obstructive airways disease

Patterns of disease

Chronic bronchitis and emphysema produce airways obstruction and frequently occur together, resulting in chronic obstructive airways disease. In the majority of cases chronic bronchitis is the major cause of obstruction but in some cases emphysema is predominant. Thus there are two patterns of chronic obstructive airways disease which can be distinguished clinically although the majority of patients show a mixture of both. In one pattern the patient is 'blue and bloated' whereas in the other the patient is 'pink and puffing' (Figure 13.1).

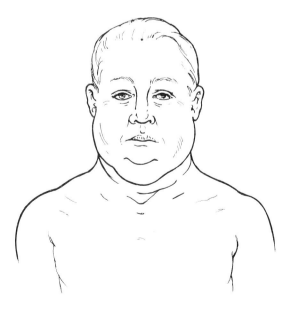
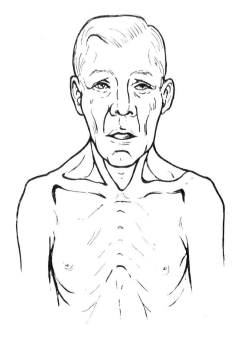

Figure 13.1 Blue bloater and pink puffer

'Blue and bloated'

Patients with this syndrome have:

1. Obesity.
2. Comparatively mild dyspnoea.
3. Copious sputum which may become infected.
4. Low Po_2 and high Pco_2 because they tend to underventilate and are insensitive to CO_2.
5. Central cyanosis with cor pulmonale.
6. Peripheral oedema due to sodium retention.
7. An increased residual volume but normal total lung capacity.

'Pink and puffing'

Patients with this syndrome have:

1. An anxious expression and are generally thin. Severe breathlessness.
2. Little or no sputum production.
3. Relatively normal Po_2 and Pco_2 because they hyperventilate and have normal sensitivity to CO_2.
4. Central cyanosis, no cor pulmonale until the late stages of the disease.
5. Generally no peripheral oedema until the late stages of the disease.
6. An increased total lung capacity due to hyperventilation.

Physiotherapy

Physiotherapy must be directed towards identifying the patient's problems by examination and assessment followed by the planning and implementing of an appropriate treatment programme. This will vary according to the predominating clinical features. Although chronic bronchitis and emphysema frequently occur together, for descriptive purposes they will now be considered separately.

Chronic bronchitis

Definition

Chronic bronchitis is a chronic or recurrent increase above the normal in the volume of mucus secretion sufficient to cause expectoration when this is not due to localized broncho-pulmonary disease. (NB. Chronic/recurrent is further defined as being present on most days during at least 3 consecutive months of each of two successive years.)

Aetiology

This is more common in middle to late adult life and in men more than women (ratio 5:1). Atmospheric pollution (e.g. cigarette smoking or coal dust) will predispose to the development of the disease and it is more common in urban areas than in rural areas. It is more prevalent in socio-economic groups 4 and 5 and is costly in terms of working days lost annually in Britain.

Pathology

Some irritative substance stimulates overactivity of the mucus secreting glands and the goblet cells in the bronchi and in the bronchioles which causes secretion of a vast excess of mucus. This mucus coats the walls of the airways and tends to clog the bronchioles (this is functionally more important). The cells increase in size and the ducts become dilated – they may occupy as much as two-thirds of the wall thickness. This causes a chronic inflammatory process which results in mucosal oedema thus further decreasing the diameter of the airways. The ciliary action is also inhibited.

This narrowing of the lumen of the airways is further emphasized during expiration by the normal lengthening and narrowing of the airways – consequently the airways obstruction is enhanced during expiration with resulting air-trapping in the alveoli. The lungs gradually lose their elasticity as the disease progresses. They will gradually become distended permanently which eventually may cause extensive rupture of the alveolar walls. After repeated exacerbations there is widespread damage to the bronchioles and the alveoli with fibrosis and kinking occurring as well as compensatory overdistension of the surviving alveoli. This is closely allied to and contributory to the development of emphysema.

Clinical features

The four most important are cough, sputum, wheeze and dyspnoea:

1. *Cough* – The patient will complain of a cough for many years initially intermittent and gradually becoming continuous. It is increased by fog, damp or infection. The patient may also complain of bouts of coughing occasionally on lying down or in the morning.
2. *Sputum* – It is mucoid and tenacious usually becoming mucopurulent during an exacerbation. The amount will progressively increase.
3. *Wheeze* – Worse in the mornings and may be related to weather changes.
4. *Dyspnoea* – Usually this is related to effort and the patient becomes progressively more short of breath as the disease progresses.

Other signs and symptoms

5. *Deformity* – These patients often develop a barrel chest with an indrawn abdomen. The thoracic movements are gradually diminished and paradoxical indrawing in the intercostal spaces may develop.
6. *Cyanosis* – Development of cyanosis is related to the development of complications, such as ventricular failure or polycythaemia.
7. Cor pulmonale in the later stages.
8. *Lung functions tests (LFTS)* – There is reduction of FEV_1/FVC ratio and the FEV_1 is grossly reduced. The RV will be increased at the expense of the VC because of the airtrapping and alveolar distortion.
9. *Blood gases* – the P_{ACO_2} rises whilst the P_{AO_2} falls. This leaves the respiratory stimulus dependent upon the hypoxic drive NOT on the levels of P_{ACO_2}.
10. *Auscultation* – There will be inspiratory and expiratory rhonci with added coarse crepitations. The breath sounds are vesicular with prolonged expiration.
11. *X-ray* – No characteristic abnormality.

Prognosis

Chronic bronchitis is a progressive disease which has acute excacerbations. It is not usually seen until irreversible damage has occurred. The survival rate varies between 5 and 30 years but eventually cardiac and ventilatory failure will occur.

Prophylaxis

1. Control of atmospheric pollution.
2. Stop smoking.
3. Treat all acute infections promptly.
4. Maintain good general health.

Principles of treatment

1. *Decrease the bronchial irritation to a minimum* – The patient should be advised to stop smoking and avoid dusty, smoky, damp or foggy atmospheres. Occupation or housing conditions may need to be changed.
2. *Control infections* – All infections MUST be treated promptly as each excacerbation will cause further damage to the airways. The patient should have a supply of antibiotics at home and be given a 'flu' injection each winter.
3. *Control bronchospasm* – Although not a prominent feature of this disease, drugs (e.g. salbutamol) may be given to relieve the airways obstruction as much as is possible.

4. *Control/decrease the amount of sputum* – By definition these patients ALL have sputum but if this can be decreased as much as possible then their lung function will improve proportionately. To this end they will be helped by physiotherapy, with inhalations and humidification where necessary.
5. *Oxygen therapy* – This should be given with great care as oxygen can cause decrease of the hypoxic respiratory drive and thus precipitate respiratory failure. Controlled oxygen is given via a Ventimask (or equivalent) with careful monitoring of blood gas levels.

Physiotherapy

General aims of treatment

1. To facilitate the removal of secretions and relieve any bronchospasm.
2. To improve the pattern of breathing and breathing control.
3. To teach local relaxation and improve posture.
4. To mobilize the thorax and the shoulder girdle.
5. To improve the exercise tolerance.
6. To give advice.

The treatment given must be appropriate to the stage of the disease and the patient's general health.

Treatment in early stages of the disease

The most important theme is clearing the airways of secretions and establishing a correct breathing pattern.

Removal of secretions

Postural drainage is essential for all patients. The optimum position for effectiveness must be established with each individual and instructions on postural drainage at home is very important. Instead of tipping the bed, a patient may lie with the thorax over the edge of a bed or a pile of newspapers under the hips (see Chapter 12).

Breathing exercises are practised whilst the patient is in the postural drainage position. Generally patients are encouraged to carry out this treatment for 20 minutes, twice daily, but some may tolerate 30 minutes and others only 10 minutes.

Clapping and shaking over affected lung segments are helpful in loosening and moving secretions, and the patient is instructed on huffing and coughing to clear the sputum.

If the secretions are very thick and tenacious the patient may be given inhalations with either pine oil or tincture of benzoin added to boiling water, prior to postural drainage.

Breathing pattern

The patient is taught how to relax the shoulder girdle in a supported posturally correct position such as crook half lying. Breathing control is taught following clearance of secretions. Expansion breathing exercises of the basal lung segments are taught to ventilate these areas. If the patient is breathless, respiratory control is regained starting with short respiratory phases and allowing the rate to slow as the patient's breathing pattern improves (see Chapter 12).

The patient may be admitted to hospital, treated in an out-patient department, in a health centre or at home by a community physiotherapist. It is important to see the patient regularly. Advice should be given on taking regular exercises, as for example a short walk every day. Thoracic mobility exercises such as bend sitting, trunk turning side to side, and trunk bending side to side should be practised daily. The physiotherapist must also reinforce any advice given by the doctor.

Later stages

It is important to maintain independence and maximum function. Postural drainage and percussion must be continued on a regular basis. It may be appropriate to teach the patient and relatives to perform percussion to assist clearance of secretions.

Breathing control is taught to counting so that the patient can walk or climb stairs with confidence. Relaxation positions are taught for regaining breathing control after activity has made the patient breathless. If the patient becomes very disabled, a walking frame may help to retain some degree of independence as the arms are fixed and accessory muscles of inspiration may be used.

Terminal care

The main theme is to keep the patient as comfortable as possible. Treatment needs to be short and frequent. A ventilator may be provided for home use. Inhalations are used to loosen and liquefy secretions. Suction may be necessary and the general practitioner may provide drugs for the patient to use at home.

Treatment during an acute exacerbation

Acute exacerbation is associated with acute inflammation of the bronchial muscosa. This leads to obstruction of the airways, lack of ventilation, reduction in perfusion, and anoxia of the brain may result which causes drowsiness and confusion. The breathing pattern becomes shallow, erratic and inefficient.

The aims of physiotherapy are:

1. To clear lung fields.
2. To loosen secretions.
3. To help and encourage productive coughing.
4. To improve gaseous interchange in the lungs.

Treatment is required for short spells but frequently throughout the day and sometimes at night. Intermittent positive pressure breathing (see Chapter 12) is given using a mask if the patient is too drowsy to use a mouthpiece. Postural drainage is necessary together with rigorous shaking applied during the expiratory phase of the ventilator.

Suction may have to be used to remove secretions if the patient is unable to cough spontaneously. If Pco_2 is high and Po_2 is low the patient should not be given a high concentration of oxygen. Two litres of oxygen through a nebulizer with the Bird respirator driven off air gives a 25% oxygen to air mix which is generally suitable. Drugs such as mucolytic agents or bronchodilators may be provided through the nebulizer attached to the ventilator. The patient is encouraged to sip drinks because dehydration makes the secretions viscid.

As the patient recovers, treatment is directed towards that given in the 'early' stages, with special emphasis on a daily maintenance programme of regular exercise, postural drainage and breathing exercises. The community physiotherapist should visit the patient soon after discharge home.

Emphysema

Definition

Emphysema is a condition of the lung characterized by permanent dilatation of the air spaces distal to the terminal bronchioles with destruction of the walls of these airways. It is nearly always associated with chronic bronchitis from which it is difficult to distinguish during life.

Aetiology

This is probably highest in England especially in the major centres of industry. A survey carried out in 1961 showed that 17% of all men and 8% of all women aged between 40 and 60 years showed clinical symptoms of the disease. They account for the vast majority of the 30 million working days lost each year which may be attributed to chronic respiratory disease. There is often a family history of the disease.

Causes and predisposing factors

1. Congenital. Primary emphysema may be caused by antitrypsin deficiency.

2. Secondary to other factors:
   (a) Obstructive airways disease, e.g. asthma, cystic fibrosis, chronic bronchitis.
   (b) Occupational lung diseases, e.g. pneumoconiosis.
   (c) Risk factors, e.g. cigarette smoking.
   (d) Compensatory to contraction of one section of the lung, e.g. fibrous collapse or removal, when the remaining lung expands to fill the space.

Types

1. Centrilobular (centri-acinar).
2. Panacinar (pan-lobular).

Centrilobular emphysema tends to affect the respiratory bronchioles with most of the alveoli remaining normal whereas panacinar emphysema results in widespread destruction of most alveoli as well as respiratory bronchioles. Primary emphysema is usually panacinar. In centrilobular emphysema the upper zones of the lung are usually affected. This causes gross disturbance of the ventilation–perfusion relationship since there is a relatively well preserved blood supply to the alveoli but the amount of oxygen reaching the capillary is decreased owing to the damage to airways proximal to the alveoli.

Panacinar emphysema predominantly affects the lower lobes. This has a less drastic effect on ventilation–perfusion relationship since the blood supply in the damaged areas is decreased in proportion to the decreased ventilation in those areas.

Pathology and proteolytic theory

Smoking causes the clustering of pulmonary alveolar macrophages (which are the major defence cells of the respiratory tract) around the terminal bronchioles. These macrophages are abnormal in smokers and they release proteolytic enzymes which destroy lung tissue locally. Polymorphonuclear leucocytes, necessary to combat infection in the lung, release an enzyme which also destroys lung tissue. The defence mechanism against the unwanted action of these enzymes lies in the serum alpha-1-antitrypsin which is normally present in the airway lining fluids. Oxidants released by both cigarette smoke and the leucocytes tend to inactivate the antiproteolytic action of the alpha-1-antitrypsin which causes destruction of lung tissue as seen in centrilobular emphysema.

Subsequent changes

The walls of the airways become weak and inelastic owing to the damage from repeated infections. They tend to act as a one-way valve with the walls collapsing on expiration. This causes air trapping and consequent increase in the intra-alveolar pressure during expiration. The alveolar septa break down and form bullae (Figure 13.2). During expiration the pressure from the trapped air in the

NORMAL

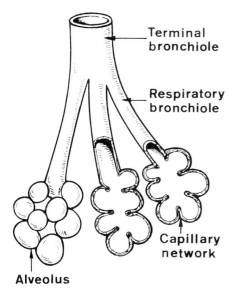

Terminal bronchiole

Respiratory bronchiole

Capillary network

Alveolus

Figure 13.2 Emphysematous changes

EMPHYSEMATOUS CHANGES

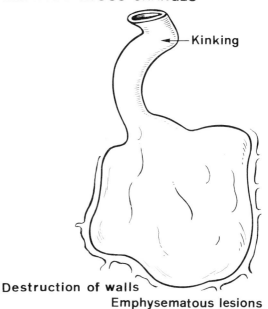

Kinking

Destruction of walls

Emphysematous lesions

bullae may compress adjacent healthy tissue thus causing occlusion and air-trapping in that tissue. The capillaries around the alveolar walls become stretched causing the lumen to decrease and atrophy to occur. This causes an alteration in the ventilation/perfusion relationship, due to the loss of surface area for gaseous exchange and the decrease in blood supply resulting from damage to the pulmonary capillary network.

Clinical features

1. *Progressive dyspnoea* – Initially this occurs on exertion but as the disease progresses it will

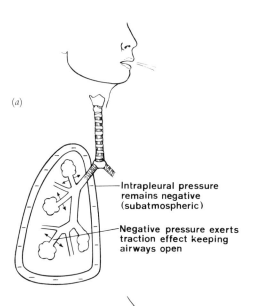

(a)

Intrapleural pressure remains negative (subatmospheric)

Negative pressure exerts traction effect keeping airways open

gradually occur after less and less activity and finally at rest. This disabling breathlessness is what prevents the patient from working and gradually transforms him into a respiratory cripple.

2. *Respiratory pattern* – The patient has a 'fishlike' inspiratory gasp which is followed by prolonged, forced expiration usually against 'pursed lips'. This creates back-pressure to try to prevent airways shutdown during expiration. Due to increased intra-thoracic pressure the jugular veins fill on expiration. A 'flick' or 'bounce' of the abdominal muscles may be seen on expiration as the outward flow of air is suddenly checked by the obstruction of the airways (Figure 13.3).

3. *Cough with sputum* – This will be present if the disease is associated with chronic bronchitis or if there is infection.

4. *Chest shape* – The chest becomes barrel shaped, fixed in inspiration with widening of the intercostal spaces. There may also be indrawing of the lower intercostal spaces and supraclavicular fossa on inspiration. This is associated with the difficulty of ventilating stiff lungs through narrowed airways. The ribs are elevated by the accesssory muscles of respiration and there is loss of thoracic mobility.

5. *Poor posture* – There is a thoracic kyphosis plus elevated and protracted shoulder girdles.

6. *Polycythaemia* – This is an increase in the number of red blood cells and may develop as a direct effect of the body's efforts to correct the ventilation/perfusion imbalance.

7. *Cor pulmonale* – This occurs in the advanced stages of the disease.

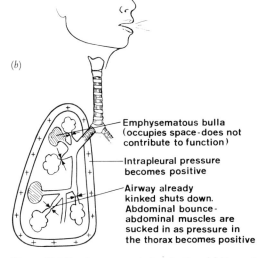

(b)

Emphysematous bulla (occupies space-does not contribute to function)

Intrapleural pressure becomes positive

Airway already kinked shuts down. Abdominal bounce-abdominal muscles are sucked in as pressure in the thorax becomes positive

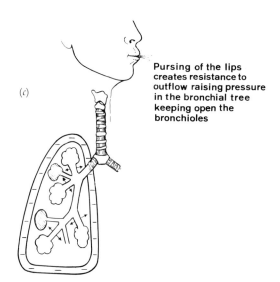

(c)

Pursing of the lips creates resistance to outflow raising pressure in the bronchial tree keeping open the bronchioles

Figure 13.3 Emphysema: end of expiration. (*a*) Normal. (*b*) Emphysema. (*c*) Pursed-lip breathing

8. *On examination* – The percussion note will be normal or hyper-resonant due to air trapping. Auscultation will reveal decreased breath sounds and prolonged expiration. Radiograph shows low flat diaphragms.
9. *Lung function tests* – FEV_1/FVC ratio is usually below 70%. RV is increased.

Prognosis

The patients become progressively more disabled, with death ultimately occurring from respiratory failure.

Complications

1. Pneumothorax.
2. Respiratory failure.
3. Congestive cardiac failure.

Principles of treatment

General

Prevention or treatment of chest infections:

1. 'Flu injections every winter.
2. Antibiotics (with a stock kept at home so that the patient can start a course as soon as possible).
3. Rehousing (if damp or cold or there are many stairs).
4. Change occupation or hobby if appropriate.
5. Stop smoking.

Improve lung function

1. Steroids are tried for 2 weeks, the effect being monitored by LFTs.
2. Bronchodilators may help the FVC although FEV_1 is irreversible.
3. Oxygen therapy is applied as necessary.
4. Surgery. If large bullae are present and compressing areas of healthy lung tissue then resection of the bullae may improve the patient's lung function. The success of this operation depends upon the severity and extent of the disease in the remaining lung tissue (for physiotherapy related to surgery see Chapter 14).

Physiotherapy

Aims of treatment

1. To teach the patient to breathe with the minimum possible effort.
2. To establish a coordinated pattern of breathing.
3. To assist in the removal of secretions.
4. To increase the range of movement of the joints of the thoracic cage.
5. To increase exercise tolerance.
6. To regain fullest possible function.

Re-education of breathing pattern

This should be started with the patient well supported in sitting or half lying. Firstly he should be taught relaxation of the shoulder girdle and the upper part of the chest by using physiological or contrast methods. Then controlled diaphragmatic breathing is taught, emphasizing relaxed expiration. The patient should be taught to shorten the expiratory phase and begin inspiration *before* the airways have a chance to close down. The patient has to learn to judge the optimum moment to begin inspiration and this requires perseverance and training. Lower lateral costal and posterior basal expansion is taught to increase thoracic mobility and coordinated movement of the thorax.

Removal of secretions

Postural drainage techniques usually need to be modified as a patient becomes more dyspnoeic. Positions generally have to be lower than normal for the basal and middle areas of the lungs. Shaking should be applied during expiration and coughing restricted to 1–2 coughs per breath. Often the patient has distressing paroxysms of coughing which is ineffective due to closure of the airways. Intermittent positive pressure breathing (IPPB) may be used at a low pressure provided no bullae are present (seen on radiograph). This may help expectoration and relieve any bronchospasm if given with a bronchodilator.

Alternatively a bronchodilator may be administered with a nebulizer.

Thoracic mobility

Free active exercises for the whole spine are important and require daily practice because the thorax tends to become fixed in inspiration with a kyphosis in the thoracic spine. The exercise programme must be interspersed with relaxation and breathing control.

An important exercise to include is sitting, trunk turning with loose arm swinging, for rotation with relaxation. It is also important to emphasize postural awareness so that the patient practises shoulder girdle retraction and lateral rotation of the arms.

Increasing exercise tolerance and function

Breathing control is taught in the positions of relaxation progressing from half lying to standing. A further progression is to teach breathing control in relation to activities of daily living, e.g. walking and climbing stairs and related to particular problems a patient may have. The patient should be encouraged to have outdoor activities such as walking or gardening. Someitimes a patient may require portable oxygen to retain independence and mobility for as long as possible.

Advanced stages of the disease

As the disease progresses there is increased stress on the heart giving rise to congestive cardiac failure. The fluid retention associated with this can be treated by diuretics. The patient may become drowsy and unable to cooperate with breathing exercises and coughing. At this stage it may become necessary to put the patient on to a ventilator to relieve the work of breathing, and secretions have to be removed by suction.

Asthma
Definition

Asthma is a clinical syndrome characterized by attacks of wheezing and breathlessness due to narrowing of the intrapulmonary airways. Remission may be spontaneous or as a result of treatment.

Types of asthma

There are two distinct types: extrinsic and intrinsic.

Extrinsic (atopic) asthma occurs in the younger age groups among those who readily form antibodies to allergens. Patients are usually sensitive to different factors (e.g. pollen, housemites, feathers, food, fur and, occasionally, food or drugs) and also have a family history of similar sensitivities. Exposure to the precipitating factor causes a mucosal inflammatory allergic reaction. This type of asthma tends to be episodic.

Intrinsic (non-atropic) asthma tends to occur in the older patient as a chronic condition. It has no apparent allergic cause or family history. This type of asthma is precipitated by, or associated with bronchial infections, chronic bronchitis, strenuous exercise, stress or anxiety.

Aetiology

The condition can occur at any age but is commonest in children, especially boys. Approximately 10% of children under 10 years of age in the United Kingdom have bouts of coughing and wheezing related to narrowing of the airways. Childhood asthma generally remits after puberty but it may return in later life. Asthma that starts in middle age is more common in women than men. Remission in this age group is rare. The majority of cases of asthma are mild although the course of the disease is unpredictable. The mortality rate is low but is higher in adults than in children.

Pathology

The main pathological changes occurring during an asthmatic attack are:

1. Spasm of the smooth muscle in the walls of the bronchi and bronchioles.
2. Oedema of the mucous membrane of the bronchi and bronchioles.
3. Excessive mucus production.

These changes result in airways obstruction. The bronchial walls become infiltrated with eosinophils and there is thickening of the epithelial basement membrane. At the end of an attack these changes are almost totally reversible but if the attacks occur frequently long-standing changes will occur. Such changes are hypertrophy of the smooth bronchial muscle, which increases the effect of bronchial spasm during an attack; permanent thickening of the mucous membrane with an increase in the number of goblet cells and mucous glands; overdistension of the alveoli due to trapping of air; and atelectasis of alveoli when a bronchiole, already narrowed, becomes blocked by mucus.

Where the predominant factor precipitating asthma is an allergic reaction there is antigen-mediated bronchoconstriction. This means that the antigen (allergen or precipitating factor) binds to two IgE molecules (immunoglobulin antibodies) on the membranes of mast cells present in the bronchial lining. This binding releases mediators which act on receptor sites on smooth muscle cells, causing changes in intracellular cyclic AMP levels which result in muscular contraction. The mediators histamine, neutrophil chemotactic factor (NCF-A), platelet activating factor (PAF) and eosinophil chemotactic factor (ECF-A) are stored in granules within the mast cells as preformed mediators. This antigen–antibody reaction is part of the body's immune response, and previous exposure to the antigen results in greater bronchoconstriction.

Clinical features
Extrinsic asthma

Onset is sudden and paroxysmal, often at night. An attack starts with chest tightness, dryness or irritation in the upper respiratory tract. Attacks may

GRAPHS SHOWING FEV₁ AND FVC

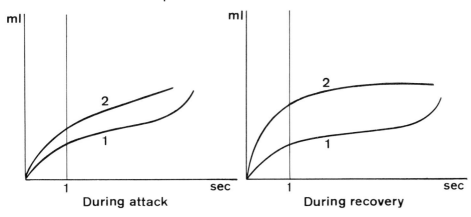

Figure 13.4 Asthma: FEV$_1$ and FVC reversibility during attack and recovery. 1 = Before bronchodilator; 2 = after bronchodilator

be episodic, often occurring several times a year. Their duration varies from a few seconds to many months and the severity may be anything from mild wheezing to great distress.

Wheeze and dyspnoea – The dyspnoea is intense and chiefly occurs on expiration, which becomes a conscious exhausting effort with a short gasping inspiration. Wheezing always occurs on expiration but may also be present on inspiration.

Cough is unproductive and 'barking' in nature. It causes an increase in bronchospasm and dyspnoea. As the attack subsides the cough becomes productive of casts or plugs of sputum containing eosinophils.

Posture – The patient sits upright with the shoulder girdle fixed (by grasping a table or bed) to assist the accessory muscles of respiration. The chest is held in inspiration.

Pulse is rapid and may be paradoxical.

Tachycardia is present.

Cyanosis may occur centrally but not usually until the later stages of the disease.

Breath sounds are vesicular with prolonged expiration and high-pitched ronchi.

Percussion note may be hyper-resonant.

Radiograph – The chest looks over-inflated.

Lung function tests (LFTs) – FEV$_1$ and FVC drop during a severe attack with little sign of reversibility (Figure 13.4). However, if FEV$_1$ is measured before and after giving bronchodilators there is a 15% increase in FEV$_1$ – which amounts to significant reversibility. The FEV$_1$ may be less than 30% of FVC. TLC, FRC and RV may be increased due to over-inflation of the lungs. Recovery is associated with a reduction in these lung volumes. PEFR dips

in the morning (Figure 13.5), especially during the recovery phase. If the dip is severe then respiratory arrest may occur. In a severe attack the PEFR drops below 100 litres/min^{-1}.

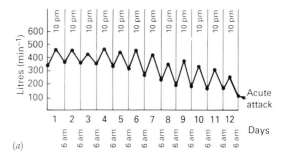

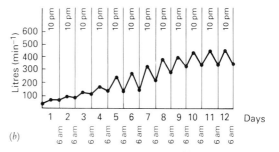

Figure 13.5 Dipping charts in asthma. (*a*) Recording of peak flow at home showing deterioration before onset of acute attack. Intervention when there is a chart like this can prevent the attack. (*b*) During recovery there is still diurnal variation. These patients are at risk and should have long-term monitoring

Blood gases – Hypocapnia (reduced P_{ACO_2}) results from the hyperventilation of the alveoli. In severe asthmatic attacks, hypercapnia may occur (increased P_{ACO_2}) because the hyperventilation fails to compensate for the fact that there are many underventilated alveoli which are distal to the blocked bronchioles. Hypoxaemia (reduced P_{AO_2}) occurs owing to the ventilation perfusion mismatch.

Between attacks

No abnormality should be detectable although children with severe asthma may develop a pigeon chest or have a persistent, low-pitched wheeze with a productive cough.

Intrinsic (chronic) asthma

This is less paroxysmal in character and is often associated with chronic bronchitis.

Clinical features are similar to those described above for extrinsic asthma, but wheeze and dyspnoea tend to be continuous and worse in the morning, cough produces mucoid sputum, respiratory infections occur with increasing frequency and radiographs may show emphysematous changes.

Status asthmaticus

This is a term sometimes used to describe a severe progressive acute attack of asthma present for 24 hours and unresponsive to bronchodilators. Such an attack is potentially life threatening.

Mortality

Ashtma causes approximately 1000 deaths each year. The deaths are most common among early morning dippers, especially in the younger age groups.

Treatment

General management of asthmatic patients comprises prevention of attacks, maintenance of general fitness and treatment during an attack.

Management between attacks and prevention of onset

This comprises identifying and removing the cause, if known. For example, a patient may have to avoid certain foods, damp-dust the home environment regularly, vacuum bedding frequently, use synthetic fibres in place of feathers for pillows and quilts and avoid certain domestic animals. Desensitization may be possible by injection of mild doses of the allergen, which will have been identified by a skin test.

Prevention of infection is important. The patient should have plenty of fresh air, avoid smoky atmospheres and keep away from people with infections such as bronchitis and influenza. Stress or anxiety must be minimized as these can precipitate an attack.

Drugs may help to prevent an attack. These are most successfully administered by aerosol because the effects are long lasting and are localized to the lungs. Sodium cromoglycate (Intal) can be used regularly to reduce attacks in patients with allergic or exercise-induced asthma. Initially, the dosage is one capsule four times daily for 4–6 weeks. Additional doses may be taken before exercise. Bronchodilators given by pressurized aerosol may be used during mild attacks of wheezing to prevent them deteriorating into severe attacks. Corticosteroids, also given by aerosol, may be necessary when bronchodilators are ineffective. The dosage is kept to a minimum compatible with effectiveness.

When drugs are administered by aerosol/inhaler it is important that the patient is taught how to use the device correctly. The technique for a metered dose inhaler in which the drug is suspended in a propellant is as follows:

1. Shake the inhaler.
2. Hold inhaler upright and direct into the mouth.
3. Start inspiration and press the activating mechanism.
4. Breathe in slowly through the mouth to allow penetration of the drug into the bronchial tree.
5. Hold the breath at maximum inspiration for 5–10 seconds to allow particles of the drug to settle on the airway walls.
6. Relax and allow easy expiration.

Rotahalers and spinhalers deliver the drug in a dry powder form. The technique is similar to the above but preparation of the device comprises inserting a capsule which is then pierced or opened within the inhaler to release the drug.

Provision of a home peak flow meter can enable the patient to identify deterioration in the PEFR and to seek assistance from a doctor before an attack develops.

Physiotherapy

The aims of treatment are to:

1. Assist in the removal of secretions.
2. Gain relaxation of the neck, shoulder girdle and upper chest muscles.
3. Teach the patient breathing control.

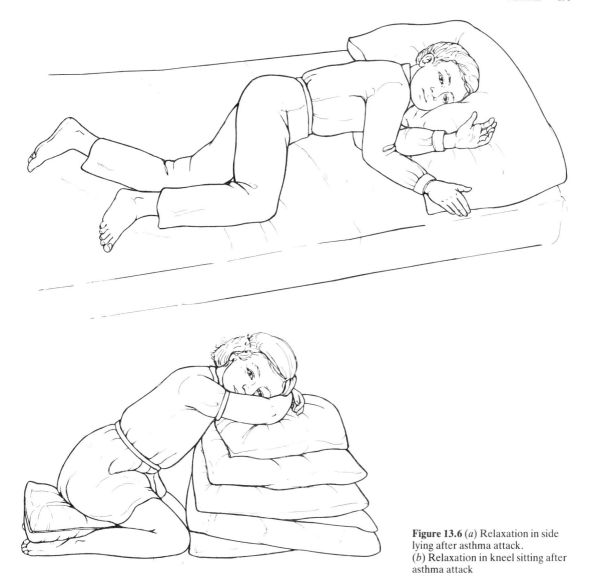

Figure 13.6 (*a*) Relaxation in side lying after asthma attack.
(*b*) Relaxation in kneel sitting after asthma attack

4. Maintain mobility of the neck, shoulder girdle, thoracic spine and thorax.
5. Educate postural awareness.
6. Maintain or improve exercise tolerance.
7. Encourage a full, active lifestyle.

Removal of secretions

Some patients, especially children, have constant excessive secretions and may require postural drainage on a daily basis. Vibrations may be necessary and relatives may have to be taught how to perform this technique. Effective coughing with minimum effort is especially important. It may be essential to teach forced expiration technique (see Chapter 12) for clearing secretions without increasing bronchospasm.

Relaxation

If the patient is able to practise relaxation it may be possible to ward off an attack when there has been exposure to an allergen. The onset of an attack is often preceded by a 'tickle' in the throat or a sensation of tightness in the chest. Relaxation and breathing control in an appropriate position (Figure 13.6) may prevent an attack developing. 'Appropriate position' depends on where the patient is and may have to be against a wall or the back of a chair (see Chapter 12).

Breathing control

Encouraging a longer expiratory phase is helpful but neither inspiration nor expiration should be forced. This may be helped by counting, e.g. 'in 1–2, out 1–2–3', and by manual pressure just under the xiphisternum to encourage basal expansion. The patient must breathe at a rate and rhythm that suits him or her. Children may be taught to breathe to a nursery rhyme.

Mobility exercises and postural awareness

To ensure ventilation of the basal alveoli the patient must be encouraged to adopt a balanced relaxed posture. Thoracic, neck and shoulder mobility exercises should be performed daily together with strengthening exercises for weak muscles (e.g. shoulder girdle retractors, abdominals and thoracic spine extensors).

Exercise tolerance

The essential aim in developing a patient's exercise tolerance is to gain breathing control during all daily activities and to increase the patient's ability to perform exercises which produce breathlessness without bringing on an asthmatic attack. Progression of exercises is made by increasing the speed of performance so that the patient gains confidence in performing activities with the knowledge that breathlessness need not produce an attack. The breathlessness is overcome by the patient using breathing control, gradually increasing the expiratory phase with relaxation.

Full active lifestyle

People with asthma should be encouraged to keep fit, avoid smoking, eat sensibly and to live a normal life in relation to work (or school), hobbies and social activities. Swimming helps to gain relaxation and improve breathing control and as such is an excellent activity. For people who suffer mild attacks an exercise programme should be developed and they should be encouraged to attend keep fit classes. Children may attend group work. After exercises requiring exertion, breathing control is practised. Jerky, quick movements should be avoided as should activities involving keeping the arms above the head for long periods. Children with chronic asthma may benefit from residential courses offering activities such as weight training, skipping, football, static bicycle, swimming and water polo. Very young children like made-up games such as mimicking different zoo animals to include relaxation, hopping, blowing out and waving arms.

Advice to parents

Children can outgrow asthma because as the airways increase in size there is less bronchospasm and constriction. Advice and education from the physiotherapist includes:

1. Avoid discussing asthma in front of the child to minimize the child's fear of having something special.
2. Encourage daily breathing exercises, trunk mobility exercises and postural drainage if necessary.
3. Ensure that the child has a constant supply of bronchodilators.
4. Encourage an active lifestyle.

Management during an attack

The patient may be treated at home (by the GP) or, if the attack is severe, may be admitted to hospital. Drugs used may be bronchodilators, steroids or antibiotics. Bronchodilators (salbutamol, aminophylline) may be given intravenously. Salbutamol may also be administered with a nebulizer or a ventilator giving intermittent positive pressure breathing (IPPB). The steroid prednisolone may be given daily to reduce the inflammatory reaction and antibiotics may be prescribed to counteract any infection. Antihistamine drugs help to counteract the allergies. Oxygen therapy may be necessary during an acute severe attack to compensate for the ventilation perfusion mismatch and may be continued for 2–3 days. Administration is by nebulizer, nasal cannulae, face mask or in an oxygen tent. The last two methods are used for young children.

Physiotherapy

Aims of treatment are to:
1. Relieve bronchospasm.
2. Assist removal of secretions.
3. Improve breathing pattern and control.

Relief of bronchospasm

The physiotherapist can help by positioning the patient in high side lying or half-lying with pillows to obtain full support. This is important because the patient is easily tired and expends much energy in breathing. Bronchodilators are given by IPPB, e.g. 1 ml 0.5% salbutamol solution added to 4 ml saline put in the nebulizer of the ventilator. The patient is encouraged to close the lips round the ventilator mouthpiece and to breathe through the mouth (a mask may be necessary if he is unable to hold the mouthpiece). The sensitivity of the ventilator is set so that it is triggered with very little inspiratory effort from the patient. The machine then delivers air and bronchodilator to the lungs while the patient relaxes. In this way, the work of breathing is relieved and the machine is used until the nebulizer is empty (10–15 minutes). This treatment may be repeated up to 6 times daily. Monitoring of the patient's PEFR should be carried out as soon as the patient can blow into the meter, measurements being taken just before and 15 minutes after the bronchodilator inhalation.

Removal of secretions

When it is evident that the bronchodilator has taken effect, the physiotherapist may give vibrations with expiration. Forced expiration technique (see Chapter 12) may then be encouraged to produce the thick sputum which patients usually have at this stage. As the secretions are loosened and the patient recovers, postural drainage may be instituted to clear the lung fields.

Improving breathing pattern and control

The patient should be encouraged to practise relaxation and breathing control. As the attack subsides, the dosage of bronchodilator may be reduced, e.g. 0.5 ml 0.5% salbutamol solution in 2 ml saline added to the nebulizer. When IPPB is no longer needed the bronchodilator may be inhaled from a simple nebulizer with basal breathing. Gradually, the patient regains confidence and starts to dress and walk while incorporating breathing control and rests between activities. Before discharge from hospital a home programme based on the principles of treatment between attacks should be worked out for the patient. PEFR should be steady (not dipping in the morning) and around 380–400 litres min^{-1}.

Bronchiectasis

Definition

Bronchiectasis is an abnormal dilatation of the bronchi associated with obstruction and infection.

Aetiology

Types

Congenital

Very rarely this occurs in *Kartagener's* syndrome. This consists of a classical triad of frontal sinusitis, bronchiectasis and complete visceral transposition.
   Congenital hypogammaglobulinaemia will predispose to the development of bronchiectasis.

Acquired

Bronchial obstruction and bacterial infection are the principal factors responsible for this disease. Obstruction of a bronchus which may be due to a tumour or foreign body will cause collapse of the lung tissue supplied by that bronchus. Bronchiectasis may also occur following an infection which causes the production of sticky sputum leading to obstruction of multiple small bronchi. Classically this is associated with whooping cough, measles and pneumonia in childhood, when the airways are smaller and therefore more easily 'plug' with sputum. Very occasionally bronchiectasis may occur as a late complication of TB which has affected the right middle lobe causing that segment to collapse. Allergic bronchopulmonary aspergillosis which is associated with an autoimmune response, can cause formation of mucus plugs resulting in bronchiectasis of the medium-sized bronchi.

Prevalence

The prevalence of bronchiectasis following a childhood infection is decreasing dramatically since these infections are treated with antibiotics, but bronchiectasis is a common feature of cystic fibrosis.

Site

The condition most commonly affects the lower lobes, the lingula and then the middle lobe. It tends to affect the left lung more than the right although 50% of cases are bilateral. The upper lobes are least affected since they drain most efficiently with the assistance of gravity.

Pathology

Bronchial obstruction will cause absorption of the air from the lung tissue distal to the obstruction and this area will therefore shrink and collapse. This causes a traction force to be exerted upon the more proximal airways which will distort and dilate them. If the obstruction can be cleared and the lung re-expanded quickly then the dilatation is reversible. Secretions may collect distal to the obstruction if it is not relieved quickly and these easily become infected. This causes inflammation of the bronchial wall with destruction of the elastic and muscular tissue. These infections occur repeatedly with the walls becoming weaker and weaker. They will eventually dilate owing to the negative intrapleural pressure. As the disease advances, the bronchi become grossly dilated and pockets containing pus are formed. The elastic and muscle tissue is destroyed and the mucous lining is replaced by granulation tissue with loss of cilia. Passage of

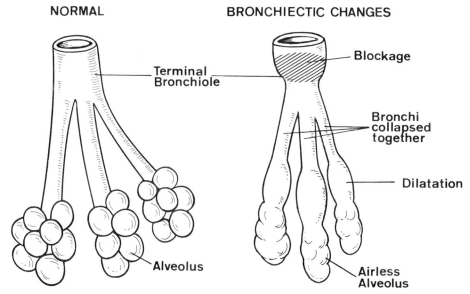

Figure 13.7 Changes of bronchiectasis

mucus out of the lungs is therefore hindered. The arterial vessels within the bronchial walls anastomose with the pulmonary capillaries and this results in the common feature of haemoptysis. Loss of aerated lung tissue results in the bronchi coming together (Figure 13.7).

Clinical features

1. *Onset* – Although symptoms often begin in childhood, diagnosis is not usually made until adult life.
2. *Cough and sputum* – These patients complain of persistent cough with purulent sputum since childhood. Initially it would only be present following colds or influenza but if the disease is allowed to progress in its severity the affected segments continually accumulate purulent secretions resulting in cough and sputum production. The sputum is usually green, often foul smelling and it is present in fairly large volume. The cough is particularly troublesome on a change of position and on rising in the early morning.
3. *Dyspnoea* – Only noticeable if the disease is particularly severe and widespread.
4. *Haemoptysis* – This occurs quite commonly usually associated with an acute infection.
5. *Recurrent pneumonia* – Characteristically this will affect the same site.
6. *Halitosis* – The breath is fetid.
7. *Chronic sinusitis* – Occurs in approximately 70% of the patients.

8. *General ill health* – e.g. pyrexia, night sweats, anorexia, malaise, weight loss and lassitude.
9. *Clubbing* – In about 50% of the patients fingers and toes become clubbed.
10. *Thoracic mobility* – Gradually decreases as do shoulder girdle movements.

Investigations

Bacteriology – Initially the sputum culture will isolate *Haemophilus influenzae* and Staphylococcus. In the later stages of the disease *Pseudomonas aeruginosa* and Klebsiella may be isolated.

Chest radiograph – Initially this will be normal but the patient gradually develops increase in the bronchovascular markings and sometimes multiple cysts with fluid levels.

Bronchography is used for the accurate localization of area affected.

Prognosis

The vast majority of these patients can lead normal lives with a nearly normal life expectancy provided the medical care is adequate.

Complications

1. Recurrent haemoptysis.
2. Pleurisy and empyema.
3. Abcess formation (lung/cerebrum).

4. Emphysema.
5. Respiratory failure.
6. Right ventricular failure.
7. Pneumonia.

Principles of treatment

1. *Relieve obstruction* before permanent damage occurs.
2. *Control infection* – Antibiotics given prophylactically in all but very mild cases. Dosage or drug is altered if an acute infection occurs.
3. *Promote good health* with good diet and fresh air.
4. *Surgery* may be indicated in young patients with localized disease. Operation of choice would be segmental resection or lobectomy (see Chapter 14).

Physiotherapy

Aims of treatment

1. To remove secretions and clear lung fields.
2. To teach good coughing technique.
3. To gain patient's confidence.
4. To maintain mobility of the thorax and good posture.
5. To promote good general health.
6. To teach the patient how to fit in home treatment within the life-style.

Treatment

Clearing secretions

Postural drainage is essential and the position must be accurate for the areas of lung affected. Accuracy is judged by production of sputum and by identification of the affected areas on a chest radiograph. If the disease is in the lower lobe the order of positioning should be:

1. Prone lying with 45 cm tip.
2. Side lying with most affected side uppermost and 45 cm tip.
3. Supine lying with 45 cm tip.
4. Side lying on other side with 45 cm tip.

This minimizes the danger of secretion overspill into the least affected side which could cause spread of the disease or pneumonia. Percussion, shaking and vibrations are also necessary and must be accurately applied over the affected area of the lungs. The patient may be taught forced expiration technique (FET) (see Chapter 12). Localized expansion breathing exercises are also taught and in these ways mucous plugs and pus are moved to the trachea from where they are cleared by coughing.

A combination of these treatments must be performed 2–3 times daily by the patient. It is important to ensure that the patient has disposable sputum pots and polythene or paper bags to dispose of the infected sputum without the risk of re-infection or endangering other members of the family.

Mobility of the thorax, good posture and good general health are achieved by the patient performing a daily exercise programme. This comprises general deep breathing and two or three exercises. Also, the patient should be encouraged to partake in sports, such as jogging, walking, cycling, tennis or swimming. Following this regimen the patient should have a full active life. Should the patient develop a cold or influenza antibiotics must be readily available together with physiotherapy so that infection and secretions can be cleared promptly.

In a young patient where the disease is localized an area of the lung may be removed in a segmentectomy or lobectomy, but this process is now rare.

Cystic fibrosis

Synonyms – Mucoviscidosis, fibrocystic disease of the pancreas.

Cystic fibrosis is a disorder of exocrine glands, with a high sodium chloride content in sweat and pancreatic insufficiency resulting in malabsorption. There is hypertrophy and hyperplasia of mucus-secreting glands resulting in excessive mucus production in the lining of bronchi which predisposes the patient to chronic bronchopulmonary infection.

Aetiology – It is the commonest hereditary disorder, being transmitted by a recessive gene which is estimated to be present in 1 in 20 in the United Kingdom. The disease was first recognized in the late 1930's. Amongst Caucasians, the incidence is approximately 1 in 2000 live births but the disease is rare in Asians and Africans.

Prognosis – With early diagnosis and good management, the life expectancy of patients with cystic fibrosis is increasing and survival may be to the third or fourth decade. The majority, however, die before 40 years of age from respiratory failure related to pulmonary infection or from absorption and nutrition problems.

Pathological changes

Pulmonary changes

1. *Excessive mucus* – There is excess mucus production especially in the small bronchi and bronchioles. These respiratory passages are structurally normal at birth but become blocked by mucous plugs.
2. *Viscid mucus* – The abnormality in the mucous glands results in production of mucus with a

reduced water content so that the secretions produced are very viscid and stick to the bronchial walls.

3. *Infection* – The accumulated mucus provides a medium for growth of bacteria and so the secretions become infected and purulent. This leads to irritation of the bronchial wall tissue which then becomes inflamed.

4. *Bronchiectasis* – Inflammation leads to weakening of the bronchial walls and dilatations occur as in bronchiectasis.

5. *Lack of development of lung tissue* – Mucus and inflammation resulting in airway obliteration inhibits the development of normal lung tissue.

Other changes

Fibrosis of the pancreas causes digestive malfunction and may lead to development of diabetes.

Intestinal obstruction may occur owing to gallstones or faecal impaction. In newborn babies, there is intestinal obstruction – known as meconium ileus because there is excess meconium (a greenish black viscid discharge from the bowel of newborn babies) which plugs the small intestine necessitating an emergency operation. Right ventricular hypertrophy occurs owing to pulmonary congestion which develops as fibrosis and thickening of the pulmonary arterial walls takes place.

Clinical features

Children

1. Meconium ileus present in approximately 10%.
2. Failure to thrive and gain weight.
3. Cough producing copious, often purulent, sputum.
4. Dyspnoea.
5. Wheezing (50%).
6. High level of sodium in sweat.
7. Frequent, foul-smelling stools.

Adolescents and adults

1. Progressive breathlessness.
2. Reduced FEV_1 as chronic airways obstruction develops.
3. Continued wheezing and productive cough with purulent sputum from which may be cultured strains of pseudomonas or staphylococcus.
4. Haemoptysis.
5. Chest radiograph shows hyperinflation.
6. Finger clubbing.
7. Puberty delayed.
8. Infertility of males occurs owing to blockage of the vas deferens.

Terminal features

1. Respiratory failure.
2. Cyanosis.
3. Cor pulmonale.

Complications

1. Haemoptysis.
2. Spontaneous pneumothorax.
3. Lung abscesses, bronchiectasis.
4. Meconium ileus equivalent in adults.
5. Liver disease.
6. Psycho-social disturbance. The essential daily postural drainage can create stresses in the family for both parents and siblings. Loss of schooling leads to impairment of intellectual development.

Management

General

Diet

A low-fat high-calorie diet is recommended supplemented with vitamins. Pancreatic enzymes are given before each meal to improve absorption.

Drugs

Antibiotics are essential and the patient is on one form or another for life.

Bronchodilators – These may be useful when there is airways obstruction which is reversible.

Oxygen – Oxygen therapy may be appropriate in the terminal stages when there is persistent hypoxaemia.

Physiotherapy

Daily physiotherapy for life is an essential part of the treatment of the pulmonary features of cystic fibrosis, and must begin as soon as the diagnosis is made. Parents, relatives and friends have to become involved in assistance with postural drainage and percussion.

The aims of physiotherapy are:

1. To clear the lung fields.
2. To maintain mobility of the shoulder girdle and thorax.
3. To train postural awareness and relaxation.
4. To encourage activities for maintaining physical fitness.

Principles

Clearing lung fields

This is achieved by the use of postural drainage, breathing exercises, percussion, shaking, inhalations, coughing and huffing.

Prior to these techniques it is useful to have an active game with a child so that he or she laughs, producing deeper respiration and then becomes breathless.

Postural drainage

This is required twice a day – every day even when the patient is apparently well. During exacerbations, or when the patient has an upper respiratory tract infection, postural drainage has to be increased up to as much as six times per day. Each session requires up to 20 minutes.

A baby is positioned on a pillow on the knee of either the physiotherapist or parent. The physiotherapist has to work out the most effective position for each individual patient and relate the treatment to the home situation. As the child grows, there comes a stage where it is necessary to position for drainage using cushions, or a newspaper parcel. A tipping frame (see Figure 12.13, page 179) which supports the patient totally is more comfortable for draining the anterior and lateral segments of the lower lobes, and middle lobe or lingula. Adolescents and adult patients may have blocks made so that their own bed may be tipped. Postural drainage should be programmed to avoid mealtimes. Early morning and late evening are suitable times for most adults but children may be treated early evening.

Breathing exercises

Localized expansion exercises for the area being drained should be practised during postural drainage to help loosen secretions.

Percussion

Clapping should be given over the segment which is being drained. To be comfortable and effective this must be skilfully applied. It is essential to emphasize to the parents the following points:

1. The technqiue is given over clothes or a blanket to minimize skin stimulation.
2. The hands must remain cupped with the fingers extended and the metacarpo-phalangeal joints flexed and the thumb tip held on the lateral side of the index finger.
3. Practising the technique on one's own thigh helps to acquire the correct wrist and arm movement so that there is no stinging or discomfort.
4. Under no circumstances whatsoever should a whole arm, flat handed action be used. The technique is clapping, NOT bashing or slapping.
5. Incorrect percussion is ineffective and cruel, causing as it does distress to the patient and it may well contribute to difficulties with parent–child relationships.

Self-percussion can be taught, using firm adduction movements of the arms with the elbows held in flexion. This is useful for adults and some children can be taught.

On a very young baby, percussion is applied with the fingertips.

Shaking and vibrations

These techniques are applied to the area being drained. Again relatives must be taught how to give these techniques with the expiratory phase. For a baby, two fingers can apply sufficient force.

Inhalations/humidification

Some form of humidification is useful to reduce the viscosity of the mucus, and may be applied using a mouthpiece and nebulizer. For babies and children a mask may be necessary. Saline acts as a mucolytic agent. For home use patients may have an electric compressor with a nebulizer.

Coughing and huffing

This is the natural way to clear secretions. Patients need to be taught to breathe in deeply, prior to coughing so that a force is generated behind the secretions. Huffing is a particularly useful technique for moving secretions towards the trachea while the patient is in a postural drainage position. The patient is instructed to take a short breath in then breathe out with force through the open mouth. A programme of thoracic expansion exercises, diaphragmatic breathing control and huffing in a postural drainage position should be developed to the individual patient's needs.

Removal of secretions

When the sputum reaches the mouth, the patient must spit into a disposable container or a pot which can be sterilized and from which the sputum may be emptied down a toilet. For children under 3 years and babies the sputum needs to be cleared by a tissue. Disposal of infected sputum must be discussed with parents, relatives or patient as it is essential to avoid reinfection. They should *NOT* swallow the sputum as this may cause an exacerbation of the abdominal symptoms.

Mobility of the shoulder girdle and thorax

This is achieved by free active exercises, activities and expansion breathing exercises.

Suitable free active exercises are:

1. Sitting: arms circling backwards.

2. Bend sitting: elbows circling backwards.
3. Sitting: trunk bending backwards.
4. Under bend sitting: trunk bending side to side.
5. Sitting: trunk turning with loose arm flinging.

Activities for children may include:

1. Windmills – for alternate arm circling.
2. Passing a ball overhead to a partner behind.
3. Passing a ball overhead and behind back from one hand to the other.

Suitable activities for adults or children may be: netball, basketball, volleyball, swimming.

Expansion breathing exercises for the basal areas help to maintain the mobility of the thorax. Localized expansion of the apical areas is necessary only if there is accumulation of secretions in the upper lobes and should be avoided if, as the disease progresses, there is hyperinflation of these areas.

Postural awareness and relaxation

Children should be encouraged to join in physical education activities at school. At home parents should be taught to recognize the poor posture of head forward, rounded shoulders and kyphosis of the thoracic spine and encourage the patient to stretch 'tall as a house' or 'straight as a guardsman'. Localized shoulder girdle relaxation may be taught as 'push your shoulders down and back then leave them there'. Diaphragmatic control is taught for the patient to regain quiet respiration after becoming breathless.

Maintenance of physical fitness

This is achieved by encouraging the parents to treat the child as normally as possible so that the child joins in physical activities at school and with friends at weekends. It is helpful for the parents to meet the child's teachers so that they know to encourage the child to participate fully in school life. Adults may benefit from regular swimming, or short sessions of jogging.

Physiotherapy for these patients is related to the stages of the disease. Initially, the physiotherapist at the specialist hospital where the condition is diagnosed will devise a programme and teach the parents. During exacerbations of infection, patients may be admitted to their local hospital where intensive physiotherapy is essential. A community physiotherapist should visit the patient's home at regular intervals and will become very well known to the involved family. The patient has to attend regular follow-up clinics to be seen by a chest specialist as well as being taken care of by the general practitioner.

Complications
Haemoptysis

If this occurs, postural drainage should continue but percussion is stopped. It is also important to ensure that the patient is using huffing and avoiding strain with coughing.

Pneumothorax

The management of pneumothorax involves insertion of a drainage tube and this makes percussion and drainage difficult, but although there may be a short interruption, physiotherapy is quickly restarted with the use of analgesics if necessary.

Socio-psychological

The disease carries with it some unfortunate social and psychological problems. Coughing and spitting is antisocial, therefore people in avoiding the patient are unwittingly unkind. The parents feel guilty as they are carrying the gene. They have to spend a lot of time with the patient which creates resentment in siblings. The patient on reaching adolescence may become resentful of treatment and increasing inability to participate in a full active life. Clearly this is only a brief mention of the total picture of which the physiotherapist must be aware.

Terminal stages

This is a distressing time as the patient becomes very ill and recognizes that death is imminent. The principal theme is to keep the patient comfortable which usually means sedation. Physiotherapy is reduced to breathing exercises with some shaking if the patient wants it.

Lung abscess
Definition

A lung abscess is the localized formation of pus, usually surrounded by a fibrous capsule, within lung tissue.

Aetiology

Antibiotics and improved anaesthesia have reduced the incidence of lung abscess and the condition tends now to occur secondary to bronchial carcinoma particularly in patients who are over 40.

Causes

A variety of bacteria may enter the lungs by one of the following routes:

1. Through the air passages due to broncho-pneumonia or following inhalation of a foreign body.
2. Through the open chest wall following a wound from a knife stab or bullet.
3. From the bloodstream.
4. Secondary to bronchial carcinoma an abscess forms where secretions accumulate distal to the tumour.

Pathology

The invading organisms cause inflammation of the lung tissue and suppuration occurs. At the centre of the area there is necrosis of lung tissue with liquefaction and suppuration. The area becomes distended and fibroblasts lay down fibrous tissue around the area until there is complete encapsulation. The capsule contracts and the abscess bursts, resulting in the production of foul smelling sputum. Sometimes the pus drains into the pleura, causing empyema, and if drainage spills into adjacent lung tissue there is a danger of bronchiectasis. Toxins from the pus can be absorbed into the bloodstream and there is then a danger of septicaemia.

Healing occurs with the formation of a fibrous scar.

Clinical features

There is:

1. Malaise.
2. Fever.
3. Dyspnoea.
4. Pain sometimes.
5. Cough which is at first irritable and unproductive then is productive of foul smelling sputum accompanied by a bad taste in the mouth.
6. Haemoptysis.
7. Halitosis.
8. Radiograph shows a fluid level.

Prognosis

With prompt treatment the patient should recover but if untreated the patient can be very ill.

Management

Antibiotics are administered for at least 6 weeks to ensure that there is no recurrence.

Surgery may be necessary if antibiotics are not successful and is carried out on patients where a tumour is discovered.

Physiotherapy

The main aim is to promote drainage.

The site of the abscess is ascertained on the radiograph and the patient is positioned accurately for 10–15 minutes every 4 hours. Shaking is applied to the chest wall and breathing exercises are taught to regain breath control after coughing. Deep inspiration should not be encouraged because the increase in negative pressure may move the pus through healthy lung tissue. It is important to adjust the patient's position to obtain maximum effective drainage and to ensure that precautions are taken to avoid any danger of cross-infection.

Pneumonia

Definition

Pneumonia is an inflammation of the lung tissue, i.e. alveoli and adjacent airways.

Classification

The disease may be classified anatomically as lobular, lobar or segmental. Bilateral lobular pneumonia is termed bronchopneumonia.

Aetiology

Pneumonia is a common disease which affects all age groups and may be fatal in the very young and elderly.

Predisposing factors

These are: winter or springtime, overcrowding where bacteria and viruses are easily transmitted, alcoholism, smoking, atmospheric pollution, lower socio-economic groups.

The disease may also occur secondary to: impaired consciousness, malnutrition, obstruction by a foreign body or tumour, influenza, chronic bronchitis, and chicken pox.

Causes

The commonest cause is infection by bacteria such as *Streptococcus pneumoniae* or *pyogenes, Staphylococcus pyogenes* and *Klebsiella pneumoniae,* mycoplasmal pneumoniae. *Legionella pneumophia* causes pneumonia known as legionnaires' disease.

Pathology

The invading organism causes inflammation in the bronchioles and alveoli. The exudate spreads into neighbouring alveoli providing a medium for rapid spread of bacteria. The alveoli become filled with red blood cells, leucocytes, macrophages and fibrin and there is congestion throughout the lobe. Resolution occurs when the leucocytes engulf the bacteria and macrophages clear the debris by phagocytosis. The inflammation can spread to the pleura and cause a fibrinous pleurisy. In lobular or bronchopneumonia the inflammation is scattered irregularly in the lungs whereas in lobar pneumonia the inflammation is spread throughout but contained within one entire lobe.

Clinical features

Onset

This may be sudden (lobar pneumonia) or gradual (bronchopneumonia or lobular pneumonia) and is associated with:

1. Malaise.
2. Fever (temperature of 38°–40°C).
3. Rigors.
4. Vomiting.
5. Confusion due to hypoxaemia, especially in the elderly.
6. Tachycardia.

Cough

This is dry at first but after a few days purulent sputum is produced.

Breathlessness

Blood passing through the affected alveolar membranes is inadequately oxygenated so the Pao_2 falls. Hyperventilation cannot compensate for this hypoxaemia because blood passing through the normal lung tissue is almost saturated. The inflammation also makes the lung stiff and compliance is reduced with the result that the effort of breathing is harder. Respiration therefore becomes rapid and shallow.

Pain

If inflammation spreads to the pleura there is a sharp pain aggravated by taking a deep breath or coughing.

Radiograph

Consolidation can be seen as an opacity especially in lobar pneumonia.

Auscultation

Bronchial breathing can be heard (especially in lobar pneumonia) because the consolidated lung tissue conducts the sounds of air movement in the trachea. *Vocal resonance* – whispering pectoriloquy and increased vocal resonance can be heard.

Prognosis

This depends on predisposing factors, the virulence of the bacteria and age and fitness of the patient. Improvement starts within 3–4 days of the patient having antibiotics, and within 10 days the sputum should be less in quantity and mucoid in nature by which time the patient is better. In an otherwise fit person, the radiograph should be clear in 6 weeks. Generally lobar pneumonia resolves and the patient recovers. This tends to be in people who are generally fit and are between the ages of 20 and 50 years. Bronchopneumonia is more serious, is often secondary to other problems and may be the terminal illness in patients who are elderly. The disease may be fatal in the very young because the secretions readily block the narrow, underdeveloped airways.

Management

1. General.
2. Antibiotics are given to control infection.
3. Adequate fluids must be taken to ensure fluid balance.
4. Analgesics are given to relieve pleuritic pain.
5. Oxygen therapy may be necessary.
6. Bed rest at home may be sufficient but a desperately ill patient has to be admitted to hospital.

Physiotherapy

Physiotherapy is indicated when the inflammation has begun to resolve. The aims of treatment are to:

1. Clear lung fields of secretions.
2. Gain full re-expansion of the lungs.
3. Regain exercise tolerance and fitness.

Clearing lung fields

Humidification may be necessary to moisten secretions. The method will vary according to the severity of the illness and may be by steam inhalation, neubulizer or IPPB. Clapping, shaking, and breathing exercises may all be necessary in a postural drainage position appropriate to the area of the lung affected. Sometimes suction is required for the very ill patient who cannot cough or expectorate. If there is an underlying bronchospasm then a bronchodilator may be given.

Re-expansion of the lungs

Expansion breathing exercises local to the affected area help to encourage ventilation of the alveoli when secretions have been cleared.

Exercise tolerance and fitness

As soon as possible, the patient should perform graded active exercises for the limbs and trunk and start walking short distances which are progressively increased in length.

Complications of pneumonia

These may be:

1. Spread to other lung areas.
2. Delayed resolution.
3. Pleural disease resulting in pleural effusion or empyema.
4. Lung abscess.
5. Cardiac failure.
6. Septicaemia.
7. Pneumococcal meningitis.

Acute bronchitis

This is acute inflammation of the bronchial tree.

Causes

Secondary to viral, chemical, physical irritation, e.g. colds, 'flu', irritant gases. Rarely presents a problem in the young fit adult. Population at risk includes the very young and the very old, those with existing history of diseases such as leukaemia. In these patients acute bronchitis could result in further complication such as respiratory failure or pneumonia.

Signs and symptoms

1. Irritating unproductive cough which becomes productive after a couple of days.
2. Upper retrosternal pain which increases on coughing.
3. Raw feeling in throat.
4. Pyrexia and malaise.
5. Wheezing and dyspnoeas (if previous lung disorder is present).
6. Usually clears within 7–14 days.

Treatment

1. Antibiotic – usually tetracycline or ampicillin.
2. Drugs to relieve pain and suppress cough, e.g. codeine lincuts, aspirin. THESE MUST NEVER BE GIVEN TO A PATIENT IN RESPIRATORY FAILURE FROM THE ACUTE BRONCHITIS.
3. Humidification – e.g. benzoin tincture inhalants may be helpful.
4. Bronchodilators if necessary.
5. Physiotherapy:
   (a) Postural drainage.
   (b) Breathing exercises.
   (c) Coughing.
   Associated with IPPB or nebulizer.

Pulmonary tuberculosis

In 1882 Robert Koch isolated the tubercle bacillus of which there are two types, one human and the other bovine. Since then the disease has been controlled by inoculation, mass radiography, drugs and pasteurized milk.

Types of TB other than pulmonary:

1. *Acute miliary* – Blood affected with spread of the disease to spleen, liver, kidneys, meninges and lymph nodes.
2. *Surgical* – Bones or joints affected.
3. *TB adenoma* – Lymph nodes affected.
4. *Lupus vulgaris* – Skin affected.

Aetiology

The disease is still very common in countries like Africa and Asia. In Europe the commonest affected age group is middle age but it also often occurs in elderly men. In Britain, the disease occurs mainly in the immigrant population from India and Pakistan.

Predisposing factors

These are: environment, poor hygiene, overcrowding, lower socio-economic groups, malnutrition, smoking and alcoholism. Diseases such as diabetes mellitus, congenital heart disorder, leukaemia, Hodgkin's disease, long-term corticosteroids or immunosuppressive drugs.

Causes

Mycobacterium tuberculosis is the bacillus responsible for the disease. It is spread by droplets so that a person can be infected from a patient's sputum.

Pathology

The bacillus causes irritation of the mucous lining in the bronchioles or alveoli and inflammatory changes take place. The bacilli are ingested by leucocytes and then absorbed by macrophages. More leucocytes form a barrier round this collection of cells and the complete mass is known as a tuberculous follicle. The centre of the area undergoes necrosis and becomes soft and cheesy in consistency, the process being known as caseation. This material may be moved into a bronchus and coughed up leaving a cavity behind. Fibroblasts lay down a capsule around the tubercle in which lime salts become deposited and healing takes place. Cavity formation and calcification are the features of TB with the calcified lesion remaining a potential source of infection. The bacillus may be reactivated and cause postprimary pulmonary tuberculosis. The danger then is that the disease may spread to other areas of the lungs including the pleura and through the bloodstream to other parts of the body.

Clinical features

These are:

1. Malaise
2. Lassitude.
3. Irritability.
4. Loss of appetite and loss of weight.
5. Pyrexia and tachycardia.
6. Night sweats.
7. Productive cough – bacillus can be cultured from the sputum.
8. Haemoptysis.
9. Diminished respiratory movements with possibly some dyspnoea.
10. Pain if there is pleural involvement.
11. Radiograph – cavity formation and calcification can be seen.

In children these clinical features may be present to a mild degree and the disease can pass undetected.

Treatment

Prevention

Vaccination of people who are at risk greatly reduces the incidence of the disease. These people may be in contact with a patient who has active TB, e.g. relatives, friends, teachers, doctors, nurses, physiotherapists. Pasteurization of milk prevents transmission of the tubercle to humans from cows.

Drug therapy

This together with rest is the treatment for curing TB. Drugs used are rifampicin, isoniazid, ethambu-tol, para-aminosalicylic acid (PAS) which are anti-TB and must be taken every day for up to 18 months. Streptomycin may also be prescribed.

Surgery

This is appropriate only in a very small proportion of patients. If a patient has a resistant tubercle a lobectomy may be performed but the patient must still be on a programme of drugs.

Physiotherapy

This is not usually indicated during the rest stage. Once the patient is ambulent, a graded programme of exercises may be required. If it is necessary to give breathing exercises, the physiotherapist should stand behind the patient to avoid droplet infection as the patient coughs. Sputum must be disposed of very carefully so that cross-infection is prevented.

Bronchial and lung tumours

These may be benign or malignant. The majority are malignant growths which may be primary or secondary.

Aetiology of malignant tumours

Incidence

In the United Kingdom, there are approximately 35 000 deaths from carcinoma of the bronchus each year. Men are more commonly affected than women.

Smoking

There is a direct relationship between smoking and development of the disease in that people who smoke have a much greater risk of developing the disease than those who do not.

Environment

The disease is more prevalent in urban dwellers than in rural dwellers. There is also evidence that exposure to substances termed carcinogens either at work or leisure can result in development of the disease. Carcinogens may be radioactive materials, asbestos, nickel, chromates, or industrial arsenic.

Pathology

The majority of tumours originate in the large bronchi and spread by direct invasion of the lung, chest wall and mediastinal structures. The tumour grows to occlude the lumen of the bronchus and then atelectasis distal to the growth will occur.

There are different histological types, the commonest is squamous cell carcinoma which is late to metastasize. Others are anaplastic or oat cell which metastasizes early and carries a poor prognosis; adenocarcinoma which arises in the periphery of the bronchi; and alveolar cell which arises from the alveolar type 2 cell and is the rarest form.

Clinical features

The onset is insidious, and the clinical features may present in a variety of ways:

1. *Cough* – This is the commonest feature which is often ignored by the patient who may associate it with smoking. Initially the cough is dry and irritating but may become productive if infection occurs in accumulated secretions.
2. *Haemoptysis* – There are recurrent small spots of blood in the sputum.
3. *Dyspnoea* – This is highly variable and may be severe when there is pulmonary collapse or pleural effusion.
4. *Pain* – Dull, deep-seated pain is common but it may be pleuritic in nature or intercostal when there is rib disease.
5. *Malaise and weight loss* are associated with late stages of the disease.
6. *Radiograph* – This often detects a tumour developing with no clinical features and reveals the site of the tumour.
7. *Bronchitis, pneumonia or lung abscess* may arise as a result of a tumour.

Prognosis

This depends on the type of tumour but overall the average length of survival after diagnosis is around a year. Surgery can prolong the life of some patients.

Treatment

This may be surgery, chemotherapy, or radiotherapy.

Surgery

This comprises removing the lobe or lung whilst the tumour remains localized and in the absence of metastases.

Chemotherapy

Cytotoxic drugs are used with increasing regularity. Results are mixed but anaplastic tumours tend to respond to this type of treatment.

Radiotherapy

Radiotherapy is used symptomatically particularly to relieve pain.

Drug therapy is essentially symptomatic and includes analgesics and antibiotics.

Physiotherapy

Physiotherapy may be related to three aspects of management of the disease:

1. *Pre/post operative* – Physiotherapy is essential for patients who have a lobectomy or pneumonectomy as described in Chapter 14.
2. *During/after radiotherapy* – Once the tumour begins to decrease in size the patient will begin to expectorate sputum. Postural drainage with vibrations may be required. Percussion and vigorous shakings should not be used where there is a danger of pathological fractures in ribs or vertebrae in which metastases may be developing nor should they be used in the presence of haemoptysis.
3. *During terminal stages of the disease* – Where accumulation of secretions is causing distress, modified postural drainage and vibrations with breathing exercises may help to make the patient more comfortable. If coughing is ineffective suction may have to be used. An active daily programme which fits the patient's requirements may need to be devised in which case the physiotherapist works in close collaboration with the health care team.

Pneumothorax

This is air in the pleural cavity. There are two different types: spontaneous and traumatic.

Spontaneous

This can occur at any age but is commonest in young men who are otherwise apparently healthy. It may also be associated with emphysema and chronic bronchitis in men over 50 years of age.

Aetiology

Causes

1. Rupture of a pleural 'bleb' in the region of the apex of the lung. A 'bleb' is like a cyst filled with air and is thought to be caused by a congenital defect in the alveolar wall.
2. Rupture of an emphysematous bulla which lies just below the pleura in widespread emphysema.

3. Rupture of a lung abscess or tuberculous lesion into the pleural cavity. If pus enters the pleural cavity as well as air, it is termed pyopneumothorax.

Pathology

As the air escapes into the pleural cavity, reducing the subatmospheric pressure (i.e. less negative) the lung collapses. The hole in the pleura closes, the air becomes absorbed and the lung gradually re-expands. Sometimes this does not happen and the hole in the pleura becomes like a valve. Air then enters the pleural cavity on inspiration but cannot escape during expiration. The lung remains collapsed and as air accumulates in the pleural cavity there is displacement of the heart together with compression of the other lung and great vessels. This is termed a tension pneumothorax and has to be treated as an emergency by needle aspiration and thereafter by insertion of a drain connected to an underwater seal.

Traumatic

Aetiology

Causes

1. Penetrating rib fractures.
2. Penetrating wounds, e.g. from bullet or knife stab.
3. Accidental opening of pleural cavity during abdominal surgery.
4. Penetration of the pleura during insertion of a central venous pressure catheter.
5. Crush injuries to the chest wall.

When the chest wall remains intact the condition is termed a closed pneumothorax but if the chest wall is opened the term used is open pneumothorax. In the presence of an open wound the emergency treatment is the applicaiton of a large dressing pad over the chest wall.

Clinical features

1. Onset is often sudden with severe chest pain and progressive breathlessness.
2. Diminished chest movement unilaterally.
3. Absence of breath sounds often over the apex of the affected side.
4. Radiograph has absence of lung markings and the edge of the collapsed lung can be seen.
5. Other clinical features may be related to the underlying pathology, e.g. emphysema.

Treatment

A small pneumothorax requires no treatment apart from a few days' bed rest until it resolves. A large pneumothorax (i.e. more than 25% of the pleural space is filled with air) is treated by needle aspiration or by an intercostal drain which connects the pleural cavity to a drainage bottle creating an underwater seal (see Chapter 14). The drain is removed when there are no more bubbles in the drainage bottle indicating that the pleural cavity is air free. Surgery is indicated for a recurrent pneumothorax. Pleurodesis comprises the insertion of a powder into the pleural cavity. This acts as an irritant to the pleural surfaces causing them to adhere to each other. Pleurectomy is the removal of the parietal pleura from the chest wall leaving a raw surface to which the visceral layer sticks. A hole in the visceral pleura may have to be stitched.

Physiotherapy

A patient who has an underwater drainage system requires expansion breathing exercises to re-expand the lung. Also, full-range shoulder movements are necessary to maintain shoulder, shoulder girdle and thoracic mobility. This treatment is generally given 3–4 times daily until the drain is removed.

Following pleurodesis, expansion breathing exercises are essential to ensure that when the adhesions form between the layers of the pleura, the lung is fully expanded. The patient must be taught to practise the breathing exercises so that thoracic mobility is maintained, otherwise there may be sharp pleuritic pain if the intrapleural adhesions become too contracted. Sometimes Entonox (nitrous oxide and oxygen) is provided for the patient to reduce the pain after the operation. If the lung does not re-expand within 36 hours then a second operation is required. Physiotherapy after a pleurectomy follows the same principles as for any thoracotomy (see Chapter 14).

Pleurisy

Definition

Pleurisy is inflammation of the pleura. Three types may be considered:

1. Dry pleurisy.
2. Pleural effusion.
3. Empyema thoracis.

Dry pleurisy

Aetiology

This condition is common in town dwellers where there is dust and grit in the atmosphere. It may also be secondary to tuberculosis or lobar pneumonia.

Pathological changes

Infection or irritation of the pleura causes inflammation. There is vascular congestion. A fibrinous exudate is formed within the pleural cavity and the pleural surfaces are roughened. The inflammation may resolve or develop into a pleural effusion, depending upon any underlying conditions. When resolution occurs fibrin laid down within the exudate tends to form adhesions between the two layers of the pleura.

Clinical features

Pleuritic pain aggravated by inspiration due to stretching of the inflamed pleura. Limited thoracic expansion at the affected area.

Pleural rub – A creaking or grating sound heard through a stethoscope on both inspiration and expiration localized to the affected area. This disappears when an effusion develops.

Cough, tachycardia and pyrexia may be present depending on associated conditions.

Radiograph – The diaphragm may be raised on the affected side.

Treatment

Identification and treatment of any underlying conditions is essential. Analgesics are given to relieve pain and possibly sedative linctus may be given to reduce coughing. Rest is important to allow the inflammation to subside and to minimize the pain.

Physiotherapy

This is not usually appropriate in the early stages. During the recovery stage, the aims are:

1. To regain full thoracic expansion.
2. To minimize adhesion formation between the pleural layers.
3. To mobilize the thorax.

Thoracic expansion is regained by teaching the patient localized expansion exercises with manual resistance over the affected area both to guide rib movement and relieve pain. General deep breathing exercises and mobility exercises such as sitting trunk bending side to side are important to regain mobility of the thorax and thoracic spine.

Pleural effusion

This is accumulation of fluid in the pleural cavity.

Aetiology

This may follow unresolved dry pleurisy. It is often secondary to conditions such as:

1. Malignancy of the lungs or bronchi.
2. Pneumonia.
3. Tuberculosis.
4. Pulmonary infarction.
5. Bronchiectasis.
6. Lung abscess.
7. Blockage of lymph vessels.
8. Rupture of blood vessels.

Pathological changes

Fluid accumulates in the pleural cavity. The composition varies according to the underlying cause. The fluid may be reabsorbed naturally or removed by surgical intervention. As the pleural layers come together they may become adherent owing to organization of fibrin if the fluid contains plasma proteins.

Fluid may accumulate in the pleural cavity as transudate or exudate. Transudate occurs when there is an increased pulmonary capillary pressure (as in congestive cardiac failure) or a decreased osmotic pressure (as in hypoproteinaemia associated with malnutrition) across the pleural membrane. Exudate occurs when there is inflammation resulting in increased permeability of capillaries and visceral pleura together with impaired lymphatic reabsorption (as in pneumonia or malignancy). Exudate is cloudy with a high protein content as opposed to transudate which is clear with a low protein content. Consequently exudate tends to become consolidated whereas transudate can be reabsorbed if the underlying condition is treated.

Clinical features

1. Breathlessness – Owing to pressure of fluid reducing lung expansion.
2. Cyanosis – May be present in a large effusion.
3. Pyrexia.
4. Lethargy.
5. Pain is less than in dry pleurisy because the fluid stops the inflamed surfaces of the pleura rubbing together.
6. Thoracic expansion is restricted.
7. Radiograph – A fluid level can be identified.

Treatment

If the fluid does not become reabsorbed naturally, then it should be aspirated. Oxygen therapy may be necessary.

Physiotherapy

The aims of physiotherapy are:

1. To assist the absorption of the fluid.
2. To prevent the formation of disabling adhesions between the two layers of pleura.
3. To obtain full expansion of the affected lung.
4. To increase ventilation of the lungs.
5. To maintain or increase the mobility of the thorax.

The treatment must be modified to take into account any underlying condition.

Following aspiration, breathing exercises to encourage localized expansion of the affected side are given. The patient is encouraged to practise these exercises possibly with the aid of a belt. If the patient has difficulty in localizing the expansion, it may be helpful to lie on the unaffected side over a firm pillow to help stretch the affected side. Breathing exercises may also be practised in this position several times a day.

When the patient has regained lung expansion the treatment programme should be expanded to include thoracic mobility exercises.

Some malignant pleural effusions may require a pleurodesis – the insertion of a powder such as tetracycline into the pleural cavity (see Chapter 14).

Empyema thoracis

This is pus in the pleural cavity.

Aetiology

The condition usually arises secondary to pre-existing lung disease such as:

1. Bacterial pneumonia.
2. Tuberculosis.
3. Lung abscess.
4. Bronchiectasis.

It may arise as a result of a stab wound or as a complication of thoracic surgery.

Pathological changes

Infected material enters the pleural cavity. Both layers of pleura become covered in thick inflammatory exudate within which fibrous tissue is laid down. As this fibrous tissue contracts it acts as a physical barrier to lung expansion. The pressure of the fibrous tissue on the pus may cause rupture of the pleura and lung tissue and the pus may then be coughed up. Alternatively, an abscess may form. Healing occurs when the pus has been surgically removed or the infection has been overcome by the patient's natural antibodies assisted by antibiotics.

The layers of the pleura come together and adhesion formation may take place, restricting lung movement.

Clinical features

1. Pyrexia.
2. Lassitude and loss of weight.
3. Tachycardia.
4. Dyspnoea.
5. Pleuritic pain severe at first then decreasing in severity.
6. Diminished thoracic movements.
7. History of pneumonia or other associated condition.
8. Radiograph – the empyema can be seen as a D-shaped shadow, the straight line of the D being on the lung surface.

Prognosis

This depends on the cause, but untreated infection can make the patient very ill from toxins absorbed into the bloodstream (toxaemia).

Treatment

Antibiotics are given to combat infection. Aspiration through a needle inserted into the cavity may remove sufficient pus to relieve the condition but continuous underwater drainage may be necessary.

Physiotherapy

The aims are:

1. To minimize adhesion formation within the pleura.
2. To regain full lung expansion.
3. To clear the lung fields.
4. To maintain good posture and thoracic mobility.

Good posture should be encouraged whenever physiotherapy is being given. The tendency is for the patient to protect the affected side. Therefore the patient should be taught to take weight evenly on both buttocks, to keep the shoulders level and to practise stretching to the opposite side from the lesion as well as stretching backwards. Breathing exercises to expand the lung on the affected side need to be carried out three or four times daily. Postural drainage may be indicated to clear the lungs if secretions are accumulating. As the patient recovers, general leg, arm and trunk exercises should be taught. Walking should begin as soon as possible with breathing control practised over progressively longer distances and going down then up stairs incorporated. If the patient has a drainage tube inserted the physiotherapy is similar to that following a thoracotomy (see Chapter 14). If the condition results in fibrosis of the pleura which severely limits lung expansion then a rib resection may be performed and the pleura stripped off the lung (decortication). Again physiotherapy is indicated following similar principles to those in Chapter 14.

Respiratory failure

This term denotes reduction of function of the lungs due to lung disease, skeletal or neuromuscular disorder and is defined in terms of the gas tensions in the arterial blood. Normal levels are Pao_2 13.0 kPa (97 mm Hg) and $Paco_2$ 6.1 kPa (46 mm Hg) (see Chapter 12). There are two types of respiratory failure:

1. Pao_2 of less than 8.0 kPa (60 mm Hg) associated with a $Paco_2$ which is either normal or below 6.7 kPa (50 mm Hg).
2. Pao_2 of less than 8.0 kPa (60 mm Hg) associated with a raised $Paco_2$ above 6.7 kPa (50 mm Hg).

Causes

Type 1

Lung disease, resulting in hypoventilation of the alveoli which produces a ventilation/perfusion mismatch. The blood supply is normal but there is inadequate oxygen uptake from the affected alveoli. Diseases associated with this type are: early chronic bronchitis and emphysema, pneumonia, asthma, acute pulmonary oedema, pulmonary embolism, pulmonary fibrosis.

Type 2

As a result of failure of the skeletal or neuromuscular components of the respiratory system there is loss of the pump mechanism essential for ventilation of the lungs as a whole. Therefore, there is a reduced tidal volume or a reduced respiratory rate producing a rise in $Paco_2$ and a fall in Pao_2.

Disorders associated with this type are: head injuries, polyneuropathies, cervical cord injuries, advanced chronic bronchitis and emphysema, status asthmaticus, crushed chest, muscular dystrophy, myasthenia gravis.

Clinical features

Type 1 due to hypoxaemia

Restlessness, confusion, central cyanosis, tachycardia, renal failure, pulmonary hypertension. Accurate diagnosis is dependent upon arterial blood gas measurements.

Type 2 due to hypercapnia

Flapping tremor of the hands, confusion, headache, warm peripheries, tachycardia. Again, diagnosis cannot be accurate until arterial blood gases are measured.

Treatment

This must be directed towards treating the cause. In Type 1, the main problem is the hypoxaemia, therefore it is important to raise the Pao_2 by giving oxygen therapy. A Ventimask giving 35% or 40% inspired O_2 may be applied. In these patients, however, there is a danger of reducing the respiratory drive which is dependent on the anoxic state of the blood stimulating the chemoreceptors in the carotid and aortic arteries. The danger then is that the patient's respiration slows or stops and the $Paco_2$ rises resulting in confusion and coma.

Physiotherapy

It is vital to clear the lung fields of secretions. Intermittent positive pressure ventilation is applied through an endotracheal tube to assist the patient's breathing. A bronchodilator (e.g. salbutamol) is administered through the ventilator. Postural drainage modified to take account of the patient's condition is used with clapping, shaking and vibrations to loosen secretions. If the patient is too weak to cough, suction has to be used. A respiratory stimulant drug such as aminophylline or doxapram may be helpful because as the blood gases improve the patient is more able to cooperate with breathing exercises and coughing. Treatment has to be for short spells at 1 or 2 hourly intervals.

All treatment is monitored by regular blood gas analysis.

In Type 2, it is again necessary to raise the Pao_2 and this is achieved by oxygen therapy using a Ventimask delivering 24% O_2. If this is not sufficient to raise the Pao_2 the Ventimask may be changed to one delivering 28% O_2, providing that the $Paco_2$ is not rising from the already high level. If the $Paco_2$ starts to rise this is indicative of hypoventilation usually because the patient is becoming exhausted and assisted ventilation is necessary. Generally, patients with lung disease are given positive pressure ventilation whereas patients with musculoskeletal disorders and respiratory muscle paralysis are given negative pressure ventilation with a cuirass or tank respirator. Physiotherapy follows similar principles to that for Type 1 where the patient has lung disease. The patient with musculoskeletal disorder requires physiotherapy should there be accumulation of secretions and re-education of breathing as the muscles recover.

Chapter 14

Pulmonary surgery

Definitions

A thoracotomy is an incision into the thoracic cavity to gain access to lungs, bronchi, heart or oesophagus. The position of the incision relative to the thorax may be lateral (postero-lateral, antero-lateral) or anterior (transverse, vertical).

Lateral incisions

Posterolateral (Figure 14.1)

This follows the vertebral border of the scapula and the line of a rib (numbers 5, 6, 7, or 8) to the anterior angle or costal margin. The muscles cut are trapezius, latissimus dorsi, rhomboids, serratus anterior, intercostals and erector spinae. A rib may be removed so that when the other ribs are retracted there is sufficient space for access to the thorax. This incision is commonly used for lung operations.

Antero-lateral

This starts close to midline in front, follows along the line of a rib below the breast to the posterior axillary line. The muscles cut are pectoralis major and minor, serratus anterior, internal and external intercostals. This incision is used for mitral valvotomy and pleurectomy.

Anterior incisions

Transverse (submammary)

This passes across from one side of the 4th intercostal space to the other. The muscles divided

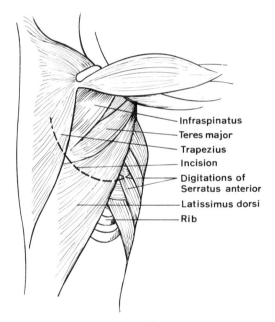

Figure 14.1 Thoracotomy incision

- Infraspinatus
- Teres major
- Trapezius
- Incision
- Digitations of Serratus anterior
- Latissimus dorsi
- Rib

are pectoralis major, internal and external intercostals. The sternum is divided transversely. It is not very often used.

Vertical (median sternotomy)

This involves splitting the sternum down the middle with no muscles cut, other than the interweaving aponeuroses of pectoralis major (see Figure 15.17). This is used for open heart surgery (see Chapter 15).

Thoraco-laparotomy incision

This is along the line of the 7th or 8th rib and there may be an abdominal incision as well. It is used for access to the oesophagus.

Indications for surgery

The indications for surgery are:

1. *Malignancy* – Primary bronchial carcinoma.
2. *Trauma* – Wounds from road traffic accidents, gunshot or knifestab.
3. *Diseases/infections* – Bronchiectasis, tuberculosis, lung abscess, large bullae.

Types of operation

1. Pneumonectomy.
2. Lobectomy.
3. Segmental or wedge resection.

Pneumonectomy is the removal of the entire lung, often with mediastinal lymph nodes or part of the thoracic wall. Lobectomy is removal of an entire lobe sometimes with a section of the thoracic wall. A sleeve resection (Figure 14.2) is removal of an upper lobe together with the section of the main bronchus from which the lobar bronchus arises (the two ends of the bronchus are sutured together). Segmental resection is the removal of a bronchopulmonary segment. Wedge resection is the removal of a small part of lung tissue.

Complications of pulmonary surgery

1. Respiratory:
   (a) Infection of lung tissue.
   (b) Consolidation/collapse of remaining lung tissue.
   (c) Pneumothorax.
   (d) Broncho-pleural fistula: This occurs when the stump of the bronchus from which the lung tissue has been removed breaks down. Fluid from the space left by the removal of the section of the lung drains into the bronchus (Figure 14.3(a)). It is more likely to occur following a pneumonectomy than a lobectomy or segmentectomy and tends to arise 8–10 days after the operation. Clinical features are tachycardia, spiky temperature and cough productive of filthy blood-stained fluid. Treatment is by antibiotics, possibly repair of the stump and/or insertion of a drainage tube into the cavity. Physiotherapy is necessary to prevent the fluid entering the remaining lung tissue. This means that the patient is treated lying on the operated side (Figure 14.3(b)) and has to be taught to keep the unaffected side uppermost (Figure 14.3(c)).
2. Circulatory:
   (a) Deep vein thrombosis.
   (b) Cardiac arrhythmias.
   (c) Tamponade (see Chapter 15).
   (d) Haemorrhage.
3. Wound:
   (a) Infection.
   (b) Failure to heal.
   (c) Adherent scar.
4. Joint stiffness:
   (a) Shoulder and shoulder girdle.
   (b) Thoracic spine.
   (c) Costo-vertebral joints.
5. Muscle weakness:
   (a) Latissimus dorsi.
   (b) Serratus anterior.
   (c) Other divided muscles.
   (d) Leg muscles if unexercised.
6. Postural deformity: Tendency to protect the scar leads to a scoliosis (concave on scar side) and forward flexion.

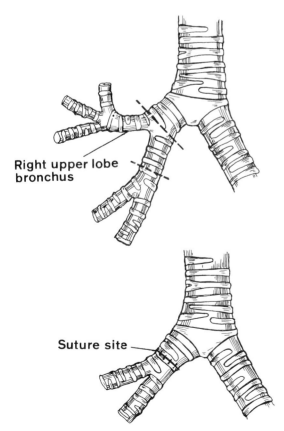

Right upper lobe bronchus

Suture site

Figure 14.2 Sleeve resection

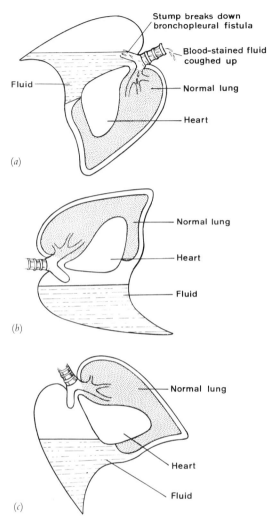

(a)

(b)

(c)

Figure 14.3 Broncho-pleural fistula. (*a*) Lying on sound side. (*b*) Lying on operation side. (*c*) Acceptable position

Drains and tubes

Two types of drains may be used – open and closed.

Open

A small tube may be inserted into a pocket of pus which then drains out onto a dressing.

Closed

These are used to drain air or fluid from the pleural cavity. Air is drained to enable the lung to re-expand following a pneumothorax or lobectomy.

Fluid is removed after any surgery that has opened the thorax to prevent a consolidated pleural effusion except after a pneumonectomy when the fluid fills in the space of the missing lung. Equipment used comprises a tube, a bottle with sterile water and possibly a suction pump. The tube passes from inside the pleural cavity down through a tight-fitting cap at the neck of the bottle to below the level of the water. This constitutes an underwater seal (Figure 14.4(a)). Air may be allowed to escape freely from a

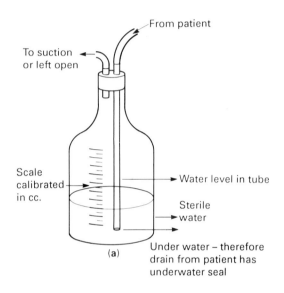

(a)

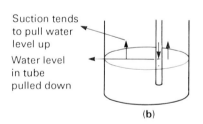

(b)

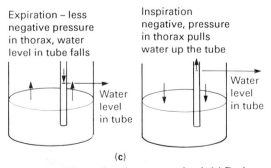

(c)

Figure 14.4 Effects of suction on water level. (*a*) Drainage bottle. (*b*) Effect of suction on water level. (*c*) Effect of patient's breathing

second tube positioned high above the water in the neck of the bottle or a suction machine may be attached to this tube. Points to be noted are:

1. Amount and type of drainage.
2. Air leak.
3. Swing of water.
4. Suction.
5. The tubes.
6. Clamps.

Amount and type of drainage

The amount of drainage is measured on a calibrated scale on the bottle, 200 ml of fluid being usual in the first 24 hours. Air drainage can be seen as bubbles in the water. If the bubbles stop, this may be because all the air in the pleural cavity has been removed or because the tube is kinked or blocked. A bottle draining either fluid or air must never be placed higher than the chest because the water would pour into the pleural cavity.

Air leak

If bubbles continue after the lung is re-expanded this is due to an air leak arising from a hole in the tube. If the patient is asked to take a deep breath then cough, bubbles appear if there is an air leak.

Swing of water

When suction is used the water level remains the same (Figure 14.4(b)). If there is no suction the water level in the bottle falls on inspiration and rises on expiration (Figure 14.4(c)). If swing stops, the lung is fully expanded or the tube is kinked or blocked.

Suction

This tends to pull the water level up in the bottle creating a negative pressure which pulls the water in the tube down thus creating a suction effect on the air or fluid in the pleural cavity.

The tubes

These are fixed to the thoracic wall by a stitch and should not become detached from the patient. If a tube becomes detached from the bottle, it should be clamped and reconnected.

A patient may be able to walk around with tubes *in situ* (not connected to a suction pump) if the bottles are placed in a small trolley which can be wheeled around.

Clamps

These are used on the tubes when the bottle is to be changed or moved above the level of the patient's chest.

Pneumonectomy

This involves the removal of an entire lung. A radical pneumonectomy includes excision of the mediastinal glands with dissection from the chest wall or pericardium. Part of the chest wall may have to be removed. There may be unavoidable damage to the phrenic nerve resulting in paralysis of half the diaphragm or to the recurrent laryngeal nerve (a branch of the vagus nerve) resulting in inability to approximate the vocal cords. Both these complications impair respiration and coughing.

Indications – carcinoma, bronchiectasis and tuberculosis.

Incision is usually postero-lateral thoracotomy.

Preoperative physiotherapy

This should begin as soon as possible after the patient is admitted. The main aims are to:

1. Gain the patient's confidence.
2. Clear the lung fields.
3. Teach respiratory control and inspiratory holding.
4. Teach posture awareness.
5. Teach arm, trunk and leg exercises.
6. Teach mobility about the bed.

Patient's confidence

An explanation of the aims of physiotherapy helps the patient's understanding. Teaching the exercises to be undertaken post-operatively and answering the patient's questions helps to allay some of the fears of the operation.

Clearing lung fields

The patient must be discouraged from smoking. Shaking, clapping and vibrations with postural drainage if necessary must be used to clear secretions from the sound lung. Huffing is taught as this is used in preference to coughing post-operatively. The patient is instructed on how to support the wound during coughing or huffing. The arm of the unaffected side is placed across the front of the thorax and round the affected side just below the incision site giving firm pressure with the forearm and hand. The upper arm of the affected side reinforces the pressure and the hand fixes the opposite elbow (Figure 14.5).

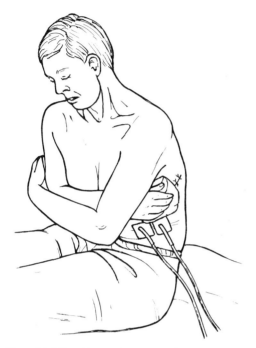

Figure 14.5 Coughing: patient supporting wound

Teaching respiratory control

Inspiratory exercises are taught for the sound lung together with inspiratory holding. This means that the patient is asked to take a deep breath in, hold, then breathe in a little further, hold, then breathe out.

Breathing control has to be practised after secretions have been cleared.

Postoperative physiotherapy

It is important to note whether the patient is on oxygen therapy, and whether there is a drain in the thorax. This drain may be used to control the amount of fluid in the cavity left by the lung. If there is too much fluid, the mediastinum is shifted to the unaffected side but if there is too little fluid the shift will be to the affected side with over-inflation of the lung. In both instances there is loss of breath and a danger of the heart being compromised.

Rate and depth of respiration are recorded. The patient must avoid straining with coughing as this can put at risk the sutures of the bronchial stump. Analgesia may be administered but must not depress the respiratory centre or cough reflex. Inhalations of, for example, benzoin tincture help to loosen secretions.

The aims of physiotherapy are to:

1. Clear secretions from the remaining lung.
2. Retain full expansion of remaining lung tissue.
3. Prevent circulatory complications.
4. Prevent wound complications.
5. Regain arm and spinal movements.
6. Maintain good posture.
7. Restore exercise tolerance.

A suitable programme may be as follows.

Day of operation (surgery am, treat pm)

Patient in half-lying with pillows arranged behind the neck and back and possibly both forearms on a pillow on the lap.

Expansion breathing exercises for all areas of the lung. Foot and ankle exercises.

Day 1 post-operation

Half-lying – segmental expansion exercises, shaking or vibrations as necessary, huffing and expectoration with wound support from the physiotherapist (Figure 14.6).

By the end of the day, the patient should be huffing with self-support. Foot and ankle exercises. Correct posture should be emphasized to prevent a scoliosis on the scar side.

Short, frequent sessions are better than few long ones. In the afternoon the patient may sit out of bed. This allows better excursion of the diaphragm. During two of the sessions the arm on the affected side must be moved:

1. Into full elevation.
2. Hand behind head.
3. Hand behind back.
4. Hand touch opposite shoulder.

A rope ladder should be provided so that the patient can pull on it to move around in bed and sit up (Figure 14.7).

Day 2 post-operation

Treatment is continued as above plus on two sessions:
1. Sitting on the edge of the bed:
   (a) Trunk turning.
   (b) Trunk bending side to side.
   (c) Trunk stretching backwards.
2. Sitting in chair – bilateral breathing exercises.
3. Walk round bed with trunk erect and arms swinging.

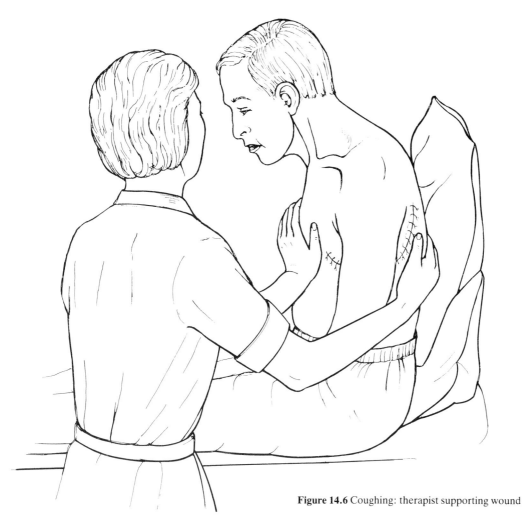

Figure 14.6 Coughing: therapist supporting wound

Day 3 post-operation

Breathing and huffing are continued as necessary. Other activities continue twice in the day. The patient may join in group therapy.

Day 4 post-operation to discharge

The patient continues with group therapy, gets dressed, walks further and, after the 7th day, practises going up and down stairs with breathing control. Bilateral breathing, trunk and arm exercises are essential.

Stitches come out usually 7–10 days after operation. Two weeks after the operation the patient is generally discharged with strict instructions to continue the exercise regimen.

Modifications to this programme

Postural drainage may be necessary if the remaining lung does not clear satisfactorily. This involves positioning the patient on the operation side. Tipping must not be used because of the danger of a broncho-pleural fistula due to the fluid bathing the bronchial stump.

If the air entry to the remaining lung is not adequate intermittent positive pressure breathing (IPPB) may be used to improve ventilation.

Oxygen therapy and humidification may be necessary. If the recurrent laryngeal nerve is injured, breathing exercises and huffing should clear the secretions. IPPB may be used with caution at low pressure and only after consultation with the surgeon.

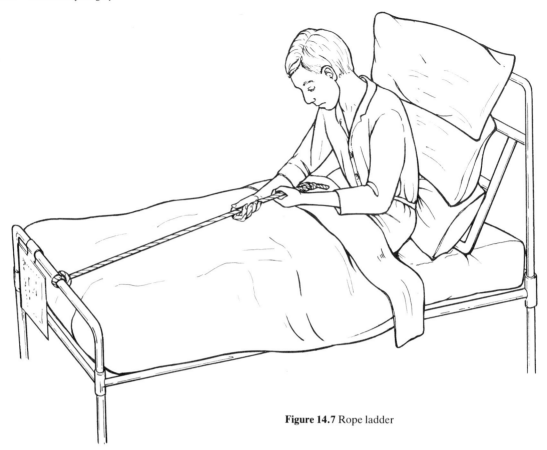

Figure 14.7 Rope ladder

If the phrenic nerve is damaged coughing can be ineffective because there is paradoxical movement of the diaphragm. IPPB can be used to mobilize secretions and increase air entry.

Incentive spirometry may be helpful to improve the patient's inspiratory capacity.

Incentive spirometry

This is a technique used to encourage a patient to take a deep breath in when there is hypoventilation after thoracic or high abdominal surgery due to pain or secretion retention. The patient breathes in through a tube which is attached to a device that illustrates the volume of the inspired air. For example, at low lung volume a plastic ball rises to the top of a column, at mid-lung volume a second ball rises and at high lung volume a third ball rises. So long as the patient holds a deep breath the balls remain at the top of the columns. Some devices operate by a light coming on when the volume of breath reaches a pre-set level. Some devices work on the expiratory phase rather than the inspiratory phase.

Long-term management

The patient generally has three monthly check-ups. On these vistis to the surgeon it is helpful to have the physiotherapist check exercise tolerance, posture, trunk and shoulder mobility so that the patient may have the home activity programme adjusted. The fluid in the cavity left by the removal of the lung gradually fills up but must not reach the level of the stump before it has healed in 10–14 days. Slowly it will fill the whole cavity and become organised and fibrosed from the base to the apex over a 2 year period. It is important, therefore, that the patient continues thoracic mobility exercises on a regular daily basis for at least this period of time.

Lobectomy

The indications are:

1. Bronchiectasis.
2. Tuberculosis.
3. Lung abscess.
4. Carcinoma.

Incision used may be a posterolateral or antero-lateral thoracotomy at the level of the 5th or 7th rib.

Preoperative physiotherapy

This begins 48 hours to a week before surgery and is the same as for pneumonectomy. The only variation is that breathing exercises will be taught to expand the lung tissue on the affected side which will still be present after the operation.

Postoperative physiotherapy

Again the treatment is similar to that following pneumonectomy. The main difference is that the patient has two underwater seal drains. Both come out of the chest wall below the incision. The air drain is usually anterior to the fluid drain (Figure 14.8). There is usually a drip in one arm. Oxygen therapy and humidification are generally used for up to 24 hours. Benzoin tincture inhalations are used if there are sticky secretions. The patient may have papaveretum (Omnopon) or aspirin as analgesia and physiotherapy should be timed if possible to coincide with the maximum effect of analgesia.

A suitable programme may be as follows.

Day of operation (given after analgesia)

Half-lying:

1. Breathing exercises to expand all segments of remaining lung tissue.
2. Vibrations over the unoperated side.
3. Huffing with the incision supported by the physiotherapist (see Figure 14.6).
4. Foot and ankle exercises.

Day 1 (treat 3–4 times as necessary)

1. Analgesia is given as necessary before treatment.
2. Inhalations may be given.

Half-lying:

3. Breathing exercises as above but add inspiratory holding.
4. Add vibrations to the operated side plus percussion as required.
5. Side-lying on the unoperated side.

When positioning the patient, check that the drains are free and that the upper arm is supported by a pillow. The underneath shoulder should not be on the pillow supporting the head. It is often helpful for the patient to have a pillow under the top knee (Figure 14.8).

Expansion breathing exercises are given for the remaining lung tissue with vibrations and percus-

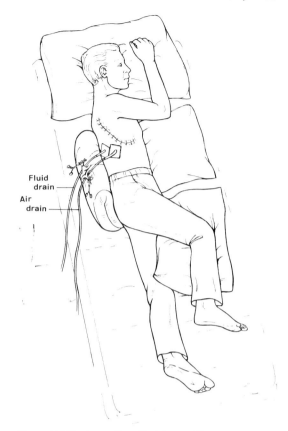

Figure 14.8 Postoperative side-lying position

sion. If necessary the foot of the bed may be raised to give postural drainage.

Return the patient to half lying and check the position so that the shoulders are level and weight is taken equally on both buttocks.

Exercises for the arm on the operated side:

1. Assisted arm elevation.
2. Assisted arm movements to touch the back of the neck and opposite shoulder.

Leg exercises are given:

1. Foot and ankle movements.
2. Quadriceps contractions.
3. Alternate hip and knee bending and stretching.

During the afternoon the patient will sit out of bed and it is important to ensure that the drains are not in danager of being kinked or blocked.

Day 2

1. As first day.
2. Add self-supported huffing (see Figure 14.5).
3. Arm exercises should be full range – auto-assisted. Elevation should be practised hourly.

4. Add trunk exercises in sitting:
   (a) Hands on shoulders bend side to side.
   (b) Hands-on shoulders turn side to side.
   (c) Abdominal contractions.

Discourage the patient from sitting crosslegged because this occludes the popliteal artery and vein and may result in a deep vein thrombosis.

Both drains are usually removed by the end of the second day. The fluid drain may be left in if there is less than 200 ml drained in 24 hours. The patient should have a short walk with, if necessary, the drainage bottle on a trolley.

Days 3 and 4

Treatments may be cut down to one or two per day.

Trunk and arm exercises should be continued and walking extended. The patient should be encouraged to dress in normal clothing and to go up and down stairs.

Formal treatment may stop and the patient should join in group therapy.

Subsequent treatment

This continues as above. Bilateral breathing exercises are encouraged. Stitches are taken out between 7 and 10 days.

Discharge is between 10 and 12 days after operation.

Notes/modifications to this programme

Expansion of the remaining lung tissue on the operated side is essential to ensure that the parietal and visceral pleura become adjacent and there is maximum surface area for perfusion.

If secretions accumulate in the intact lung the patient may be treated lying on the operated side. This should be delayed until the drains are out and then used only if really necessary.

Long-term management

As with pneumonectomy, the patient will have regular check-ups at which time it is helpful if the physiotherapist checks thoracic mobility, ensures that the scar is not adherent and that all areas of the lungs are expanding.

Thoracoplasty

This operation is performed to produce permanent collapse of a lung. It may be used in pulmonary tuberculosis or chronic empyema and is very rare.

The operation consists of resection of a varying number of ribs, leaving the periosteum in position. Four to ten ribs may be removed.

The two main complications of this operation are:

1. Deformity.
2. Paradoxical breathing.

Deformity

If the first rib is removed, the distal attachment of the scaleni is removed and this results in the muscles of the opposite side pulling the head and neck over to the sound side. The shoulder is raised on the affected side and rotated medially because the rhomboids are cut. The trunk leans to the affected side to balance the head displacement, and the spine goes into a long C curve concave to the sound side.

Paradoxical breathing

The flaccid area of the chest wall is sucked in on inspiration and blown out on expiration. This can be prevented by strapping over a cotton-wool pad to support the chest wall until it has become firmer.

Preoperative physiotherapy

The patient has to be taught breathing control, expanding the remaining lung, forced expiration technique and coughing, posture correction, shoulder girdle and shoulder exercises.

Postoperative physiotherapy

Day of operation

Treatment is given after analgesia. Half-lying. Breathing exercises to expand the lower areas of the lungs bilaterally. The physiotherapist applies firm pressure over the apical areas of the thorax, and the patient is encouraged to cough or huff.

Day 1

Posture correction must be started with the physiotherapist instructing the patient to push the head sideways against manual resistance, towards the affected side and to push the shoulder down and back.

Active assisted arm movements are practised on both sides.

Day 2

Continue with breathing exercises and coughing. Posture correction is progressed so that the patient has to align the head and shoulder and thoracic spine with scapular retraction without the guidance of the physiotherapist.

Day 3

The patient will be up and about. Manually resisted exercises for the shoulder girdle and arm on the affected side should be included.

Day 4

Trunk exercises in sitting are added.

Days 5–7

Trunk exercises in standing should be included. Posture correction in walking should be practised.

Day 8 to discharge from hospital

The patient must practise exercises to maintain trunk mobility, thoracic cage mobility and a good posture which have to be continued at home for at least 3 months after discharge.

When the patient attends for check-up with the surgeon the physiotherapist should check the patient's posture and thoracic expansion.

Operations on the pleura

These are:

1. Pleurectomy.
2. Abrasion pleurodesis.
3. Decortication of the lung.

These all require a thoracotomy and therefore the principles of physiotherapy follow similar lines to those for lobectomy.

Pleurectomy is the removal of the parietal layer of pleura from an area of the chest wall leaving a raw surface to which the visceral layer sticks and is performed for pneumothorax. It is particularly important to emphasize expansion breathing exercises for the affected side so that as the visceral layer of pleura sticks to the chest wall the affected lung is fully expanded. It is also important that the drainage tubes run freely and that clamps are not used on them so that the air or fluid in the thorax will not impede the expansion of the lung.

Pleurodesis is the insertion of a powder into the pleural cavity. This acts as an irritant to the pleural surfaces, causing them to adhere to each other. It is performed for spontaneous pneumothorax or malignant pleural effusions. As with pleurectomy, expansion exercises are essential. The patient is positioned to enable the powder to reach all areas of the pleural surface for up to 10 minutes in each position. Expansion breathing exercises are performed in each position and the patient is encouraged to practise these exercises throughout the day.

Decortication of the lung is the stripping off of layers of pleura that have become thickened due to chronic inflammation from pleurisy which restricts movement of the chest wall and expansion of the lung. Where empyema is not resolving, the whole pleura is removed to clear away the chronic pus-filled area plus surrounding fibrous tissue. Expansion breathing exercises for all areas of the lung are essential. The patient must practise expanding different areas of the lung using auto-resistance for apical and anterior, lateral and posterior basal segments.

After these operations the patient is generally up on day one and walking about on the second day.

Chapter 15

Diseases of the heart

Diseases of the heart

Before considering the pathology of disorders and diseases of the heart, a brief résumé of the anatomy and physiology of the normal heart will be given.

Gross structure (Figure 15.1)

The heart is a hollow, muscular organ divided into four chambers and enclosed in a two-layered sero-fibrous sac – the pericardium. It is lined with a

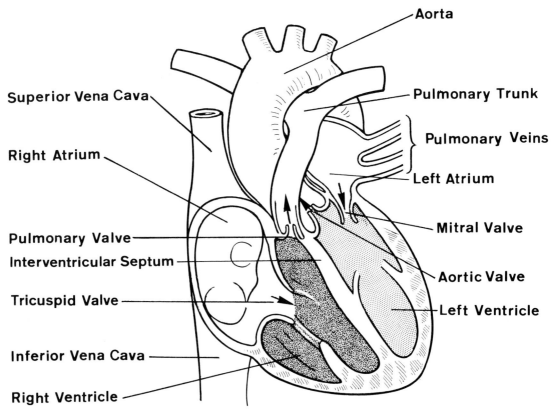

Figure 15.1 Features of the normal heart

222

membrane known as the endocardium from which the valves are formed. The two upper chambers are the right and left atria which are separated from each other by the interatrial septum. Their functions are:

1. To receive blood – the left atrium from the pulmonary circulation via the pulmonary veins, and the right atrium from the systemic circulation via the superior and inferior venae cavae.
2. To pump the blood into the ventricles.

The lower two chambers are the right and left ventricles which are separated by the interventricular septum. Their functions are: (1) to receive blood from the atria and (2) to pump the blood out of the heart. From the left ventricle, oxygenated blood is pumped throught the aorta to the systemic circulation and from the right ventricle deoxygenated blood is pumped through the pulmonary trunk to the pulmonary circulation.

Valves of the heart

The atrioventricular valves lie between the atria and the ventricles with the tricuspid on the right and the mitral on the left.

The pulmonary valve is between the right ventricle and the pulmonary trunk.

The aortic valve is between the left ventricle and the aorta.

The only other complete valve is at the entry of the coronary sinus to the right atrium.

Blood supply to the heart

The heart is supplied by the right and left coronary arteries which branch off the aorta just as it emerges from the heart. Blood is supplied to the heart mainly

during diastole. Venous drainage is into the coronary sinus which opens into the right atrium.

Circulation through the heart

Deoxygenated blood enters the right atrium, passes through the tricuspid valve to the right ventricle and leaves through the pulmonary trunk to the pulmonary circulation. Oxygenated blood enters the left atrium through the pulmonary veins, passes through the mitral valve to the left ventricle then leaves through the aorta to the systemic circulation. The superior and inferior venae cavae receive deoxygenated blood from the systemic circulation and drain into the right atrium.

The cardiac cycle (Figure 15.2)

This is the name given to the sequence of events which takes place during a single beat of the heart. The heart beats about 70–75 times per minute and each beat lasts approximately 8/10ths of a second. The contraction of the atria (atrial systole) lasts for 1/10th second and the contraction of the ventricles (ventricular systole) lasts for 3/10ths second. During the remaining 4/10 of the cycle the whole heart relaxes, this period being known as total diastole.

During atrial systole

The contraction of the atria closes the openings of the superior and inferior venae cavae, pulmonary veins and coronary sinus, so that no blood enters the heart. The contraction raises the pressure of the blood in the atria such that the atrioventricular valves are forced open and blood enters the ventricles.

During ventricular systole

The atria relax so that blood again begins to enter from the great veins. The rising pressure in the contracting ventricles closes the atrioventricular valves and at the same time opens the semilunar valves of the aorta and the pulmonary trunk so that blood is pumped into these vessels. The first heart sound (lubb) occurs during ventricular systole and is caused by the contraction of the ventricular walls and the vibrations of the chordae tendineae which, by their tension, prevent the rising pressure in the ventricles from forcing the tricuspid and mitral valves backwards into the atria. Disease of either of these will therefore alter the nature of this sound.

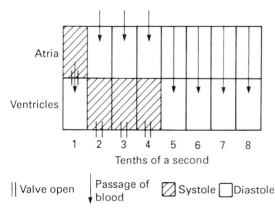

Figure 15.2 The cardiac cycle. || = valve open; ↓ = passage of blood; ▨ = systole; ☐ = diastole

During total diastole

The whole heart relaxes. The aortic and pulmonary valves close, because the pressure in the great vessels is higher than in the relaxing ventricles. They remain closed until the beginning of the next ventricular systole, thus preventing regurgitation of the blood. The atrioventricular valves open as the ventricular pressure falls so that blood trickles from atria to ventricles, as well as entering the atria from the veins.

The second heart sound (dup) takes place at the beginning of diastole and is caused by the closing of the aortic and pulmonary valves. This sound is altered by disease of these valves.

Contraction of the heart

The impulse of contraction of the heart passes from base to apex originating in a mass of specialized tissue known as the sinu-atrial node situated in the right atrium at a point near the opening of the superior vena cava. From the sinu-atrial node (also known as the 'pacemaker' or SA node) the impulse passes downwards through the atrial muscle tissue to the atrioventricular node (AV node) which is a mass of specialized tissue situated in the right atrium – near the interatrial septum and right ventricle.

The impulse is transmitted from this node to the ventricle by the atrioventricular bundle – which runs down the ventricular septum before dividing into two parts, one for each ventricle. The atrioventricular bundle consists of specialized muscle tissue known as Purkinje fibres.

Regulation of the heart beat

Contraction is an inherent property of cardiac muscle tissue and occurs independently of impulses from the nervous system but the rate of contraction is regulated by the autonomic nervous system through the parasympathetic system by the vagus nerve and through the sympathetic system by sympathetic nerves. The vagus nerve endings are concentrated near the SA node, and the sympathetic nerve endings are around both nodes and in the cardiac muscle tissue. When the vagus nerve is active the SA node sends out fewer impulses and the heart rate slows down. When the sympathetic nerves are active the SA node sends out more impulses and the heart rate increases. The two components of the autonomic nervous system are under the control of the cardio-accelerator centre (sympathetic) and the cardio-inhibitor centre (parasympathetic) which are situated in the medulla.

The rate of contraction is also influenced hormonally. Adrenaline or noradrenaline, released from the medulla of the adrenal glands during emergencies associated with anxiety, fear or anger, increase the rate and strength of the heart beat.

Electrocardiography

Preceding and during each contraction, a wave of electrical depolarization spreads through the heart, producing an electrical field which extends to the body surface. An electrocardiograph records these electrical changes, indicating rate and rhythm of the heart.

The normal pattern (Figure 15.3)

Some abnormal patterns

Heart block (Figure 15.4)

Variable P-R interval because atria and ventricles are working independently.

Ventricular tachycardia (Figure 15.5)

The ventricles are out of control of the SA node. The patient is very ill.

Extrasystole (Figure 15.6)

This occurs where a small infarct in the myocardium disrupts the normal electrical conductivity of the heart.

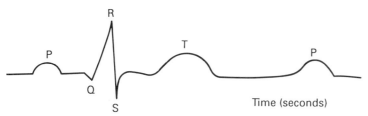

Figure 15.3 The normal ECG. P = atrial contraction due to stimulation of the SA node; P-Q = impulses pass over the AV node to the AV bundle; Q = apex of ventricles contract; R = main ventricular contraction; S = final ventricular contraction; T = change from contraction of heart to relaxation during which there is repolarization

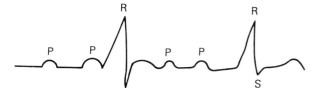

Figure 15.4 Heart block

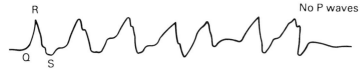

Figure 15.5 Ventricular tachycardia

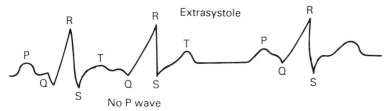

Figure 15.6 Extrasystole

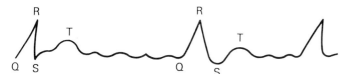

Figure 15.7 Atrial fibrillation

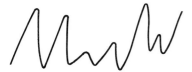

Figure 15.8 Ventricular fibrillation

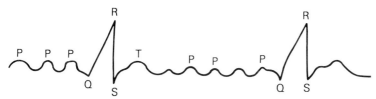

Figure 15.9 Atrial flutter

Figure 15.10 Asystole

Atrial fibrillation (Figure 15.7)

QRS normal but irregular. No P waves.

Ventricular fibrillation (Figure 15.8)

No QRS. Patient is in arrest or dead.

Atrial flutter (Figure 15.9)

P waves regular but QRS is half or quarter the atrial rate.

Asystole (Figure 15.10)

No electrical changes, therefore no contraction of the myocardium – the patient is dead.

Diseases and disorders of the heart

These may be considered as follows:

1. Pericarditis.
2. Myocarditis.
3. Endocarditis.
4. Rheumatic fever – resulting in valve disorders.
5. Ischaemic heart disease.
6. Coronary valve disease.
7. Congenital disorders.
8. Cardiac arrest.

1. Pericarditis

This is inflammation of the pericardium and may be acute or chronic.

Acute pericarditis

This is acute inflammation of the pericardium caused by viral or bacterial infections, malignancy or post-myocardial infarction. Patients usually recover with rest and anti-inflammatory drugs. Steroids or antibiotics may be necessary. Physiotherapy is not normally indicated.

Chronic pericarditis

This is a condition where there is fibrosis of the pericardium which results in restriction of heart expansion during diastole. Main signs and symptoms are a raised jugular venous pressure, fatigue and enlarged liver and ascites. Treatment is by surgery to mobilize and remove parts of the pericardium. The incision may be left thoracotomy or median sternotomy. Physiotherapy is, therefore, indicated pre- and post-operatively (see cardiac surgery).

2. Myocarditis

This is inflammation of the cardiac muscle. It usually occurs in association with pericarditis or rheumatic fever.

3. Endocarditis

This is inflammation of the lining and valves of the heart. In *subacute bacterial endorcarditis (SBE)*, there is bacterial invasion of a valve or other area of the endocardium. SBE is a serious condition treated by antibiotics. Endocarditis may also occur in rheumatic fever (see below).

4. Rheumatic fever

This disease is characterized by polyarthritis and carditis.

Aetiology

Sex – Males and females are about equally affected.
Age – Most common in children aged 4–18 years.
Incidence – Severity and incidence are decreasing in the Western world.

Cause

The disease develops in some people following infection with group A haemolytic streptococcus, but the inflammation is aseptic and so it may be that the body's own antibodies participate in the causative mechanism.

Pathological changes

Acute inflammation in the synovial membrane, primarily of the knee, shoulder, wrist, ankle and elbow joints. It is a particular feature of the disease that a joint may be acutely inflamed one day and appear normal the next.

Acute inflammation of the endocardium, myocardium and pericardium:

1. The valves become hyperaemic and swollen.
2. Fibrin and platelets are deposited along the margin of the cusps.
3. Thickening of the cusps occurs as the fibrin is converted into fibrous tissue, which spreads to the chordae tendineae.
4. Fibrous tissue contracture leads to stenosis or incompetence of the valves.

Clinical features

1. Gradual onset often following a sore throat.
2. Pyrexia – sudden rise in temperature (102–104°F, 38°C).
3. Tachycardia – increase in pulse rate.
4. Raised erythrocyte sedimentation rate.
5. General malaise.
6. Subcutaneous nodules – firm painless nodules on the extensor surfaces or elbows, wrists, knees, the occiput and spinous processes of lumbar and thoracic regions.
7. Pink rash on trunk and limbs.
8. Chorea occurs 2 months after infection.

Features of carditis in rheumatic fever

1. Heart murmurs – endocarditis.
2. Cardiac enlargement – myocarditis.
3. Friction rub – pericarditis.

Features of polyarthritis in rheumatic fever

1. Pain.
2. Swelling.
3. Tenderness.
4. Heat.

These features move from one joint to another.

Management

Management may be divided into the acute, subacute and chronic stages.

Acute stage

Bed rest is essential until there is no fever. Antibiotics, analgesics and anti-inflammatory drugs are administered. Physiotherapy is not usually appropriate.

Subacute stage

The patient is progressively mobilized at this stage. Physiotherapy is directed towards:

1. Relief of pain.
2. Regaining mobility of joints.
3. Strengthening of muscles.
4. Restoring the patient's confidence.

Methods of treatment

Ice to relieve pain, applied in towels round the affected joints.

Radiant heat to relieve pain and warm the muscles prior to exercise.

Wax may be used to apply warmth to the wrists and hands or ankles and feet.

Free active exercises designed to move each joint through full range are taught, in a non-weight-bearing position. The patient should then move each joint in a daily pattern of, for example, five movements twice daily. As recovery continues, the exercise regimen should be progressed to gravity-resisted movements so that the effect is more strengthening than mobilizing.

Pool therapy is of particular value because the warmth and support of the water can relieve pain and encourage movement. Walking re-education may begin in the pool.

Restoration of confidence is achieved by a progressive scheme of exercises which incorporates dressing, walking and going up and down stairs. Group work in a gymnasium or ward may be of value.

Prognosis

The majority of patients make a complete recovery. A small number have permanent damage to the heart valves, resulting in stenosis or incompetence.

Significance in physiotherapy

1. It is important that a physiotherapist treating a patient who has a history of rheumatic fever checks that there is no cardiac impairment, as it may be necessary to modify the treatment programme.
2. Physiotherapy is required before and after operation where a valve defect is treated surgically.

5. *Ischaemic heart disease (IHD)*

This is the term used as a diagnosis where the coronary blood flow is insufficient for the needs of the heart as a result of coronary artery disease.

It is one of the leading causes of death in affluent populations. In England and Wales it has been estimated that it causes 160 000 deaths per year (Hampton, 1983). Many are under the age of 65 years.

Terms used

Heart attack is the lay term used for the collapse of a person due to failure of the heart to maintain an adequate circulation.

Myocardial infarction (MI) – This is necrosis, with resultant loss of function, of part of the heart muscle due to ischaemia, which may be caused by occlusion or spasm of the coronary arteries and can occur in anaemia, shock or haemorrhage.

Coronary artery disease

Coronary thrombosis

Development of occlusion of the coronary arteries is serious, not only because of the damage to heart muscle but also because there is very little anastomosis and very little development of collateral circulation.

The heart can overcome the effects of diminished blood supply – up to a point – by compensation which will be explained later.

Platelets are trapped on the blood vessel walls where they break down and fibrinogen is formed which leads to further accumulation of blood cells and a thrombus is created. This usually leads to sudden occlusion.

Free embolus

Vegetation from an aortic valve – Calcified scar tissue may break off from a diseased aortic valve under the pressure of blood from the left ventricle, enter a coronary artery and become lodged in it, causing sudden occlusion.

Vegetation from mitral valve – A piece of scar tissue may break free from a diseased mitral valve, pass through the aortic valve and into a coronary artery – again causing sudden occlusion.

Endocarditis, especially in association with rheumatic fever, is a common cause of the valvular disease which leads to occlusion many years after the initial damage.

Atherosclerosis

The term cardiosclerosis may be used where the disease affects the coronary arteries.

There is hardening of the vessel walls due to calcium deposits and loss of elasticity, and lipid material is deposited on the tunica intima. There is, therefore, gradual loss of lumen of the arteries and the ventricles become hypertrophied as a result of the extra force required to push the blood through the narrowed vessels.

The degenerate patches on the arterial walls may lead to platelet entrapment, and a thrombus develops. (See Chapter 16 for more detail on arteriosclerosis.)

Aortitis

Inflammation of the aorta may result in narrowing of the mouths of the coronary arteries. This could occur in syphilitic aortitis.

Aetiology of ischaemic heart disease

It is more common in men than in women.

Age – From 45 years although it can occur in much younger age groups.

Site – The left coronary artery is more commonly affected than the right. This results in diminished blood supply to the left ventricle, apex, interventricular septum, and anterior surface of the atria.

Predisposing or 'risk' factors

1. Hypertension.
2. Cigarette smoking.
3. High level of serum cholesterol.
4. Obesity.
5. Stress, anxiety.
6. Heredity.
7. Western world living conditions or lifestyle – the disease is rare in the Eastern world.
8. Occupation, e.g. long-distance drivers of heavy goods vehicles (HGV).
9. Lack of regular exercise.
10. Diabetes mellitus.

These factors appear to contribute to the likelihood of a person developing IHD.

Sudden unaccustomed exercise precipitates a 'heart attack' where there is already some coronary artery disease or ischaemia of the myocardium and the heart cannot cope with the extra demand.

The incidence of heart disease in Finland is one of the highest in the world, and in the United Kingdom there is a high incidence in Glasgow.

Pathological changes

Sudden occlusion

If a large embolus or thrombus blocks the left coronary artery, the myocardium of the left ventricle cannot pump blood with an adequate force to maintain the systemic circulation. The inadequate blood supply to the brain and vital centres in the brain-stem leads to unconsciousness and death.

Death within 2 minutes to 2 hours occurs in a fairly high percentage of patients with this condition. In those who survive and in those where the blockage is in a smaller artery, the heart can recover function in proportion to the degree of damage. Hypertrophy of the remaining heart muscle takes place, and blood pressure is maintained.

Gradual occlusion

A collateral circulation may be established and the heart function could remain normal for many years.

If a collateral circulation does not develop, the heart muscle may hypertrophy to compensate but eventually there would be heart failure. People with this disease may have an episode of severe chest pain or minor collapse; and on investigation, blockage is detected in the main arteries.

Coronary artery grafting gives these people a much greater chance of survival.

Complications

1. Disorders of cardiac rhythm.
2. Heart block.
3. Heart rupture.

1. Disorders of cardiac rhythm

Every area of infarction of cardiac muscle is inactive forever both as contractile tissue and in impulse conduction. This results in disruption of the smooth transmission of contraction through atrial and ventricular muscle and produces arrhythmias.

2. Heart block

The coronary arteries supply the interventricular septum, the atria and the ventricules, therefore infarction can occur at these sites. Impulses travelling through the muscle tissue of the right atrium from SA node to AV node may, as a result of infarction, be interrupted partially or completely. Also, impulses transmitted by the atrioventricular bundle may be disrupted by infarction of the interventricular septum. This disruption of impulse transmission is known as heart block. The result is that the ventricles contract independently of the atria and control by the SA node is impaired.

3. Heart rupture

If there is a severe infarct with large areas of heart muscle replaced by fibrous tissue, then this tissue may rupture under the pressure of the blood. This can happen around 2 weeks after the initial infarction.

Compensation and cardiac failure

The normal heart has a large reserve of extra power which is not in use under normal circumstances. In health, fatigue of the musculo-skeletal system enforces rest before the heart is excessively stressed.

If the heart is diseased, the blood pressure falls, some of the reserve power is utilized, the blood pressure is restored and compensation has taken place.

Compensation is a relative term. A severely affected heart may compensate in lying but not in sitting whereas a less severely affected one may compensate in sitting but not in standing. In coronary artery disease and myocardial infarction, compensation takes place by hypertrophy of the remaining normal muscle. (The mechanism in valve disease will be explained in the section on valves.)

Clearly, there comes a limit when all the reserve has been utilized and no more compensation can take place – the heart then fails.

Cardiac failure

This may be acute or chronic.

Acute failure

This is the sudden inability of the heart to maintain an adequate circulation. It occurs when a main artery is suddenly occluded or where there is reduced blood pressure due to reduced peripheral resistance or haemorrhage.

Chronic failure

As the term implies, this means a gradual process whereby the compensatory property of the heart is used up and there is increasing inability of the heart to maintain circulation. If the left coronary artery is diseased, the function of the left ventricle diminishes and there is left ventricular failure (LVF).

Once this occurs a series of changes takes place backwards through the circulatory system.

As the left ventricle fails to pump on all the blood, the left atrium cannot empty fully; there is, therefore, a back-pressure through the pulmonary veins which causes congestion in the pulmonary circulation (Figure 15.11). This leads to back-pressure through the pulmonary artery to the right ventricle, to the right atrium and thence to the systemic circulation. Thus there is a gradual reduction of nutrition to the tissues, fluid collects in areas such as the feet and ankles and in the lungs.

Congestive cardiac failure

This is said to be present when there is failure in both ventricles. Right ventricular failure is often secondary to left ventricular failure.

Signs and symptoms of ischaemic heart disease

These vary in severity according to the size of the infarct:
1. *Pain*:
   (a) *Angina pectoris* – This may be retrosternal or spread across the anterior chest wall. It may radiate to both arms but more often affects the left arm (Miller, 1972). The nature of the pain is described as tight and band-like. It is aggravated by physical exertion, eased by rest, and is possibly due to lack of blood supply, leading to accumulation of metabolites stimulating nerve endings in or around the myocardium.

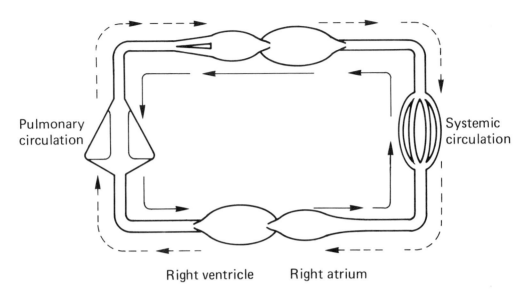

Left atrium   Left ventricle

Pulmonary
circulation

Systemic
circulation

Right ventricle   Right atrium

Figure 15.11 Back-pressure on the heart. --→ = normal
blood flow; → = back-pressure

(b) *Pain of myocardial infarction* is more severe, and longer lasting, but otherwise has a similar distribution and quality to angina pectoris.

2. *Dyspnoea* – Breathlessness, on exertion at first, and later, as pulmonary oedema occurs, present at rest. People with severe myocardial ischaemia cannot sleep flat because the abdominal organs push the diaphragm up and this increases the effect of the oedema and congestion in the lungs. Dyspnoea is also due to anoxia of the tissues.

3. *Alteration of skin colour* – Colour may be grey, white or blue especially over the face, hands and feet. The bluish colour is termed peripheral cyanosis and is due to excess deoxygenated blood because of diminished cardiac output. The grey/white colour is due to poor arterial supply.

4. *Clamminess and sweating* – This occurs particularly in the palms and face, and is a sympathetic nervous system reaction.

5. *Decreased blood pressure* – As the cardiac output diminishes so must the blood pressure.

6. *Altered pulse* – Bradycardia means reduced rate, tachycardia means increased rate. The pulse may be thin, 'thready', 'racy' or impalpable because of the diminished cardiac output. A rate of below 40 beats per minute can occur in heart block.

7. *Pyrexia* – The temperature is raised for one or two days after an occlusion leading to infarction because of the necrotic process in the myocardium.

8. *Pericardial rub* – If the infarct affects the pericardium, there is a pericardial rub – a sound heard through a stethoscope due to inflamed surfaces of the pericardium rubbing together.

9. *Radiograph* – The heart can be seen to be enlarged owing to the hypertrophy of the myocardium (the normal heart takes up half the width of the chest). If there is arteriosclerosis of the coronary arteries or aorta there may be a line of calcium visible.

10. *Oedema* – As the heart fails, there is retention of sodium and water by the kidneys. There is then excess tissue fluid which moves to dependent parts such as the feet and ankles, or the sacral area in bedfast patients.

11. *Haemoptysis* – Blood may be coughed up when a pulmonary blood vessel ruptures because of the congestion in the pulmonary circulation causing distension of the vessels.

12. *Cerebral symptoms* – Cerebral anoxia leads to faintness, giddiness and sometimes irritability and depression. The term cardiac syncope is used to denote loss of consciousness caused by reduction of the blood supply to the brain.

13. *Abdominal symptoms* – Venous congestion, anoxia and lack of arterial supply to the

abdominal organs can produce nausea, indigestion and constipation.

14. *Altered blood gases* – There is decreased oxygen and increased carbon dioxide in the blood because there is diminished gaseous interchange in the pulmonary circulation and greater interchange in the systemic circulation because of the sluggish flow.
15. *Disorders of rate and rhythm* – These may be detected by electrocardiography. Disorders in ischaemic heart disease may be heart block, ventricular tachycardia, extrasystole or ventricular fibrillation (see above).
16. *Cardiac asthma* – When left ventricular failure produces pulmonary congestion there is increased pressure in the pulmonary capillaries, and fluid passes into the alveoli – pulmonary oedema results. The patient is usually worst at night-time. The patient wakes gasping for breath with a feeling of suffocation and coughs up pink, frothy sputum.

Treatment of ischaemic heart disease

This may be considered under the headings:

1. Prevention.
2. Medical.
3. Surgical.
4. Physiotherapy.

Prevention

There is a growing need for general health education. Prevention of ischaemic heart disease means reducing the predisposing, or risk factors. People who are at risk should stop smoking, lose weight, reduce animal fat intake, eat polyunsaturated fats of vegetable origin and reduce egg consumption. They should be advised to take regular, moderate exercise and to reduce work-related stress (Christie, 1972). Physiotherapy should have an expanding role in prevention, particularly in group-work related to education in relaxation, reduction of tension and stress and in advice on regular exercise.

Medical

1. Rest in bed, probably in a coronary care unit for up to 2 days, to reduce the work of the heart.
2. Drugs, for example:
   (a) Analgesics and sedatives – morphine, pethidine.
   (b) Anticoagulants – heparin, warfarin, phenindione (Dindevan).
   (c) Defibrillating – lignocaine.
   (d) Increasing contractility of heart – digitalis.
   (e) Diuretics – chlorothiazide, frusemide.

   (f) Vasodilators – glyceryl trinitrate relieves pain of angina.
   (g) Antiarrhythmia – quinidine.
   (h) Beta blockers – propranolol (Inderal), oxprenolol (Trasicor); counteract beta effects of noradrenaline and adrenaline (Miller, 1972).
3. Oxygen – especially in pulmonary oedema.
4. Diet – a light diet puts less load on the heart during digestion.

Surgical

1. Pacemaker.
2. Coronary artery bypass graft. The graft is taken from one of the saphenous veins (Figure 15.12).
3. Heart transplant.

Physiotherapy in relation to medical management

Physiotherapy in the rehabilitation of a patient with ischaemic heart disease, coronary artery disease or myocardial infarction depends on several factors. Two of the most dominant of these are the cardiac specialist's philosophy and experience, and availability of physiotherapists with the enthusiasm and opportunity to investigate the literature and work on the subject.

Exercise programme

It is an essential theme in cardiac rehabilitation that exercise programmes are geared to the requirements of the individual patient's specific needs. Factors to be taken into account in the development of a programme include:

1. Age.
2. Occupation.
3. Previous history.
4. Mental well-being.
5. Heart size.
6. Severity of disease.

Complications

Complications that may arise during rehabilitation requiring alteration in a programme are:

1. Tachycardia.
2. Bradycardia.
3. Ventricular arrhythmias.
4. Angina.
5. Congestive cardiac failure.
6. Infection of the lungs or bronchi.

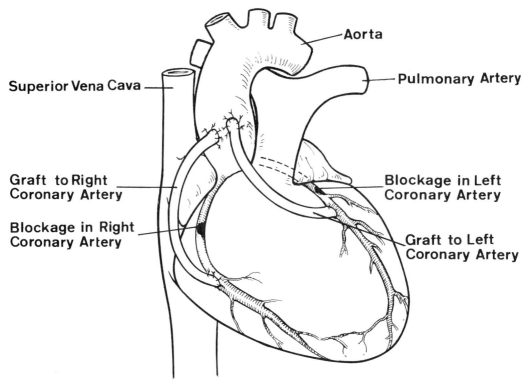

Figure 15.12 Coronary artery bypass

Warning signs and symptoms

Warning signs and symptoms of possible onset of complications are:

1. Dyspnoea.
2. Pulse rate:pulse ratio.
3. Chest pain.
4. Fatigue.
5. Dizziness.
6. Cramp.
7. Abnormal electrocardiogram recordings.

It is important that the significance of these signs and symptoms is explained to the patient and the progression of exercise or activity is altered accordingly.

1. Dyspnoea

This is a state of disordered breathing in which the patient has an unpleasant awareness of difficulty in breathing. During exercises, respiratory rate increases and depth decreases. This must return to the patient's normal within 2 minutes after the end of the exercises.

2. Pulse rate

Pulse rate must be back to the patient's resting pulse within 2 minutes after ending the exercises.

McCoy (1978) stated that tachycardia of over 100 beats per minute is an indication for stopping exercise in the early stages. A guide for safety in pulse rate increase is indicated in the work of Astrand and Rodahl (1977) and is useful in the later stages of rehabilitation (Table 15.1).

Table 15.1 Heart rate increase related to age

Age (years)	*Suggested maximum safe rate* (beats/min)
20–29	170
30–39	160
40–49	150
50–59	140
60–69	130

Pulse ratio (PR) – This is taken in relation to a test exercise which is the hardest for the stage of the patient. The pulse is taken before the exercise. Then immediately on completion, the pulse is counted for two consecutive minutes. The pulse after exercise is then divided by the resting pulse to give the pulse ratio.

Examples of calculation:

1. Pulse before
   exercise   80 (Resting pulse = RP)

   Pulse after   First minute   100
   exercise   Second minute   85
                                  ‾‾‾‾‾
                                  185 (Working
                                       pulse, WP)

   Ratio $= \dfrac{185}{80} = \underline{2.3}$

2. Pulse before
   exercise   80

   Pulse after   First minute   105
   exercise   Second minute   90
                                  ‾‾‾‾
                                  195

   Ratio $= \dfrac{195}{80} = \underline{2.4}$

The ratio should not, as a rule, exceed 2.3 in heart valve disease or 2.1 in ischaemic heart disease.

If the patient is on bed rest then there may not be an appropriate test exercise. The following is a useful guide in this case:

Pulse before one of the active exercises = 82
Pulse first quarter of a minute after the exercise = 22; 22 × 4 = 88
Pulse has been raised 6 beats which is likely to be safe.

3. Chest pain

Patients must be educated to report chest pain and to rest immediately there is any onset of a sensation of tightness in the chest.

4. Fatigue

Patients are educated to recognize fatigue. This is applicable where a patient may be repeating an exercise, say, 10 times. Then one day, on the eighth time, it seems to require more effort or the patient feels tired. The patient must stop the exercise at that point and rest.

5. Dizziness

Any onset of dizziness or faintness must be reported and the patient should rest.

6. Cramp

If cramp develops in any of the muscles working during an exercise, the exercise is stopped for the day.

7. Electrocardiogram

The exercise programme will be progressed slowly, or stopped altogether, where there are ECG abnormalities.

Recordings that may be taken during an exercise programme

1. Respiration rate.
2. Pulse rate.
3. Blood pressure.
4. Electrocardiogram monitoring.

Physiotherapy

Physiotherapy in cardiac rehabilitation may be considered under five themes, which are:

1. Complete bed rest – up to 2 days.
2. Partial bed rest – up to 4 days.
3. Up and about – in hospital from third or fourth day for up to 2 weeks.
   Total in hospital: 2–3 weeks.
4. After discharge from hospital: 3 weeks to 12 weeks.
5. Outpatient rehabilitation: 3–9 months.

Complete bed rest

Aims of physiotherapy

1. To prevent accumulation of secretions in the lungs.
2. To prevent deep vein thrombosis.
3. To prevent pressure sores.
4. To teach and encourage relaxation.
5. To explain the purpose of an active rehabilitation programme.

Techniques

1. Relaxation.
2. Breathing exercises.
3. Relaxed passive movements.
4. Free active exercises.

Example of programme. Twice daily

1. *Relaxation* – Lying (or half-lying), conscious relaxation 10 min approximately (not contrast relaxation because the exercise would put a load on the heart). Modified physiological relaxation may be indicated. For example, the patient is instructed to 'push the shoulders' down then stop pushing, to gain relaxation of the shoulder girdle muscles; or stretch the fingers and feel the bed supporting the hand then stop pushing and leave the hands on the bed. If the patient can learn to relax, the heart rate is reduced and this aids

recovery by easing the load on the heart (Mitchell, 1977).

2. *Breathing exercises* – Bilateral basal breathing, encouraging the patient to use the bases of the lungs within the normal pattern of respiration – three times. There must be no forcing of breathing in or out as this increases heart load. Teaching the patient to use the bases in quiet respiration improves the oxygenation of the blood and therefore reduces the demand on the heart.
3. *Free active movements* – lying (or half-lying):
   (a) Toes and ankles bending and stretching, × 5.
   (b) One foot turning in and out, × 5.
   (c) Repeat with other foot, × 5.
   (d) Fingers bending and stretching, × 5.
   (e) Wrists bending and stretching, × 5.
4. *Breathing exercises* – Anterior basal expansion within patient's normal pattern, × 3.
5. *Passive movements* – Patient in lying (or half-lying):
   (a) One hip and knee bending and stretching, × 1.
   (b) One leg turning in and out, × 1.
   (c) One leg carrying sideways and in, × 1.
   Repeat with other leg.
   (a) One elbow bending and stretching, × 1.
   (b) One arm raising sideways and lowering, × 1.
   Repeat with other arm.
   These movements maintain range of movement and are performed slowly in as full a range as possible.
6. *Breathing exercises* – Posterior basal exercises in the patient's normal pattern, × 3.
7. *Passive movements* – Patient in lying if possible: one hip and knee bending and stretching, × 5. Repeat with other leg.
   These movements are for maintaining circulation and may help prevent deep vein thrombosis.
8. *Relaxation* – Relaxation is repractised as at the beginning of the programme. On the second treatment of the day the passive movements may be increased by one repetition each and/or free active movements may be similarly increased.

Next day the programme is repeated with the passive and active movements increased by one repetition each.

Variations on bed-rest programme

1. Passive movements may be × 10 at first.
2. Hip and knee movements or arm movements may be active from the first day.
3. Active foot movements may be × 10 from day one.
4. Static contractions for quadriceps and gluteal muscles may start from day one (Ireland and Taylor, 1982).

Partial bed rest

The patient is up to sit for 1–2 hours per day. Feeding, washing, and using the commode are allowed.

Aims of physiotherapy

1. To maintain clear lung fields.
2. To increase the load on the heart such that there is hypertrophy of the myocardium.
3. To educate the patient to recognize signs and symptoms of excess exercise.
4. To begin rebuilding the patient's confidence.
5. To train postural awareness.
6. To strengthen leg and trunk muscles.

Example of a programme

1. Half-lying. Relaxation, × 5 minutes.
2. Posterior basal breathing exercises, × 3.
   This should be within the patient's pattern but the inspiratory and expiratory phases may be increased slightly.
3. Half-lying or lying:
   Alternate foot pulling up and pushing down, × 5.
   Feet circling, × 5 each way.
   Quadriceps contractions hold for count of 5 × 3.
   Gluteal contractions hold for count of 5 × 3.
4. Diaphragmatic breathing (anterior basal breathing).
5. High sitting; posture training.
6. High sitting; arms bending, stretching up, bending and stretching down, × 10.
7. Half-lying; lateral basal breathing.
8. Lying; one hip and knee bending and stretching, × 3.
   Repeat with other leg, × 3.
   Lying; one leg carrying sideways and in, × 3.
   Repeat with other leg.
9. Lying; relaxation + posture training.
10. Crook lying; head and shoulders pushing back hold for 5 × 3 (these may have to be in crook, half-lying).

Progress

Progress is achieved by:

1. Adding one repetition to each exercise.
2. Asking patient to repeat toe and foot exercises × 4 daily.
3. Add more exercises: for example, *bend high sitting*, trunk turning side to side.
   Sitting, alternate knee straightening and bending.
4. Add in short walks within the ward.

During the programme, between exercises, the physiotherapist continues to explain the purposes of the progressive exercises. Before and during the programme the patient is educated to recognize the warning signs of excess work (chest pain, fatigue, dizziness, cramp).

Up and about in hospital

The patient is allowed to wash, feed, go to the toilet and have a bath – with supervision. At some time during this stage the patient should dress in everyday clothes.

Aims of physiotherapy

1. To continue promoting hypertrophy of the heart muscle to strengthen trunk and leg muscles.
2. To continue rebuilding patient's confidence.
3. To improve exercise tolerance.
4. To teach awareness of exercise capacity.

Programme

1. Stop formal relaxation practice but remind the patient of the need to relax the neck and shoulder girdle and to develop posture sense of this area.
2. Stop localized breathing exercises.
3. Stop localized arm and leg exercises but the patient should perform foot and ankle movements, × 2 daily.
4. *Stride standing* (holding bedrail or chair). Knees and hips bending and stretching, × 5.
5. *Bend standing.* Elbow circling, × 5.
6. *Standing.* Arms raising forwards and upwards and lowering, × 5.
7. *Walk standing* (holding bedrail or chair). One hip and knee bending forward and stretching backwards, × 5.
   Repeat with other leg, × 5.
8. *Standing.* Posture checking – walk short distance in ward gradually increasing this until walking round ward at easy walking pace with arms swinging freely, × 3.
9. *Sitting.* General deep breathing exercises, × 3.
10. *Bend sitting.* Trunk bending side to side, × 3.
11. *Bend sitting.* Trunk turning side to side, × 3.
12. Progress each exercise × 1 each day.
    By about the middle of the second week:
    (a) Walk up and down one flight of stairs. Progress – two flights.
    (b) Dress and walk to hospital garden or shop.
13. *Improving confidence*:
    (a) The patient feels more normal dressed all day in everyday clothes.
    (b) The patient is allowed to participate in ward activities, e.g. go to hospital shop, do errands for other patients.

Awareness of capacity for exercise

Discuss with the patient the indications for stopping and resting:

1. Dyspnoea.
2. Chest tightness/pain.
3. Tachycardia.
4. Dizziness.

After discharge from hospital

The patient should leave the hospital with instructions on home management by the cardiac specialist. For example, a patient may be advised to have rest at night of 8–10 hours and in the afternoon of 1–2 hours. A week to 10 days after discharge from hospital the patient may start taking progressively longer walks every day.

Usually patients are advised not to drive a car before a review appointment 4–8 weeks after leaving the hospital. It is usually wise to avoid flying for 3–4 months but the patient could start light work around this time. In some cases a change of occupation may be necessary – for example, airline pilots and drivers of heavy goods vehicles are not allowed to continue in their occupation.

Out-patient rehabilitation

This is usually in the form of a group or circuit activity in a gymnasium. Patients benefit from meeting fellow patients in the group.

Equipment required

It is advisable to have the following equipment in a gymnasium used for cardiac rehabilitation:

1. Defibrillator.
2. Suction apparatus.
3. Oxygen.
4. Electrocardiograph.

Staffing

A cardiac team of trained doctors and technicians should be within calling distance (i.e. on bleep or telephone).

It is desirable to have a minimum of two physiotherapists in the gym and they must be trained in the recognition and treatment of cardiac arrest.

Aims of physiotherapy

1. To increase exercise tolerance.
2. To maintain/improve confidence.
3. To provide support and encouragement.
4. To help reduce risk factors and thereby possibly reduce recurrence.

Criteria for selection

These will depend upon the experience of the physiotherapist, cardiac specialist and possibly the patient's general practitioner, and it is impossible to lay down rules. However, the following points should be considered when patients are to be accepted:

1. Concurrent disease or disability, pulmonary congestion or oedema, diabetes, hypertension, general arthritis, peripheral vascular disease. (In the ideal situation, patients with these disorders should be seen at home by a community physiotherapist.)
2. *Age* – The greater the age, the greater is the risk of another episode. Generally, the upper age limit is 65.
3. *Distance and mode of travel* – These circumstances may be such as to make a patient unsuitable because the effort required to attend would not be justified.
4. *Personality* – Nixon (1972) stated that patients may be addicted to work and tension. Muldoon (1972) stated that physiotherapy should not be started unless the patient has mastered his aggression and addiction to tension and tiredness.
5. *Radiograph showing enlargement of the heart* – It may be illogical to aim to hypertrophy a heart that is already enlarged.

Examples of exercises to improve exercise tolerance and self-confidence

Group: Warm-up exercises, one or two of which precede the general exercises:

1. Bend sitting; elbow circling, × 10.
2. Sitting; arms swinging forward and back, × 10.
3. Sitting; alternate knee straightening and bending, × 5 each leg.
4. Sitting; trunk turning with loose arm flinging, × 5 each side.

General exercises:

1. Half-yard grasp standing; one leg swinging forwards and backwards, × 10.
   Repeat with other leg.
2. Half-yard grasp standing; knees and hips bending and stretching, × 5.
3. Yard standing; arms circling backwards, × 20.
4. Yard stride standing; trunk bending and turning to touch left knee with right hand and straightening.
   Repeat opposite way, × 10 each way.
5. Lying; alternate hip and knee bending and stretching, × 10.

6. Sitting (facing partner, holding light ball); throwing and catching ball between partners, × 2 minutes.
7. Standing; (low stool) stepping up and down, × 2 minutes.
8. Standing (arms stretched forwards palms on wall); arms bending and stretching, × 20.
9. Wing stride standing; trunk bending side to side, × 5 each side.
10. Sitting; standing up and sitting down, × 10.
11. Standing (grasping ball); passing ball overhead and behind back, × 10.
12. Stride standing (grasping ball); bouncing ball, × 5 each hand.
13. Stride standing (grasping ball); throwing ball against wall, × 2 minutes.
14. Sitting (holding pole across back of shoulders), trunk turning side to side, × 10.
15. Sitting; trunk bending to pick up pole, arms stretching up, arms lowering, trunk bending to replace pole, × 5.
16. Crook lying; pelvis raising and lowering, × 5.

These exercises require very simple equipment and can be readily adopted for a home programme. As a general guide, a suitable number of exercises is 8–10 in any one session, and they should be chosen to move all parts of the body.

Where there are sufficient physiotherapists to supervise, patients may perform individual circuits instead of group work. The exercises may again be simple and progressed for the individual requirement in the following ways:

1. Increase number of repetitions.
2. Increase the length of time for each exercise.
3. Increase speed, i.e. greater number of repetitions in same or reduced time.
4. Add weights.
5. Alter range, e.g. higher stool for stepping on and off.

Support and encouragement

Patients may attend 2–3 times per week and gradually reduce to once a week. Every patient should have time at each attendance to discuss progress.

Pulse rate is taken before and after the exercises. The patient may participate in the pulse taking by using a pulse meter. Pulse ratio and its significance is discussed so that the patient is actively included in the decisions to progress the exercises.

Walking is encouraged – on a level surface for 3–4 miles. Jogging may replace walking in some cases (McCoy, 1978).

Golf is a suitable sport to recommend.

6. Coronary valve disease

Stenosis and incompetence are two disorders of valve function that result from disease.

Stenosis

This is narrowing of the opening and results in reduced blood flow through the valve and back-pressure into the chamber behind the valve.

Incompetence

This means that the valve does not fully close; therefore, when the chamber that receives blood through the valve is contracting there is regurgitation of blood back to the chamber behind.

Causes of valve disorders

1. Rheumatic endocarditis (see rheumatic fever).
2. Syphilis – aortic valve affected.
3. Trauma – chest compression injuries.
4. Arteriosclerosis of the valve – aortic especially.

Changes, signs and symptoms of valve disorders

Mitral valve changes

Stenosis

When the left atrium contracts it cannot force all the blood through the narrowed opening into the left ventricle. Less blood reaches the ventricle and in turn less blood enters the systemic circulation. Cardiac output is therefore reduced.

Compensation takes place in two ways: (1) the left atrium hypertrophies, and (2) later the left atrium dilates.

Gradually the left atrium cannot cope with the extra volume and pressure of blood and there is back-pressure into the pulmonary veins. This causes increased movement of fluid from pulmonary capillaries into interstitial tissues, lymph vessels and alveoli, producing pulmonary oedema. The pressure is transmitted backwards to the right ventricle which hypertrophies but ultimately fails.

Incompetence

When the left ventricle contracts most of the blood goes into the aorta but some regurgitates back through the partially open valve. Less blood reaches the systemic circulation.

The left atrium dilates to accommodate the extra blood, then hypertrophies to increase the force behind the blood going into the ventricle. As with stenosis there is an increased volume of blood in the atrium which causes back-pressure through the

pulmonary veins to the pulmonary circulation to the right ventricle which then hypertrophies. Again this ventricle eventually fails.

As the process continues, there is back-pressure through the tricuspid valve to right atrium, through the venae cavae to the systemic circulation, and back to the left ventricle which then hypertrophies with failure later.

Signs and symptoms: stenosis and incompetence

Mainly due to back-pressure in the pulmonary circulation:

1. *Cyanosis* – Especially of the face.
2. *Dyspnoea* – Due to pulmonary congestion.
3. *Cough and haemoptysis* – Due to pulmonary congestion and oedema.
4. Palpitations.
5. *Radiograph* – Right ventricular hypertrophy (and eventually left ventricular hypertrophy).
6. *Oedema* – Ankles, feet, abdominal area.

   Stenosis
   First heart sound loud (lubb)
   Diastolic heart murmur

   Incompetence
   First heart sound weak
   Systolic heart murmur (lubb-shoosh-dup)

Heart murmurs are heard either when blood flow is under increased pressure (as when it is passing through the narrowed stenotic valve) or where there is turbulent flow (as when there is back-flow through the incompetent valve).

Complications

The main complication of a mitral valve disorder is that of embolus formation. Part of the diseased tissue may break off and enter the aorta. It may then pass into a coronary artery causing sudden occlusion or through a carotid artery into the cerebral circulation causing hemiplegia.

Aortic valve changes

Stenosis

Some of the strength of contraction of the left ventricle is used in overcoming the resistance of the narrowed opening; therefore, there is less force behind the blood in the systemic circulation and blood pressure falls. The left ventricle hypertrophies.

Incompetence

Blood flows back through the valve into the left ventricle. Blood pressure falls because of the reduced volume. The left ventricle dilates then hypertrophies.

Signs and symptoms: stenosis and incompetence

These are due to the poor arterial supply to all parts of the body and are more severe when there is incompetence.

1. *Pallor* – Pale, greyish white.
2. *Cerebral anaemia* – Headaches, faintness, giddiness, insomnia, irritability, depression.
3. *Chest pain* – Due to ischaemia of the heart.
4. Oedema later.
5. Dyspnoea, less than in mitral disease.

Stenosis
Systolic murmur
Weak pulse

Incompetence
Diastolic murmur
Left ventricular failure
Waterhammer pulse

Waterhammer pulse

If the radial artery is palpated with the patient's arm vertical, the pulse beat is felt suddenly with great force and then is suddenly impalpable.

The great force is due to the ventricular contraction, and loss of pulse is related to the regurgitation of the blood.

Tricuspid valve changes

Stenosis

The right atrium cannot force all the blood into the ventricle and less blood goes into the pulmonary circulation. The atrium cannot accommodate all the blood and there is back-pressure in the systemic circulation.

Incompetence

There is excess blood in the right atrium because of regurgitation during right ventricular contraction. Again there is back-pressure in the systemic circulation.

Signs and symptoms: stenosis and incompetence

1. Throbbing in the head on stooping due to back-pressure in superior vena cava.
2. Abdominal discomfort due to distension of the liver.
3. *Fatigue* – Due to diminished oxygenation of the blood.
4. *Ankle swelling* – Due to back-pressure in inferior vena cava.
5. *Pulsation in the jugular vein* – Due to increased venous pressure.

Pulmonary valve

Pulmonary stenosis is nearly always congenital – see Fallot's tetralogy.

Pulmonary incompetence can occur after endocarditis but more commonly regurgitation is due to pulmonary congestion leading to back-pressure, which causes engorgement of the pulmonary artery and stretches the pulmonary valve. Signs, symptoms and treatment are therefore those of the cause of the pulmonary congestion.

Treatment of valve disorders

This may be medical or surgical.

Medical

In mild cases, or where surgery is contraindicated, treatment is by rest and drugs and is similar to the management of the patient with ischaemic heart disease.

Surgical

1. Valvotomy.
2. Annuloplasty.
3. Valvuloplasty.
4. Replacement.

Valvotomy

1. A closed valvotomy is used for mitral and pulmonary stenosis. An instrument is inserted through a ventricle, passed up through the valve and dilated within it.
2. In an open valvotomy, the heart is opened and the cusps of the valve mobilized under direct vision.

Annuloplasty

This is used for incompetence of, for example, the tricuspid valve. The valve ring is plicated to reduce its size, allowing the cusps to come together.

Valvoplasty

This is used for incompetence; the cusps may be partially stitched together or repaired if they are split.

Physiotherapy

Pre- and postoperative physiotherapy is an essential part of the management of patients treated by surgery. (See physiotherapy in cardiac surgery, page 243.)

7. Congenital disorders of the heart and great vessels

1. Outside the heart:
   (a) Patent ductus arteriosus.
   (b) Coarctation of the aorta.
2. Inside the heart:
   (a) Atrial septal defect.
   (b) Ventricular septal defect.
   (c) Pulmonary stenosis.
   (d) Transposition of great vessels.
   (e) Fallot's tetralogy.
   (f) Tricuspid atresia.

Patent ductus arteriosus (Figure 15.13)

The ductus arteriosus is a vessel which, during fetal life, connects the aorta with the pulmonary artery. Normally, it closes within a few hours of birth.

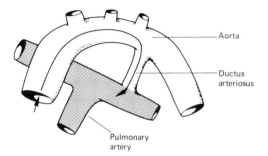

Figure 15.13 Patent ductus arteriosus

When it remains open, blood from the aorta flows through to the pulmonary artery resulting in two main effects:

1. Reduction of blood flow to the systemic circulation.
2. Overfilling of the pulmonary circulation.

Signs and symptoms

1. The child is prone to respiratory infection and bacterial endocarditis.
2. The child is undersized.
3. Heart failure if the duct is very large.

Treatment

When the child is 3 or 4 years old surgery is undertaken to ligate the vessel.

Coarctation of the aorta (Figure 15.14)

This is the name given to a constriction of the aorta just distal to the origin of the left subclavian artery.

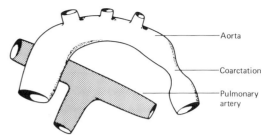

Figure 15.14 Coarctation of the aorta

The common site of constriction is in the region of the ductus.

Main signs and symptoms

1. The blood pressure is high in the upper part of the body (supplied by the vessels given off before the constriction) but low in the lower part of the body with poor circulation.
2. Hypertrophy of the left ventricle.

Treatment

Surgery is performed to remove the restricted portion and either sew the ends together or put in a Dacron graft.

Atrial septal defect and ventricular septal defect

As the name suggests, in these cases there is an opening in the interatrial or interventricular septum ('hole in the heart'). Blood passes between the two sides of the heart. This is the most common form of congenital heart defect.

Main signs and symptoms

Children with moderate defects often do not develop signs and symptoms until late teens. The chief signs and symptoms are:

1. Failure to thrive.
2. Tendency to develop chest infections.
3. Untreated patients develop pulmonary hypertension in their late twenties to thirties.

Treatment

Surgical repair is necessary unless the defect is very small.

Pulmonary stenosis

This is congenital narrowing of the pulmonary valve, resulting in diminished blood flow to the pulmonary circulation.

Signs and symptoms

1. Dyspnoea.
2. Cyanosis.
3. Fatigue.

Treatment

Pulmonary valvotomy.

Transposition of the great vessels (Figure 15.15)

The aorta and pulmonary arteries are reversed, so that venous blood circulates round the body and oxygenated blood circulates round the lungs. This is incompatible with life unless there is a left to right shunt as in patent ductus arteriosus or a septal defect. Where there is no such shunt, surgery is essential. A channel is formed to connect the aorta and the pulmonary veins.

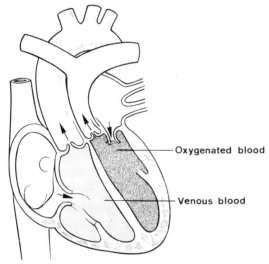

Oxygenated blood

Venous blood

Figure 15.15 Transposition of the great vessels

Fallot's tetralogy (Figure 15.16)

This consists of the following:

1. Pulmonary stenosis.
2. Ventricular septal defect.
3. Dextra-position of the aorta so that it receives blood from both ventricles (Figure 15.16).
4. Hypertrophy of the right ventricle.

Signs and symptoms

1. Cyanosis.
2. Syncope.
3. Squatting.
4. Dyspnoea on exertion.

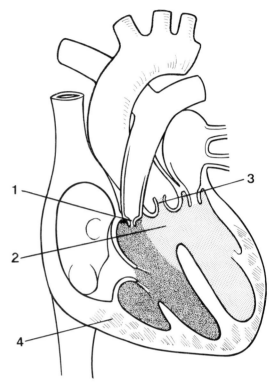

Figure 15.16 Fallot's tetralogy. 1 = Pulmonary stenosis; 2 = ventricular septal defect; 3 = dextra-position of the aorta; 4 = hypertrophy of the right ventricle

Cyanosis

This is due to venous blood:

1. Entering the left ventricle through the septal defect.
2. Entering the aorta from the right ventricle and circulating in the systemic arterial circulation.

Syncope

This occurs because of cerebral anoxia, especially during emotional upsets.

Squatting

The child tends to adopt a squatting position. This compresses the abdominal aorta and femoral arteries and raises the resistance in the systemic circulation which decreases the shunt of blood from right to left through the septal defect.

Dyspnoea on exertion

This is due to the diminished oxygen content of the blood in the systemic circulation.

Treatment

This has to be some form of surgery. There are a number of different operations that may be performed. For example, a Blalock–Taussig operation which connects a subclavian artery with its corresponding pulmonary artery, may be performed on a child of a few weeks to 5 years. Then, for patients between 5 and 10 years, the septal defect is repaired and the pulmonary stenosis released.

Tricuspid or pulmonary atresia

The tricuspid or pulmonary valve is deficient. Pulmonary flow occurs via other defects such as ventricular or atrial septa deficiency or patent ductus arteriosus.

Cardiac surgery

The introduction of the cardio-pulmonary bypass machine has led to major advances in cardiac surgery. The machine performs the pumping action of the heart and the gas exchange function of the lungs, thus enabling surgeons to open the heart or operate on the coronary arteries and aorta.

Operations usually requiring the bypass machine are:

1. Valve repairs or replacements.
2. Coronary artery bypass grafts.
3. Grafting or repair of coarctation of the aorta.
4. Closure of atrial or ventricular septal defects.
5. Correction of Fallot's tetralogy.
6. Heart transplant.

Operations not normally requiring the bypass machine are:

1. Valvotomy.
2. Pacemaker insertion.
3. Ligaturing of patent ductus arteriosus.
4. Blalock–Taussig operation.
5. Pericardectomy.

The physiotherapist treating cardiac surgery patients must be aware of the position of incisions, the complications and their danger signals and the nature of the lines, tubes or drains that may be used.

The incisions

These are median sternotomy (or sternal split), lateral thoracotomy and submammary.

Median sternotomy (Figure 15.17)

This is a commonly used incision for heart operations and includes division of the sternum. No muscle fibres are cut but the sternal attachment of the pectoralis major can be impaired. Post-operatively, patients feel that the two margins of the healing sternum are grating together. Therefore, when the patient is moved, care must be taken to ensure that the shoulder girdles are kept level in all planes. The commonest postural fault with this incision is shoulder girdle protraction. The physiotherapist must teach the patient to retract the shoulder girdles to avoid shortening of the anterior thoracic structures because this can result in aching or pain.

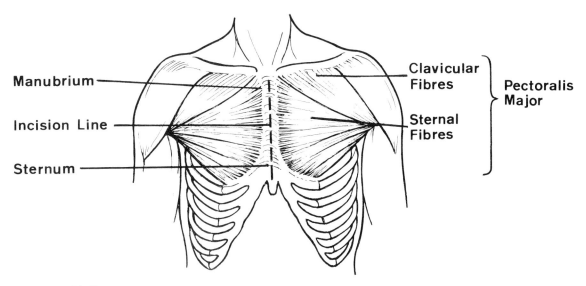

Figure 15.17 Median sternotomy

Lateral thoracotomy

This incision goes through an intercostal space on one side of the thorax – for heart operations the level is usually left fourth or fifth intercostal space. The muscles cut and postural faults associated with this incision are discussed in Chapter 14. Although a left thoracotomy is usual, a right thoracotomy may be used for some heart operations.

Submammary incision

This is an incision through the fourth intercostal space with the sternum divided transversely. The muscles cut are the intercostals and pectoralis major. It is not very commonly used.

Complications

The likely complications are:

1. *Respiratory*:
   (a) Infection of lung tissue.
   (b) Consolidation or collapse of whole or part of a lung.
   (c) Pneumothorax.
   (d) Haemothorax.
2. *Cardiovascular*:
   (a) Deep vein thrombosis, with resultant danger of pulmonary embolus.
   (b) Cardiac arrest.
   (c) Cardiac arrhythmias.
   (d) Tamponade – collection of blood in the pericardial cavity which compresses the heart, reducing its capacity to fill with blood during diastole and leading to cardiac arrest.
   (e) Emboli from diseased valves may break off, lodge in a cerebral vessel and cause a stroke.
3. *Wound*:
   (a) Infected.
   (b) Unhealed.
   (c) Adherent.
4. *Joint stiffness*:
   (a) Shoulder and shoulder girdle.
   (b) Thoracic spine.
   (c) Costovertebral joints.
   The shoulder/shoulder girdle complex is especially prone to stiffness unilaterally following a lateral thoracotomy and bilaterally following a median sternotomy.
5. *Muscle weakness*:
   (a) The muscles affected by the incision will be weak.
   (b) Leg and abdominal muscles become weak during bed rest.
6. *Postural deformity*:
   (a) Protraction ('rounding') of the shoulder after median sternotomy.
   (b) Scoliosis, concave on the operation site after a lateral thoracotomy.

The danger signals

Monitoring of the patient by the various machines connected to the lines or tubes used post-operatively is under the control of the surgeons and nursing staff. A physiotherapist working on a cardiothoracic unit, or intensive care unit, must be familiar with the functions of the machines, their danger signals and with the action to be taken according to the policy of the unit.

The physiotherapist may be the first to detect diminished chest expansion which predisposes to consolidation of the underlying lung tissue. She is also likely to be the team member to detect developing joint stiffness or postural deformity.

Lines, tubes and drains

1. *Endotracheal tube* – This is a tube which extends from the mouth to the trachea. It allows attachment of a ventilator and facilitates suction of secretions from the trachea.
2. *Humidifier* – There are a number of types of humidifier, but the function of them all is to moisten the air or gas mixture entering the patient's lungs, so that secretions do not become encrusted in the trachea or on the endotracheal tube. There is always a humidifier when a patient is on a ventilator.
3. *Oxygen* – This may be delivered by mask or nasal cannulae or via endotracheal tube where one is *in situ*.
4. *Drainage tubes* – There may be one to drain fluid and/or one to drain air from the pleural cavity (see Chapter 17). There may be mediastinal and pericardial drains to Redivac bottles. Where the great saphenous vein is removed to provide material for coronary artery grafting or valve replacement, there will be a drain in the affected leg.
5. *Drip* – There may be one drip in the arm or leg to provide blood transfusion saline or plasma, i.e. fluids to maintain fluid and electrolyte balance. There may be a tube in a jugular vein passing to the right atrium for administering drugs.
6. *Central venous pressure recording* – CVP recording is used to monitor the force of venous return and can detect the onset of cardiac failure. The line passes from the recording instrument through a vein, such as the internal jugular, through the superior vena cava, to the right atrium. (The same tube may be used for CVP recording and drug administration.)
7. *Arterial pressure* – A tube in an arm artery may be used to record arterial pressure or may be used to obtain blood samples.

8. *Ryle's tube* – This is a tube that passes through the nose to the stomach. It enables aspiration of gastric juices to be performed and can help to prevent vomiting.
9. *Pacemaker leads* – The patient may be linked up to an external pacemaker with leads attached to the chest.
10. *Electrocardiography* – Usually four leads connect the patient to an electrocardiograph for continuous monitoring (see page 225 for traces).
11. *Urinary catheter* – This may be placed in the urethra to prevent urinary complications.

Tubes or lines inserted into the patient are referred to as 'invasive' and there are hazards to the patient with them all. Surgeons, engineers, electronics experts and a large number of scientists are always searching for useful non-invasive techniques. Blood gases, blood flow and pH of the blood can now be assessed with non-invasive techniques using sensors placed on the patient's chest.

Physiotherapy in cardiac surgery

A patient for cardiac surgery is admitted at least 2 days and often 7 days prior to the operation. This enables him to meet all the staff, find his way around the unit and to have tests. During this time the aims of the physiotherapist are as follows:

1. To gain the patient's confidence.
2. To ensure that the lung fields are clear and that all areas of the thorax are expanding.
3. To explain where the incision site will be and how it will be supported during coughing or moving.
4. To teach coughing or huffing.
5. To teach the patient general leg and trunk exercises.
6. To teach shoulder and shoulder girdle exercises.
7. To train position sense.

Procedure

Introduction, explanation

The physiotherapist on a cardiothoracic unit should have a quiet, competent manner and be able to adapt her instructions, explanation and sympathy according to each individual patient's needs.

During her first visit she should explain the purpose of the physiotherapy that the patient will receive. She must also examine and assess the patient along the following lines:

1. Check that all areas of the thoracic cage are expanding.
2. Note the type of sputum the patient is producing – if any.

3. Check that there is full range movement at the joints of the spine, shoulder/shoulder girdle, and both lower limbs.
4. Observe the patient's posture, noting any deviation from normal, especially of trunk, neck and shoulder girdle.
5. Read the patient's notes to determine results of tests, e.g. exercise tolerance, chest X-ray.

A suitable pre-operative programme is then developed according to the examination findings.

Lung fields and thoracic expansion

If there are secretions in the patient's lungs, then action must be taken to clear them as the operation may have to be delayed. The physiotherapist will give breathing exercises, shaking, clapping, postural drainage and intermittent positive pressure breathing modified to take into account the condition of the patient's heart. Short, numerous treatment sessions may be necessary. On the other hand, if the lungs are clear then the patient need only be taught expansion breathing exercises for lower lateral costal, anterior basal and posterior basal areas.

The importance of maintaining thoracic expansion in prevention of lung collapse is explained. Bilateral exercises are used when there is to be a sternotomy. Unilateral exercises may be used where there is to be a lateral thoracotomy.

Incision site

The physiotherapist must know which incision site is to be used so that she can teach the patient how support will be applied during moving, coughing or huffing (Figure 15.18).

Coughing and huffing

The patient must be taught that coughing or huffing is essential for removing secretions from the lungs. The incision has to be supported and the patient taught to cough at the beginning of expiration after a deep inspiration.

Huffing should also be taught so that the patient is practised in both methods of lung clearing. Relaxation and diaphragmatic breathing are encouraged after coughing.

Exercises

It is important to teach the patient shoulder, trunk and leg exercises because these must be started on the first day after the operation. The number of repetitions of each movement must be geared to the patient's tolerance.

One movement in each direction may be sufficient for teaching foot, knee and hip movements.

However, for the arms, elbow circling backwards, shoulder girdle circling backwards, and arm elevation are important enough to be repeated two or three times, with assistance if necessary. Bilateral movements are important following a median sternotomy.

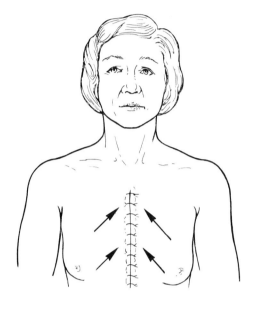

Position sense training

Throughout the preoperative programme, the patient's position must be corrected so that the shoulders are level, back and down, and weight is taken evenly on both buttocks. No breathing exercises, coughing, relaxation or exercises should be taught while the patient is out of alignment. In this way the patient's position sense is educated to recognize postural faults and how to correct them.

Moving and turning

The patient is taught how to move into side lying and lying because these positions may be used postoperatively. It is important to remember that postural drainage is contraindicated by cardiac arrhythmias or pulmonary oedema.

Where the policy of a hospital is such that the patient will be looked after by more than one physiotherapist, it is important that he should meet them all before the operation. On the whole, it is more reassuring for the patient if the same physiotherapist can attend to him at least for the first 48 hours after the operation.

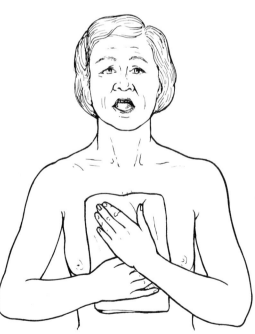

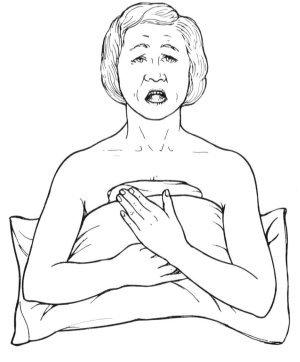

Figure 15.18 (a) Support for wound during coughing. (b) Cough pad in position. (c) Pillow support for coughing

Post-operative treatment

For the first 48 hours after cardiac surgery, the patient will be in an intensive care unit, because he can be under continuous supervision and skilled personnel are immediately on hand to deal with any emergency.

Aims of physiotherapy

The aims of physiotherapy are as follows:

1. To maintain a clear airway.
2. To prevent lung collapse and consolidation.
3. To help the patient to maintain good posture.
4. To ensure that mobility of the shoulder, neck, trunk and legs is maintained.
5. To prevent deep vein thrombosis later – i.e. after 48 hours up to 2 weeks.
6. To restore the patient's confidence.
7. To increase the patient's exercise tolerance.
8. To teach the patient a home exercise plan.

Outline of an uncomplicated recovery following an operation using the cardiopulmonary bypass machine

Day of operation

The physiotherapist must note the position of drips, tubes and lines. She must check recordings such as temperature, blood pressure, ECG, pulse rate, respiration rate, time of administration of analgesic drugs. She will know, from discussion with the staff, of any complications during surgery.

If the patient does not require artificial ventilation and there are no excessive pulmonary secretions, physiotherapy may be delayed until the endotracheal tube has been removed.

The patient is helped to sit forwards from half-lying and the physiotherapist listens to the breath sounds, especially in the posterior basal areas. With the incision supported, the patient is encouraged to take three deep breaths and to try one or two huffs. He is then repositioned in half-lying with full support for his head and trunk from pillows.

Day 1

Treatment is given four times during the day. Diaphragmatic and bilateral basal breathing exercises are practised with huffing and then coughing when the patient can manage. Each treatment session is a mixture of treatment and assessment in that, as the physiotherapist instructs the patient in breathing exercises, she can assess thoracic expansion at the same time. Position sense training is incorporated because the shoulders, head and neck should be aligned before breathing exercises are performed and relaxation encouraged after coughing.

If the patient has had a lateral thoracotomy, the arm of the operation side should be assisted into elevation at two of the treatment sessions. Foot movements – five times in each direction must be encouraged and one hip and knee bending and stretching should be performed 3–4 times at two of the treament sessions.

At the end of this day most of the drips and drains will be out and the patient will be beginning to feel more human.

Day 2

The physiotherapy will be the same as for day 1. A rope ladder may be tied to the end of the bed to enable the patient to sit up himself, but not all patients like this after a median sternotomy. Arm movements should be full range on the side of a lateral thoracotomy. Where the incision has been a median sternotomy, the patient may start bilateral shoulder movements.

By the fourth treament session the patient may be up to sit beside his bed, and breathing exercises are given in this position.

Day 3

The patient will be clear of all drips, drains and lines and will be back in the ward of the cardiothoracic unit. Physiotherapy may be reduced to three visits. Breathing exercises and huffing should continue. General arm and trunk exercises will be included in at least one session and the patient may be taken for a short walk (within the ward) on another session. Posture correction and arm swinging should be incorporated into the walking practice.

Day 4

The patient should be up and about independently and allowed to go to the toilet on his own. The physiotherapist must assess chest expansion once at least. Arm, trunk and leg activities may be performed with other patients in a ward class.

Days 5–14

Activities until the day of discharge – usually 2 weeks after the operation – must be geared to the individual patient. Around days 5–7 the patient should be able to walk upstairs (about 8–10 stairs) and an exercise programme may be developed along the lines of a patient recovering from a myocardial infarction.

Before discharge

The patient should be confident that he will be able to cope with his home situation, otherwise he may go to a recovery unit if the hospital has one. He must have full thoracic expansion and know how to practise breathing exercises every day. He must also have full joint mobility. The progression of length of walking and daily activities, and the date of return to work, is for the surgeon to decide at follow-up appointments.

Variations

Ventilated patients

Some patients may be on a ventilator for the first 12–24 hours after cardiac surgery. Physiotherapy may be required if there is evidence of collection of secretions in the patient's lungs. Vibrations and suction may then be given but the vigour and length of treatment are dictated by the patient's overall condition, especially in relation to the stability of the cardiovascular system.

Operations not using the cardiopulmonary bypass machine

The physiotherapy is similar to that already described but patients usually progress more quickly.

Pacemaker insertion

This is comparatively minor compared with other cardiac operations. A pacemaker is an electrical device used to treat patients with heart block. The incision may be simple in that the device is placed under the skin of the axilla but a thoracotomy may be necessary. Physiotherapy should be given to prevent chest complications.

Development of complications

Lung collapse due to accumulation of secretions may have to be treated with vibrations and manual hyperinflation. If the patient is on a ventilator, then vibrations are given during the expiratory phase after which suction is given, to remove the secretions.

Wound infection may be treated by ultraviolet rays – E4 dosage from a water-cooled mercury vapour burner. A slow-healing wound may be treated by application of an E2 dosage.

Joint sitffness may require treatment by specific techniques such as hold–relax or repeated contractions. Muscle weakness can be treated by graduated exercises.

Children

Children aged over 4 years follow the same sort of postoperative recovery as adults. They need more encouragement to practise breathing exercises and general activities with games rather than formal exercises. Patients under 4 years old are cared for in a special children's unit where, although the principles of treament are the same, techniques must be modified. Vibrations are finer than those used for adults using, for example, only two fingers. Activity is encouraged, only where necessary, as when the child is not moving enough naturally.

Cardiac arrest

Cardiac arrest may be defined as the failing of heart action to maintain adequate cerebral circulation in the absence of causative irreversible disease.

Diagnosis

Diagnosis of cardiac arrest is based on the following signs and symptoms:

1. Sudden collapse.
2. Apnoea or cessation of respiration.
3. Loss of consciousness.
4. Absence of pulse – the carotid pulse is the best to use because it is the strongest. The radial pulse is next best.
5. Dilatation of the pupils. If the patient is alive the pupils constrict in response to light.

Once the diagnosis of cardiac arrest is made, resuscitation must start immediately, since the maximum length of time for which the brain can survive without oxygen is 4 minutes. If the oxygen supply is restored to the brain within 2 minutes there should be no brain damage at all. If 2–4 minutes elapse then there may be some brain damage. These times are related to normal body temperature.

Procedure

1. Place the patient in supine lying on a hard surface.
2. *Clear the airway*:
   (a) Put a finger in the mouth and remove any material that may obstruct the airway, including dentures.
   (b) Extend the head and lift the jaw forwards and upwards to avoid obstruction from the tongue – this position is very important and must be retained throughout resuscitation.

3. *Inflate the lungs by mouth-to-mouth resuscitation*:
   (a) Pinch the nose to close the nostrils with one hand.
   (b) Take in a deep breath, place the lips over the patient's mouth so that no breath can escape and blow sharply into the patient's mouth. If the thorax does not expand re-check the airway.
4. *Apply external cardiac massage* – Place the heel of one hand, reinforced by the heel of the other hand, over the lower half of the sternum (Figure 15.19) and give a short, sharp anterior–posterior thrust. This squeezes the heart between the sternum and vertebral column, pushing the blood out into the pulmonary and systemic circulations. The heart then refills with blood when the thrust is released.
   Repeat the thrust another 4–5 times at a rate of approximately one per second.
5. Check the carotid pulse.
6. If the heart and breathing restart, turn the patient on to one side because vomiting often follows cardiac arrest, and if this does occur while the patient is supine the vomit can cause choking.
7. If the heart and breathing do not start, then a rhythm has to be established of one breath into the patient's mouth, five thrusts on the sternum, check the pulse. This coordinated rhythm should obtain 50–60 cardiac thrusts and 12 breaths per minute. **This pattern is continued until the heart and breathing restart, a resuscitation team takes over, the operator's stamina runs out or common sense dictates that the procedure should be abandoned.**

Variations on this theme

Lung inflation

1. A Brook's airway may be used to blow through.
2. An Ambu bag may take the place of the person blowing.
3. Inflating through the nose is easier than through the mouth because less pressure is required to inflate the lungs.
4. The technique includes holding the patient's mouth closed and applying the operator's lips over the patient's nose.

External cardiac massage (ECM)

When the patient is a child one hand is used for ECM instead of two, and one finger is sufficient for a baby.

Points to note

1. If ECM is performed correctly the carotid pulse should be palpable and a systolic pressure of 60 mmHg is attainable at each thrust.
2. Figure 15.19 illustrates the surface marking of the heart – to be borne in mind when applying ECM.
3. Turning the patient may be facilitated by using the following procedure to turn to the right side:
   (a) Stand or kneel beside the patient's right side.
   (b) Straighten the right arm down by the patient's side so that the trunk will roll over it.
   (c) Turn the patient's head to the right.
   (d) Bend the patient's left leg and carry the knee over to lie in front of the right thigh.

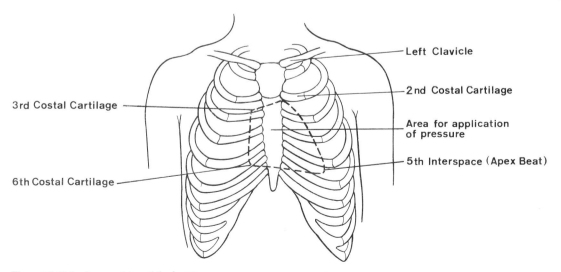

Figure 15.19 Surface marking of the heart

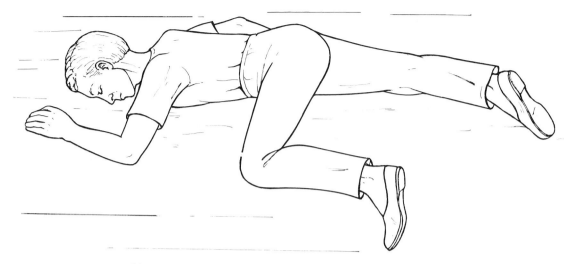

Figure 15.20 Recovery position

(e) Place the patient's left hand in front of the face.
(f) Turn the patient by holding behind the left shoulder girdle and hip bone.
(g) The patient should then be in the position shown in Figure 15.20.
4. Action must be taken to send for a resuscitation team. Methods by which this team are called vary according to hospital procedure. An ambulance must be called as soon as possible in the event of an arrest occurring other than in a hospital.

Transplant surgery

Heart transplants are performed for end-stage cardiac disease, resulting from irreversible myocardial damage. There is at present no alternative to transplantation for patients at this stage of the disease. Lung transplants are performed for irreversible lung disease (e.g. pulmonary fibrosis).

Heart and lung transplants are performed where there is extensive disease of both lungs (e.g. cystic fibrosis). Studies by Buxton *et al*. (1985) and O'Brien *et al*. (1988) have shown that following these operations there is a marked improvement in the quality of life of the patients. Physical mobility is particularly improved.

Preoperative management

Prior to the operation the patient undergoes several tests, such as ECG, chest X-ray, tissue typing, pulmonary function tests, exercise tests and blood tests. The patient is also introduced to members of the transplant team and shown round the appropriate ward. It is also helpful for the patient to meet people who have had a similar operation. Depending on the unit, the patient may be admitted for a few days during which these tests and meetings may be arranged. Following this the patient is on the waiting list and has to be available at short notice (i.e. a few hours).

Physiotherapy at this stage

This consists of teaching the patient breathing exercises and effective coughing, together with an explanation of the postoperative exercise and activity programme. The patient is assessed for physical mobility and exercise tolerance.

Postoperative management

The patient is nursed in an intensive care unit (ICU) with a barrier nursing procedure for 12–48 hours which is designed to prevent infective organisms being transmitted to the patient. Usually, the patient is up, out of bed on the second day postoperatively, and is encouraged to become increasingly active. For heart-alone transplants the patient may go up and down stairs from the sixth day onwards, and discharge home is usually 10 days after the operation. This period is 3 weeks for heart and lung transplants.

Physiotherapy at this stage

1. Treatment usually starts within an hour of the endotracheal tube being removed – 6–8 hours after return from the theatre.

2. Breathing exercises are given with the patient in half-lying.
3. Vibrations may be applied if there are intrapulmonary secretions, and effective coughing is encouraged.
4. Exercises are given such as:
   (a) Leg exercises – toe and foot pulling up and pushing down, foot circling, repeated 3–5 times.
      This programme may be performed 2–3 times on day one.
   (b) On day two, depending on how well the patient is, for example if he or she is allowed out of bed the programme may be: Breathing and leg exercises as for day one. A pedal cycle is used for 1–2 minutes at the lowest resistance and low revolution rate (e.g. 35 revs per minute). The following exercises are performed – once in the day:
      Sitting – stand up sit down, 2–3 times.
      Standing – knees bend a small way, 3 times.
      Standing (holding bed rail) – heels raising, 3 times.
      Arm exercises are also added – repeated 3 times:
         Hands on shoulders – elbows circling.
         Hands on shoulders – arms stretching upwards and bending.
   (c) Once all drains and drips have been removed walking is added to the programme and the patient dresses in everyday clothes. The exercise cycle programme is increased, for example by 1 minute each day.
   (d) On the fifth or sixth day the patient may go to the physiotherapy gym, depending on local arrangements. It is important to remember that the new heart has no nerve supply and response to exercise is much slower than normal (e.g. 5 minutes instead of 1 minute). An exercise programme is worked out, starting with warm-up exercises, e.g. as already performed on day 1, adding in adduction and abduction of the legs. Then there is a peak activity on the exercise bicycle:
      1 minute 0 resistance, 35 revs per minute.
      2 minutes 0 resistance, 50 revs per minute.
      1 minute 0 resistance, 35 revs per minute.
   (e) Over the next 5 days, the patient learns to progress the exercise programme so that he or she is confident to go home and continue progressing. Walking is encouraged and before discharge the patient should be confident in climbing a full flight of stairs.

Throughout the postoperative recovery period relatives are encouraged to be with the patient and to help with the recording and monitoring of the exercises.

Follow-up management

The patient has to attend for blood tests, ECGs and biopsies at regular intervals. This may be 2–3 times a week at first, then once a week up to 3 months and then perhaps reduced to fortnightly. These tests are necessary to monitor rejection and therefore ensure that the immunosuppressive drug therapy is correct. Regular check-ups continue during the first 2 years and then as necessary to monitor the drug therapy and health status. The main drugs that the patient has to take for life are immunosuppressives to prevent rejection (e.g. cyclosporin A or azathioprine (Imuran)) together with others to reduce the viscosity of the blood and reduce the recurrence of coronary artery disease (e.g. aspirin or dipyridamole (Persantin)).

The patient has to avoid danger from infection because the immunosuppressive drugs, necessary to reduce the risk of rejection, also depress the reticuloendothelial system so that antibody production is diminished. This necessitates rigorous cleaning of the house and a high standard of personal hygiene. Socializing is curtailed, especially for the first 2 months, to reduce the risk of meeting people with infections. Pets may be kept but birds must be avoided. Sexual activity may be resumed as soon as the patient wishes. Driving a car has to be delayed until at least 6 weeks after operation, and the DVLC at Swansea must be informed of the operation. A diet low in fat and cholesteral and high in fibre is recommended. Alcohol may be taken in moderation but smoking is absolutely contraindicated.

After 6 months, the patient can begin to go out and about on public transport and in public places. As stated already, the quality of life is much better than before the operation, and survival rate is improving with each operation.

Physiotherapy during the follow-up stage

The patient has to record the cycling exercises, and walking is performed daily. The bicycle exercises are progressed gradually up to 20 minutes. Then the revolution rate may be increased. Resistance may be increased but is not appropriate for every patient.

Depending on proximity to the hospital in which the transplant was performed, the patient may attend for outpatient physiotherapy after 3 months. This enables the patient to have a monitored, progressive exercise programme and to join in with other patients following the same operation. Exercise tolerance and stress tests continue at 9-, 12- and 18-month intervals, and the patient is encouraged to live an active lifestyle which is conducive to a 'healthy heart'. If the patient lives too far away to travel to the hospital then arrangements should be made for attendance at a local physiotherapy department.

Within 6 months after the operation the patient should be able to resume everyday activities such as work, gardening, shopping and sport.

Complications

The major complications are rejection and infection. Others are aches and pains.

Rejection

This is monitored principally by blood tests and biopsies. If a patient feels excessively tired or does not feel up to the exercises one day, the physiotherapist must determine in discussion with other members of the team whether this is a sign of rejection or perhaps depression. If tests indicate rejection, clearly the exercise programme is curtailed and drug therapy adjusted (rejection episodes do occur during a normal post-operative recovery). If on the other hand it is a spell of depression (this also occurs during a normal recovery) then the patient should be encouraged to perform the exercises he or she likes best, e.g. walk to the hospital garden. The company of a relative is very beneficial during this period, and arrangements should be made for the relative to stay in hospital accommodation as necessary.

Infection

The precautions already described are essential to reduce the risk of infection. The patient is generally instructed by the nursing staff to wear a face-mask for the first few weeks – particularly when he or she is out and about in the hospital. Daily weight and temperature measurements are recorded by the patient. If there is a rise in temperature sustained over two measurements then the patient should contact the appropriate doctor.

Aches and pains

The healing sternum and neighbouring tissues are painful for some time and there may be back, shoulder and chest pains from time to time. This gradually diminishes but the patient does need to be reassured that full functional arm, shoulder girdle and thoracic spine movements should be performed every day within the limits of comfort. These exercises should be performed slowly, with control, and for the first few days may be assisted either by the physiotherapist or a relative.

Children

The principles of rehabilitation are the same as for adults. The parents play a very large part in encouraging activity and monitoring weight and temperature.

A tricycle is more appropriate for a small child than an exercise cycle.

Heart and lung transplants

The principles of rehabilitation are again as outlined above. The main differences are slower progression and more emphasis on clearing the lung fields. It is important to remember that the new lungs do not have a nerve supply and the presence of secretions is not detected by the patient. Daily postural drainage as a routine is often, therefore, necessary. Adults require postural drainage and vibrations twice daily until discharge from hospital. Relatives should be taught how to position the patient for postural drainage at home. They may also be taught to apply vibrations. Parents of young children must be taught how to give postural drainage by positioning the child on the lap and to encourage activity by play.

References

Astrand, P.O. and Rodahl, K. (1977) *Textbook of Work Physiology*, 2nd edn. McGraw Hill, New York

Buxton, *et al.* (1985) In *Costs and Benefits of the Heart Transplant Programmes at Harefield and Papworth Hospitals*, DHSS Research Report Number 12 (eds Acheson, Caine, Gibson and O'Brien), HMSO, London

Christie, D. (1972) The prevention of heart attacks. *Physiotherapy*, **58**, 348

Hampton, J.R. (1983) *Cardiovascular Disease*, Heinemann, London

Ireland, G. and Taylor, D.J.E. (1982) The effect of exercises starting within 24 hours of infarction. *Physiotherapy*, **68**, 191

McCoy, P. (1978) Rehabilitation after uncomplicated myocardial infarction. *Physiotherapy*, **64**, 183

Miller, H.C. (1972) The medical and surgical treatment of angina pectoris. *Physiotherapy*, **58**, 344

Mitchell, L. (1977) *Simple Relaxation*, John Murray, London

Muldoon, D.E. (1972) Physiotherapy in rehabilitation of the coronary patient. *Physiotherapy*, **58**, 338

Nixon, P.G. (1972) Rehabilitation of the coronary patient. *Physiotherapy*, **58**, 336

O'Brien, B.J., Banner, N.R., Gibson, S. and Yacoub, M.H. (1988) The Nottingham Health Profile as a measure of quality of life following combined heart and lung transplantation. *Journal of Epidemiology and Community Health*, **42**, 232–234

Chapter 16

Diseases of the blood and lymph vessels, ulcers and scar tissue

Anatomy
Investigations in arterial disease
Diseases of arteries
Arterial surgery
Amputations

Diseases of veins
Ulcers
Pressure sores
Lymphoedema
Scar tissue

Anatomy
Structure of blood and lymph vessels

Arteries have three coats:

1. *Tunica adventitia* – An outer coat composed mainly of fibrous tissue which prevents overdistension.
2. *Tunica media* – A middle coat composed of muscle and elastic tissue. In the large arteries this coat is mainly elastic but in the smaller arteries it is mainly muscular to control the lumen.
3. *Tunica intima* – An inner coat composed of epithelial cells providing a smooth lining which helps to prevent clotting.

Veins also have three coats. These are similar to the arteries but there is much less muscle and elastic tissue in veins. The tunica media, therefore, is thin. The tunica intima is reduplicated at intervals to form valves which aid venous return by allowing the blood to flow in one direction only, i.e. towards the heart. Valves are numerous in the veins of the lower limbs.

Lymph vessels

These consist of a thin layer of endothelium similar to blood capillaries but much more permeable. This allows the drainage of tissue fluid which cannot be re-absorbed directly into the bloodstream either because there is an excess amount or there are particles that are too large to enter the blood capillaries.

Structure of the arterial system

The arterial system begins on the left side of the heart with the ascending aorta. The aorta continues as an arch and then descends through the thoracic and abdominal cavities before dividing into common iliac arteries. Each common iliac artery divides into an internal iliac artery which supplies the pelvis and an external iliac artery which continues as the femoral artery to the lower limb. The femoral artery continues as the popliteal artery which divides into anterior and posterior tibial arteries. The anterior tibial artery continues as the dorsalis pedis artery and the posterior tibial artery divides into medial and lateral plantar arteries before ending in the foot as a series of arches.

From the arch of the aorta, the brachiocephalic trunk on the right side gives off the subclavian and common carotid arteries but on the left side these arteries are given off directly from the arch. The subclavian artery continues as the axillary and then brachial arteries before dividing into radial and ulnar arteries which end in the hand in a series of arches.

The common carotid artery divides into an external carotid artery supplying the head and neck and the internal carotid artery which supplies the brain through the cerebral arteries. The brain is also supplied by the vertebral artery. Both vertebral arteries (from the subclavian arteries) join to form the basilar artery which forms an anastomosis with the cerebral arteries.

Structure of the venous system

This is divided into two main sets of veins, deep and superficial.

Deep veins

These accompany the arteries. The smaller arteries, for example brachial and tibial, each have two sets of veins – venae commitantes – accompanying them but the larger arteries have a large single vein, usually of the same name (for example popliteal and axillary), following the same course. In the lower part of the body the common iliac veins unite to form the inferior vena cava and in the upper part of the body the subclavian veins and the internal jugular veins unite to form the brachiocephalic veins which in turn form the superior vena cava. The two venae cavae drain into the right atrium of the heart.

Superficial veins

In the lower limb there are two main veins:

1. *The great (long) saphenous vein* – This begins as a continuation of the medial marginal veins of the foot, passes up in front of the medial malleolus, behind the medial tibial and femoral condyles, up the medial side of the thigh to pass through the saphenous opening and ends in the femoral vein in the femoral triangle.
2. *The small (short) saphenous vein* – This begins as a continuation of the lateral marginal vein of the foot, then passes behind the lateral malleolus up the lateral border of the tendo calcaneus. It pierces the deep fascia, passes between the two heads of gastrocnemius and ends in the popliteal vein in the popliteal fossa.

In the upper limb there are two main veins:

1. *The cephalic vein* – This begins on the lateral side of the dorsal venous network of the hand and passes on to the anterior aspect of the lateral side of the forearm. In front of the elbow joint it passes between biceps and brachioradialis, up the lateral border of biceps and then passes between deltoid and pectoralis major. In the infraclavicular fossa it pierces the clavipectoral fascia, crosses the axillary artery and ends in the axillary vein.
2. *The basilic vein* – This begins on the medial side of the dorsal venous network of the hand and passes up the posterior aspect of the medial side of the forearm. Just below the elbow it passes anteriorly up the front of the elbow between biceps and pronator teres and along the medial border of biceps. It becomes deep at the middle of the upper arm and ascends along the medial side of the brachial artery to the lower border of the teres major where it continues as the axillary vein.

Structure of the lymphatic system

This is a network of lymph vessels and nodes (glands) which is responsible for draining tissue fluid from the tissue spaces and returning it to the venous network near the heart.

The lymph vessels accompany blood vessels and are found in the skin, subcutaneous tissue, muscle, fascia, viscera and intestines. Along the course of the vessels are situated lymph nodes. Lymph, therefore, passes along lymph vessels through a series of nodes before entering the venous circulation.

In the upper limb lymph flows through vessels to the axillary lymph nodes from where it passes to the subclavian trunks.

In the lower limb lymph flow passes through popliteal and inguinal nodes to iliac nodes and then to the lumbar trunk.

The lumbar trunk and the left subclavian trunk drain into the thoracic duct which is the main vessel of the lymphatic system. The right subclavian trunk drains into the right lymphatic duct. Both these vessels end by draining into the junction of the jugular and subclavian veins.

Investigations in arterial disease

1. Chest X-ray and ECG to determine the state of the blood supply to the heart and lungs.
2. Blood glucose values and urine analysis to determine the presence of diabetes mellitus.
3. Blood tests are used to determine the presence of fat which can increase the blood viscosity which in turn inhibits blood flow. Haemoglobin count is taken for evidence of anaemia which exacerbates arterial disease. Polycythaemia, clotting and platelet abnormalities should also be investigated.
4. *Arteriography* – Radio-opaque fluid is injected into the arteries and this outlines the vessels. The lower limb arteries are investigated through a lumbar aortogram or a femoral arteriogram and carotid and cerebral arteries are investigated through a carotid arteriogram. The state, lumen and course of the arteries can be detected.
5. *Ultrasound scanning* – This can be used to detect abnormalities in the size and position of vessels, e.g. aneurysms. As a non-invasive procedure it is safer and less distressing for the patient than other procedures.
6. *Arterial pulse* – Palpation or auscultation of arterial pulses provides a guide to the level of the occlusion. Complete occlusion results in absent pulses distally, and partial occlusion may result in a weakened pulse. Increased pulsation with a murmur is due to an aneurysm.

7. *Skin changes* – Charts may be made of the distribution of loss of sensation and of skin temperature. These can be used to determine the extent and progress of the disease as it affects the skin.
8. *Doppler tests* – Ultrasound is used to detect the rate of blood flow in an artery. When the sound wave is reflected there is a change in frequency which is a function of the blood flow rate. Flow patterns vary with the degree of occlusion.
9. *Radio-isotopes* – These can be used to measure blood flow by means of a Geiger counter.
10. *Pressure changes* – These can be measured by inserting a needle into the vessel and reading the level on a manometer or by measuring the pressure with a sphygmomanometer cuff placed round the leg and the Doppler flow probe.
11. *Exercise tolerance* – This is tested by the patient stepping up and down two steps at a set rate or on a treadmill which gives a standardized test. The number of steps without pain or discomfort gives an indication of the patient's exercise tolerance.
12. *Thermography* – This is a non-invasive technique which gives a picture of the skin temperature variation of the whole limb.

Diseases of arteries

Arteriosclerosis

This is a degenerative process during which elastic tissue is replaced by fibrous tissue and the tunica media becomes thickened. It is part of the normal ageing process.

Pathology

Degenerative changes begin in the tunica media of medium-sized arteries with destruction of muscle and elastic tissue. These changes spread later to affect the tunica intima. Calcium is deposited in the tunica media replacing the degenerated tissues.

There is therefore loss of elasticity which leads to increased peripheral resistance and raised blood pressure.

Atherosclerosis

This is the most common occlusive arterial disease and is characterized by an abnormal mass of lipid material (atheroma) in the intima layer of an artery.

Atherosclerosis and arteriosclerosis may exist independently but frequently occur together.

Aetiology

Atherosclerosis becomes increasingly common with age. The majority of patients are aged over 50 and the disease is rarely found in people aged under 30. Males are affected more than females.

Vessels affected are the aorta, large arteries and some medium-sized vessels particularly the cerebral, renal, femoral and coronary arteries. The smaller arteries are not so commonly affected. When the disease is found in one vessel other arteries are likely to be affected and it may well be widespread. A number of factors are known to predispose to the condition. These are:

1. *Diet* – A diet rich in animal fat raises the serum cholesterol level. This occurs in the affluent societies of North America and Europe and not in the underdeveloped countries.
2. *Hyperlipidaemia* – A high level of lipids in the bloodstream.
3. *Diabetes* – This is associated with arteries being narrower than normal.
4. *Cigarette smoking* – When nicotine is absorbed into the bloodstream it causes vasoconstriction of the small peripheral vessels.
5. *Hypertension* – This may accelerate vascular disease.
6. *Other factors* – These may be obesity, lack of exercise, high alcohol intake.

Pathology

1. Lipid material is deposited on the tunica intima.
2. Fibrin is laid down over the lipid material causing patches of raised areas on the intima.
3. Thrombocytes tend to become caught on these areas and this leads to thrombus formation.
4. These lesions gradually increase in size whilst the underlying intima becomes softened and the areas become ulcerated.
5. This ulceration leads to inflammation which spreads to the other arterial walls and neighbouring veins.
6. As thrombus formation continues, the lumen of the affected vessel becomes occluded. A collateral circulation may become established (Figure 16.1) and this can be adequate to supply the needs of the tissues.

Clinical features

These depend on the site of the affected artery. Coronary artery disease causes angina and leads to ischaemia of the cardiac muscle (see Chapter 15). Cerebral artery disease causes ischaemia of the brain and clinical features depend on the area of the

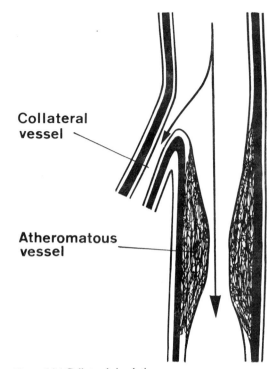

Figure 16.1 Collateral circulation

brain affected (see Chapter 19). Vertebral artery disease may cause dizziness, faintness or impaired vision.

The iliac, femoral and popliteal arteries are commonly affected, and the clinical features are as follows:

1. Intermittent claudication.
2. Rest pain.
3. Cold limbs.
4. Sensory changes.
5. Skin changes.
6. Loss of pulses.

Intermittent claudication

The patient complains of severe cramp-like pain, commonly in the calf muscles, which develops during exercise, particularly walking. At first, the pain ceases when the exercise stops but as the disease progresses the pain is provoked by less exercise and takes longer to subside. It is due to the circulation being inadequate to meet the demands of the working muscles. Other muscles affected may be the glutei, quadriceps, and anterior tibialis.

Rest pain

This is a severe burning pain in the foot or toes which occurs most commonly at night. The patient is frequently wakened by the pain which may be relieved to a certain extent by the leg being suspended over the side of the bed.

Cold limbs

The toes and feet feel cold both to touch and to the patient.

Sensory changes

Pins and needles, tingling or complete anaesthesia may be present especially in the hands or feet and is increased by exercise.

Skin changes

Owing to ischaemia there may be dryness, scaling, brittle nails and loss of hair. The skin may have a white, shiny appearance or be discoloured with a delay in the return of colour after blanching.

Gangrenous changes resulting in death of tissue may be present in the toes or heels and trophic ulcers may be formed on the skin.

Loss of pulses

There may be partial or complete loss of one or more peripheral pulses depending on the severity of the condition and the site of the occlusion.

Complications

Aneurysm – especially in the arch of the aorta.

Rupture of an artery from a trivial cause such as a slight blow or injury or a sudden rise in blood pressure.

Treatment

Medical

Advice is given to stop smoking, avoid cold, wear warm loose clothing, keep the skin clean and free from infection or pressure, avoid using hot water bottles, avoid sitting with the legs crossed, avoid wearing tight shoes, socks, garters or belts. Shoes should be inspected for stones or nails and trauma of all kinds to the legs avoided. It may be necessary to use padding to keep the heels off the bed and blocks to keep the pressure of the sheets off the feet.

Analgesics are prescribed to relieve pain. Anti-coagulants may be given to patients with diffuse occlusive disease.

Diet should be low in animal fat and cholesterol and patients suffering from obesity must start a reducing diet.

Regular exercise is important, and the patient should undertake to walk a stated distance each day.

Physiotherapy

This is usually given postoperatively and will be considered with surgery later. Some patients on medical treatment may be referred for physiotherapy. This may mean teaching the patient a good walking pattern and monitoring a walking programme – teaching the patient how to chart the intensity of pain on a scale of 0–10, to record the distance walked and the time taken for the pain to settle with rest.

Buerger's exercises may be indicated. This is a pattern of positions designed to encourage the development of a collateral circulation in the legs. The procedure is as follows:

1. The patient lies supine with the legs supported in elevation (at an angle of 45° to the horizontal) until the skin blanches – about 2 minutes.
2. The patient sits up with the legs dependent until the skin colour is bright red – about 3 minutes.
3. The patient lies with the legs horizontal until the skin colour returns to normal – about 5 minutes.

This pattern of positions is repeated four or five times for three times daily. Improvement is determined by the decreasing times required for the changes in skin colour.

Trophic skin ulcers may be treated following principles similar to those for venous ulcers.

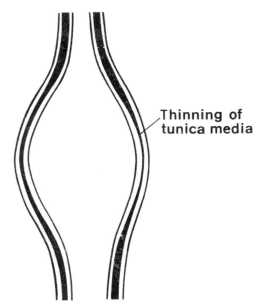

Figure 16.2 An aneurysm

Aneurysm

An aneurysm is a dilatation of the wall of an artery forming a sac in communication with that vessel. A true aneurysm is a dilatation of one or more layers of its wall caused mainly by atherosclerosis and sometimes by syphilis or acute infections. The weakened arterial wall produces a sacular or fusiform dilatation with resultant thinning of all coats (Figure 16.2). Most commonly affected vessels are the aorta and popliteal arteries. Since atherosclerosis occurs most commonly in men over 60 years of age the incidence of aneurysms is greatest in this age group.

A dissecting aneurysm is formed by a split in the tunica media producing an inner and outer wall with blood passing through two channels (Figure 16.3).

A false aneurysm results from an accident to an artery due to trauma or surgery. Blood escapes from the damaged vessel and forms a haematoma adjacent to the arterial wall.

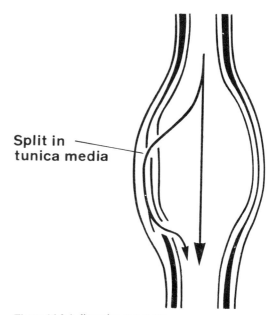

Figure 16.3 A dissecting aneurysm

Clinical features

Many aneurysms are asymptomatic and may be diagnosed on examination for another condition. When symptoms do occur they are usually caused by pressure on neighbouring structures and depend upon which artery is implicated. The following may occur:

1. Ischaemia, gangrene in the foot (popliteal artery).
2. Lumbar backache or central abdominal pain (abdominal aorta).
3. Pulsating mass in the abdominal cavity (abdominal aorta).

4. Difficulty in swallowing due to oesophageal pressure (thoracic aorta).
5. Paraplegia due to pressure on nerve roots or spinal cord (aorta).

If untreated, aneurysms may rupture and this can be life threatening in that the patient may bleed to death.

Treatment

Resection of the aneurysm and replacement with a prosthetic graft or a by-pass graft.

Thromboangiitis obliterans (Buerger's disease)

Aetiology

This is a disease of unknown aetiology which is precipitated by cigarette smoking. Cessation of smoking improves the outcome of the disease. It affects males between the ages of 20 and 40. There does not appear to be any marked racial bias although originally it was thought to be more common in Jews. The arteries of the upper limb and viscera are affected as well as those in the legs but the distal arteries of one leg are usually affected first unlike atherosclerosis where the larger proximal arteries are initially affected.

Pathology

Lymphocytes invade the arterial wall. The wall becomes inflamed and clots form which obstruct the lumen of the artery. Ultimately, the vessel may degenerate and fibrous tissue formation further reduces the lumen. The process is slowly progressive and extends to the collateral vessels.

Clinical features

These are mainly in the legs. There is rest pain and the feet are cold, sweating and often have fungal infections. On elevation, the foot becomes pale and on dependency red. The two principal symptoms are intermittent claudication and gangrene. As the digital arteries are affected the toes may be completely ischaemic but the foot has a good blood supply and the foot pulses are present. (In atherosclerosis the gangrene is the result of proximal arterial disease and the pulses are absent.) The pain associated with the onset of gangrene is severe and may prevent sleep.

Treatment

Smoking is forbidden because it causes vasocon-striction. Drugs may be prescribed in the form of analgesics and vasodilators. Skin hygiene is essential to prevent wound infection.

Physiotherapy

The aim is to improve the circulation to increase the blood supply to the affected limbs thus delaying the onset of gangrene. Buerger's exercises may be given to assist the establishment of a collateral circulation. In the early stages of the disease the patient is encouraged to exercise without producing the pain.

Surgery

1. Upper thoracic or lumbar sympathectomy to relax arterial muscle and increase the vessel lumen thereby improving the blood supply to the extremities.
2. Amputation, initially of gangrenous toes, may be performed but amputation higher up the limb is usually necessary later due to the progressive nature of the disease. Reconstructive surgery of the arteries is difficult because the smaller distal vessels are affected.

Raynaud's disease

This is a vasomotor disorder characterized by intermittent spasm of the digital arterioles.

Aetiology

The disease occurs in women more than men and between the ages of adolescence and middle age. The hands are primarily affected, usually bilaterally, and the feet may also be affected. Exposure to cold precipitates the disease and in some cases emotional disturbances have similar effects.

Pathology

Spasm of the digital arterioles reduces blood flow to the skin of the fingers which become white and numb. When the spasm wears off the blood returns to the fingers. Initially the fingers are blue because the blood quickly loses its oxygen to the ischaemic tissues but then they become red, swollen and painful as the blood fills all the dilated arterioles. As the disease progresses there may be permanent spasm resulting in necrosis of the fingers or toes.

Clinical features

The attacks are intermittent, affecting both hands. On exposure to cold, the fingers feel numb and appear white and shiny. On rewarming they become pink with a burning sensation. Severe cases show ulceration and atrophy of the fingers. The wrist and ankle pulses can be palpated. Similar features are present in other vascular disorders such as Buerger's disease and atherosclerosis as well as in cervical rib. These are known as secondary Raynaud's phenomena.

Treatment

Medical

Advice is given to avoid cold extremities by wearing thick, loose-fitting gloves, woollen socks and fur-lined boots. Also the hands should not be immersed in cold water. Working and living conditions should be in a warm atmosphere. Smoking must be stopped because nicotine in the blood causes vasoconstriction of the blood vessels, especially the small peripheral ones.

Vasodilator drugs have been tried but have limited success because the normal vessels tend to dilate rather than the diseased vessels.

Physiotherapy

Active exercises may be given to increase the flow of the general circulation.

Contrast baths may help. The patient is instructed to place the hands or feet in a hot bath for 3 minutes and then a cool bath for 1 minute. This can help to accelerate the rate of blood flow in the peripheral vessels.

Connective tissue massage may provide a symptomatic improvement in the condition. The sacral and lumbar basic area should be treated first and then the extremities. This reduces tension in the back and the patient often feels the extremities becoming warmer. A course of connective tissue massage is often of benefit prior to the advent of winter.

Surgery

Sympathectomy – In the dorsal region for the hands and in the lumbar region for the feet. The vasoconstrictor action of the sympathetic system on the blood vessels is released resulting in vasodilatation. The effect tends to wear off after a few months although some permanent benefit can be obtained. Again the operation should be performed at the beginning of winter.

Arterial surgery

This involves reconstruction of arteries.

Indications

Arteriosclerosis, thrombosis, aneurysm, congenital abnormalities, trauma.

Types of operation

1. Sympathectomy.
2. Direct suture.
3. Embolectomy.
4. Endarterectomy.
5. Arterial grafts.

When arterial surgery has failed or it is not possible to revascularize a limb, amputation is the only treatment.

Sympathectomy

This involves removal of the sympathetic nerve supply to a part of the body causing selective vasodilatation (increased activity of sympathetic system causes vasoconstriction).

A sympathectomy produces a local increase in blood supply to skin but its effect is not permanent. (Vasodilator drugs have a general effect.) The sympathetic system does not affect muscle arterial circulation and it is of no benefit in the treatment of intermittent claudication.

Direct suture

This is the rejoining of an artery after a part is removed.

Embolectomy

This is direct removal of an embolus through an opening in the artery. A Fogarty catheter with a balloon at the end is passed beyond the embolus. The balloon is then inflated and the catheter is withdrawn, removing the embolus and clearing the vessel.

Endarterectomy

This is the removal of an atheromatous occlusion by stripping it out together with the tunica interna and part of the media.

Arterial grafts

A graft may be used to replace an aneurysm or obstructed segment of an artery in larger arteries. A graft may also be used to construct a bypass round an obstructed artery. A bypass will be successful provided there is no significant arterial disease proximal or distal to the bypass.

For a general artery bypass the next suitable material is a saphenous vein which has a thick muscular wall and can withstand arterial pressure. As the vein has valves to aid venous blood flow the vein used for grafting must be reversed so that arterial blood flow is not obstructed. The cephalic vein in the arm can also be used.

A number of synthetic materials have been tried for grafting but the most commonly used is Dacron (terylene) which is inert, flexible and strong. Dacron grafts remain patent in aortic or iliac regions, and it is the material of choice because saphenous veins are not wide enough. It does, however, show a tendency to thrombose when used in the femoral or popliteal arteries and is used only when a saphenous vein graft is not possible or has failed.

An arterial bypass graft is described by the proximal and distal anastomoses, for example:

1. A femoro-popliteal graft is from the femoral artery to the popliteal artery (Figure 16.4).

2. An aorto-bifemoral graft is from the aorta to both femoral arteries (a trouser graft).
3. A femoro-femoral graft is from one femoral artery to the other (cross-over graft) and is used when one iliac artery is healthy and the other diseased.
4. An axillo-femoral graft is from the axillary artery to the femoral artery and is used to revascularize the lower limb when the aorta is blocked.

Complications of surgery

These can be general as in any major surgery or local around the site of operation.

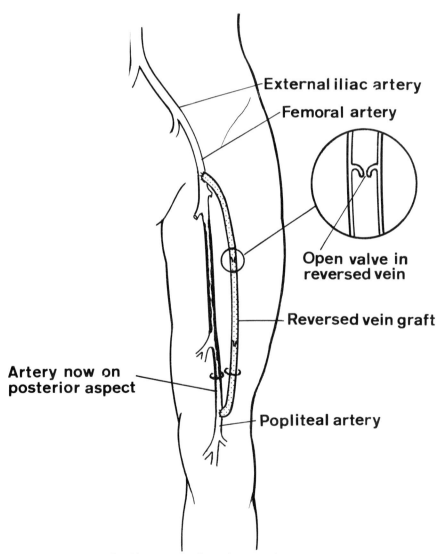

Figure 16.4 Femoro-popliteal bypass graft using saphenous vein

General

Circulatory complications are more likely to arise in arterial surgery than in other forms of major surgery because of the nature of the disease, the site of surgery and the age of patient:

1. *Coronary thrombosis or cerebrovascular accident* – If a thrombosis dislodges it may block one of the blood vessels supplying the heart or the brain.
2. *Deep vein thrombosis* – A thrombosis may form in the deep veins particularly of the calf due to sluggish venous circulation and increased release of thromboplastin at the operation site which may be near veins.
3. *Respiratory complications* – Secretions may accumulate because the patients are often smokers. The operation may take a number of hours and the patients may have limited respiratory function.

A pulmonary embolus may result from deep vein thrombosis.

Local

1. *Infection* – This is more likely to arise with a Dacron graft because it has no natural antibodies. Infection leads to breakdown of the anastomosis and leakage of blood into the neighbouring tissues.
   Signs of graft breakdown:
   (a) Excessive loss of blood from redivac drain.
   (b) Swelling at operation site.
2. *Haemorrhage* – This results from immediate leakage at the suture line.
3. *Graft obstruction* – This may arise due to thrombosis formation from slowing of the blood flow or irritation of the arterial wall.
   Signs of graft obstruction: The following signs may be present distal to the operation site:
   (a) Diminished or lost pulses.
   (b) Limb feels and/or appears cold.
   (c) Pain and numbness.
   (d) Colour becomes mottled, pale.
4. *Peripheral neuropathy* – Peripheral nerves may be damaged resulting in weakness of the muscles supplied by the damaged nerve.

Management

Preoperatively

All patients except those for acute emergency surgery, bleeding aneurysms or sudden total blockage of a main artery will be admitted before surgery. Investigations are carried out on the arterial and respiratory systems (see above). Drug therapy is reviewed, e.g. antibiotics and anticoagulants (heparin or warfarin).

Physiotherapy

This involves an explanation to the patient of the treatment and teaching the postoperative exercises to prevent complications.

Respiratory care

1. The patient is strongly advised to give up or at least reduce smoking.
2. Expansion breathing exercises and breathing control are taught.
3. Effective coughing or huffing is practised with the patient shown how to support the wound particularly if there is an abdominal incision.
4. More vigorous treatment may be required if lung infection is present.

Circulatory care

The importance of foot exercises must be explained and the patient practises them except where there is evidence of gangrene in the foot. General deep breathing is also taught so that the diaphragmatic movement will aid venous return.

Postoperatively

The patient may spend 24 hours in the intensive care unit, particularly for aortic grafts.

The patient wears antiembolitic stockings and lies supine with a bed cradle to allow the feet to move freely. This also enables observation of skin colour and arterial pulses. The lower limbs should be flat and not supported on a pillow.

A redivac drain remains *in situ* until drainage is minimal.

Physiotherapy

Breathing exercises

These are given when the patient recovers consciousness to the basal areas of the lungs combined with huffing to encourage expectoration with minimum effort by the patient. Thoracic incisions must be supported by the patient with the help of the therapist.

Foot exercises

These are given immediately to prevent deep vein thrombosis.

Active toe and ankle movements of both legs, particularly full-range dorsi- and plantar flexion are encouraged with all levels of graft. The patient must do the exercises vigorously every hour.

The therapist should note the skin temperature and colour of the lower limbs for signs of postoperative complications. The temperature chart should be read daily because a raised temperature is indicative of infection in the chest, urine or wound. Pain and swelling in the calf is indicative of deep vein thrombosis.

Blood-stained sputum, together with chest pain, should be reported in case a pulmonary embolus is developing. All arterial surgery has the same basic physiotherapy but following an embolectomy or endarterectomy the patient can move all joints of the lower limbs and is discharged after a few days.

Following arterial grafts no undue strain must be put on the graft and kinking must be avoided. The joints over which the graft passes must not be bent, e.g. avoid knee movements in femoral popliteal grafts and hip movements in ilio-femoral grafts.

The patient begins walking in 2–3 days following a femoral popliteal graft and knee movements are gradually encouraged. With more proximal grafts the patient must be encouraged to stand straight. The walking pattern is corrected daily and the distance is gradually increased before discharge in 7–10 days. The patient should walk up and down stairs.

In surgery where an arm vein has been used for grafting all movement of the upper limb joints should be encouraged postoperatively. Patients do not normally require physiotherapy after discharge from hospital.

Advice to patients

1. Avoid restrictive clothing which may interfere with the circulation, e.g. tight belts or bands.
2. Stop smoking or reduce it as much as possible.
3. Avoid positions which cause pressure on the graft, e.g. knee flexion beyond 90°, sitting back on heels, or crossing one leg over the other in femoral popliteal grafts.
4. Avoid prolonged standing (but if this is unavoidable then practise marking time). However, a daily walk should be encouraged.
5. Avoid exposure to excessive cold and take care with application of heat, e.g. hot-water bottles.
6. A gradual return to normal function and increasing the amount of physical activity is to be encouraged.

Amputations

Amputation is performed when arterial reconstructive surgery has failed or is not technically possible. It is also performed when the state of a limb is such that good function cannot be obtained.

Aetiology

Causes

1. *Congenital* – Deformities in infants (1% of all cases).

2. *Acquired*:
   (a) Peripheral vascular disease (arterial disease, usually atherosclerosis of the lower aorta and its branches) – majority of patients are elderly (64%).
   (b) Trauma – majority of patients have been in RTAs and are young adults (8%).
   (c) Malignancy (4%).
   (d) Metabolic – diabetes giving rise to ulcers and gangrene (21%).
   (e) Infection – bone disease (2%).
   (Department of Health statistics, 1985)

Amputations due to malignancy are decreasing whilst those due to peripheral vascular disease are increasing.

Site

Amputation of the lower limb is more common (24:1) and due mainly to peripheral vascular disease. That of the upper limb is due mainly to trauma.

Level (Figure 16.5)

Lower limb

1. *Toes.*
2. *Transmetatarsal* – Difficulty in healing but no prosthesis required – only an adapted shoe.
3. *Symes (through ankle)* – Rarely used for vascular patients but suitable for trauma and infection. Again, can walk without prosthesis.
4. *Below knee (BK)* – Ideal amputation site. Stump length 12.5–15 cm from knee joint. If the stump is too long, no muscle bulk is left for myoplastic flap. This level retains the knee joint, giving more mobility with lower energy requirements. The main problem is poor healing, particularly in vascular disease.
5. *Through-knee disarticulation* – No bone section is involved and the stump is strong with no muscle imbalance but the knee is cosmetically poor and prosthetically difficult. It is unsuitable in the presence of arthritis at the knee and a hip flexion deformity.
6. *Gritti–Stokes (femoral condyles)* – Good healing qualities but unsightly prosthesis.
7. *Mid-thigh (above knee, AK)* – Very good healing qualities but mobility is reduced due to loss of knee joint and higher energy requirements for function. The prosthetic knee mechanism must have 12 cm clearance; therefore, the soft tissues of the stump should be at least 12 cm above the knee joint.
8. *Hip disarticulation* – This is used in trauma or malignancy, not for peripheral vascular disease.

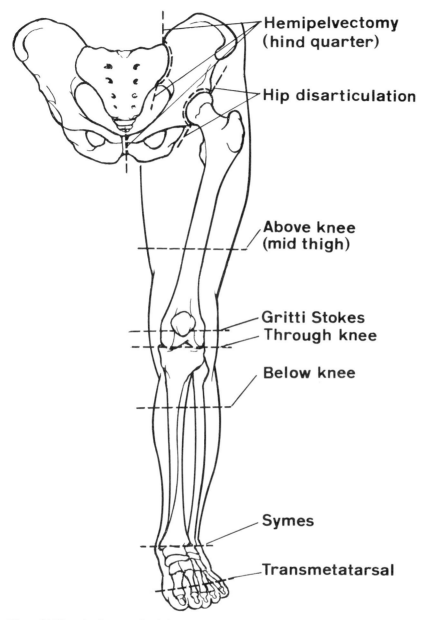

Figure 16.5 Levels of amputation in leg

The hip joint is disarticulated and the pelvis is intact.

9. *Hemipelvectomy (hindquarter)* – Removing the lower limb and half the pelvis with a muscle flap covering the internal organs. This level is used mainly in malignancy.

Over 90% are above or below knee in approximately equal numbers because these levels provide stumps suitable for a good functioning prosthesis. Below knee is the level of choice because energy requirements are less and functional independence is greater.

Sex

Male to female 2:1 – all amputations.

Prevalence

In the UK there are 132 amputees per 100 000 of the total population, resulting in 4500 per health region.

Prognosis

This is poor for those with peripheral vascular disease. Approximately 30% of unilateral amputees become bilateral amputees within 2 years and 50% die within 5 years. For the young adult amputee following trauma to the lower limbs the prognosis is excellent.

Management

These patients are most successfully managed in specialized units using a team approach. A typical team will consist of the surgeon, physiotherapist, prosthetist, occupational therapist, social worker, nurse, and the GP on discharge.

After an amputation the patient must have the rehabilitation programme and what can be achieved with cooperation explained For the elderly the main aim is to achieve independence but for the young adult a high level of physical activity can be attained.

Rehabilitation of lower limb amputations

The rehabilitation programme can be divided into:

1. The preoperative period.
2. The post-operative period:
   (a) Pre-prosthetic stage.
   (b) Prosthetic stage.

Preoperative period

If possible the patient should be assessed and treated by the physiotherapist before surgery. The longer the preoperative treatment the greater its value. An assessment of the physical, social and psychological states of the patient should be made.

Physical assessment

Assess the:

1. Muscle strength of the upper limbs, trunk and lower limb apart from affected limb below the level of amputation.
2. Joint mobility, particularly the joint proximal to the amputation level.
3. Respiratory function.
4. Balance reactions in sitting and standing.
5. Functional abilities.

The examination findings should be recorded for comparison at a later date.

Social assessment

The patient's social circumstances should be noted: family and friend's support, living accommodation (stairs, ramps, rails, width of doors, wheelchair accessibility), proximity of shops.

Psychological assessment

Note the patient's psychological approach to amputation and the motivation to walk.

Following assessment

A treatment programme should include:

1. Breathing exercises to clear secretions in the lungs because many vascular patients are smokers.
2. Strengthening exercises for the shoulder extensors and adductors, elbow extensors, hand grip, abdominals and trunk extensors, hip extensors, adductors and abductors (and quadriceps for below-knee level).
3. Mobilizing exercises for hip extension (and knee flexion and extension for BK level).
4. Bed mobility – bridging, moving up and down the bed, rolling to prone and back to supine.
5. Transfers from bed to chair and back.
6. Wheelchair mobility – the ability to stop, start, turn and control the wheelchair. The patient should have a wheelchair supplied preoperatively because it will be necessary for at least a few weeks post-operatively.
7. Stabilizations for the trunk in sitting and standing.

Postoperative period

Preprosthetic stage

The patient's bed should have a firm mattress and be adjustable in height with a rope ladder or monkey pole and a cradle. Postoperatively the patient requires regular and adequate analgesics to combat pain which may arise from the wound site or the phantom of a limb. Uncontrolled pain may limit the rehabilitation programme.

Aims of treatment

1. To prevent post-operative complications.
2. To prevent deformities.
3. To control stump oedema.
4. To maintain strength of whole body and increase strength of muscles controlling the stump.
5. To maintain general mobility.
6. To improve balance and transfers.
7. To re-educate walking.
8. To restore functional independence.
9. To treat phantom pain.

Prevention of postoperative complications

Breathing exercises and brisk foot exercises for the unaffected leg to prevent respiratory and circulatory complications are given on the first post-operative day and continued until the chest is clear and the patient is ambulant.

Prevention of deformity

Postoperatively there is a tendency for knee flexion in BK and hip flexion, adduction or abduction in AK amputations. Deformities arise due to pain, unopposed muscle action and the patient sitting for long periods in a wheelchair. They can be prevented by the following.

Positioning in bed – The stump should be parallel to the unaffected leg without resting on pillows. The patient should lie as flat as possible for short periods during the day and progress to prone lying when the drains are out and the patient's condition allows. The time should be progressed from 10 minutes to 30 minutes three times daily. If the patient has cardiac or respiratory problems or if the prone position is too uncomfortable he should remain supine for as long as possible.

Exercises. Strong isometric work to counteract the deformity:

1. For the quadriceps in a BK amputation.
2. For the hip extensors and adductors in a high AK amputation.
3. For the extensors and abductors in a low AK amputation.

These are begun when the drains are out in 2–3 days. Progress is made to free active and then resisted stump exercises. Initially the stump is very sensitive and the patient should be encouraged to handle it as much as possible to reduce the sensitivity. This also helps the patient to begin to overcome the shock of realization that the leg has actually gone.

Stump board – In a BK amputation the stump must rest on a stump board when the patient is sitting in a wheelchair (Figure 16.6). Long periods with the knee flexed must be avoided.

Control of stump oedema

A swollen stump is slow to heal and will make fitting a prosthesis difficult. The stump exercises and stump board will help to control oedema. In addition the bed end should be elevated 30°.

Controlled environment treatment (CET)

This may be applied to slow healing and swollen BK stumps and remains in place until swelling is reduced, and the stump is healed. The 'dressing free' stump is placed in a clear, sealed plastic sleeve which is attached to a pressure-cycled machine blowing sterile warmed air over the wound. The temperature, pressure and humidity are all controlled giving the ideal environment for the healing of

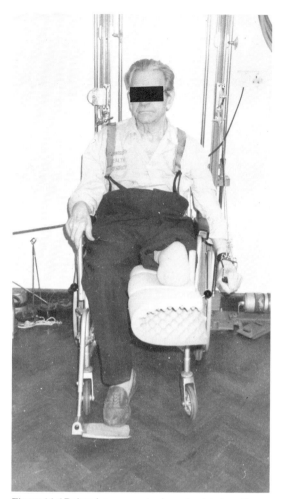

Figure 16.6 Below-knee amputee in a wheelchair resting on a stump board strengthening upper limb muscles

the stump, the progress of which can be easily seen. The patient can continue exercises and walking while attached to the machine.

Pressure environment treatment (PET)

This is a simpler version of the CET because the air is not sterilized, has no temperature control and limited pressure control. It is used on oedematous but healed stumps for up to 2 hours per session, e.g. in a physiotherapy department.

Flowtron

The stump is placed in an invaginated plastic bag. The air pressure in the bag varies rhythmically, compressing and relaxing the stump to reduce the oedema.

Stump compression socks or bandaging

The wound is covered in a non-stick dressing and fixed with a loose crêpe bandage to avoid constriction and ischaemia to the stump. Sutures are removed 2–3 weeks post-operatively.

Elasticated stump compression socks (Juzo socks) are a convenient method of reducing any oedema and conditioning the stump for all-round pressure which the patient experiences when wearing a prosthesis. They come in different widths and sizes and should be applied with a Seton Tubigrip frame for the first 3–4 days to stop rubbing of the skin, wound breakdown and pain. Bandaging is a controversial method of controlling stump oedema particularly in vascular patients where poor bandaging can cause stump damage. When the sutures are removed an Elset 15 cm (6 in) wide for an above-knee amputation and 10 cm (4 in) wide for a below-knee amputation can be applied (Figure 16.7). The pressure should be even and firm, decreasing towards the groin. Diagonal rather than circular turns prevent a tourniquet effect. The bandage should be reapplied at least three times a day and worn day and night but removed when wearing a prosthesis. The patient and relatives should be shown its application. When the patient is wearing a definitive limb all day and the stump fits it comfortably in the morning, the application of pressure to the stump can stop unless the patient is confined to bed for more than a day. Bandaging usually begins when the sutures are removed but Juzo socks can be applied after a week. Regular inspections of the skin must be undertaken and both the socks and bandage must be washed frequently.

If the stump does not heal or breaks down, ultraviolet radiation may be given. For an infected wound an E4 or double E4 is given to the open area only and for an uninfected wound an E1 can be given to both the open area and the surrounding skin.

Maintain body strength and strengthen muscles controlling stump

The extensors and adductors of the shoulder and elbow extensors can be strengthened by working against weights or springs attached behind to the bed. For example:

1. Grasp stretch lying; shoulder extension and adduction (against springs or weights).

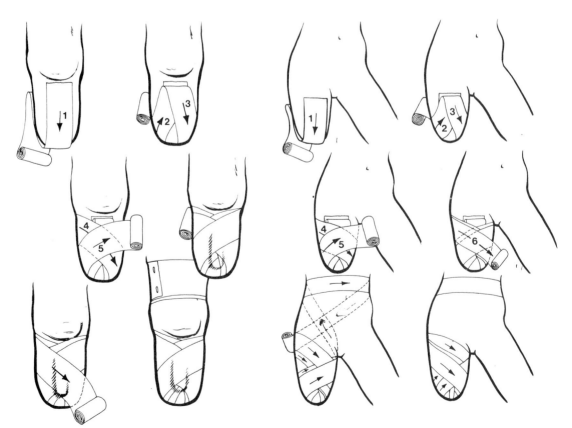

Figure 16.7 Stump bandaging (Courtesy Seton Healthcare Group.)

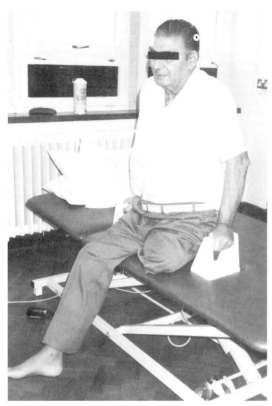

Figure 16.8 Amputee lifting buttocks

2. Grasp lying (elbows bent); straighten elbow (against springs).
3. Lying; slow reversals – flexion, adduction, lateral rotation – extension, abduction and medial rotation.
4. Sitting; push down on hands, raise buttocks (Figure 16.8).

Strong arm muscles are necessary for crutch walking;

5. Trunk muscles can be strengthened by crook lying; bridging (Figure 16.9).
6. Lying; rolling.
7. Sitting; stabilizations to trunk.
8. Crook lying; knee rolling side to side.

Exercises for the unaffected leg:

1. Lying; static quadriceps.
2. Lying; static gluteal.
3. lying; leg carrying sideways and in.
4. Lying; leg lift and lower.
5. Lying; one hip and knee bend and stretch.

These exercises can be started on the first day post-operatively and gradually progressed by adding manual resistance or increasing the spring resistance.

Stump exercises begin when the drains are out and are gradually progressed from static exercises to free active and then resisted exercises (Figures 16.10–16.12). In a BK amputation progress to knee

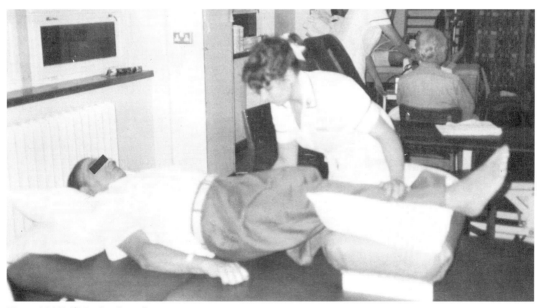

Figure 16.9 Bridging by above-knee amputee

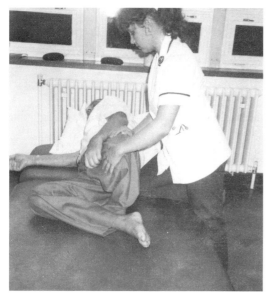

Figure 16.10 Stump exercises for above-knee amputee

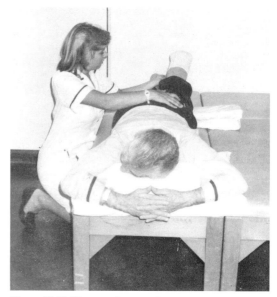

Figure 16.12 Hip extension exercises

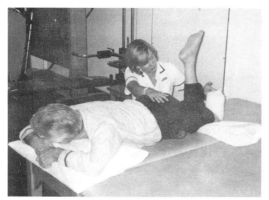

Figure 16.11 Knee flexion exercises

straightening against resistance and in AK amputation prone lying leg lifting and lower against resistance. The hip extensors can be strengthened using springs, weight and pulley circuit and manual resistance.

Maintain general mobility

Exercises which move the shoulder joint in all directions will maintain its mobility. Trunk movements in lying and sitting will improve trunk mobility which is essential for good function of the lower limbs.

Improve balance and transfers

The patient is allowed to sit in a wheelchair from the first day provided that he is alert and cooperative.

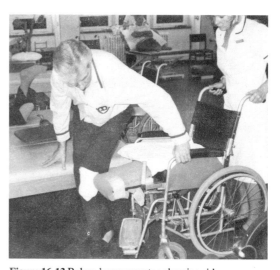

Figure 16.13 Below-knee amputee showing sideways transfer

Transfer to the wheelchair from the bed may be achieved by a backward or a sideways transfer (Figure 16.13) with the help of a sliding board. A sideways transfer is easier to the side of the remaining leg. Double amputees transfer forwards to the bed or toilet because a sideways transfer requires much more strength. Once the method of transfer has been determined, all team members must use the same method to reinforce it. Following transfers the patient is taught how to manoeuvre the wheelchair. This will enable him to move around the ward and give the patient a sense of freedom.

Balance in sitting can be improved by encouraging balance reactions (Figures 16.14 and 16.15), by tapping the patient in all directions, or by trunk stabilizations if the patient is unsteady. Later, use can be made of a balance (wobble) board for advanced balance work.

Re-educate walking

Partial weight bearing is commenced in the parallel bars using the pneumatic post-amputation mobility aid (PPAM aid) 5–10 days post-operatively (Figure 16.16). The patient should wear normal dress and a good walking shoe on the unaffected leg. The PPAM aid consists of outer and inner plastic cuffs, a rigid metal frame in different sizes and an air-pump. The outer cuff for the above knee is shorter with the air inlet proximally and the below knee outer cuff is longer with the inlet distally.

Application of PPAM aid

Slightly inflate the inner cuff and apply by folding it in half or invaginating it over stump. The outer cuff is then slipped over stump and inner cuff to reach the groin and buttock. Ease the metal frame over

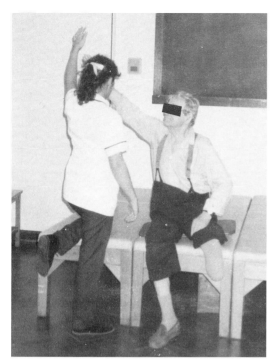

Figure 16.14 Balance re-education for below-knee amputation in lateral direction

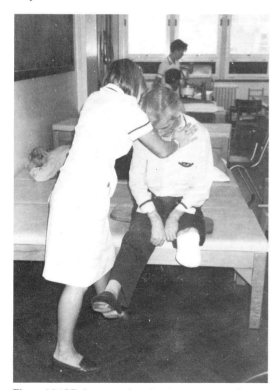

Figure 16.15 Balance re-education in antero-posterior direction

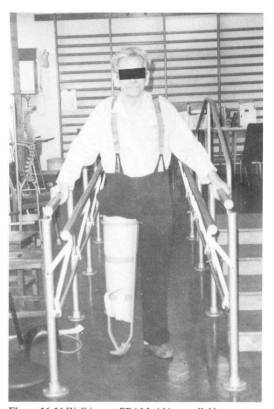

Figure 16.16 Walking on PPAM aid in parallel bars

both cuffs and measure length by comparing it with the unaffected leg. The frame should be 7–10 cm below the tip of the outer cuff. The webbing straps are fixed to support the distal end of the outer cuff. Inflate the outer bag which presses against metal frame. Progress is made by increasing the pressure registered on the pump:

Begin with   10 mm Hg for 10 min ⎤
             20 mm Hg for 10 min ⎬ Day 1
             20 mm Hg for 20 min ⎦

             30 mm Hg for 20 min ⎤
             30 mm Hg for 30 min ⎬ Day 2
             40 mm Hg for 30 min ⎦

Once the patient is comfortable at 40 mmHg he stands up and the leg length is checked before starting partial weight bearing in the parallel bars (small, slim patients may begin partial weight bearing at 30 mmHg). Before beginning walking apply the PPAM aid with the patient in bed and progress to sitting on a chair between the parallel bars. Walking progression is made to elbow crutches but never to sticks and the patient should not attempt stairs, steps or slopes. The patient must hip hitch and not swivel on the rocker while using a good gait pattern. Until the sutures are out the aid is used for short periods of time and only walk up the parallel bars once. Later the PPAM aid can be worn for 1–2 hours with some rest periods to check the skin. The wound should be inspected after each application and if there are many marks or wound leakage the use of the PPAM aid should stop immediately.

For added suspension in above-knee amputations use a shoulder strap which passes from the frame over the patient's opposite shoulder and back to the frame. Avoid using the PPAM aid for 1–2 days when the sutures are removed, particularly with BK amputations. The PPAM aid allows early weight bearing through the affected leg, helps to reduce oedema, provides all-round pressure on the stump similar to a prosthesis and can be used to assess a patient's ability to walk with a prosthesis. It cannot, however, replace a prosthesis because it cannot be applied by the patient himself or worn constantly all day and knee flexion is not possible when sitting down.

Bilateral amputees may use the PPAM aid if they can wear a prosthesis on the other leg.

Walking without a prosthesis

When the wound is healed the patient has the stump firmly supported with compression socks or a bandage and gait training can be done in the parallel bars. The patient can progress to a frame or crutches depending on stability. This form of mobility may be useful for the patient to move around the home because it may be easier and faster than using a prosthesis and all rooms may not be accessible to a wheelchair.

Restore functional independence

This begins the first day post-operatively by encouraging bridging with the stump in extension and rolling together with bed mobility. The patient is taught to move up and down the bed by pressing on the sole of the remaining leg which may require protection with a sheepskin boot if the cause is vascular disease. Sitting up from lying by pushing down with arms can begin when the drips are removed. Good trunk rotation will make this function easier.

As soon as the patient is able, functional training should be carried out in the physiotherapy department approximately 4–6 days post-operatively. The patient is encouraged to dress each day and propel himself in a wheelchair to the department.

The exercise programme should now consist of resisted pulley work, mat exercises, slow reversal and repeated contractions to the trunk and limbs, spring resistance. During this time the occupational therapist will help the patient with any dressing difficulties, teach bath transfers and provide cooking practice.

The patient must be encouraged to be as independent as possible.

Phantom pain

This is pain or sensation in the stump or 'phantom limb' and its incidence is higher in patients with a severely painful limb preoperatively. It should be explained to the patient that it is due to memory of the amputated part in the cortex and nerve impulses still travelling through nerve fibres in the part, but the pain is only temporary and will gradually fade within a year. Persistent severe phantom pain may be helped by non-invasive treatment. The patient should be given adequate analgesics preoperatively and be encouraged to handle the stump postoperatively to reduce its sensitivity. A number of modalities can be tried such as transcutaneous nerve stimulation (TNS) (Figure 16.17), interferential, acupuncture, ultrasound and percussion manually or electrically.

Prosthetic stage

The patient is referred to a Limb Fitting Centre for assessment when the stump is healed 2–3 weeks post-operatively. Not all patients are automatically fitted with a prosthesis.

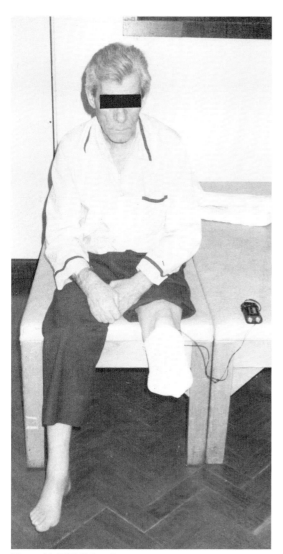

Figure 16.17 TNS for phantom pain

Factors to be considered before supplying a prosthesis

1. *Age and physical condition* – The old and frail may be unsuitable.
2. *Mental condition* – Well motivated and not confused.
3. *State of stump* – Must be well healed and not constricted or swollen.
4. *Level of amputation* – Bilateral above-knee amputees are not suitable for prosthetic rehabilitation but almost all unilateral below-knee amputees are suitable.
5. *General condition* – Patients with cardiac, cerebral, respiratory, or other limb problems may be unsuitable.

If prosthetic rehabilitation is not possible the patient may be supplied with a prosthesis for cosmetic purposes only.

Prostheses

1. Temporary prosthesis.
2. Definitive prosthesis.

Temporary prosthesis

This takes approximately 2 weeks to make and is supplied because it is:

1. Quick and easy to manufacture.
2. Cheaper, lighter and relatively simple to apply.
3. Allows time for stump shrinkage to take place.

Definitive prosthesis

Measurements are taken when stump shrinkage is complete and the definitive prosthesis takes 2–3 months to manufacture.

Structure of a prosthesis

All prostheses have:

1. A socket into which the stump fits.
2. Suspension to fix the stump securely to the prosthesis during the swing phase.
3. A complete prosthetic foot (for amputations from the ankle proximally).
4. Joints to replace those amputated.
5. Endoskeletal or exoskeletal design.

Sockets are made of felt, metal or plastic. The definitive prostheses fit better than temporary.

Suspension – A patellar tendon bearing (PTB) is suspended by leather supracondylar straps (male) and an elastic stocking and suspender belt (female). Both an above knee (AK) and an above-knee below-knee (AKBK) may be self-suspending, have a rigid pelvic band or soft suspension. A shoulder strap may give additional suspension.

Prosthetic feet

There are two main types:

1. Solid ankle cushion heel (SACH) which has a rubber heel with cushion properties providing mobility and making an ankle joint unnecessary.
2. A uniaxial or polyaxial ankle joint in a wooden or plastic foot.

Joints

Knee joints may be uniaxial or polyaxial, free (controlled by patient's muscle power) or with a locking mechanism built in. This gives a stable joint

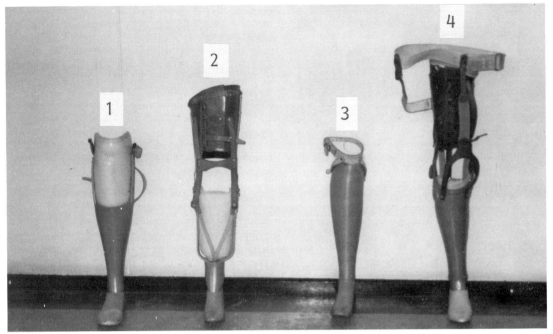

Figure 16.18 (1) Temporary PTB. (2) Temporary AKBK. (3) Definitive PTB. (4) Definitive ischial weight bearing

during weight bearing but unlocks to allow knee movement to permit easy sitting.

Ankle – Mentioned in prosthetic feet.

Design

Endoskeletal prostheses have a rigid central support (metal or carbon fibre) surrounded by a soft cosmetic covering.

Exoskeletal prostheses have two rigid metal bars forming part of the cosmetic cover.

Types of prosthesis for amputation levels

1. *Transmetatarsal* – Special shoes with cushion-made insoles or toeblocks.
2. *Below knee* – A temporary prostheses may be:
   (a) *PTB* where weight is taken through the patellar tendon and other pressure-tolerant areas. A soft Pelite liner is surrounded by a hard socket. This is the prosthesis of choice (Figure 16.18(1)).
   (b) *AKBK* – Where the weight is taken through the ischium. It consists of a leather thigh corset and a felt socket which accommodates an unhealed or poorly shaped stump (Figure 16.18(2)).

   Definitive prostheses are of similar design but more cosmetically acceptable, and the AKBK has a rigid socket (Figure 16.18(3) and (4)).

3. *Mid-thigh*:
   (a) The temporary prosthesis has a metal or plastic socket with a rigid pelvic band and is ischial weight bearing (Figure 16.19(1)). A shoulder strap can give additional support. The knee mechanism is locked during weight bearing and released for sitting.
   (b) The definitive prostheses has a similar design to the temporary prosthesis but can have increased movement at the hip and ankle and a soft suspension.
   (c) A variety of knee mechanisms exist which control the joint in the stance or swing phases.
   (d) In the stance phase the knee may be manually fixed or free or may automatically lock in extension (Figure 16.19(2) and (4)). In the swing phase a wheel mechanism can adjust the freedom of knee movement (Figure 16.19(3)).
   (e) A suction prosthesis may be given to patients with good muscle control and a stable stump. There is no pelvic band and the stump muscles contracting against the socket together with the vacuum produced by a valve provide the necessary suspension.

Application of a prosthesis

Stump socks help to provide an efficient fit of the stump to the socket. There are three types:

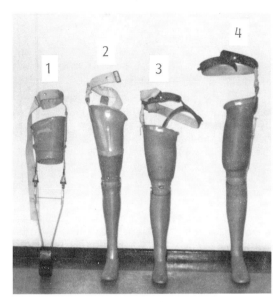

Figure 16.19 (1) Temporary AK. (2) Definitive AK with small lever at knee. (3) Definitive AK with wheel mechanism. (4) Definitive AK with high lever at knee

1. *Nylon* – Very thin and allows free sliding surface between stump and socket.
2. *Wool* – Thick material which absorbs perspiration. Extra socks can be worn to compensate for stump shrinkage.
3. *Cotton* – Three cotton socks are equivalent to one wool and are used to make finer adjustments in the fit of the stump to the socket.

When more than three wool socks are required the socket should be relined at the limb fitting centre.

PTB

The patient sits and applies stump sock (socks). Place Pelite liner firmly over stump and sock until patella tendon bar rests on tendon. The hard outer socket is applied over the liner as proximal as possible so that on weight bearing, the stump will not sink any further. The supracondylar straps or elastic stocking suspension are firmly fastened.

To remove the prosthesis the process is reversed, but the socket, liner and sock usually all come off together. On removal, the skin of the stump should be checked for any abnormal pressure areas.

AKBK temporary prosthesis

The patient is sitting or half-lying with stump bandage or compression socks applied. The leather thigh corset is loosened, and the prosthetic knee joint is fixed in extension. The stump sock is applied, and the stump slips into the felt socket until the patient's knee joint is 1–5 cm below the prosthetic knee joint. The pelvic band followed by the leather socket is fastened. A shoulder strap, if present, is adjusted in standing.

To remove the prosthesis the patient sits down, keeps the prosthetic knee joint in extension and unfastens the pelvic band and leather corset. The stump slips out of the felt bucket and all socks and bandages are removed. The patient's skin must be checked for areas of redness or rubbing.

Mid-thigh temporary prosthesis

The patient sits on a firm surface with the prosthetic knee joint unlocked in flexion and the foot laterally rotated. The stump sock is applied and the stump slips into the socket. The rigid pelvic band followed by the shoulder strap are loosely fastened, and the stump sock is pulled up over the rim of the socket.

The prosthetic knee joint is locked in extension and the patient stands up, securely fixing the pelvic band which brings the joint into mid-position. The shoulder strap is then adjusted. Some young patients may apply the prosthesis in standing.

To remove the prosthesis, the patient sits down, loosens the pelvic band and shoulder strap, slips the socket off the stump and inspects the skin as with all prostheses.

Suction prosthesis

The patient stands up and a bandage is loosely applied to the stump, from proximal to distal. The distal end of the bandage is passed through the inside of the socket and out through the valve hole. The stump is slipped into the socket and the bandage is pulled through the valve, easing the stump into the socket. When the stump is correctly positioned in the socket, the valve hole is closed.

A suction prosthesis can be eased off the leg by opening the valve hole.

Correct fitting of a prosthesis

Before application of a prosthesis – The therapist must check that it is correct for the patient, the shoes are a pair and are the original ones given to the prosthetist (or have exactly the same heel height).

After application of a prosthesis – The therapist must check that:

1. The socket fits correctly. In standing the patient is asked to transfer weight onto the prosthesis. The patellar bar must remain firmly on the patellar tendon in a PTB. In an ischial weight-bearing prosthesis the therapist palpates the patient's ischial tuberosity, and asks the patient

to transfer weight onto the prosthesis. If the tuberosity slides down into the socket, it is too large or the stump has shrunk. If the tuberosity stays above the weight-bearing shelf, the stump is too large or the socket is too small. If the socket is too large, extra stump socks may be worn (up to three woollen) and if the socket is too tight thinner stump socks may be worn, or the stump volume reduced by bandaging or mechanical pressure.

2. The prosthesis is the correct length. In a PTB the length is correct if the heel and toe are on the ground. A fixed-knee prosthesis should be 1–2 cm shorter than the remaining leg to enable the patient to hip hitch.

3. There is no discomfort in the adductor region in an ischial weight-bearing prosthesis.

4. The suspension is correctly adjusted.

5. The patient fully understands the mechanism of the prosthesis and is taught how to apply and remove it.

Gait training

This begins in the parallel bars and the patient transfers weight first in stride and then in walk standing. This should be achieved by shifting the pelvis and not by bending the trunk.

Hip hitching is taught if the patient has a prosthesis with a locked knee. The prosthesis should not be allowed to abduct, or shoot forwards. Walking is taught using a three- or four-point gait according to the patient's ability. Begin with weight transference to the prosthetic leg, and swing the unaffected leg forwards by pushing the pelvis forwards and extending the stump back against the socket. The patient is encouraged to take short, even steps with an upright posture, and to turn by taking short paces without swivelling round. Progress is made by using one stick and one parallel bar, and then two sticks first within the bars and then round the department. For greater stability some patients may require tetrapods instead of sticks, and a frame may be used if the patient requires even greater support.

When the patient can walk with a reasonable gait progress is made by walking with one stick in the appropriate hand, until this may be discarded altogether. As the patient's ability improves, other activities can be introduced to the treatment programme:

1. Walking sideways and backwards.
2. Walking on different surfaces, carpets, tiles, gravel, grass, rough ground.
3. Standing up and sitting down in a chair.
4. Ascending stairs (unaffected leg first) and descending stairs (prosthesis first).
5. Ascending a slope (long stride with unaffected leg, short stride with prosthesis) and descending slope (strides reversed).
6. Getting up from the floor – roll over to unaffected side, extend prosthesis, push up on unaffected leg with hands on chair or stick.
7. Picking up objects from floor.
8. Clearing obstacles.

Gait training should be carried out in front of a full-length mirror to enable the patient to observe and correct any faults.

Increase the walking time each day, and inspect the stump at the end of each treatment.

Young, fit amputees will require a week's gait training, but elderly patients will require 2 weeks or more.

Patients with PTBs will use a normal walking pattern without hip hitching. When the patient is supplied with a definitive limb, a further period of gait training may be needed.

Some patients may progress from a prosthesis with a fixed knee to one with a free knee. Gait training will particularly emphasize the swing phase with the prosthesis. The prosthesis is brought forwards with hip flexion (not hip hitching) and the stump is strongly extended on heel strike.

Home visit

A home visit should be made prior to discharge from hospital and another may be necessary at the end of gait training. An assessment should be made of floor coverings, stairs, slopes, door widths necessary for ramps, additional rails or structural changes, access to bathroom, facilities in kitchen for cooking and washing.

The occupational therapist will help with the home visit, dressing, transfers, wheelchair provision if necessary and contacting the patient's local social services.

Final rehabilitation involves the patient returning to a normal, active everyday life including, in the case of the young, participation in sports such as squash, tennis and golf, and in the case of the elderly to functional independence.

Hemipelvectomy and hip disarticulation

These are extensive amputations, often due to malignancy, and the patients require special psychological support. The preprosthetic stage follows a similar pattern to that of the lower levels, but as the prognosis is poor this stage should be as short as possible. These patients are supplied with definitive prostheses from the beginning and emphasis is put on functional re-education. Details of the prostheses are beyond the scope of this book.

Bilateral lower limb amputations

Patients with peripheral vascular disease who initially have a unilateral amputation often become bilateral amputees. They will follow a similar programme to that already described, except for standing and walking. Physiotherapy will emphasize strengthening the upper limb and trunk, re-education of sitting balance and independence in a wheelchair which is needed for such patients.

Initially these amputees are supplied with rocker pylons, with back extensions. These pylons are much shorter than the patient's own legs, so that the patient's centre of gravity is lower, making balance and walking easier. Very few bilateral above-knee amputees become functionally independent on prostheses, but may use them cosmetically.

Upper limb amputations

The amputations are acquired mainly due to trauma or malignancy, but some may be the result of congenital deformity. Physiotherapy is similar to that in the lower limb amputations, but the occupational therapist plays a greater part in functional rehabilitation. In the preprosthetic stage, mobilizing the shoulder and shoulder girdle is vital preparation for using a prosthesis. Prevention of a flexion, adduction and medial rotation deformity in the above elbow and a flexion deformity in the below elbow is important.

When the stump is healed and oedema is controlled by bandaging, the patient is assessed for a definitive prosthesis. Many patients can become functionally independent without a prosthesis, and use one only cosmetically. Working prostheses can be powered by the patient's muscles, or electronically. A number of terminal devices can be supplied to meet the needs of individual patients, but the split hook is the most versatile.

Diseases of veins

Superficial venous thrombosis (phlebitis or thrombophlebitis)

This is an inflammation of the inner walls of superficial veins – mainly of lower limb.

Causes

1. Trauma to the vessel wall – a drip needle or pressure externally due to tight garments or position of limb.
2. Circulating toxins from septic wounds.
3. Association with deep venous thrombosis.

Pathology

Irritation produced changes in the tunica intima, causing a thrombus to form. The thrombus becomes attached to the vein wall and rarely produces an embolus.

Clinical features

There is a localized, reddened, warm area with hard, cord-like swelling along the course of the affected superficial vein. Pain may be present at rest and is aggravated by movement of the limb. As the condition resolves the skin becomes pigmented (brown) along the course of the vein.

Treatment

1. Firm elastic bandaging or stockings from the toes to beyond the upper limit of the affected area.
2. Drug therapy:
   (a) Antibiotics in cases of infective phlebitis.
   (b) Analgesics to relieve pain.
   (c) Anti-inflammatory, e.g. indomethacin to reduce the inflammation.
3. Exercise – The patients should be encouraged to carry out foot exercises with the legs elevated and to remain ambulant to maintain venous circulation. In severe cases the patient may be confined to bed for a short period.
4. It is important that the physiotherapist recognizes the condition in a patient so that treatment can be instigated and physiotherapy modified if necessary.

Deep venous thrombosis (DVT)

This is blocking of a deep vein by the formation of a thrombus – most commonly in the lower limb.

Predisposing factors

1. Venous stasis due to a paralysed or immobile limb, prolonged bed rest or during surgery.
2. Injury to the vessel wall – during surgery or trauma.
3. Increased coagulability of the blood. An increase in the number of platelets is common after surgery or childbirth.
4. Middle-aged to elderly patients, particularly those who are obese.
5. Drugs – notably the contraceptive pill.
6. A previous history of DVT or people with vascular or blood disorders.

Pathology

Damage to the intima causes platelets to be deposited on the vein wall. Venous stasis increases the accumulation of platelets which adds to the size of the thrombus resulting in occlusion of the vessel lumen. There is further extension of the thrombus (propagated thrombus) along the vessel to the next junction with a vein. A portion may break off giving rise to a pulmonary embolus or the thrombus may become organized and firmly attached to the venous wall. Gradually it is recanalized and the circulation is re-established but the valves are often destroyed leaving chronic venous insufficiency. This is a particular disadvantage in the lower limb.

Clinical features

1. Aching or cramp-like pain at site of thrombus.
2. Tenderness on deep palpation over the area.
3. Oedema around the joint distal to the area.
4. May be symptomless.
5. Unexplained systemic features, e.g. mild pyrexia, pleuritic pain, tachycardia in a patient recovering from surgery.
6. Severe pulmonary embolus giving signs of extreme distress, breathlessness and shock may be the first indication of DVT.
7. Increased pain in the calf on passive dorsiflexion of the foot (Homans' sign) is suggestive of DVT in lower leg.

Treatment

Prevention is better than cure and early diagnosis is important for effective treament.

Diagnosis

Phlebography is used for establishing the diagnosis in doubtful cases.

A Doppler probe can assess venous flow. If a distal vein is blocked no flow will occur in a proximal vein, e.g. thrombosis in calf results in no flow in the femoral vein.

Prevention (lower limb DVT)

1. Inpatients confined to bed with a cradle under the bedclothes and the bed end elevated 15–22 cm.
2. TED (anti-embolitic) stockings should be worn by all patients who are confined to bed post-operatively.
3. General breathing exercises and active movements of the hips, knees and particularly foot and ankle for patients on prolonged bed rest.
4. Early ambulation and not sitting with the legs dependent is important.
5. Passive movements of a paralysed limb.
6. Any risk factors should be minimized, e.g. stop the contraceptive pill before planned surgery.

7. Anticoagulant therapy, e.g. low-dose heparin may be given preoperatively in high-risk cases or dextran during surgery.

Treatment

1. Bed rest with a cradle and the end of the bed elevated until all the local signs subside – maybe up to 7 days. This helps the thrombus to adhere to the venous wall.
2. Foot and leg exercises while in bed and a gradual increase in mobility. The patient must walk and not stand or sit with the legs dependent and must wear support on the legs at all times even in bed.
3. Anticoagulant therapy. This is begun immediately with heparin given intravenously (heparin inhibits the conversion of prothrombin to thrombin).

    Oral anticoagulants are then started, e.g. warfarin which slows down the formation of vitamin K necessary in the formation of thrombin. This may be continued for up to 6 months to reduce the risk of further DVT

Pulmonary embolism

This is a complication of deep venous thrombosis. If a thrombus breaks off in a deep vein it travels in the venous system to the right side of the heart where it enters the pulmonary artery and passes into the pulmonary circulation where it blocks a vessel, the lumen of which is too narrow to let it pass through. The factors that predispose to a deep vein thrombosis also predispose to a pulmonary embolism.

Pathology

A large embolus causes complete occlusion of the pulmonary artery causing blockage of the blood flow from the right ventricle, usually resulting in death.

Smaller emboli cause occlusion of pulmonary circulation to a segment of a lung.

Clinical features
Large embolus

1. Sudden collapse.
2. Severe retrosternal pain and shock.
3. Dyspnoea and distension of neck veins.
4. Reduced air entry and scattered wheeze.

Smaller embolus

1. Sudden onset of severe chest pain.
2. Dyspnoea.
3. Haemoptysis and pleuritic pain.

Treatment

1. Drugs: anticoagulants. Streptokinase – dissolves thrombus.
2. Surgery – pulmonary embolectomy.
3. Bed rest with the end of the bed elevated. Patient is allowed up when all symptoms have disappeared.

It is important that the physiotherapist can recognize the signs of a pulmonary embolus so that treatment can be instigated early. Physiotherapy in the form of active exercises to the lower limb and early ambulation are important preventative measures.

Varicose veins

Varicose veins are dilated, lengthened and tortuous with incompetent valves. Superficial varicose veins can be seen through the skin.

Aetiology

Age – any age, but commonest 40–50 years.
Sex – Female more than male.

Predisposing factors

1. Compression of pelvic veins during pregnancy.
2. Occupation necessitating constant standing, e.g. shop assistant.
3. Tight corsets or garters.
4. Heredity may be a factor.
5. Secondary to deep venous thrombosis.
6. Basic weakness of vein wall.

Pathology

The vein wall dilates at weak areas and the valves become incompetent. Normally as the calf muscles contract there is pressure on the deep veins which forces the blood proximally. This pressure is not transmitted to the superficial veins because of the valves in communicating veins. When these valves become incompetent the pressure pushes the blood into the superficial veins which dilate and lengthen. A vicious circle is set up, the ineffectual valves permitting regurgitation and the increased amount of blood thus left in the veins still further dilating them and making the valves more incompetent.

During standing the force of gravity tends to keep the blood in the lower parts of the body, aggravating the condition.

There is loss of elastic tissue, muscle atrophy of the media layer and hypertrophy of the outer layer.

Clinical features

1. Superficial veins appear as tortuous 'knotted' structures.
2. May be only cosmetically troublesome or the patient may complain of pain, aching and fatigue in the legs with difficulty in walking.
3. Cramp in calf muscles, especially at night.
4. Calf muscles weaken, lose their pumping action and support for the veins accentuating the venous changes.
5. Skin of leg may be pigmented, indurated and show signs of ulceration.
6. There is congestion and oedema of the ankles due to the dilated veins and the abnormally high pressure in the capillaries which results in increased exudation of lymph.

Complications

1. Bleeding following rupture of vein.
2. Venous ulcer due to devitalized skin.
3. Superficial venous thrombosis.
4. Oedma, particularly of the foot and ankle.

Treatment

1. Conservative.
2. Surgical.

Conservative

The aim of treatment is to improve venous return:

1. Elastic support which increases efficiency of calf muscles as a pump. This may be elastic stockings or elastic bandages which may be more effective.
2. Encourage walking but avoid standing especially for long periods.
3. Elevation of lower legs for 10 minutes three times a day and sleep with end of bed raised.
4. Injection of sclerosant solution into the vein followed by firm bandaging of the leg for 6 weeks. The sclerosant produces inflammation in the vein causing its lumen to be obliterated so that no blood can pass through.

Physiotherapy – The patient is encouraged to practise foot and ankle exercises in elevation and instructed to walk 1–2 miles a day, in support stockings if necessary, to keep blood flowing through the deep veins. The correct pattern of walking must be emphasized.

Surgical

This is carried out when the patient is in severe pain or is in an occupation which involves prolonged standing. The aim is to remove as many dilated veins as possible and ligate others.

Physiotherapy

Post-operatively the legs are bandaged and elevated to promote blood flow in the deep veins. When resting, the knee should be straight but the patient must practise leg exercises hourly as soon as possible. For example: foot and ankle 'pumping' exercises, hip and knee flexion and extension, quadriceps and gluteal contractions.

First day post-operatively – The patient is helped out of bed and walking is commenced with the legs well bandaged. The patient is encouraged to move the ankle and knee joints together with the correct 'push off' with even timing and stride length patterns.

Second day post-operatively – The distance walked is progressed (avoid standing still) and a flight of stairs attempted.

The patient is discharged within 48 hours with clear instructions on the wearing of support stockings for several weeks and the continuation of the exercises at home.

Physiotherapy may also be given for any venous ulcers or oedema.

Ulcers

An ulcer is a loss of epithelial cells causing exposure of the underlying tissue.

Types

1. Venous.
2. Arterial (ischaemic).
3. Pressure sores.

Venous ulcers

Aetiology

Sex – Women more than men.

Age – Most common in 50–70 year age group.

Site – Lower two-thirds of the lower leg (slightly higher on the anterior and medial aspects) and on parts of the foot not supported by the shoe.

Size – This varies but 18–20 cm^2 on the lower leg is quite common. In some cases an ulcer can become very large and encircle the leg.

Predisposing factors

1. Venous and lymphatic congestion associated with varicose veins or deep venous thrombosis.
2. Occupations demanding prolonged standing.
3. Poor personal hygiene and malnutrition.

Precipitating factors

Local trauma – often very slight – breaks the weakened skin.

Pathology

Due to failure of the venous pump as a result of valve incompetence, binding down of deep fibrous tissue, and lack of pumping action by the calf muscles there is chronic venous congestion. This results in increased exudate and slowing down of the blood flow. Nutrition of the tissues is diminished and the skin is devitalized. The cells necrose and the skin breaks down. There is insufficient oxygen and nutrition to promote healing and the area remains open. Bacteria may invade the area or the dead cells may irritate the normal tissue, causing inflammation and the ulcer spreads. If the chronic venous congestion is reduced and the circulation, bringing oxygen and nutrition to the area, is improved together with the removal of any infection and the mobilizing of the soft tissues the ulcer will heal with the formation of scar tissue.

Clinical features (Figure 16.20)

1. The floor of the ulcer (part showing loss of tissue, exposing underlying tissues – even bone if severe) may be:
   (a) Pale and anaemic with watery discharge – indolent (static, unhealing) ulcer.
   (b) Green or yellow discharge – infected ulcer.
   (c) Pink, bubbly with red spots – granulating ulcer.
2. The edge of the ulcer (boundary between floor and surrounding skin) may be:
   (a) Well defined, straight or undermined, red and shiny – ulcer spreading.
   (b) Hard, oedematous, overhanging floor – ulcer chronic.
   (c) Shallow, sloping out from floor with bluish tinge – ulcer healing.
3. The base of the ulcer (zone of tissue immediately surrounding and underlying the ulcer) may show:
   (a) Gross induration (hardening), the extent of which varies according to the severity and duration of the ulcer.
   (b) Pigmentation due to breakdown of red blood cells.
   (c) Poor circulation.
   (d) Coarse skin texture with heavy scaling or papery thin and eczematous tissue.
   (e) There may be partial scar tissue.
4. Oedema of base of ulcer and foot and ankle to shoe line.
5. Considerable pain around the ulcer, especially if infected. Pain increased on walking.

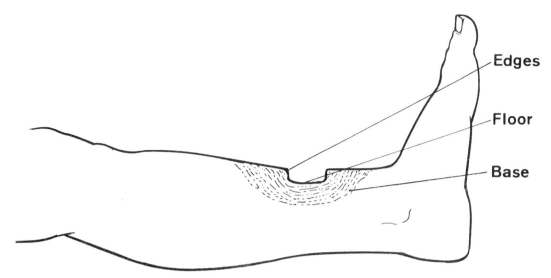

Figure 16.20 Components of an ulcer

6. Limited movement of the foot and ankle.
7. Muscle weakness and atrophy – mainly of calf muscles with loss of pumping action.
8. Walking pattern poor with no push-off.

Treatment

1. Conservative.
2. Surgical.

Conservative

The *general* aims are to:

1. Relieve pain.
2. Relieve congestion and reduce oedema.
3. Improve general circulation to lower limb.
4. Soften induration of lower leg especially around ankle area.
5. Mobilize joints of lower limb especially foot and ankle, and strengthen lower limb muscles especially calf.
6. Improve condition of skin of lower leg.
7. Teach home care and management.

The *local* aims are to:

1. Increase circulation to ulcer to promote healing.
2. Clear any infection.
3. Reduce oedema and induration around ulcer.
4. Free adherent ulcer from underlying tissues.

Methods of treatment

Soft-tissue techniques

Remove all bandages and dressings, clean wound and cover with gauze swabs during general techniques.

The leg is elevated to an angle of 45° at the hip to aid venous drainage.

Deep manipulations are given to the whole limb to reduce oedema and congestion, beginning with the thigh and continuing down the limb. Slow, deep kneading (squeezing kneading if necessary) followed by slow, deep strokes of effleurage. Progress to picking up and wringing on the thigh. Special attention should be paid to the dorsum of the foot, the region of the tendo-calcaneus and behind the malleoli. Thumb kneadings over the anterior tibialis muscles, finger or thumb kneadings over above areas and deep kneading to the foot followed by deep effleurage can be given.

The region of the ulcer is next treated with finger and thumb kneadings to soften the induration, working inwards from the periphery to the edges of the ulcer itself. Care is necessary if the skin is thin when the techniques must be stationary. Support one side at a time if the ulcer is very painful.

The ulcer can also be moved from side to side, the physiotherapist placing her fingers on one side and her thumbs on the other, to free it from the underlying tissues and improve the circulation.

This can be progressed to wringing as the mobility of the tissues improves.

Local techniques are better avoided when the ulcer is infected.

Ultraviolet rays

For infected ulcers

This can be given to destroy micro-organisms and increase circulation to the area. The Kromayer lamp is most commonly used (for very large ulcers the air-cooled mercury vapour lamp). A large dose (fourth degree (E4) or double fourth degree (E4 × 2)) is given to the base of the ulcer, the edges being screened with damp, sterile gauze. This is repeated two or three times a week until the ulcer is clear of infection. If the edges are clear of infection a first-degree (E1) or suberythema (E0) may be given to the edges and surrounding skin to promote healing. This can be repeated daily.

For healing ulcers

As the ulcer heals it grows inwards from the edges or outwards from islands in the middle. The ultraviolet rays are given to promote granulation tissue. An E1 (for shallow ulcers) or an E2 (for deep ulcers) is given to the floor of the ulcer and an E1 or E0 is given to the surrounding skin. The E0 or E1 is repeated daily and an E2 is given twice weekly.

These dosages can be given with blue uviol or Cellophane filters which cut out the abiotic (UVC) rays and stimulate growth of granulation tissue. With these filters the E1 of the lamp is considerably more, therefore a test dose with the filter is necessary.

For indolent ulcers

The ultraviolet rays are given to stimulate the circulation. Absorption of the rays produces hyperaemia in the congested area and produces an increased exudate. An E3 is given to the floor with the edges screened and an E1 or E2 to the edges and surrounding skin. As the ulcer improves the base should become pink and vascular when the E3 can be reduced and treatment given as for a healing ulcer.

Ultrasound

This can be given with coupling cream to the surrounding skin or in a sterile saline bath to the ulcer itself as well as the surrounds.

The ultrasound will promote healing of the ulcer, soften the induration and increase the vascularity in the surrounding tissues. The 3 MHz head using a low dosage, e.g. $0.25-0.5 \, W/cm^2$ is applied for 5–10 min. A pulsed beam is used if the area covered is small but a continous beam is used if the area is large. The dosage can be increased up to $1.0 \, W/cm^2$ for chronic indurated areas in the lower leg. Ultrasound is contraindicated in the presence of superficial or deep venous thrombosis.

Pulsed electromagnetic energy (PEME)

PEME is the production of short bursts of high frequency currents. Continuous high frequency currents at sufficient intensity produce heat in tissues. If PEME is applied to tissues there is a relatively long 'rest' period and during this time heat is dispersed by the circulation thus producing non-thermal effects. When wounds are treated with PEME there is increased organization of connective tissue and growth of epithelial tissue thus promoting healing. A pulse duration of 65 microseconds (µs) set at a frequency of 400 pulses per minute (ppm) given for up to 30 minutes daily would be suitable for treating wounds.

Ionozone therapy

This is the production of steam which is ionized, by being passed over a mercury vapour arc, into a mixture of ionized water, ozone and oxygen. It is applied at approximately 35 cm from the ulcer and surrounding area for 10–20 min. This will reduce pain, overcome infection and promote healing. The steam is directed horizontally with the patient appropriately positioned. It is useful where the patient cannot be positioned satisfactorily for screening for treatment with ultraviolet rays. All grease should be removed from the ulcer and surrounding areas. If the surrounding skin is thin the area should be screened with a waterproof material or the distance should be increased up to 50 cm. The treatment is applied daily to infected ulcers and reduced to two or three times a week as healing occurs.

Light amplification by stimulated emission of radiation (laser)

Beams are in the visible and infra-red part of the electromagnetic spectrum (600–950 nm). Due to their ability to increase vasodilatation, the number of fibroblasts and the size of cells at wound margins which divide quicker, laser beams can be used.

The wound should be as dry as possible and oil free. Any oil-based dressings must be cleaned off. A cluster probe with a number of wavelengths is most effective for ulcers. The energy dosage should be $1 \, J/cm^2$ which is less than the normal $2-4 \, J/cm^2$ because there is no skin. This is achieved by applying the probe at 30 mW for 33 s. A higher power for a shorter time is more effective.

The probe is held at 90° to the wound just off the surface of the ulcer. In painful ulcers longer pulses are used at a lower frequency and extensive ulcers are treated in sections. Treatment should be given on alternate days.

Pneumatic compression

A double-layered plastic sleeve which may have zip or Velcro fastenings is applied to the lower limb. It can cover dressings and provides intermittent or sequential compression where the ankle, knee and thigh are compressed in turn. This is followed by a rest period for approximately 1 minute. Pressure can be varied up to 100 mm Hg but is normally between 35 mm Hg and 55 mm Hg. Some machines blow cool air over the leg to make it more comfortable. The sleeves are worn up to 24 hours per day. The veins are compressed for relatively short periods of time which greatly reduces venous stasis, improves venous circulation and promotes healing. Due to the mechanical compression and relaxation there is reduction in oedema.

Support and pressure

Graduated compression which reduces from distal to proximal increases venous blood flow and prevents dilatation of the leg veins. The support enhances the muscle pump and aids reduction of oedema round the ulcer and in the limb generally. A 2 cm sorbo pad or gauze compress is applied over the dressing, of a size corresponding to the ulcer and the oedematous area round it.

Wool or felt padding is placed in the grooves behind the malleoli and round the lower leg and foot. It is kept in position by a gauze bandage. Over this an elastic bandage, Tubigrip or elastic stocking is applied from the metatarsal heads to the tibial tubercle. The elastic bandage starts from the inner border of the foot level with the metatarsal heads (Figure 16.21(a)) and is carried straight round the foot for 1½ turns (Figure 16.21 (b)). It is then taken over the dorsum, round the back of the heel to just above the starting point (Figure 16.21(c)). Hold the bandage here while continuing outwards and downwards across the dorsum, under the sole and upwards (near the heel) across the front of the ankle (Figure 16.21(d)). These two turns must be accurately applied in order to give the essential support and pressure round the tendo-calcaneus and malleoli. The heel must be covered completely, otherwise there will be pain and swelling. Hold the ankle turn so that it is fixed by the first spiral turn (Figure 16.21(e)). It is then continued as a simple spiral to the tibial tubercle (Figure 16.21(f)). The tension should be half-full stretch of the bandage. When using Tubigrip, two layers should be used, the inner one extending to the bulk of the calf muscles and the outer to the tibial tubercle. The support can be removed at night when the leg is elevated but is worn throughout the day for at least 3 months after the ulcer is healed. The patient is taught to reapply the pressure bandage a few times a day to maintain tension and vary the pressure areas of the bandage on the skin.

Exercises

Active exercises of the ankle, subtalar, and mid-tarsal joints are essential to improve venous circulation and mobilize the joints. The exercises should be carried out with the elastic support removed to emphasize joint mobility and against the resistance of the support to increase circulation and muscle strength especially the calf muscles. Re-education of walking with emphasis on the 'push-off' must be given. Functional activities which particularly work the ankle should be practised, for example:

1. A treadle machine.
2. Cycling.
3. Foot power loom.
4. Walking a dog.

If the joints of the knee and foot do not regain full range with active exercises, mobilizations (passive oscillatory techniques), both physiological and accessory movements may be applied.

The exercises must be carefully taught and explained to the patient who must practise them frequently throughout the day.

Advice

When sitting, the patient must elevate the legs with support under the knees and avoid standing still for any length of time. Any increase in pain must be reported.

Cleaning and dressing the ulcer

The ulcer is cleaned prior to applying electrical techniques or local massage and is dressed before giving exercises. The cleaning and dressing should be carried out using a 'non-touch' technique with sterile packs, instruments and lotions. Cotton wool balls soaked in saline (clean ulcer) or hydrogen peroxide or Eusol (infected ulcer) are used for cleaning. If the ulcer is very painful it may be irrigated instead of cleaned with cotton wool. Sterile gauze swabs soaked in saline can be used for screening the ulcer for UVR. A great variety of ointments, solutions and preparations are available for dressing the ulcer and surrounding skin. A desloughing agent may be applied to a very infected ulcer and specific antibiotic creams may be necessary for specific infections. Paraffin gauze is useful to protect the floor of a granulating ulcer. A soothing cream, e.g. calamine, may be used if surrounding skin is irritable, painful and eczematous but arachis oil is better for dry, scaly skin.

A gauze compress covering up to 2 cm of the ulcer surrounds may be used if the ulcer is shallow and granulating at the edges. For deep ulcers Silastic foam (a silicon-based fluid which sets to the shape of the ulcer) may be used during the granulation stage but for infected ulcers ribbon gauze soaked in Varidase packed into the cavity ensures that the lotion is in contact with the floor (Figure 16.22). Finally the ulcer is dressed in a non-absorbent dressing, e.g. Melolin or Perfron.

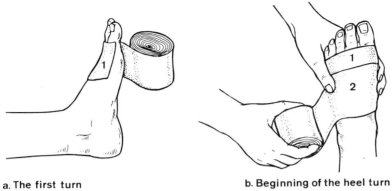

a. The first turn

b. Beginning of the heel turn

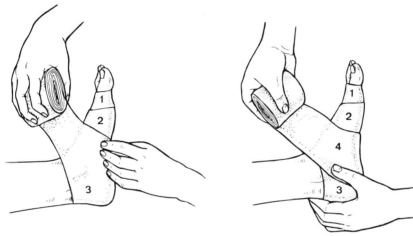

c. Fixation of the heel turn

d. The stirrup turn

e. Holding the fixation of the
   stirrup turn

f. Bandaging up the leg

Figure 16.21 Compression bandage

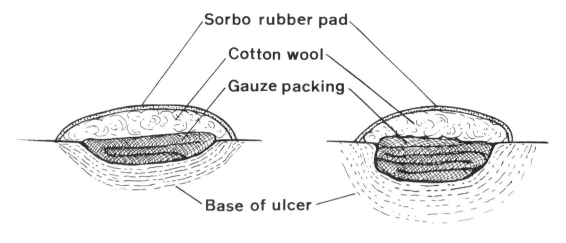

SHALLOW ULCER   DEEP ULCER

Figure 16.22 Dressing of shallow and deep ulcers

If the ulcer has a copious discharge, cotton wool padding will absorb the exudate. A sorbo-rubber pad or white felt 2 cm thick can be applied if the ulcer is overgranulating, or there are persistent patches of local oedema (and induration).

An ulcer often responds to one solution or dressing for 1–2 weeks and then slows up. When this happens it is useful to change the solution or dressing.

Prognosis

With good treatment the majority of ulcers will heal but some take many months. Recent ulcers heal quicker than long-standing ones: oedema, obesity, arthritis and lack of nutrition are factors which delay their healing. Ulcers tend to heal quicker with intelligent and cooperative patients. Without adequate care ulcers will break down again.

Complications

1. Superficial venous thrombosis.
2. Deep venous thrombosis.

Records

1. Tracings and graphs

Tracing show changes in the shape but not in depth of an ulcer. A sterile glove (two layers of Cellophane) is placed over the ulcer and a tracing is made on the top layer. The underneath layer (next to the ulcer) is thrown away and the tracing is transferred to graph paper for easy comparison (Figure 16.23).

The tracing should be taken at the first attendance and at regular intervals thereafter.

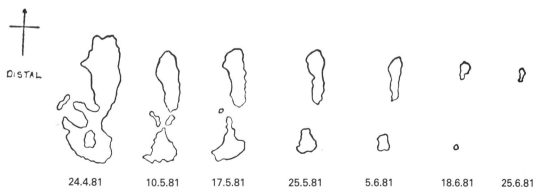

| 24.4.81 | 10.5.81 | 17.5.81 | 25.5.81 | 5.6.81 | 18.6.81 | 25.6.81 |

Figure 16.23 Tracings of an ulcer

2. *Photography*

Photographs of the ulcer taken at regualr intervals give an indication of its state and depth in addition to its area but are more expensive than graphs.

Surgical

The healing of large venous ulcers may be hastened by surgical intervention. This may include:

1. Ligation of veins.
2. Debridement and skin grafting.

Ligation of veins is usually necessary to improve the venous return of the lower limb which is the predisposing cause of the ulcer.

Debridement and grafting – If an ulcer is infected it must be cleaned before applying a skin graft. This may be done by local application of antiseptic lotions or UVR. Various types of split skin grafts may be carried out. Mesh grafts are more successful particularly if the ulcer is large (Figure 16.24). The skin is normally taken from the thigh and passed through a mesher which makes multiple slits enlarging the graft. The slits enable the circulation to move freely through the graft and therefore 'take' readily.

For physiotherapy following the graft, see Chapter 18.

Arterial (ischaemic) ulcers

Aetiology

Sex – Men more than women.
  Age – Elderly.
  Site – More commonly on toes, foot and heel but may be found on lower leg.
  Cause – Lack of nutrition to the skin due to inadequate arterial supply.
  The floor of the ulcer is pale, anaemic and liable to infection.
  The surrounding skin may be normal or ischaemic.

Treatment

The ulcer will not heal unless the blood supply is improved and usually surgery is necessary. After surgery local treatment as for a venous ulcer will reduce infection and promote healing.

Pressure sores

Pressure sore is a term used to describe any pressure injury which may vary from an area of erythema to a deep-seated ulceration exposing the underlying bone.

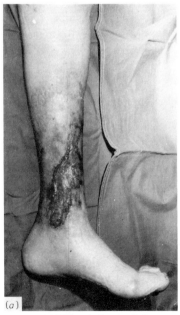 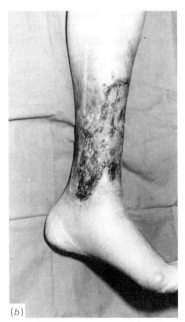 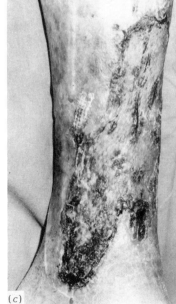

Figure 16.24 Ulcer before and after a mesh graft. (*a*) Prior to grafting. (*b*) 10 days after application. (*c*) Close-up view

Aetiology

Age – Can occur at any age but is more commonly found in the elderly (75% found in over-seventies).

Sex – Sexes equally affected.

Site – Found in pressure areas, e.g. heels, buttocks, hips, elbows.

Condition – More commonly affects patients with neurological disorders, e.g. paraplegia and Parkinson's disease.

Cause

This can be external factors (in the environment) or internal factors (in the body itself).

External factors

Prolonged and constant pressure causing deficiency of blood supply. The tissue damage will depend on the amount and type of pressure – shear or friction. In shear pressure the skin remains stationary and the underlying tissues move forward, destroying the circulation but in friction the skin surface moves over the bed surface causing a superficial abrasion.

The pressure may be caused by immobility of the patient due to:

1. Post-operative pain.
2. Immobility in a plaster of Paris.
3. Unconsciousness.
4. Loss of sensation where the patient does not feel pain.
5. Prolonged bed rest.

Internal factors

1. Bony prominences, e.g. sacrum or greater trochanter, cause pressure to build up internally.
2. Increased muscle tone results in the patient remaining in a fixed position with increased pressure.
3. Illnesses reducing the nutritional state of the body.
4. Incontinence results in skin breakdown due to moisture.
5. Weak or wasted muscle bulk causes poor protection for the underlying tissues.
6. Diabetes may lead to trophic ulcers.

Pathology

There are two types of pressure sores – superficial and deep.

Superficial type – This begins with breakdown of the skin surface resulting in destruction of the epidermis, dermis and possibly subcutaneous tissues. The resultant ulcerated area may become infected with a yellow or green exudate.

Deep type – This begins in the subcutaneous tissues overlying bony prominences. It results in necrosis of the subcutaneous tissue, fascia and possibly muscle tissue. The only sign may be a slight reddening of the skin surface. In severe cases the destruction may spread superficially through the dermis and epidermis until a deep cavity is exposed.

Superficial pressure sores are three times as common as deep sores but deep sores occur in seriously ill patients and are associated with a very high mortality rate.

In both types the pressure compresses the tissues, occludes the blood supply and the nutrition is cut off. If the pressure is prolonged acute changes of inflammation take place with necrosis of tissue, suppuration, and healing by second intention.

Clinical features

There is an open area of varying size on a pressure site. The floor of the sore may be pink and vascular or filled with infected exudate. The cavity may be shallow or deep with loss of subcutaneous tissue and exposure of bone.

Around the cavity the skin is red or blue.

The patient will complain of pain if sensory nerve endings are not destroyed.

Prevention of pressure sores

Prevention of pressure sores is better than cure.

Aims of prophylactic treatment – To relieve pressure and prevent breakdown of skin.

Medical

1. Turning the patient every 2 hours day and night and avoiding pressure on the sore, e.g. for a trochanteric sore change from lying to side lying on the unaffected side.
2. Use of a special mattress or bed designed to relieve pressure:
   (a) Water bed which provides even pressure over all parts of the body.
   (b) Ripple mattress which continually alters the pressure points.
   (c) Net bed – an open mesh net provides reduced pressure and is suspended between two wooden rollers allowing easy turning of the patient.
   (d) Air fluidized bed – air is pumped through a sand medium giving complete flotation. The fluidization can be switched off giving a solid surface for ease of handling.

(e) Low-air-loss bed – consists of waterproof sections filled with air to different pressures providing even pressure distribution.

(f) Sorbo packs which can be positioned to keep susceptible areas pressure free.

3. Sheepskins can help to keep skin dry and reduce friction but are not suitable for incontinent patients. They can vary in size from a small square to one which protects the whole body. Boots lined with sheepskin help to prevent pressure sores on the feet.

4. 'Roho' cushion – an air-filled cushion which moulds to any shape and spreads pressure evenly.

5. Encourage patient to be mobile as soon as possible and encourage short walks.

6. The patient is instructed to inspect pressure sites for signs of pressure and taught methods of self pressure relief.

7. Treatment of associated diseases will help to prevent skin breakdown. Incontinence must be treated, oedema reduced and anaemia corrected.

8. A balanced diet to maintain patient's general health is essential.

9. Good instructions in turning and lifting to the patient, the patient's relatives and carers is necessary if prophylactic measures are to be completely successful.

10. Dermalex spray.

Physiotherapy

This may include:

1. Exercises for strenghthening muscles to enable patient to lift himself/herself in bed or chair for pressure relief.

2. Active exercises to encourage mobility in bed and walking, assisted if necessary, as soon as possible.

3. Ice massage over a reddened area for a few minutes several times a day will increase circulation and reduce oedema, thereby preventing tissue breakdown.

4. Relaxed passive movements to paralysed limbs aid circulation and prevent contractures which might produce pressure sores.

Management of pressure sores

The aims of treatment are to: relieve pressure, reduce infection, improve circulation and promote healing.

Medical and surgical

1. Turning and positioning the patient, together with the use of suitable beds and cushions as described in prophylactic treatment.

2. Aseptic cleaning to reduce infection if necessary followed by the application of a dressing to promote healing, e.g. non-stick Perfron, semi-permeable Op-Site, Silastic foam for deeper granulating sores, Bactigras for infected sores or paraffin gauze for large granulating sores.

3. A high-protein, high-calorie diet including all vitamins and iron improves the patient's general health and promotes healing.

4. Surgical excision and grafting. If the sore is infected debridement (excision of infected tissue) is necessary first. When a large sore is healing and unlikely to be subjected to further pressure a skin graft may be sufficient but a rotation flap may be necessary if there is any danger of further breakdown. In a rotation flap there is rotation of muscle and skin flap to cover the defect and an additional skin graft to cover the area left by the flap. Following the flap, pressure must be relieved until the wound begins to heal.

Physiotherapy

The methods of treatment are similar to those advocated for venous ulcers: massage round edges of sore, ultrasound to surrounds, UVR to the floor and edges, Ionozone, ice, PEME and laser. Unlike ulcers oedema of the surrounding tissues and limited joint movement are not features of pressure sores, therefore compression and support bandaging are not used.

Tracings can be used to show decrease in the size but not the depth of a sore.

The response of the sore to the different modalities is very variable and the choice will depend on the state and progress of healing.

The prevention and treatment of pressure sores includes a good team approach by nurses, physiotherapists, doctors, dietitians, carers, relatives and not least the patient who must ensure pressure relief.

Lymphoedema

This is the collection of lymph in the subcutaneous tissues due to an abnormality of the lymphatic system.

Types

Primary – There is an inherent abnormality in the lymphatic system.

Secondary – The lymphatics have been damaged causing obstruction of lymph flow.

Aetiology

Primary

Sex – Females more than males.
> *Age* – It can occur at any age. For example:

1. At birth due to lymph vessels being small and few or dilated and tortuous.
2. At puberty due to the lymphatic system being unable to cope with hormonal changes.
3. Later in life – due to deterioration of the lymphatic system.

Secondary

This is caused by obstruction of the lymphatic system due to:

1. Malignant disease, e.g. breast cancer in upper limb or pelvic tumour in lower limb.
2. Radiotherapy to pelvic or axillary regions, e.g. after mastectomy.
3. Chronic inflammation leads to fibrosis and occlusion of lymph vessels.
4. Filariasis caused by infection through mosquito bites.

Pathology

Owing to obstruction or anatomical abnomalities protein molecules escape into the surrounding tissues. The fluid stagnates and coagulates because of its increased protein content. Fibrosis then occurs with later thickening of the skin. The changes are localized to the subcutaneous tissues by the deep fascia.

Clinical features

1. Mainly lower limbs affected.
2. Gradual increase in swelling of affected part usually unilateral. Primary lymphoedema begins distally and spreads proximally but secondary lymphoedema may begin proximally.
3. Initially the oedema 'pits' on pressure but later it becomes solid.
4. Enlargement of regional lymph glands in secondary lymphoedema.

Management

1. Conservative.
2. Surgical.

Conservative

The majority of patients are treated conservatively.

Apparatus

Machine – This consists of a pneumatic pump with:

1. Pressure control measured in mm Hg or kilopascals. The scale may be deflection of a needle or a knob round a scale.
2. On/off switch.
3. Maybe a time control which varies the ratio of inflation/deflation.

Sleeves – Consisting of a double layer of sealed polyurethane. These can be full upper limb, full lower limb or below knee only. The upper limb cuff is straight but the lower limb has a foot shape at the end. All cuffs taper, the broader end being proximal to allow for the limb being larger at this part. Some have zips or Velcro fastening to make application easier.
> Sleeves with more air entry holes give more even pressure.

Pneumatic compression

The compression may be:

1. *Intermittent* – The whole sleeve is alternately inflated and deflated.
2. *Sequential* – Sections of the sleeve inflate and deflate in turn giving compression to the limb from distal to proximal.

Application

All clothing and jewellery must be removed to avoid restricting the circulation. The limb should be well supported and elevated during treatment. The sleeve which is applied on top of a layer of Tubigauze (thin cotton gauze) must include all the hand and foot otherwise the circulation is restricted and the patient complains of pins and needles.

Assessment

Before beginning treatment the joint range and muscle strength of the limb should be recorded. Palpation of the oedema should be made and the mobility of the tissues noted. Limb measurements must be made at the set levels and ideally repeated by the same person (Figure 16.25). These measurements are taken in:

1. The upper limb at:
   (a) Axilla.
   (b) 8 cm proximal to olecranon.
   (c) 11 cm distal to olecranon.
   (d) Wrist.
   (e) Level with web of thumb.
2. The lower limb at:
   (a) Groin.
   (b) 15 cm above base of patella.

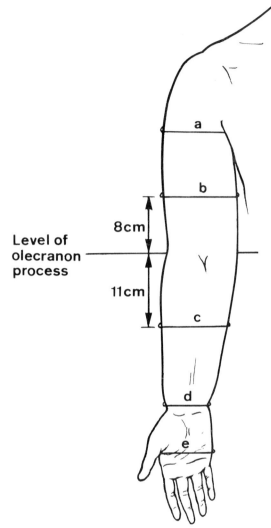

Level of olecranon process

8cm

11cm

a

b

c

d

e

Figure 16.25 Levels of measurement of upper limb in lymphoedema

(c) 15 cm below apex of patella.
(d) Ankle (malleoli).
(e) Middle of metatarsals.

Both the affected and unaffected limbs must be measured for comparisons immediately after treatment, 1 hour later and in the evening.

Treatment

The pressures for the upper limbs and lower limbs are the same. The pressure cycles may be:

1. Fixed – 30–45 s inflation 15 s deflation.
2. Variable – inflation time can be increased up to 60 s.

The machine should provide the same physiological conditions as a normal muscle contraction.

Suitable outline plan

Begin with 40 mm Hg for 30 min and assess immediately and 1 hour later. Repeat treatment twice daily.

Pressure is kept the same and time is gradually increased until at the end of a week the dosage is 40 mm Hg for 1 hour.

In the second week increase the pressure by 5 mm Hg per day until 65 mm Hg (maximum) is reached. Treat for 1 hour twice daily. If patient complains of pain use a lower pressure and treat more frequently,

e.g.   45 mm Hg three times per day
or   30 mm Hg four times per day.

Treatment should be carried out 7 days per week.

Variations

If the patients' condition allows treatment can begin with 40 mm Hg for up to 2 hours and repeated up to three times daily. The pressure can be increased during the first week.

Treatment can be given as an inpatient, outpatient, by the community physiotherapist, or machines may be loaned for home treatment usually for a month and then reassessed.

Soft-tissue manipulation

Before applying pneumatic compression give massage round each shoulder region because the sleeve does not extend to the shoulder region and it helps to promote circulation proximally. Begin with deep kneading or squeezing, kneading if the tissues are stretched followed by clearing effleurage to the axilla. As the tissues become more mobile picking up and wringing are used in addition to kneading. Finger or thumb kneading is used for localized thickenings.

Exercises

The aim of the exercises is to aid removal of tissue fluid from the subcutaneous tissues. The exercises are performed slowly but firmly with the limb in elevation. This can be achieved by the limb resting on three or four pillows with the distal joints higher than the proximal joints.

The exercises should be done three times a day and each one repeated 15–20 times. For example, for upper limb:

1. Fingers bend and stretch.
2. Wrists bending forwards, backwards and circling.
3. Elbow bend (fingers to shoulder) and stretch.
4. Sitting; arms place behind neck and behind waist.

Support

Lymphoedema sleeves or stockings should be worn 24 hours a day because the effects of treatment last longer. They come in different sizes and extend from the bases of the fingers and toes to the shoulder and groin respectively.

The support should be removed for treatment with the compression machine. If sleeves or stockings are not available an elastic bandage can be applied with the pressure gradually decreasing from distal to proximal. Poor bandaging aggravates rather than improves the condition.

Advice to patient

1. Use the limb as normally as possible.
2. Avoid minor injuries such as scratches which provide an entry for infection. Should they occur treat with an antiseptic. If the area becomes red, swollen or hot seek medical advice as soon as possible.
3. Avoid injections on the affected side.
4. Do not take hot baths since the limb will swell further – cool baths are allowable.
5. Do not wear tight bands (garters) or jewellery (rings) on the swollen limb.
6. Elevate the limb by putting the lower limb on a chair during the day and raising the foot of the bed at night. Support the upper limb in a sling or sit for short periods with the hand on the head.
7. Do not carry heavy shopping or cases with an affected upper limb.
8. Wear footwear that supports the foot.
9. Wear a thimble when sewing.

Surgery

A minority of patients require surgical treatment for gross swelling of the limb and recurrent episodes of infection. Some surgeons remove excess tissue while others in addition attempt to create communication between superficial and deep lymphatics. Preoperative treatment is similar to conservative treatment and post-operative treatment aims to improve lymph flow and function of the affected limb. The limb is supported in elevation and active movements to stimulate the circulation are encouraged. In the lower limb the patient is ambulant as soon as possible and is given gait re-education to improve function. Ultrasound or pulsed electromagnetic energy may be used to mobilize the tissues.

Scar tissue

Scar tissue gives rise to:

1. Pain which can be caused by:
   (a) Nerve tissue becoming involved in the scar.
   (b) Venous congestion in deep scars.
   (c) Traction on the neighbouring structures when the scar is adherent.
2. Limitation of movement which arises when the scar is over a joint line.
3. Impaired blood supply when the scar constricts blood vessels.

Common sites of scars requiring treatment

1. Palm of hand following release of Dupuytren's contracture.
2. Knee and elbow after surgery
3. Ankle after an internally fixed fracture.
4. Hip surgery.
5. Burns and skin grafts.

Treatment

This varies according to the age of the scar.

Recently healed scars (up to 3 weeks)

The aims are to:

1. Prevent contractures and loss of joint movement.
2. Mobilize the scar.

Massage

This may include stroking round and towards the scar with the thumb. Thumb kneading on one side of the scar while the other side is supported avoiding stretching which could split the fibrin.

Wax baths – improves the condition of the skin and makes it more supple.

Active exercise – to move the joints through full range without stretching the scar transversely.

Adherent scar (over 3 weeks)

The aims are to:

1. Mobilize the scar.
2. Stretch adhesions and contractures.
3. Regain normal function.

Massage

Stroking and thumb kneading can be applied deeply and vigorously. Modified picking up and wringing between thumb and index finger and skin rolling are useful for mobilizing the scar. If the tissue is tough and thick transverse frictions may be applied to the scar.

Ultrasound

Applied over the scar this increases tissue length and the mechanical movement of tissues makes the scar tissue more pliable. It also mobilizes the scar from the underlying tissues. The frequency used should be 3 MHz. An intensity of $1 \, W/cm^2$ for 4 minutes increasing up to 10 minutes has been found to be effective. Pulsed mode is suitable for small scars, continuous for large scars.

Passive stretching

Once the scar tissue has been mobilized and lengthened with massage and ultrasound passive stretching may be applied if the scar is near a joint. A slow continuous stretch may be used or an oscillatory technique may be applied or (often) a combination of both is effective. Active exercise should follow passive stretching and the patient should continue with this at home.

Other modalities

Serial splinting for a contracted scar. Whirlpool baths which soften scar tissue may be applied by immersing the affected part in a hot bath through which an air stream is passed to agitate the water molecules.

Chapter 17

Skin disorders and diseases

The structure of the skin

The epidermis

This is the superficial part of the skin. It consists of five layers which are:

1. Stratum germinativum – growing layer.
2. Stratum spinosum – layer with bridges.
3. Stratum granulosum – cells and nuclei disintegrating.
4. Stratum lucidum – clear cells.
5. Stratum corneum – keratin flakes.

The keratin flakes are constantly rubbed off and replaced from cells below.

Melanin is a pigment produced by melanocytes which are present in the stratum germinativum (Figure 17.1).

The dermis

This is thicker and deep to the epidermis.

It consists of fibrous tissue and contains blood capillaries, sweat glands, sebaceous glands, hair follicles and nerve ending (Figures 17.2–17.4).

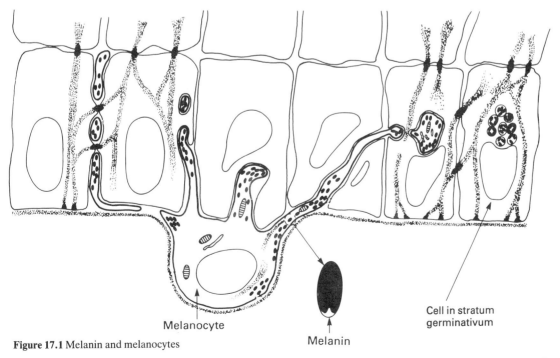

Melanocyte

Melanin

Cell in stratum germinativum

Figure 17.1 Melanin and melanocytes

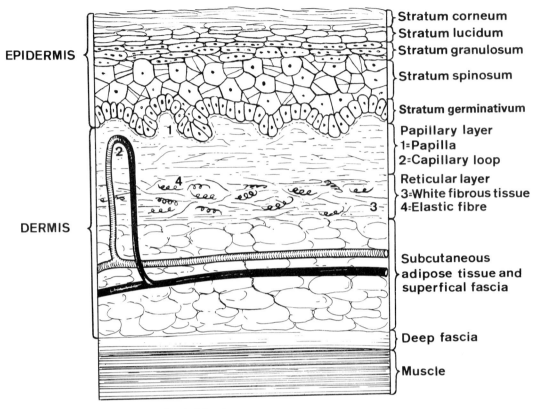

EPIDERMIS {

- Stratum corneum
- Stratum lucidum
- Stratum granulosum
- Stratum spinosum
- Stratum germinativum
- Papillary layer
  1=Papilla
  2=Capillary loop
- Reticular layer
  3=White fibrous tissue
  4=Elastic fibre

DERMIS

- Subcutaneous adipose tissue and superfical fascia
- Deep fascia
- Muscle

Figure 17.2 Structure of the skin and underlying tissues

Functions of the skin

The functions of the skin are:

1. *Protection* – The skin prevents water, bacteria and harmful objects from entering the body.
2. *Absorption* – substances applied to the skin are absorbed.
3. *Temperature regulation* – To lose heat, the sweat glands produce sweat which evaporates from the surface and the blood vessels dilate. To conserve heat, the blood vessels contract and the arrector pili muscles produce 'goose pimples'.
4. *Fluid and electrolyte balance* – Water, sodium chloride and urea are lost in sweat. The skin also prevents excess loss of body fluid, thereby contributing to homoeostasis.
5. *Sensory* – Nerve endings provide information on the environment, body position, impending damage (by pain, thermal and pressure receptors) and constitute an essential component of the body's defence mechanism.
6. *Self-concept* – The skin is very important psychologically. Appearance is important to self-image and therefore self-confidence. It identifies us as who we are and to some extent where we belong (family likeness, race and culture). The facial skin particularly expresses state of health and contributes to non-verbal communication, as does hand skin. Destruction, disease or disfigurement involving skin causes severe difficulties for the patient and for the people he or she meets in society.

Introduction to disorders and diseases

The patient with skin disease needs a great deal of sympathy and support from the physiotherapist. Unsightly skin lesions do not attract sympathy and support from the public; indeed there tends to be rejection or revulsion of psoriatic patients, and acne can be the subject of very hurtful taunting. People stare at bad skin and children can be heard to say

'Why has that lady got spots, Mummy?' A 5 year old with psoriasis on her palms and soles cannot find a partner at school – no one wants to hold her hand because 'it feels horrid'. When a young woman's psoriasis breaks out her husband moves into the spare room and she has to be treated immediately in the physiotherapy department. The distress suffered by these patients is equal to the disability of arthritis or paralysis but is not often seen as such.

Conditions treated by physiotherapy

By ultraviolet radiation (UVR):

1. Psoriasis.
2. Acne vulgaris.
3. Mycosis fungoides.
4. Polymorphic light eruption.
5. Vitiligo.
6. Pityriasis rosea.
7. Alopecia.

By iontophoresis: hyperhidrosis.

Examination of patients with skin conditions

Subjective

The history is taken before the patient undresses. Questions asked are:

1. Duration of lesions.
2. Recurring – ? intervals.
3. Severity – ? variable.
4. Medication:
   (a) Systemic.
   (b) Topical.
   (c) Effects of these.
5. General health.
6. Occupation, hobbies, lifestyle.
7. Family history of skin diseases.
8. Patient's views/expectations/previous treatment by physiotherapy.
9. Skin reaction to UVR.
10. Skin type (see under Psoriasis).
11. Rule out contraindications.

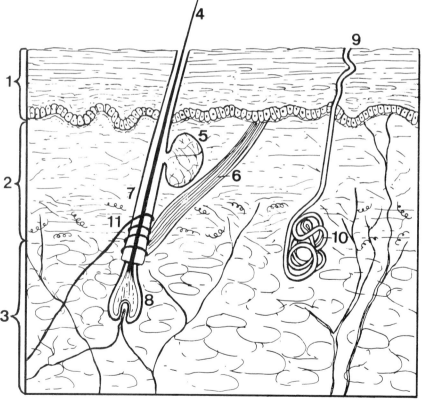

Figure 17.3 Hair follicle and sweat gland. 1 = Epidermis; 2 = Dermis; 3 = Subcutaneous adipose tissue; 4 = Hair; 5 = Sebaceous gland; 6 = Arrector pili muscle; 7 = Hair follicle; 8 = Hair follicle bulb; 9 = Duct and opening of sweat gland; 10 = Sweat gland; 11 = Nerve supply to hair follicle (sympathetic)

Objective

Observation

1. Chart lesions on body chart.
2. Use different colours or numbers for large patches.
3. Show these to the patient so that both patient and physiotherapist can recognize progress or regression.

Palpation

If appropriate, note swelling, heat, skin texture. Psoriatic lesions are proud of the skin at first and flatten on first signs of improvement.

Before treatment

1. All ointment, make-up and perfume should be removed.
2. Alcohol should be avoided as it can alter skin sensitivity.
3. A skin test with UVR is appropriate if the Theraktin or mercury vapour air-cooled burner are used.

Record keeping

This is essential for safety and repetition of treatment. The following records should be kept:

1. Distance of patient from UVR source.
2. Time given.
3. Screening if any.
4. Joules per cm^2 of body surface (for PUVA treatment. See below).
5. Reaction obtained.
6. Patient's reports, e.g. itching/burning.
7. Equipment used (the same source of UVR should be used at each attendance).

Ultraviolet rays

These are electromagnetic rays with a wavelength between 400 and 100 nm. Conventionally they are divided into three bands:

1. Long, UVA (320–400 nm).
2. Medium, UVB (290–320 nm).
3. Short, UVC (180–290 nm).

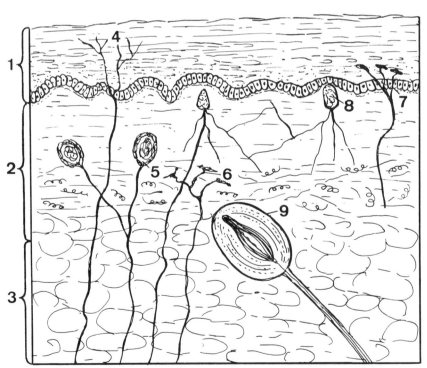

Figure 17.4 Nerve endings in the skin. 1 = Epidermis; 2 = Dermis; 3 = Subcutaneous adipose tissue; 4 = Free nerve endings; 5 = Krause's end organs; 6 = Ruffini's end organs; 7 = Merkel's discs; 8 = Meissner's corpuscles; 9 = Pacinian corpuscle

Sources

UVA: fluorescent tubes in a special cabinet.
UVB: Theraktin – fluorescent tubes. High-pressure
ultraviolet mercury vapour burner (HP UV burner),
air cooled.
UVC: HP UV burner, air cooled; and water cooled
(Kromayer).

Dosage with UVR

Reaction to UVR depends on:

1. Skin type (see Table 17.2, page 296).
2. Skin distance from source (shorter distance,
   greater reaction).
3. Time of exposure.
4. Age of source – output diminishes with use.

Recording of individual treatment is therefore
essential together with reaction obtained if any.
Times/dosages suggested in the text must be taken
as a guide only.

Minimal erythema dose (MED) is the time taken
at a set distance to produce a faint pinking of
average skin which fades in a few hours. MED is
related to the equipment used. A first-degree
erythema (E1) is a reaction of a patient's skin where
there is faint pinking which fades within 24 hours of
exposure. MED and E1 are essentially the same
thing. A suberythema dose does not produce
pinking of the skin except on prominent parts (e.g.
buttocks), and this fades in a few hours.

An E2 is a deep pink clearly defined area, which
lasts for 2–3 days and is followed by mild peeling.

An E3 is a red, clearly defined area which may be
slightly oedematous. It lasts for 5–7 days and is
followed by free peeling.

Mode of action of UVR

UVR stimulates synthesis of epithelial cells in the
stratum germinativum of the epidermis. In acne this
is desirable. An E2 produces accelerated growth of
the skin through to the keratin layer, which peels off
and clears acne. In PUVA the UVA activates
psoralen, which slows down the rate of growth of
skin which is desirable in psoriasis. The use of UVR
from the Theraktin for psoriasis is an apparent
contradiction because it stimulates growth where the
problem is that of accelerated growth. Patients
undoubtedly get better with UVR given at suberythema dosages, and although this cannot be
explained at present this is no reason for denying
patients Theraktin treatment where no UVA
equipment is available.

Psoriasis

This is one of the commonest and most intractable
disorders of the skin.

Definition

Psoriasis is a chronic imflammatory disease of the
skin characterized by clearly defined dry, rounded
red patches with silvery scales on the surface.

Aetiology

Age:

1. Common age of first occurrence is 15–30 years.
2. Can occur as young as 2 years.
3. Can start as late as 80 years.

Sex – Both sexes are equally affected.
Climate – The condition is worse in damp, cold
climates. It has been known to clear if a patient who
suffers quite badly in the UK goes to a sunny
climate.

Predisposing/precipitating factors

A number of factors appear to predispose or
precipitate an exacerbation of the condition. These
are as follows:

1. *Heredity* – There is an inherited defect in the skin
   which results in psoriasis developing in certain
   circumstances; 30% of patients have blood
   relatives with the condition.
2. *Infection* – Psoriasis has been known to develop
   after, for example, an upper respiratory tract
   infection.
3. *Trauma* – Lesions tend to develop at sites of
   potential or actual trauma, e.g. mechanical
   friction, cuts, stings.
4. *Anxiety* – Psoriasis often appears in relation to
   mental stress, e.g. bereavement, exams.
5. *Drugs* – Some drugs, e.g. chloroquine, may
   precipitate the condition.
6. *Diabetes* – Some patients with diabetes develop
   the condition.
7. *Arthropathy* – Sero-negative arthritis develops in
   some patients (See Chapter 9).

Cause

The membrane of the skin cells in patients who
develop psoriasis contain abnormal proteins which
manifest as abnormal surface antigens. Antibodies
form in response to these 'foreign' bodies and are
carried by B-lymphocyte cells. When these antibodies lock onto the antigens, a complex reaction
takes place at the dermo-epidermal junction and
psoriatic lesions are produced.

In normal skin the maturing of epidermal cells
takes 21–29 days. In psoriasis this is accelerated to 4
days. What causes the abnormal protein to form and

what triggers the antibody–antigen reaction is not known but it is probably related to the predisposing factors already listed.

Pathological changes

Epidermis

1. There is increased reproduction in the stratum germinativum.
2. The stratum spinosum is thicker due to an increased number of cells plus oedema.
3. The stratum granulosum is absent.
4. The strata lucidum and corneum are replaced by several layers of nucleated, incompletely keratinized, soft cells (para-keratotic cells).

There is no time for the normal changes to take place through the skin layers. The cells at the surface are sticky and do not fall off like normal keratin. Accumulation of these cells forms scales which over 2–3 weeks dry out and fall off in big flakes.

Dermis (Figure 17.2)

1. Capillaries are dilated with increased blood flow.
2. Papillae are elongated.
3. There are changes of inflammation.

Healing

The centre of the patch heals first causing circular lesions. Normal skin recovery takes place without scarring.

Clinical features

1. Sharply defined red and pink areas termed plaques.
2. Silvery scales due to light reflecting from the swollen stratum spinosum.
3. Distribution:
   (a) Elbows, knees, scalp and sacrum are covered in thickly scaled patches.
   (b) Plaques of varying sizes appear anywhere on the body.
   (c) Nails become pitted, ridged or separated from the nail bed. This can be the only evidence of the disorder in some people.
   (d) Skin contact areas can be badly affected – between fingers, axillae, groin, between toes, under breast, behind ears.
   (e) The face is rarely affected.
   (f) The size of plaques and distribution varies so that different types are described. These are:
       (i) Guttate.
       (ii) Pustular.
       (iii) Erythrodermic.

Guttate

Commonest and least severe, with good prognosis. Responds well to UVR.
   Features:

1. Small multiple plaques are scattered evenly over trunk and limbs.
2. Often appears suddenly.

Pustular

This principally affects scalp and body folds, although palms and soles can be badly affected. There is more severe inflammation and pustles are formed. The fluid contained in the pustules is sterile and must not be confused with the infected pustules of acne. UVR has limited success in this type.

Erythrodermic

The plaques join up and there is extensive erythema. The excessive distribution of blood to the skin can cause cardiac failure and loss of temperature regulation.
   This type does not usually respond to UVR.

Prognosis

Psoriasis clears completely with no marks but unfortunately can recur. There can be no sign in the evening and next morning it has started. It tends to be better in summer, worse in winter and recurs if the patient is worried.

Treatment

This may be considered under:

1. General management.
2. Topical (application of creams/lotions to the skin).
3. Systemic.
4. Physiotherapy.

General management

1. A sympathetic, considerate approach is required together with reassurance.
2. Any anxiety or worry should be identified and the patient encouraged to relax or seek appropriate help.
3. Reassurance that it is not infectious or disfiguring must be given to both patient and family. Also an 'open door' system should operate so that the patient can get to a dermatologist or physiotherapist immediately there is an eruption.
4. Dieting may be tried if there appears to be any allergy factor.

Topical treatment

Many patients do well on topical treatment. Treatment may be:

1. Simple bland aqueous cream.
2. Coal tar applications with salycylic acid and zinc oxide in soft paraffin may be used alone or with UVR. The patient is usually admitted to hospital. The ointment is applied every day to the whole body except face and scalp. Every 24 hours it is washed off in a bath containing coal tar solution. If UVR is given, it must be after a bath because the yellow soft paraffin absorbs UVR. A suberythema general treatment is given daily using the Theraktin. This is the Goeckerman regimen.
3. Dithranol in Lassar's paste is used for resistant psoriasis. It is highly effective but can burn the normal skin. The patient may be admitted to hospital or treated as an outpatient. If the patient is applying the paste the physiotherapist should look out for blisters or reddish-purple stains on the skin and warn the patient of the danger. UVR with the Theraktin may be given in conjunction with dithranol as a daily suberythema dose. The paste is removed in a coal-tar bath before the UVR and is then reapplied afterwards.
4. Corticosteroid cream produces good results at first but when treatment stops the disease can return worse than before. It is useful in an acute eruption and on the face and hands because there is greater absorption in moist areas. The dangers of side-effects makes long-term use inadvisable.

Systemic

1. Retinoids – a variant of vitamin A – taken in tablet form produces marked improvement. Retinoic acid or etretinate is marketed as Tigason. Unfortunately, this produces unpleasant side-effects such as dryness and cracking of the mouth, alopecia and pruritis. It is teratogenic (produces malfunction in a fetus), therefore must be avoided in pregnancy.
2. Cytotoxic drugs such as methotrexate are sometimes used in severe cases. These have dangers such as damage to bone marrow, intestinal and liver tissue.

Physiotherapy

Psoriasis can be treated very successfully with UVR. Two sources are used: the Theraktin and PUVA.

The Theraktin

This is usually in the form of a tunnel with four fluorescent tubes. The patient lies flat for the treatment, therefore in order to treat the whole body the patient is generally naked and lies supine for half the treatment session and prone for the other half. The spectrum of UVR emitted is 390–280 nm and peak emission is around 313 nm, therefore this constitutes UVB treatment. It may be used alone or in conjunction with coal tar or dithranol.

Treatment

A sub-erythema dose is given daily or three times a week. The prominent parts of the body have a mild erythema which fades before the next treatment is due. The time is increased to maintain the reaction (e.g. 12½% every 1–2 treatments). When the lesions start to flatten and heal the same time is repeated and the frequency of treatment reduced to twice weekly, once weekly and then once a fortnight.

The course of treatment may be spread over 8–12 weeks. These patients tend to deteriorate during the autumn and need treatment in the winter or spring. About 75% of patients with guttate psoriasis respond to UVB.

PUVA

This is psoralens plus UVA and is used for resistant psoriasis. Psoralens are photosensitizing substances which occur in plants such as parsley, parsnips and celery. The one used for psoriasis is 8-methoxypsoralen (8-MOP). UVA is produced from fluorescent tubes, mounted upright in a hexagonal shaped cabinet inside which the patient stands throughout the treatment. The spectrum of UVR emitted is 330–390 nm and peaks at 360 nm – hence it is UVA. Infra-red rays are also emitted and it is essential to have a cooling fan so that the patient can tolerate up to ½ hour in the cabinet.

Method

The patient takes 3–6 tablets of psoralen preferably with milk 2 hours before exposure. Tablet dosage is according to body weight (Table 17.1). UVA is

Table 17.1 Dose of 8-MOP

Patient's weight (kg)	*Dose* (mg)
30	10
30–50	20
51–65	30
66–80	40
81–90	50
90 and over	60

calculated according to skin type in joules (Table 17.2). There is little erythema with UVA, therefore the skin type chart has to be used. (To produce an erythema with UVA requires a dosage 1000 times greater than UVB.)

Table 17.2 UVA doses in PUVA treatment

Skin type	Start (J)	Increase (J)
I: always burn, never tan	½	½
II: always burn, then slight tan	½	½
III: sometimes burn, always tan	1	1
IV: never burn, always tan	1	1
V: lightly pigmented	1½	1½
VI: black	1½	1½

The dosage is recorded in J/cm^2. An exposure meter is used to test the output and measures milliwatts/cm^2; $1\,mW/cm^2 = 1/1000\,J/s$.

Duration of treatment

This may be 5 minutes at first for skin types I and II and progressed by 1 minute up to 15 minutes. It may start at 6 minutes and progress by 2 minutes up to 20 minutes for skin types III and IV. It may start at 7 minutes and progress by 3 minutes up to 25 minutes for skin types V and VI.

A record is kept of the total joule count. This is essential because there is an undeniable risk of malignant melanoma in patients who have been exposed to between 1500 J and 2000 J.

The patient attends three times a week until healing starts, then frequency of treatment is reduced to twice weekly, once weekly, once per fortnight or monthly 'holding sessions'.

Precautions/dangers/advice to patients on PUVA

1. Do not take psoralens on an empty stomach.
2. There is a real danger of cataract, therefore protective goggles are essential during exposure. Polaroid sunglasses must be worn from the time of taking the psoralen to at least 12 hours after. The psoralen is excreted in 8 hours but the effect of photosensitizing continues. The physiotherapist should test the glasses with a Blackray metre; 90% of UVA must be screened by the glasses. Patients are advised to wear protective glasses out of doors for at least 24 hours after taking the psoralen and also whilst watching television, a VDU screen or in fluorescent lighting.
3. The skin must be covered in bright sunlight and a hat worn for 24 hours after treatment.

4. Stop using all ointments during PUVA.
5. If the skin is dry simple oil or lubricating lotions may be used.
6. Do not become pregnant or father a child – contraceptive measures are essential during PUVA treatment.
7. A check-up is essential every month after completion of treatment.
8. During treatment if the patient feels faint the physiotherapist must be called immediately.

Mechanism of action

8-Methoxypsoralen binds to DNA and is activated by UVA. The psoralen binds to DNA thiamine bases, producing cross-linking which inhibits epithelial synthesis and cell division. In essence, therefore, the accelerated reproduction of epidermis in psoriasis is reduced, hence the beneficial results.

Long-term management

It may take up to 10 weeks to clear the skin and a further 4–6 weeks of maintenance doses may be given depending on individual response. Thereafter 2–6 monthly review is necessary. Once discharged, the patient should have access to treatment as soon as there is a recurrence.

Pustular psoriasis

This may be successfully treated by PUVA when the condition is on the soles and hands. They can be treated with a special piece of equipment in which the fluorescent tubes are horizontal and the hands or feet are placed on a grid over them.

Acne vulgaris

Definition

This is a chronic inflammatory disease of the sebaceous glands.

Aetiology

Age – It starts between 9 and 17 years, is associated with puberty and is generally clear by 30 years.

Sex – Males are affected more than females although it may cause more distress to females in the age group affected.

Incidence – 80% of all adolescents have acne to some degree.

Predisposing factors

1. *Puberty* – Changes in the skin during puberty take place, the sebaceous glands secrete sebum, the hairs become coarser and sweat gland openings are wider. Some people have greater changes than others and are more likely to develop acne.
2. Lack of fitness, exercise or fresh air, poor health, constipation.
3. Diet high in butter, cream, sugar, chocolate or alcohol may have an effect.
4. Sweating, e.g. under long hair or a band around the forehead. Poor skin hygiene.
5. Endocrine abnormalities involving testosterone.
6. Anxiety.
7. Skin type – dark complexion, heredity.

Cause

Bacteria, especially *Propionibacterium acnes*, infect the sebaceous glands and the glands increase in activity so that more sebum is released on to the skin (Figure 17.3).

Pathological changes

1. There is increased sebum production.
2. The pilo-sebaceous duct and hair follicle becomes blocked with sebum and keratin. The exposed surface becomes oxidized and blackened and is termed a comedone (blackhead).
3. The blocked material irritates the walls of the follicle and inflammation takes place. This causes swelling and distension of the follicle and duct; the lesion is termed a *papule*.
4. Invasion of follicle and duct by bacteria causes pus formation known as a *pustule*.
5. Once the pus is discharged, the duct and follicle shrink and healing takes place.
6. The condition can clear completely but repeated attacks can result in scar tissue formation.
7. Inflammatory changes and pus formation may spread between sebaceous glands through the dermis causing quite large swollen areas known as *cysts*. These heal once the pus is discharged on the surface and scar tissue is formed producing small pitting surface scars.
8. These changes may take place at the same time in different areas.
9. Acne is spread by material being extruded on to the surface and infecting neighbouring hair follicles, sebaceous glands and sweat glands.

Clinical features

1. Comedones – blackheads in the surface of the skin.
2. Sebaceous white worm-like material can be squeezed out of the comedone.
3. Papules:
   (a) Reddened round raised areas with comedone in the centre.
   (b) Slight itching.
   (c) Slight discomfort.
   (d) Tenderness.
4. Pustules:
   (a) Yellow raised areas with a comedone on the summit.
   (b) Surrounded by reddish purple area.
5. Cysts:
   (a) Purple coloured area which fluctuates on palpation.
   (b) Pain.
6. Scars:
   (a) Small pitted areas, the extent varies according to the severity of the condition.
   (b) Keloid, if the patient is unfortunate enough to have this type of tissue.
7. Distribution – face, upper chest and back.

Prognosis

Usually acne clears by 30 years of age. There are good results with treatment, although the disease tends to fluctuate. The lesions can be unsightly, resulting in loss of confidence and depression. It is very important to encourage optimism and prevent scarring.

General management

An understanding approach is necessary because the patient who seeks medical help is undoubtedly suffering considerable distress and probably social isolation.

Treatment may be:

1. Topical.
2. General.
3. Physiotherapy.

Topical treatment

1. Sulphur-based ointments.
2. Salicylic-acid based ointments.
3. Resorcinol paste.
4. Vitamin A acid gel.
5. Benzoyl peroxide gel.

These substances are applied directly to the affected areas. That there is a variety reflects the way in which different patients respond to different preparations. Benzoyl peroxide gel is more cosmetically kinder than sulphur-based ointments, which produce an erythema and peeling.

General treatment

1. *Antibiotics* – These are used in pustular and cystic acne to clear infection and prevent scar formation.
2. *Oestrogen therapy* – This can help women whose acne is exacerbated just before menstruation.

Physiotherapy

This involves application of UVR and advice on fitness.

UVR

The source generally used is a high-pressure air-cooled mercury vapour burner (although success with a low-pressure burner using special shutters has been reported). This is housed in a reflector which can be angled to obtain maximum absorption of UVR with the patient supported in a comfortable position (usually modified sitting). The spectrum of UVR is 190–390 nm. The skin–burner distance is usually 45 cm.

Treatment

Two main schools of thought exist in the treatment of acne. In one the aim is to improve skin health and in the other the aim is to promote peeling.

Improvement of skin health

A first-degree erythema (E1) is given 2–3 times a week for 3–4 weeks. The theory is that the maintained increase of arterial circulation provides extra amino acids, oxygen and other nutritive substances to enable the synthesis of healthy skin. Given that epidermal cells pass from basal layer to the surface in 3 weeks, the principle is that the treatment is given over a longer period. It is safe to give an E1 to the face, chest and upper back in the one treatment session. The patient with all areas affected feels that something is being done for the whole condition.

Promotion of peeling

A second- or third-degree erythema (E2, E3) is given and repeated only when peeling has stopped.

The theory is that affected skin is removed more quickly and healthy skin will replace it. The E2 or E3 will open up the pilo-sebaceous openings causing the infected material to be discharged rather than retained within the skin. It is not very pleasant to have a peeling face so an E2 is generally the maximum reaction aimed for. An E3 may be tolerated on the chest or upper back. An E2 can be tolerated to the face, upper back and chest but if all areas are red and sore at the same time the patient has difficulty lying down to sleep. Therefore, attendances are spaced to take account of this. The condition clears with this treatment in 6–8 weeks. If there is no improvement in 12 weeks it is probably wise to abandon treatment given that there is a danger of skin cancer with excessive UVR, and unlike the PUVA method there is no means of measuring the electromagnetic energy to which the patient has been exposed.

In both approaches some benefit is probably derived from the surface bacteria being destroyed by UVR and spread of the condition is reduced. Also the patient responds to a humanitarian approach by the physiotherapist.

Fitness

The physiotherapist may give advice to the patient as follows:

1. Follow faithfully any instructions from the doctor or dietitian regarding lifestyle, drugs and diet.
2. Take part in outdoor sport and shower scrupulously afterwards to remove sweat – sweat provides a medium in which bacteria thrive.
3. Wash the affected areas at least twice a day with oil-free soap and be sure to rinse well with cool water.
4. Remember that people tend to accept you as you are – face the world with a smile and no one (who matters) will notice the spots.

Mycosis fungoides

Definition

This is a condition in which there is a slowly developing T-cell infiltration of the skin with malignant lymphoma. There is chronic antigenic stimulation.

Clinical features

1. Lesions appear on the skin which are similar to those of psoriasis.
2. Distribution is different from psoriasis – often the face, particularly around the eyes is affected.

3. Tumours may form.
4. The disease may progress to the lymph nodes and vital organs.

Treatment

Physiotherapy

The skin lesions respond well to PUVA treatment. The method is as for psoriasis. Patients wear goggles to protect the eyes so that the UVR can reach the facial lesions.

Case studies

A woman who has attended for PUVA treatment periodically over the last 7 years is settling well after a recent course of 6 J once a week for 3 months. The disease has been stable for about 2 years.

Another woman is now in remission after a course of 6 J, three times a week for 4 months. Three tumours on her scalp were successfully removed with deep X-ray therapy.

Polymorphic light eruption (PLE)

Definition

A condition in which patients have extreme sensitivity to UVR and visible light.

Clinical features

1. Itch.
2. Erythema.
3. Papules and possibly blisters.

These appear after exposure to only very mild sunlight. The patient may have to live in curtained rooms or have special filter window glass installed.

Treatment: physiotherapy

The aim is to raise the sensitivity of the skin to UVR. PUVA greatly helps these patients. A course of treatment starts in February or March at low doses of 0.25–0.5 J. This is progressed slowly over 2–3 months to 6 J. Patients who have followed this regimen have been able to enjoy Mediterranean holidays for the first time in their lives.

Vitiligo

Definition

This is a condition in which areas of the skin are depigmented owing to loss of normal melanocyte function.

Clinical features

Irregular patches of skin become depigmented and appear white against normal skin.

Treatment: physiotherapy

The aim is to produce pigmenting of the abnormal areas. PUVA is very successful. Psoralens may be taken by mouth or painted on to the affected areas topically. The psoralen used may be tri-methyl-psoralen (TMP) although 8-MOP was used for vitiligo before it was used for psoriasis. Exposure is as for polymorphic light eruption.

If a UVA source is not available, UVB from the Theraktin can be successful. A suberythema dose should be tried one or two times per week for 6–8 weeks. Note: if red spots or itching/burning sensations arise during treament of PLE or vitiligo the skin should be rested. When it has settled treatment should start again at one-half the dose and progress slowly. It is worth trying this several times because treatment can be ultimately successful even with these apparent setbacks.

Pityriasis rosea

Definition

This disease presents a rash of red or pink scaling macules on the skin of the trunk, often following viral infection.

Treatment

Usually the disease is self-limiting but if it persists the patient may be referred for UVR.

Physiotherapy

Suberythema doses of UVB with the Theraktin two or three times a week for 2–3 weeks usually obtains good results.

Alopecia

Definition

Absence or premature loss of hair.

Classification

Alopecia areata – loss of scalp hair in patches.
Alopecia totalis – loss of all scalp hair and eyebrows.
Alopecia universalis – total loss of body hair.

Aetiology

1. Age – under 30 years.
2. Sex – both sexes equally affected.
3. Predisposing factors:
    (a) General anxiety.
    (b) Fatigue.
    (c) Poor health.
    (d) Heredity (universalis is often congenital).

Cause

Alopecia areata or totalis may be treated by physiotherapy.

Pathological changes

1. Hair becomes thin and falls out of follicles.
2. Hair follicles atrophy.
3. Sebaceous glands are less active.

Clinical features

1. Onset is usually insidious.
2. Clumps of hair come away in the comb.
3. Bald patches appear in which the skin is very white.
4. The patient can be very distressed, especially when new patches appear as others are recovering.

Prognosis

Fine downy growth may reappear in 2 months. The majority of patients recover in a year. Some patients may not recover. The new hair may not be pigmented and feature as a white streak in otherwise normally coloured hair.

Physiotherapy

The aims are:

1. To improve general health.
2. To improve nutrition to hair follicles.

General health

UVR given with the Theraktin may be given as a general body treatment. A suberythema or E1 dosage is given daily for 6–8 treatments. This is appropriate only if there is evidence of poor health being a factor in the precipitation of the disorder.

Promotion of nutrition

UVR given with the Kromayer may be given to individual patches. Dosage used may be an E2 or an E3.

Two or threes patches may be treated in one session and the patient may attend one or two times a week. It is important to remember that the patient has to sleep and an area of the head must be able to take pressure, therefore there has to be a plan or order for treatment of the patches.

The patient may attend for 2–3 months. If there is no sign of recovery after this time then treatment should be stopped and the condition reviewed in 2–3 months.

As soon as hair starts to grow in a patch UVR must be stopped to that area. As with all skin conditions, sympathy and understanding are important as it is very distressing for a young person to lose hair. This must not be confused with balding where there is receding at the temples and gradual loss from anterior to posterior which may well occur in young men whose father had exactly the same problem.

Hyperhidrosis

Definition

This is a condition in which the exocrine (or apocrine) sweat glands are hyperactive (Figure 17.3).

Clinical features

Sweat pours out of the glands even during relative inactivity and in moderate atmospheric temperatures.

Distribution – palms of hands, soles of feet, axillae and trunk are affected.

It can be embarrasing and disabling, in that work with hands (sewing, baking, handling money or paper) is difficult.

Age group affected is 14–35 years.

Physiotherapy

If a patient is referred for physiotherapy, the treament requested is iontophoresis.

The principle is that the sympathetic nervous system activitates sweat glands, and the main transmitter substance is acetylcholine. Therefore introduction of an anticholinergic compound reduces the activity of the glands. Such compounds may simply be applied to the skin but their effectiveness is dependent on the amount of absorption, through the epidermis to the dermis in which the glands are situated (Figure 17.4). If a low-intensity direct current $(1-2\,\text{mA/in}^2$ of electrode) is applied so that the anode is over a pad soaked in the compound (or in a bowl of water with the compound) then the positive charge of the anode repels the positive ions in the compound into the skin and they are effective at the glands. The cathode is placed proximal to the anode to complete the circuit. The current is applied for 15–20 minutes. Morgan (1980) recommends Glycopytronium bromide as a longer-lasting anticholinergic compound.

Inevitably, there is scepticism about this treament and it may have limited effect on axillary hyperhidrosis. However, a croupier who had to handle chips at a casino was able to work by having 6–8 treatments every 9 months, until the condition cleared. In his case, the hands were placed one at a time in a water-filled plastic tray containing the anode and compound and his feet were placed one at a time in a water-filled foot bath with the cathode.

Side-effects

Patients report dryness of the mouth. If this is troublesome, the dosage should be reduced but patients tend to tolerate this for the benefit gained by the treatment. Sips of water during the treatment may help.

Reference

Morgan (1980) The technique of treating hyperhidrosis by iontophoresis. *Physiotherapy,* **66**, 45

Chapter 18

Burns and skin grafts

Burns

A burn results in loss of skin with impairment of skin functions. The effects of a burn depend on the extent and site of damage. Burns are therefore classified as follows.

Classification of burns

1. Erythema.
2. Superficial.
3. Partial thickness.
4. Full thickness.

1. Erythema

The skin is intact, the erythema lasts for a few days and the patient does not normally seek medical help – unless the problem is extensive, as can occur with sunburn.

2. Superficial

The tissue damage results in seepage of fluid in between the layers of epidermis causing a blister which is surrounded by a dark red erythema. It is very painful. A small 2–3 cm diameter burn (e.g. from an iron or cooker) heals in 7–10 days, and the patient does not normally seek medical help. A larger burn may require treatment, and if 30–40% of the body area is involved the patient may be admitted to hospital. Movement is agonizingly painful.

3. Partial thickness

The epidermis is destroyed with or without part of the dermis. There are blisters, patches of white destroyed tissue and red areas. Sensation varies according to the degree of dermal damage (see Figure 17.2(c)).

4. Full thickness

The epidermis, dermis and other underlying tissues are destroyed. The presenting surface may be black, white or yellow.

Aetiology

Causes

These are as follows:

1. Flame.
2. Chemicals.
3. Hot fluids.
4. Electrical.

Flame burns

These occur when the patient is caught by fire, e.g. in a house or car. Because the clothes catch fire, the burns are often partial or full thickness. Flash flame tends to cause partial-thickness burns. Prompt action to smother flames and cold water dousing reduces the depth of burn.

Chemicals

Caustic substances cause partial-thickness burns, the depth of which can be limited by prompt action. Again, copious quantities of cold water poured over the area reduces the depth of burn.

Hot fluids

Hot water is the commonest cause of scalds. It may be as a hot drink, or by boiling fluid from a pan or kettle (a cup of tea is hot enough 15 minutes after being poured to burn a child, and the water in a kettle remains hot enough to scald three-quarters of an hour after the water has boiled).

Electrical

A patient has burns on the skin which has been in contact with a live wire. Often this accident is complicated by cardiac and respiratory arrest.

Prevention

This is very important in the home because about 75% of burns are domestic accidents. Young children are particularly vulnerable. It is essential, therefore, to ensure that:

1. Kettles and hot pans are well away from the reach of children.
2. Electrical sockets have shutters, and electrical cables are secure with the insulation intact.
3. Sources of flame (matches, cigarette lighters) are kept safely. Guards should be positioned round electric or gas fires and cookers.
4. Fireguards are used.
5. Clothes, especially children's, are flameproof.

Parents can be prosecuted if a child is burnt due to lack of a fireguard (Children and Young Persons Act 1914).

Most of the remaining 25% of burns are industrial, caused by chemicals, electrical accidents, molten metals, friction burns and blow-backs. The Health and Safety at Work Act 1974 has gone some way to preventing such accidents by enforcing the raising of safety standards.

Pathological changes

These may be considered in three stages:

1. Stage of shock.
2. Stage of eschar (burned skin) removal.
3. Stage of healing.

Stage of shock

This lasts for 2–3 days, longer in the elderly.

There is increased capillary permeability with loss of protein and electrolytes from the blood. The main changes are:

1. Reduced plasma volume.

2. Increased proportion of red blood cells to plasma in the blood vessels – resulting in increased blood viscosity and slowing of the circulation.
3. Reduction of cardiac output.
4. Increased heart rate.

During this stage the great dangers are:

1. Pulmonary oedema.
2. Occlusion of arteries.
3. Cardiac failure.
4. Renal failure.
5. Liver failure.
6. Permanent brain and vital organ damage.

Stage of eschar removal

The burned skin becomes crusted and leathery. It separates in 3–4 weeks.

After a superficial burn the skin is healed underneath. Following a deeper burn, tissues are exposed which require skin grafting.

Stage of healing and reconstruction

After superficial burns, the skin heals and can be normal. Following burns that have destroyed the epidermis, there is scar tissue. Over a number of weeks this tissue can become contracted and bound down or may be excessive in growth as in keloid scarring.

Where there is extensive destruction, the patient undergoes grafting and reconstructive surgery which may take months. In the case of children there may have to be episodes of surgery for as long as 12 years.

Complications of burns

These are:

1. Congestive cardiac failure.
2. Left ventricular failure.
3. Cardiac arrhythmias.
4. Inhalation injuries from:
    (a) Hot steam.
    (b) Noxious chemicals from burning materials.
    (c) Carbon monoxide.
    (d) Overheated air.
5. Pneumonia.
6. Infection:
    (a) Of the wound site.
    (b) Of the urinary tract.
7. Septicaemia.
8. Paralytic ileus.
9. Renal and liver failure.
10. Neuropathies.
11. Joint effusion and periarticular swelling.
12. Calcification of periarticular tissues.

Prognosis

Factors affecting outcome are:

1. Age of patient and pre-existing disorders.
2. Extent of surface area of body surface burned.
3. Inhalation burns.

1. Age

Over 70 and under 10 years carry a poor prognosis.

2. Extent

The greater the extent, the poorer the prognosis. A formula for gauging outcome is:

Percentage chance of survival = 100 − (age + % of body area), e.g. 100 − (60 years + 30% area) = 10

Therefore, 10% chance of survival.

100 − (20 years + 30% area) = 50

Therefore, 50% chance of survival.

This formula does not apply to children aged under 10 years. A formula for gauging body surface area is 'the rule of nines'. This rule divides the body surface into 11 areas, each constituting 9% of the total (Figure 18.1). The perineum is counted as 1%.

It is interesting to note that if both legs are burnt 36% of the body surface is affected. Therefore, a 50-year-old patient with such extensive burns has (50 + 36 = 86) 100 − 86 = 14% chance of recovery.

3. Inhalation burns

A high percentage of patients with facial burns develop pneumonia. Where there are inhalation burns as well, the mortality rate is very high.

Clinical features

At the site of the burn

1. Redness – erythema.
2. Blisters.
3. Blackened skin – later leathery in nature.
4. Weeping of plasma – straw-coloured.

Inhalation injury

1. History – smoke and soot, and fire.
2. Burnt lips and nose.
3. Soot in nostrils and mouth.
4. Singed nasal and facial hair.
5. Hoarseness of the voice.
6. Sore throat.

During shock (2–3 days after burn)

1. Restlessness.
2. Coldness and paleness of the skin.

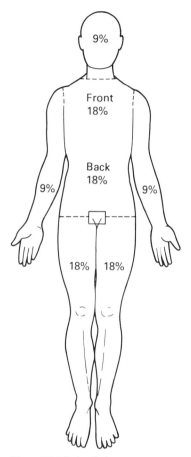

Figure 18.1 Rule of nines

3. Sweating.
4. Thirst.
5. Reduce blood pressure.
6. Tachycardia.
7. Cyanosis.

Later (about 4 weeks)

1. The burned skin (eschar) separates.
2. Scar tissue forms.
3. The scar tissue becomes contracted causing:
   (a) Pain due to traction on sensory nerve endings.
   (b) Limitation of joint movement.
   (c) Loss of function.

Long term

The severity of dysfunction and disfigurement obviously depends on the site and extent:

1. Amputation of a limb may be necessary.
2. Damage to the hands can be very disabling.

3. Facial damage makes rehabilitation of the patient and family very difficult.
4. Both patient and relatives go through severe emotional trauma and varying moods.
5. Social rejection is one of the hardest features that a disfigured person has to endure.

Management of the burned patient

First aid

Flame burns

Flames must be smothered with blankets or carpets.

Cold water applied continuously over the burnt area relieves pain and limits the depth, because heat is conducted to the deeper tissues for several minutes after the flames have been extinguished.

Charred clothing which is adherent to the skin should be left for removal at hospital.

Chemical burns

Copious quantities of running water must be applied to the area, except where the burn is due to sodium or potassium. These metals must be pushed off the skin with a matchstick or picked off with forceps.

Scalds

Again, thorough and continuous dousing with cold water can limit the extent of the damage and reduce the pain.

Electrical burns

The patient may require mouth-to-mouth respiration and external cardiac massage, before attention can be paid to a burn. Unlike heat burns these do not spread and it is sufficient to cover the area with a clean towel or sheet which has been soaked in cold water.

The patient should be transported to hospital as quickly as possible.

Hospital management

Minor burns

These are cleaned with chlorhexidine and covered with a bactericidal non-stick dressing. The patient can rest at home and, depending on local circumstances, the dressings are changed every 2–3 days by a visiting nurse, by relatives or at the hospital accident and emergency department. In 7–10 days, the burnt skin comes off either freely or by a nurse removing it with forceps and scissors. In 14–21 days, the skin should be healed.

A minor burn involves less than 10% of the body surface. Physiotherapy is not usually associated with treatment of patients with minor burns, unless the hands or feet are affected or the patient is elderly. The patient may be in the care of the community physiotherapist. In this case it is important that the advice from the doctors and nurses is reinforced (i.e. rest the part). Also, if the dressings are soaked or the patient complains of excess pain, itching or redness developing in tissues surrounding the burn (i.e. evidence of infection) then the physiotherapist must report this to the visiting nurse, or doctor.

Where physiotherapy is required to regain function after a minor burn, the principles are the same as for a major burn.

Major burn

This is a burn that covers more than 10% of the body surface. Other factors that may necessitate hospitalization are:

1. Inhalation of smoke or gas.
2. Elderly or very young patients.
3. Burns involving feet, perineum, buttocks, hands or face.
4. Associated conditions, e.g. cardiac arrest, fractures, inadequate home situation, non-accidental injuries in children.

Early management (including shock phase)

This involves:

1. Maintenance of a clear airway.
2. Pain relief.
3. Maintenance of fluid balance.
4. Removal of adherent clothing and covering of the burns with sterile cotton cloths.
5. Reassurance and explanation for the patient.
6. Transfer to a Burns Unit or admission to an Intensive Care Unit.

Management after 3–4 days

This involves care of the patient as a whole and care of the wound areas.

The patient as a whole

Fluid replacement is carried out by intravenous drip and naso-gastric tube if necessary.

A diet of high protein and calorie content is worked out by the dietitian.

Urine is measured and tested regularly. Infection is prevented by:

1. Isolation of the patient in a room with air filtering.
2. Only two visitors being allowed at a time.
3. Gowns and masks for staff and visitors.
4. Sterilization of all items that go into the patient's room.

Maintenance of respiratory function is related to injuries. Humidified oxygen, suction of bronchial secretions or mechanical respiration may be necessary.

Prevention of renal failure is achieved by intravenous fluids in the first instance and then if necessary by haemodialysis or peritoneal dialysis.

The mental stability of the patient is preserved by an optimistic, but realistic approach from all staff. The patient has to be encouraged to be active and as independent as possible.

The wound areas

Management of wound areas varies according to the experiences of the staff and facilities. The two main themes are open or closed.

Open

This method leaves the wound exposed, and if exudate is cleaned away regularly the area dries out. Bacterial growth is inhibited and this method is used for areas that are difficult to dress. Healing of the epithelium tends to be slower than with the closed method.

Closed

Dressings may be positioned on top of a bactericidal powder or gel. A few layers of gauze allows the air to get to the surface and helps the wound to dry. Silver sulphadiazine or silver nitrate may be applied with Vaseline gauze and many layers of gauze and wool applied to keep the air out. With bandages securing the dressings the patient may be able to get up and about and possibly leave the burns ward to exercise in a physiotherapy gym. When the burn affects a hand, a Polythene bag may be placed over the hand and bandaged to the forearm. The patient can exercise the hand regularly. The bags are changed twice a day at first and the hands washed in saline.

Surgical care

Escharotomy is a slit made in leathery skin which can restrict movement – especially if it is around the chest, where respiration can be impaired.

Escharectomy is removal of the dead, burnt skin. A bleeding surface is left and has to be grafted.

Grafting involves covering the open tissues with skin. This may be from a normal area on the patient (an autograft) or from another person (allograft). Sometimes pigskin is used where there are extensive areas to be covered. Grafts other than autografts do not last but provide protection for 2–3 weeks.

Donor sites take 7–10 days to heal and can be very painful during the first few days. Where there is a shortage of available donor sites on the body due to the size of the burn, the 'split-skin' that is removed for grafting purposes has to be extremely thin so that the donor area can be used again after 14 days. Unfortunately these very thin layers tend to contract more later. Extensive burns require considerable excision and grafting carried out every 1–2 weeks. This is a long, painful, distressful period for the patient who has to have repeated anaesthetics and operations.

Grafts are kept in position with tulle gras, bandages and plaster of Paris to immobilize the joints next to the grafts.

Rehabilitation

This may be relatively short (1–2 months) or over many months. Children require review for the growing years.

Physiotherapy

This is necessary for both in- and out-patients. In-patients may be in a special ward, intensive care unit or a regional burns unit. The last is best because the patient receives highly specialist attention, but it can cause difficulties for relatives undertaking long journeys to visit the patient. The physiotherapist, together with other team members, must recognize the devastating effect a bad case of burning can have on the family. It is important to recognize moods of guilt, depression, anger, bewilderment and bitterness which can arise in the patient and family. The cause of the accident clearly has a bearing on these moods. The physiotherapist has to gauge what is the appropriate reaction – sympathy, cajoling, encouragement or optimism – whilst achieving the aims of treatment. Given the long-stay nature of the recovery period, staff and patients develop a special relationship which must remain professional for the emotional well-being of all concerned.

The aims of physiotherapy are to:

1. Prevent respiratory complications.
2. Maintain joint range, and prevent contractures or deformities.
3. Maintain muscle strength.
4. Regain maximum function for the patient.
5. Help the patient return to an active lifestyle within society.

Respiratory care

Clearing secretions is achieved by shaking, clapping, postural drainage, coughing and suction. If it is very uncomfortable for the patient to have hand pressure on a chest burn, then a piece of foam may be used under the hands. Tipping is contraindicated if there is facial oedema but the patient may lie supine or on either side.

A ventilated patient usually requires suction and humidification.

A little treatment, often, is the general theme. Steam inhalations (see Chapter 12) may be necessary for the non-ventilated patient especially when there has been inhalation of smoke or fumes. Breathing (expansion) exercises are also important to maintian ventilation of all lung areas.

The physiotherapist must not be afraid to treat with the vigour required to achieve the aims even when the chest skin is burnt.

Intensive respiratory care is required in the following situations:

1. Elderly patients.
2. Burns affecting face, mouth and inhalation burns.
3. Immobile patients.
4. A history of a chronic respiratory condition.
5. Pre- and post-operatively.
6. Patients with full-thickness burns on the chest – breathing exercises to keep the eschar mobile.

Joint range, prevention of contractures and deformities

Positioning, splinting and exercise are used for maintaining and gaining joint range.

Positioning

Unfortunately for the patient, the position of comfort is the position of contracture (mostly flexion).

Positions of necessity are, therefore, as follows.

Head and neck

Small roll (towel) under the neck and/or a pillow under the shoulders to maintain extension. The patient may be in lying (chest and leg burns) or in half-lying with facial burns (because of facial oedema).

Upper limbs

Elevation (over 90°) of the limbs with the shoulder in abduction and slight flexion, elbows and wrists in extension, MCP joints in flexion, IP joints in extension and thumb in abduction.

Lower limbs

Hips in extension and slight abduction, knees in extension and ankles in 90° dorsiflexion. Elevation is obtained by raising the end of the bed, not by placing pillows under the legs which would put the hips into flexion.

Splinting

Splints may be static or dynamic.

Static

Static splints are used where it is essential to hold the position until movement can start. These are designed and made to individual requirements and changed as the patient recovers, e.g. from grafting.

Splinting may be required only at night to prevent soft-tissue tightening whilst the patient is asleep.

Sometimes joints are stabilized to facilitate the function of others.

Dynamic

Dynamic splints permit controlled movement of various joints. For example, a foam roll placed in the hand allows extension and some flexion of the fingers, so allowing damaged extensor tendons to move in a limited range but not to be overstretched.

Collars may be necessary to keep the neck positioned because the skin on the anterior aspect of the neck contracts very readily, pulling the lower jaw down to the chest. A soft material may be adequate for daytime and a firmer one used at night.

General points for splinting

1. The position has to be effective, not necessarily the position of function.
2. Joints must not be included unnecessarily in splints.
3. Tight encircling must be avoided; therefore, splints must be bandaged on evenly.
4. Bony prominences require corresponding padding in the splinting.
5. Nerve compression must be avoided.
6. Correction and prevention of deformity is essential but so too is muscular activity. Therefore, intermittent and dynamic splinting must be used where possible.

Exercises

Every joint should, where possible, be moved through full range each day. An active exercise programme must, therefore, be devised to achieve this. Assisted active exercise is necessary for the damaged limbs and free active exercise for undamaged areas. Hourly exercise should be performed to reduce oedema so that this does not consolidate and cause joint stiffness. During bathtime, the patient is immersed in plain water with baby shampoo and it is very useful to have physiotherapy incorporated. Joints can be moved through full range and the patient's sense of well-being is greatly enhanced, movement being a comforting contrast to recumbency. This can be started 2–3 days after injury and may take place every 2–3 days thereafter.

Regaining range when the surgeon decides mobility should start involves controlled passive stretching, hold–relax, repeated contractions and assisted active exercises. As soon as possible the patient must be encouraged to be independent in self-care and activities of daily living.

Muscle strength

Where joints can be moved, the patient must work the muscles for each joint through full range twice a day. Muscles working over joints which are fixed can be worked isometrically, either by having the patient feel the muscle tightening or by overflow from muscles working in the same pattern, e.g. manual resistance to the knee extensors can produce overflow into the ankle dorsiflexors – or strong work in the muscles of one leg causes work in the muscles of the other leg. Both arms can be resisted to obtain overflow into the trunk muscles. As soon as possible the patient should be up and about and following an exercise/activity programme in the gym and hospital locality.

Regaining maximum function

As soon as the wound condition is stable, the patient should go to the physiotherapy gym. Dressings are bandaged on securely and lower limb burns are supported by elastic bandages to control oedema. An individual circuit is worked out which involves free exercise and equipment work. Goals should be set, e.g. so many miles on a cycle, so many repetitions without rest on skipping, spring work or ball bouncing, jumping a height, reaching a grip strength by a given time (in weeks). This programme continues to discharge with modifications following grafting. Trips to the hospital shop and then to neighbouring shops and pubs should be included so that the patient starts to feel like a member of society again. Discharge home is arranged as soon as patient and relatives are ready.

Out-patient physiotherapy

This continues to involve gym work. Contractures must be prevented by regular passive stretching, and mobility of scar tissue is maintained by kneading with the fingers or palm of hand.

Pressure garments are fitted by the physiotherapist. These are used to reduce hypertrophic scarring which is excessive formation of collagen resulting in thick, rope-like, uneven scars which both limit function and look unsightly. Pressure by an elasticated garment worn more or less continuously for up to 2 years reduces this scarring (Figures 18.2–18.4).

Smaller burns

These may be treated by physiotherapy on an out-patient basis. Pulsed electromagnetic energy twice daily for 25 minutes has been shown to promote healing and there is some evidence that laser treatment increases the rate of wound healing and reduces pain.

Active exercise is just as important for small burns as for larger ones so that scar tissue is kept mobile and prevented from causing adhesions between fascia, tendons, muscles and periosteum.

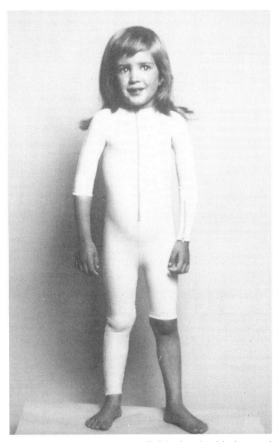

Figure 18.2 Pressure garment. Full body suit with short and long limbs and zip closures. (Reproduced by courtesy of Seton Healthcare Group.)

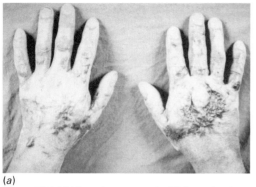 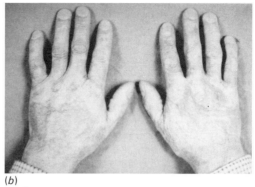

(a)   (b)

Figure 18.3 (*a*) Flame burn to hands. (*b*) Same hands 14 months later after wearing pressure gloves.

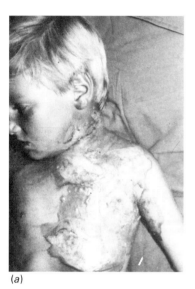 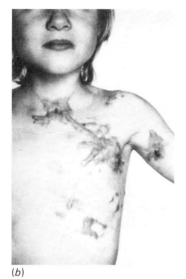 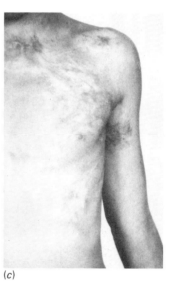

(a)   (b)   (c)

Figure 18.4 (*a*) Child with burn on upper trunk. (*b*) Same child 5 months later after wearing pressure vests. (*c*) Same child 19 months later after wearing pressure vests. (Reproduced by courtesy of Seton Healthcare Group.)

Return to active lifestyle and society

From the start, the patient's independence is encouraged, and the entire staff dealing with the patient work together to encourage, sympathize and cajole. The physiotherapist has sometimes to push the patient hard, particularly where likelihood of contractures or loss of function is high, e.g. burns of the hands, axillae, chest, feet and anterior aspect of neck. Analgesics should be timed for maximum effect when treatment is under way.

The occupational therapist has a vital role in patient management. Activities and crafts, e.g. macramé, give the patient a purpose, and can toughen the skin whilst increasing strength and mobility. Patients must get used to using equipment again, e.g. cooking, pouring from a kettle, lighting a cigarette. The occupational therapist rebuilds the patient's confidence by simulating potentially frightening situations. Patients with hand or face burns may be accompanied by the occupational therapist or physiotherapist to eat in a local pub or restaurant. Sometimes it helps to have patients meet people who have recovered from severe injuries, and self-help groups can provide invaluable long-term support. Return to work is obviously dependent on the nature of work and type of injury but generally the patient should return even if there are interruptions for release operations, follow-up appointments and pressure garment refits. Family, friends and employers have, therefore, to play a part in the restoration of a full active lifestyle.

Children

The treatment of children follows the same principles as for adults. The main differences are as follows.

The relatives require a careful and considerate approach. They need to have all the treatment methods explained and to be allowed to join in where possible, e.g. feeding, reading stories, playing games. The patient will be reviewed every year up to 10 or 11 years after the injury and relatives need to know the commitment. They also need to know that there is help at hand to allay anxiety if the burn area splits, bleeds or is becoming tight.

If non-accidental injury is suspected, nurses, social workers, general practitioner, psychiatrist and surgeons have to confer and try to devise the best outcome for patient and parents.

Skin grafts

Skin grafts may be used for any part of the body in areas where there has been extensive damage by burns, lacerated wounds, ulceration, pressure sores, or for healed contracted scars.

Types of skin graft are (1) free grafts and (2) flaps and pedicles.

Free grafts (Figure 18.5)

These consist of slices of skin removed from one part of the body and applied to a raw surface in another part.

They vary in thickness. *Split-skin (Thiersch)* varies from very thin to consisting of the whole epidermis and part dermis.

Whole-thickness (Wolfe) consists of the skin down to but excluding superficial fascia. These grafts are transferred without blood supply. For the first 48 hours nutrition is obtained from free tissue fluid of the recipient site. Capillaries grow into the graft and vascularization is generally established after 48 hours. This is a critical time because movement of

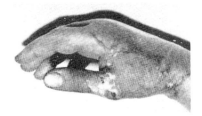

Figure 18.5 Free skin graft over first metatarsal. Note smooth scar formation at junction of graft and skin. Small areas have yet to heal. Note keloid formation on ungrafted areas on thumb and first finger

the graft destroys the capillary buds, and then the graft usually fails. Dressings fixing the graft may be kept on for up to 5 days at which time active exercise of the area may start. After about 14 days, the graft begins to contract and there is danger that it will become adherent to underlying tissues. Donor sites heal in 12–14 days depending on the thickness. A donor area used for full-thickness skin has to be covered by a split-skin graft.

Flaps and pedicles

With these, the skin to be transferred remains attached by one end to the donor area and the other end is attached to the recipient site (Figure 18.6). A pedicle may have intermediate as well as a final

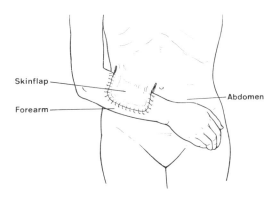

Figure 18.6 Abdomen–forearm skin flap

recipient site (Figure 18.7). A blood supply to these grafts is preserved throughout the procedure. Three weeks elapse between each stage so the patient is fixed in an awkward position for this time.

Free flaps may be used. In these, the skin is raised, together with its blood vessels which are then anastomosed with vessels of the recipient area. These operations are performed with the use of a microscope – hence the term micro-surgery. The operation is long and exacting for the surgeons but the patient is saved the distress and pain of fixation for 3 weeks at a time as required for fixed flaps and pedicles.

Physiotherapy for skin grafts
The graft

Once the grafted skin is established – at least 14 days later, finger kneading round the edges with lanolin is used to mobilize the tissues. The technique may gradually encroach on the graft. It is important to

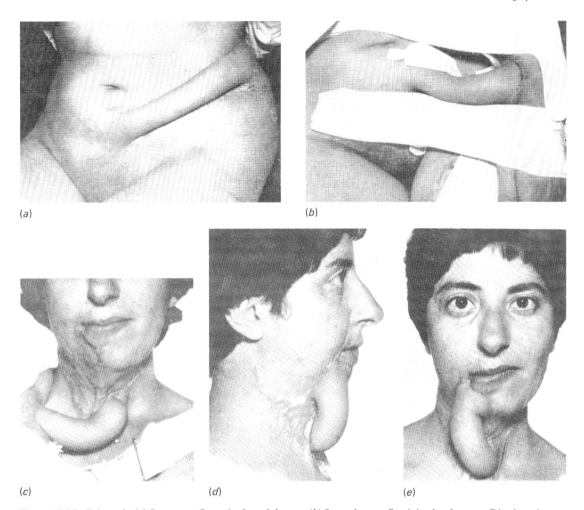

(a)

(b)

(c)

(d)

(e)

Figure 18.7 Pedicle graft. (*a*) Stage one; flap raised on abdomen. (*b*) Second stage; flap joined to forearm. Distal portion will remain attached to abdomen until proximal attachment on forearm takes. (*c*) Flap freed from abdomen and free end attached to neck. Forearm attachment will remain until graft takes on neck. Arm strapped into position to prevent movement meanwhile. When new graft takes operation will be performed. Scar tissues will be excised, forearm attachment will be freed and applied to scarred area. (*d*) and (*e*) Last but one stage of graft. It has now been detached from the arm and is in the final grafting position. Note the contraction of the scar and the hard ridged area

use small range movements, to keep the pressure superficial and at all costs to avoid sliding over the skin while applying pressure, because this can cause blistering. The aim is to soften and mobilize the grafted tissue to enable freedom of movement and improve nutrition and therefore restore function.

The donor area of a split skin graft may be treated with ultraviolet rays (UVR) to promote healing 3–4 days after operation. An E1 is given to the area (often the anterior aspect of the thigh) which is screened to within 2–3 cm of the actual site. The air-cooled mercury vapour burner is used at a distance of 45 cm and a daily treatment for 3–4 days

is usually sufficient for healing to occur. This is helpful when the donor area may be needed again.

Where a graft has 'taken' in all but one small area, the same approach may be used with UVR using either the Kromayer or the air-cooled mercury vapour burner to encourage epithelialization of the raw area. This has particular value in preventing the need for further surgery. Irradiation of the graft may or may not be considered wise – this is a matter for discussion between the surgeon and the physiotherapist. UVR is sometimes also given to an infected area to clean the surface prior to grafting (see ulcers).

Joints and muscles

Joints and muscles near the graft should be exercised through as full a range as possible and all other joints and muscles should be put through a general full-range movement programme. The muscles near the graft over the immobilized joints should be moved isometrically, e.g. five contractions per muscle every hour. This eases some of the discomfort and maintains fluid flow through the tissues. These exercises usually start 5–7 days after grafting.

When a flap or pedicle is released, heat, kneading, hold–relax or mobilizations may be used to relieve pain and relax muscle spasm. Free active exercises should start within a day or two after release. If heat is used, it must not irradiate the flap, pedicle or grafted surface, as the heat increases metabolism of these delicate tissues beyond the scope of the developing blood vessels.

Respiratory system

Breathing exercises with huffing or coughing to clear the lung fields may be necessary – especially after the long time under an anaesthetic when microsurgery is performed.

General

The physiotherapist should listen to the hopes and fears of the patient and discuss, at a case conference, the help that may be needed. A general fitness programme in a gymnasium may be appropriate – but this depends on the presence of other conditions, e.g. fractures. Physiotherapy for grafted burns and ulcers is described under those headings.

Chapter 19

Diseases of the nervous system

Introduction

The range and flexibility of the nervous system is very extensive to allow for the physical and intellectual activities of man. The system is thus very complex and is still not fully understood despite the enormous amount of study devoted to it. Clinical studies of nervous diseases have indicated that the anatomy and physiology of the nervous system is not simple and that it is not always possible to explain all the clinical features from the known facts, or pathology. Current techniques of study such as the electron microscope and microphotometry with morphological studies and clinical observations have improved knowledge in this field.

The following section gives some of the basic concepts relating to the nervous system to help the reader to understand the pathological changes occurring in the neurological conditions described. Detailed textbooks on neuroanatomy, neurophysiology and neurological conditions must be studied to give a greater depth of knowledge, which is essential for those therapists specializing in the treatment of these conditions. It is important to realize that knowledge of neuroanatomy and neurophysiology is continually changing as new techniques of investigation and the results of clinical observations give new information.

Basic concepts

The evolution of the species has resulted in the complex structure of the human body, with living cells becoming specialized and adapted to form different systems. Survival of man as a species is dependent on the ability to react to a changing environment while maintaining the physiological functions and anatomical integrity of the body. However, man is not only a creature of reaction but has the intellectual ability that allows proaction – the initiation of mental processes that can manipulate the environment. Emotional activities are developed to a higher level in the human and go beyond the basic emotions of the animal responding to pain, grief at the loss of a mate, pleasure at the sight of food, or fear. There is a very wide range of physical, intellectual and emotional activities which must be appreciated in dealing with the results of disease. A man may be physically strong but emotionally labile, or have a high intellectual ability and be physically weak, and so on. Inherited qualities of physique, intellect or the emotions may be developed or adversely affected by the environment, for example by education, by the family, by culture or by nutrition. The physical, intellectual and emotional activities can only be achieved by a central controlling system with a wide network of communications, and this is the nervous system.

Basic anatomy and physiology

The different parts of the nervous system are all integrated and so disease or injury of one part will invariably affect other parts. However, the system can be subdivided for the study of its structure and function. There is the peripheral system transmitting impulses to and from the spinal cord, and the central nervous system comprising the brain and spinal cord.

The peripheral nervous system is further subdivided into the somatic part and the autonomic part. The somatic part has afferent fibres carrying impulses from receptor organs in the skin, subcutaneous tissues, muscles, tendons and joints which transmit modalities of touch, pressure, stretch, pain, and thermal sensation. The efferent fibres transmit impulses to the effector organs in skeletal muscle, and each neuron may innervate from a few to hundreds of muscle fibres. The autonomic part has afferent fibres which carry impulses from receptors in viscera and blood vessels. Generally these afferent impulses are concerned with reflex activities which are below the level of consciousness, but certain sensations are appreciated, for example hunger, distension, nausea and visceral pain. Pain can sometimes be felt in an area of somatic distribution when the afferent somatic fibres enter the spinal cord at the same segments as the autonomic afferents. This is known as referred pain. The efferent autonomic fibres carry impulses to effectors in glands and unstriated muscle.

The somatic and autonomic sections are continued within the central nervous system and are linked with other complex activities. Although the sections can be described separately in structure and function it is important to appreciate that activity of one section may affect the other.

The autonomic nervous system is itself divided into two sections, parasympathetic and sympathetic. These two sections oppose each other in their functions and yet are complementary in controlling the activities of the body in different situations.

The parasympathetic system helps to maintain the normal activities of the body and conserve energy by its actions on the body systems such as the heart and alimentary tract. Whereas the sympathetic system prepares the body for activity by increasing the blood supply to the heart, muscle and brain, it increases the heart rate and lessens the activity of the alimentary tract. The higher centres of this system lie in the brainstem and although some centres can be identified as a collection of neurons controlling certain autonomic functions, other neurons of this system are mixed with neurons belonging to other parts of the central nervous system and cannot be structurally localized as a centre.

The sympathetic system has a chain of ganglia lying on either side of the vertebral column, and connector fibres pass from cells in the lateral columns of the thoracic and upper lumbar part of the spinal cord to these ganglia or to more peripheral ganglia and thence by effector neurons to effector organs.

The parasympathetic system has a similar two neuron efferent pathway with connector neurons passing through the cranial and sacral nerves to ganglia near the organs to be supplied, and then a short efferent neuron to the effector organs. Afferent fibres of the autonomic system pass similarly to afferents of the somatic system.

The brain comprises three main parts, the hindbrain, midbrain and forebrain (Figure 19.1). The hindbrain is formed by the medulla oblongata,

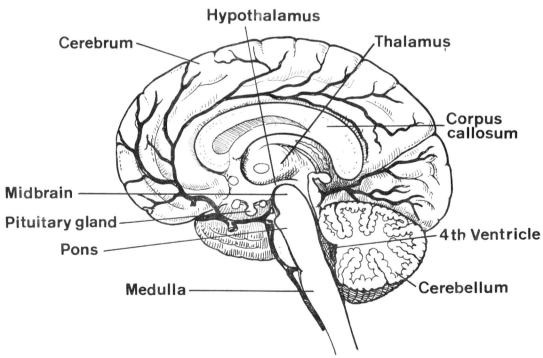

Figure 19.1 Sagittal section through the brain (midline)

pons and cerebellum. The medulla and pons contain the continuation upwards of most of the afferent tracts from the spinal cord and the efferent pathways passing down to the cord. Most efferent fibres (approximately two-thirds) cross from one side to the other in the medulla (decussation of the pyramids). There is a similar decussation of some of the afferent fibres, namely the fasciculus gracilis and fasciculus cuneatus, whereas others cross in the cord or pass straight up. The pons also contains fibres passing to and from the cerebellar hemispheres. Both the medulla and the pons contain nuclei of some of the cranial nerves and some important centres concerned with the autonomic system, for example those of the cardiovascular, respiratory and digestive systems. There are other areas of grey matter in the brainstem and this includes the part described as the reticular formation. The reticular system consists of scattered areas of grey and white matter which have diffuse connections with the cerebrum, cerebellum and spinal cord, also efferent connections to autonomic centres, and are concerned with locomotor control.

The cerebellar hemispheres lie one on either side and behind the medulla and pons. They are linked with other parts of the brainstem by three peduncles carrying impulses to and from the cerebellum. The cerebellum receives information from cutaneous receptors, proprioceptors, the eyes, the ears, the cerebral grey matter and from the reticular formation. The main function of the cerebellum is concerned with equilibrium, coordination of movement and plasticity of muscle. In contrast to the cerebral hemispheres a cerebellar hemisphere controls the same side of the body.

The mid-brain is another connecting area between parts of the brain and the spinal cord. Also it contains important areas of grey matter, part of the reticular formation, and areas linked with visual and

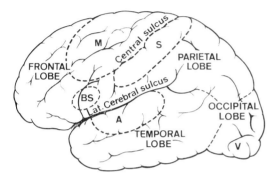

Figure 19.2 Localization of function in the cerebrum. Superolateral surface of the left cerebral hemisphere. A = Auditory area; B = Broca's speech area (if dominant hemisphere); M = motor area; S = sensory area; V = visual area

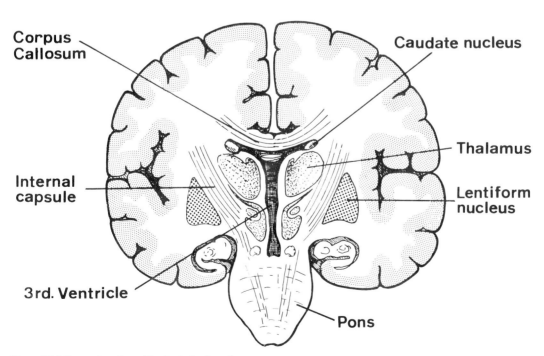

Figure 19.3 Coronal section of the brain to show the internal capsule (Section through the ventral part of the pons.)

auditory reflexes. The cerebral hemispheres, forming the main part of the forebrain, are connected to
each other by the corpus callosum, and to the
hindbrain and spinal cord by the mid-brain. The
localization of function shown in Figure 19.2 is still
used as a guide but it is no longer as simple as was
originally thought, and this probably accounts for
some of the unexpected clinical features that are
found with some lesions. There is a concentration of
fibres passing to and from the various areas of the
cortex within the internal capsule (Figure 19.3) and
for this reason circulatory problems that affect this
part can cause widespread damage to function of the
opposite side of the body. Apart from the grey
matter of the cerebral cortex there are other areas of
grey matter known collectively as the basal ganglia
because of their position. These areas are concerned
with the quality of movement, and lesions produce
unwanted or uncontrollable movements, for example athetoid, ballismic or choreiform movements.

The basic components making up these various
parts of the nervous system are the neurons, the
non-excitable supporting tissue called neuroglia,
ependyma and Schwann cells. A neuron consists of a
cell body with a varying number of branching
extensions called neurites; some of these carry
impulses towards the cell body (dendrites) and
others carry impulses away (axons). Some neurons
are concerned with receiving stimuli through a
specially adapted part at the peripheral end of the
dendrite called a receptor organ, whereas others are
concerned with transmitting an impulse by an
adapted part at the end of an axon called an effector
organ. Others are termed connector or inter-
neurones as they transmit between neurons. An
interneuron may receive stimuli from many other
neurons and transmit to many others. Some of the
main pathways in the central nervous system can be
traced and the result of interference with these
pathways can be observed, but it is difficult to
discover the effects of all the intermediate pathways
and connections. This may explain why recovery is
better than expected following some cases of
neurological damage, yet may be worse in others.

Transmission of impulses from one cell or its
fibres to another neuron takes place at a synapse
(Figure 19.4). There is no physical connection
between the cellular structures of one neuron and
another, but they are in close proximity at the
synaptic cleft. The fibre of a neuron ends in a
synaptic bag which contains a chemical transmitter.
When an impulse passes along the nerve fibre to the
synaptic bag (presynaptic membrane) the transmitter is released and diffuses across the gap to the
membrane of the adjacent cell (post-synaptic
membrane) and causes an alteration in the ionic
permeability. Some neurotransmitters are excitatory
and others are inhibitory (Figure 19.5). When
excitatory stimulus is sufficient to exceed the

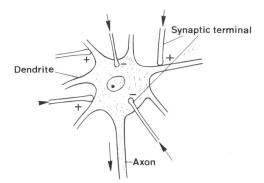

Figure 19.4 Transmission across a multipolar neurone

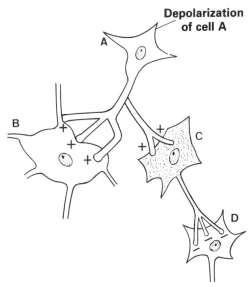

Figure 19.5 Transmission to show increased and decreased
excitatory state of neurones

threshold of excitability an action potential will be
discharged. Transmission across the synapse can
take place in one direction only.

Reflex activity

Many responses of the body to stimuli are automatic
and occur without conscious thought. Simply
explained, a reflex action requires a stimulus to a
receptor organ resulting in an impulse along an
afferent fibre to synaptic connections which will give
a reflex response through an efferent fibre to an
effector organ. For example, pain elicited by
touching a hot surface will result in a reflex
withdrawal of the hand. In reality, reflexes are not
so simple and numerous areas within the nervous
system will be involved: the posture of the body

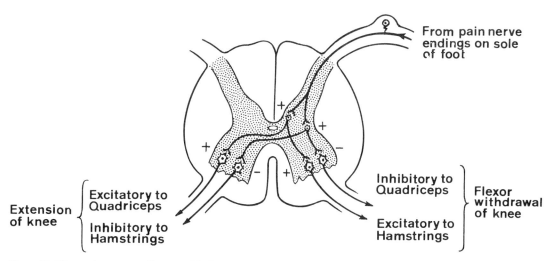

Figure 19.6 Crossed extensor reflex. + = Excitatory neurotransmitter; − = inhibitory neurotransmitter

must be adjusted as the hand is withdrawn, there will be conscious awareness of pain, and the autonomic system will respond to a degree which will depend on the nature and severity of the injury. A more complex reflex will occur in the lower limbs if a painful stimulus on the sole of one foot causes the person to lift the foot off the ground. To prevent the person falling over there is a shift of gravity over the other foot and there is an increase in the tone of the extensor muscles of the leg. This is called the crossed extensor reflex (Figure 19.6). Recent studies indicate that reflex activity of muscle spindles in relation to the length of the extrafusal fibres is, in fact, more complicated than previously thought. The spindle probably monitors the activity of the extrafusal fibres and the spindle itself can be set to respond to different thresholds of activity. Many aspects of visceral activity are under reflex control, for example changes in heart rate and blood pressure. Some lesions may interrupt reflex arcs or may result in the release of primitive reflex activity.

Aetiology

Lesions of the nervous system – whether of the brain, the spinal cord, or the peripheral nerves – may be due to injury or disease, and the principal causes are as follows.

Trauma

Head injuries may result in brain damage which may be temporary or, if there has been destruction of nerve tissue, permanent. The severity of the head injury may not correlate with the amount of brain damage as it is possible to have a fractured skull with very little damage or a blow to the head, without a fracture, which may cause severe damage. The injury may result in concussion, contusion, laceration or compression. The spinal cord may be damaged by a fracture, fracture dislocation of the vertebral column, or by protrusion of an intervertebral disc as a result of injury.

Peripheral nerves may be damaged by a fracture or dislocation, either directly, or indirectly because of accompanying soft-tissue damage. Also, a peripheral nerve can be damaged by a laceration or compression.

Disease

Infections

Micro-organisms may affect the nervous system and generally seem to have a selective affinity for a particular part of the system. The incidence of some infective diseases has decreased with advances in medical science, although they may still occur in some parts of the world. Generally the incidence of tuberculosis of the brain and spinal cord caused by the tubercle bacillus has decreased as the result of chemotherapy, better health care, and health education. Similarly, cases of poliomyelitis due to viral infection have decreased as the result of a poliovirus vaccine. However, there are other viruses that can attack the nervous system, for example meningitis can occur as the result of pyogenic organisms passing through the circulation – pneumococcal meningitis. Syphilis (a venereal disease) caused by *Treponema pallidum* may lead to infection of the nervous system and neurovascular tissue.

The peripheral nerves may be affected by viral infections, for example Herpes zoster (shingles), or acute infective polyneuropathy (Guillain–Barré syndrome) which may be a viral or post-viral infection.

Circulatory conditions

Nerve cells require a constant supply of oxygen via the bloodstream, and brain death may occur in as short a time as 5 minutes after a cardiac arrest. Circulatory disturbances affecting the brain are due largely to atheroma which may result in ischaemia, thrombus, embolism or haemorrhage. Circulatory abnormalities may affect the spinal cord but this is rare.

Congenital defects

Some children suffering from cerebral palsy have congenital defects of the brain; however, there are other causes of this condition including anoxia at birth. Spina bifida is a congenital condition affecting the vertebral column and in some instances the spinal cord.

Deficiency diseases

Deficiency of some vitamins can cause neurological damage in addition to other general changes. A lack of vitamin B can lead to beri-beri with the development of an acute polyneuritis. An inability to absorb vitamin B_{12} due to a lack of the intrinsic factor from the stomach can result in pernicious anaemia which if not treated may lead to changes in peripheral nerves and the spinal cord.

Inherited conditions

These are rare but they include Huntington's chorea, which is inherited as a dominant trait, usually developing in the third decade, and causes progressive chorea and dementia.

Neoplasms

Tumours of any type can damage the nervous system both by compression and by actual invasion and destruction of nerve tissue.

Toxic substances

These are numerous and include lead, arsenic, mercury and some agricultural insecticides. Many of these affect the peripheral nerves more severely than the central nervous tissue.

Diseases of unknown origin

One of the most common of these diseases affecting the central nervous system is multiple sclerosis. There are a number of theories concerning the cause but nothing has been proved.

Pathology

The pathological changes in nervous diseases are usually either inflammatory or degenerative. In some cases of injury there may be immediate destruction of some nerve tissue, but usually this is accompanied by inflammatory or degenerative changes, or both, in the surrounding tissues.

Inflammation

The changes of acute inflammation are similar to those described in Chapter 1. There is a dilatation of blood vessels with increased capillary permeability followed by exudation of leucocytes and plasma into the surrounding tissues. Nerve cells may be destroyed, or compressed by the exudation. Any neurons that are destroyed cannot be replaced because such highly specialized cells have lost the ability to reproduce. Pain may occur because of the pressure caused by the oedema or other irritants, but this will depend on the area affected and the presence of nociceptors. Depending on the causation, severity and extent of the inflammation it may terminate in a number of ways. The inflammation may subside and full recovery may occur, there may be a partial recovery with some permanent damage, or it could prove fatal. If there is permanent damage, the disability will depend on the extent of the damage and the particular area affected. Chronic inflammation could lead to a progressive deterioration as more damage occurs.

Degeneration

Degenerative change involves the transformation of highly specialized cells into connective tissue, which in the nervous system may be neuroglia. Sometimes the cause of the degeneration is unknown, as in the case of multiple sclerosis, or it may be due to a lack of blood supply to the area. The action of some micro-organisms or compression of nerve tissue may cause degenerative changes.

In the case of peripheral nerves recovery may take place provided that the nerve cell has not been destroyed (see Chapter 21). However, in the central nervous system recovery of nerve fibres will not take place because of the absence of the endoneural tube with the Schwann cells.

Clinical features

Clinical features of diseases of the nervous system are determined partly by the site or sites of the lesion and its extent. However, it is essential to appreciate the integrative nature and complexity of the nervous system when studying the clinical features of disease and injury as they cannot always be explained by the pathology and site(s) of the lesion.

The clinical features outlined below are general, and specific features will depend on the nature of the lesion. The physiotherapist must make an assessment to ascertain the presenting features. The clinical features presented in a textbook for a particular condition are a guide but it is unlikely that the position and extent of a lesion are the same in any two patients. Even if the lesion were very similar no two patients respond to disease or injury in the same way. Added to these problems it is very difficult to predict which other areas may be affected because of the complex integration.

Mental state

The site of the lesion may or may not affect the mental state of the patient, although in either case there are likely to be altered intellectual and emotional behaviour patterns.

Physical dysfunction

Dysfunction may occur as the result of lesions affecting the somatic motor system or the somatic sensory system, or both. Thus the following is a list of the features with the sensory/motor causation being mentioned as applicable. It is important to note that some signs and symptoms can be increased or decreased in severity by alterations in the mental state of the patient or by disturbances of autonomic function.

Incoordination of movement

Coordinated movement requires the normal activity of both somatic afferents and efferents. Some types of incoordinated movement may take particular forms, such as ataxia, and these are described below. Weakness of some muscles will give an imbalance of activity and hence the movement will be incoordinated. Similarly, if a muscle or muscles are paralysed movement may be possible because of the activity of normal muscles but it may be incoordinated. Muscles act as agonists, antagonists, fixators and synergists, and weakness or paralysis of any muscles contributing to these actions will cause an imbalance of activity and an incoordinated movement.

Paralysis of muscle (flaccidity)

This occurs if the pathway for impulses through the lower motor neuron is lost, as may happen in a peripheral nerve lesion (see Chapter 21), or in some instances if there is an interruption of supraspinal pathways to the anterior horn cell. The extent of the disability will depend on the amount of the paralysis. For example, paralysis of the dorsiflexors of one foot will result in an incoordination of movement – but the patient will be able to walk, albeit with a poor gait. However, if both legs are totally paralysed, as may occur in a cauda equina lesion, the patient will be unable to walk unless provided with special appliances. The paralysed muscles feel 'flabby' and will quickly lose their bulk (atrophy).

In some cases not all the motor neurons to a muscle are affected and the muscle will function inadequately, giving an incoordinated and weak movement (paresis).

Ataxia

This is another form of incoordination which may be due to a lesion affecting the proprioceptive pathways to the cerebellum or to a lesion within the cerebellum. Movements cannot be carried out smoothly and are irregular and jerky. There is an inability to gauge distance in carrying out a movement. This is due largely to the loss of postural control for which the cerebellum is responsible. In the case of a cerebellar lesion there is a hypotonia due to the loss of the facilitatory influence of the cerebellum on the spinal reflex circuits. Cerebellar lesions are further complicated because the visual pathways are affected which gives an incoordination of eye movement known as nystagmus.

Spasticity

This hyperexcitability of muscle (increased tone) can in part be explained as a release phenomenon, whereby the balance between the higher level excitatory and inhibitory impulses on the spinal reflex arc are upset by a release of excitatory impulses. However, increasing knowledge of neuroanatomy and neurophysiology indicate that the mechanism causing spasticity is still incompletely understood. Spasticity occurs in groups of muscles and not individual muscles, and the particular groups affected will depend on the position, level and extent of the lesions. For example, a hemiplegic patient may present with a flexor spasticity of the arm and an extensor spasticity of the leg. Some lesions may involve the release of primitive postural reflexes, such as the tonic neck reflexes.

The spasticity may be affected by various other factors including the position of the patient, the emotional state of the patient, autonomic activity, pain or irritation of the skin and touch or pressure on certain areas. When passive movements are performed a quick movement will increase the spasticity whereas a slow movement will initially meet with some resistance; however, if the pressure is maintained the spasticity will usually decrease and allow the full movement. This is known as the 'clasp knife' phenomenon.

Rigidity

This relates to a hyperexcitability of muscle but differs from spasticity in the response to stretch and in the muscle groups affected. Usually the rigidity occurs evenly in opposing muscle groups; and unlike spasticity, the resistance to passive movement continues through the range of movement in either a 'cog-wheel' or 'lead pipe' manner. The 'cog-wheel' usually occurs when there is a tremor and is due to an alternating increase and decrease in the excitation of muscle fibres, while the 'lead pipe' rigidity offers a steady resistance to the passive movement.

Involuntary movements (dyskinesias)

Athetosis

This is thought to be the result of a lesion affecting the basal ganglia. The movements produced are writhing and slow, involving gross movements of the arms and legs which are more marked distally, particularly in the legs. Usually there is a more marked activity of the muscles supplied by the cranial nerves when the lesion is bilateral, and this includes various facial distortions and abnormal tongue movements. These athetoid movements are increased by excitement, but disappear during sleep.

Chorea

This condition is characterized by quicker movements than those seen in the athetoid patient, but which also occur in the limbs and muscles of facial expression. They are made worse by attempts to produce voluntary movements but disappear during sleep. The site of this lesion also appears to be in the region of the basal ganglia. In some patients there is a mixture of athetoid and choreiform movements. Both types may be accompanied by problems with speech, mastication and swallowing.

Dystonia

This is an increased excitability of muscle which tends to affect a group of muscles and hold the limb in an abnormal position.

Ballismus

This condition is characterized by involuntary movements resulting from a lesion in the thalamic area. The movements are large and sudden, occurring at the proximal joints. The condition may affect one side only and then is called hemiballismus.

Tremor

Usually these are fine rapidly oscillating movements and there are a number of varieties which will be mentioned, as appropriate, under the different conditions. A tremor made worse by voluntary movement is called an 'intention tremor'.

Sensory problems

Some of these problems have been mentioned already because of their effect on movement, such as the loss of proprioception leading to ataxia.

Pain

This is a variable feature in nervous disease and its presence or absence will depend on a number of factors. If the disease or trauma affects the pain nerve endings and/or pathways the passage of impulses may be interrupted and there may be no pain. However, if the pain nerve endings are irritated, then there may be acute pain which may be episodic or prolonged depending on the nature of the irritant. Partial nerve lesions may cause acute pain known as 'causalgia' and this may be linked with vascular disturbances which can give trophic changes in the area. In other instances the pain may be less acute and be described as a dull ache, throbbing pain or other descriptions depending on the irritant and also on the pain threshold of the patient. Pain may be felt because of altered body positions, as may occur with spasticity or contractures, resulting in stretching of soft-tissue structures.

Referred pain has been mentioned earlier in this chapter when it occurs as the result of a visceral lesion and affects the somatic nerve distribution that emerges at the same segmental level in the spine. Also, this type of pain may occur when there is a lesion of a nerve root and the pain is felt in a more peripheral part of its distribution. For example, pressure on cervical nerve roots may give pain in the fingers relating to the peripheral parts of these nerves. Some peripheral sensory nerves have been found to be bifurcated, and so if the fibre coming from an area of skin is irritated it may affect the other part of the fibre coming from a muscle.

Disturbance of cutaneous sensation

Interruption of afferent pathways can result in a loss of sensation known as anaesthesia, or in the case of an incomplete lesion there may be altered sensation which may take the form of paraesthesia or hyperaesthesia. Paraesthesia refers to diminished sensation and there may be tingling and numbness, whereas hyperaesthesia indicates increased sensitivity. When there is a complete lesion of a peripheral nerve there will be a loss of sensation in the area supplied by that nerve; however, it must be appreciated that there is considerable overlap in the distribution of sensory nerves. The disturbance will depend on the site of the lesion and the modalities affected.

Alteration of reflex activity

An interruption of the afferent or efferent pathways in the peripheral nervous system will result in the diminution or loss of tendon reflexes related to the particular lesion. However, lesions affecting the central nervous system may result in diminished or exaggerated reflexes depending on the site of the lesion. Exaggerated lesions are evident in some lesions of the upper motor neuron pathways.

Cutaneous reflexes, as for example the abdominal reflex, will be absent if the spinal reflex pathway is interrupted. However, they are also dependent on impulses passing down the corticospinal tracts and so lesions affecting these tracts may result in diminished or absent reflexes. The extension plantar response (Babinski's sign) may also be elicited in the presence of a corticospinal lesion.

Higher lesions of the central nervous system may result in the release of primitive reflexes, such as the tonic symmetrical neck reflexes.

Perceptual defects

Central lesions affecting the sensory mechanism may cause a number of problems, one of which concerns space orientation in which the patient has difficulty in perceiving his position in relation to the environment. For example, he may not appreciate the position of furniture or people. Dressing may be a problem, as the patient may be unable to relate the position of a sleeve to the arm. Similarly, placing a leg in a trouser or stocking may be difficult. The patient may not be able to judge the position of a chair to sit on. Thus considerable difficulty is experienced with most functional activities that require to be related to an object.

Astereognosis

This sensory problem is due to a lesion in the sensory cortex, in which the patient is unable to recognize an object by its feel. The patient may be able to recognize the object if he can see it, but with the eyes closed he will be unable to determine its shape and texture.

Visual defects

There are a number of problems that can occur and it is important that these are recognized as they may affect rehabilitation. For example, there may be hemianopia in some hemiplegic patients or nystagmus in a patient with cerebellar ataxia.

Auditory defects

These may not be caused by the neurological disorder but may have a profound effect on rehabilitation. Deafness can create problems in communicating with a patient.

Speech defects

These can be very frustrating, particularly for a patient who is not intellectually handicapped. The defects include dysarthria which is an inability to articulate clearly; dysphasia which is difficulty in comprehension and expression of words; and aphasia in which there may be no speech. Speech can be affected by respiratory problems.

Autonomic disorders

Autonomic function may be upset even when there is no lesion affecting these areas because of the integrated action of the whole nervous system. For example, a patient who is frightened may show excessive sympathetic reactions. Dysfunction may also be due to lesions affecting autonomic areas or pathways.

Trophic lesions

These can occur for a number of reasons and especially when there are lesions interrupting afferent or autonomic pathways in peripheral nerves. An anaesthetic area of skin, particularly in the hands, means the patient is unlikely to notice minor traumas (mechanical, thermal or chemical) which can lead to lesions. A person will normally respond to prolonged pressure on an area by moving, but in an anaesthetic area this will not occur and a pressure sore may develop. Lesions can also occur as the result of central lesions such as syringomyelia.

Principles of management

Medical and/or surgical management is dependent on the particular condition and its effect on the individual patient. It is not possible to generalize on treatment and this will be indicated for the specific neurological disorders described. However, as the conditions given in this book are those primarily affecting physical function it is important to stress the team management. The management must be coordinated and the progression, or sometimes regression, of the patient must be carefully monitored to try to achieve optimal function. The team must have a leader who will consider the assessments and reports of the other members and evaluate the effectiveness of the measures being taken. Whenever possible, the patient should be considered as a member of the team.

Physiotherapy

The aim is for the patient to achieve optimal independence, the level of which will depend on a number of factors including the type of lesion and the extent of permanent damage. When a functional activity is impossible to achieve, then the physiotherapist will try to help the patient to compensate for this loss. For example, a paraplegic patient who is unable to walk can be taught to use a wheelchair and possibly an adapted car in order to become as mobile as possible. This will only be successful if the patient is well motivated and willing to accept a change in lifestyle. Help is required from health professionals, relatives, friends and when appropriate employers and co-workers.

The extent of recovery is often difficult to predict because of the complexity of the nervous system. It may be difficult to make an accurate diagnosis of the extent of the lesion, and in some cases the nervous system seems to have the ability to adapt and form alternative pathways. Apart from this there are other factors affecting recovery such as the motivation of the patient, the quality of care and reactions of other people in the community where the patient lives. There are some remarkable cases of good recovery when the initial prognosis has been poor and conversely some patients with a good prognosis do not make a good recovery. Good assessment and treatment is an essential part of mangement and should continue as long as the physiotherapist considers that it contributes to further functional recovery. Sometimes in the later stages of recovery treatment may not be necessary but the physiotherapist can have an important role in monitoring progress by ensuring that the patient is maintaining and if possible improving function. The physiotherapist may also have a role in cases where there is a progressive deterioration by helping to maintain independence as long as possible or helping relatives to manage.

Environmental changes can occur which will affect the rehabilitation of the patient. For example, plans for relatives to help the patient may have to be altered if the patient becomes ill or if the relatives decide they are unable to cope when they appreciate the full extent of a problem. Treatment is specific for different lesions and for every individual, but some general guidelines can be included in this section. However, it must be remembered that lesions of one system will affect other systems and so cannot be treated in isolation. Realistic goals must be set with the rehabilitation of the 'whole' patient within his environment as the key consideration.

Therapy may be carried out in the hospital and the community depending on the needs of the individual patient and the facilities available.

Assessment

Patients with neurological diseases or injuries create complex management problems. Assessments by individual members of the health-care team (doctors, nurses, physiotherapists, occupational therapists, community health care professionals and possibly speech therapists and psychologists) must be brought together at a case conference to plan the overall management. The patient is the central figure in all the planning and whenever possible should be included in the case conference. Relatives may also play a key role in rehabilitation and should be included in discussions and planning when appropriate. If good management is to be achieved each member of the team must understand the role of the others and the treatments must be linked to give an integrated plan of management. It must also be appreciated that assessment is a continuous process and so management plans will need to be altered or modified according to the changes taking place in the physical and mental state of the patient.

There are a number of important points for the physiotherapist to consider, and these are outlined below.

1. General

Whenever possible, information about the previous mental and physical state of the patient should be obtained in order to make realistic plans for the future. This also relates to his position in society and within the family.

Before commencing a specific assessment it is important to gain a general impression about the present state of the patient.

The medical history should be read to ascertain any past or present factors that could have a bearing on the assessment and future planning.

2. Specific examination

This is a very important aspect and requires careful consideration and structuring if it is to be a useful part of the assessment. In some instances the patient may not be able to give any information because he may be confused or may not be able to communicate clearly, or there is a hearing defect. If the patient is able to understand but cannot communicate because of a speech defect or a loss of hearing, then it is important to establish some form of communication. When information may be gained from the patient it is important that it is relevant to the assessment. The questioning must be carried out with sensitivity and understanding as the physiotherapist will hope to gain the cooperation and confidence of the patient, and if this is achieved the patient may volunteer some of the information required.

Some of the relevant information may have been gained from the medical notes in which case it is unnecessary to ask for it again. Part of the questioning can be integrated with the physical examination, particularly by an experienced phy-siotherapist. Principally the physiotherapist hopes to gain information about the environment of the patient – home, social activities, work – which is pertinent to rehabilitation. It is necessary to appreciate the psychological reaction of the patient to the illness and the problems that this is likely to pose regarding management. It is important to assess whether the patient can respond to instruc-tions and also his ability to concentrate.

It is very important to note the problems as perceived by the patient and to link them with those found by the physiotherapist or other members of the team.

Objective examination

Before starting on a specific examination a general impression should be gained regarding the position of the patient, any active movements that are made, and if there is any normal functional activity.

The following is a checklist of points for an objective examination, but this in no way dictates the order of events since these will depend on the disorder, the condition of the individual patient, and the physiotherapist carrying out the examination. It may be unnecessary to examine all the items in some disorders, for example tests for perception or stereognosis would be inappropriate with a peripheral nerve lesion.

Observation

Deformities – Notice any abnormal positions of the body. Deformities may differ according to whether the patient is in a lying position, or is sitting or standing.

Involuntary movement – Note the type of any movements at rest and when the patient is attempting any active movement.

Tremor – Note whether this occurs at rest or during movement.

Circulation – Abnormalities of the circulation may be particularly noticeable in peripheral parts of the body.

Skin condition – This may be linked with circulatory problems. Observe the colour, texture, scars or any trophic lesions.

Muscle bulk – There may be an observable decrease in muscle bulk particularly if one limb differs from the other. It may be possible to notice spasticity by looking at the contour of the muscle.

Palpation – This may be necessary to locate areas of pain, mobility of skin, and texture of muscles. However, it may be integrated at appropriate places through the examination rather than being taken as a separate entity.

Movement

The position of the patient will be very important in attempting any active or passive movements. For example, if a patient is in a wheelchair it might be better to see what active movements are possible from that position. However, this will depend on the disorder and the condition and mental state of the patient. On the other hand, if the patient is in a position that increases the spasticity of muscles, it may be impossible to produce any active movement and a change of position will be necessary.

Free active movement – If the patient is able to produce any activity note the character of the movements. Can the movement be taken through full range? Is it a smooth movement or is it uncoordinated, does it affect the position of other parts of the body? If the range is limited is there any observable reason? It is also important to observe whether active movement increases any involuntary movements or tremor.

Balance – The patient must be able to balance in order to perform any useful activity from a particular position. Balance should be checked in sitting and standing when possible.

Measurements – It may be useful to record ranges of movement but this will depend on the particular disorder, although generally it is not a particularly useful technique in a neurological examination. It may be necessary to record muscle action using the Medical Research Council grades which are as follows:

0 = No contraction.
1 = A flicker of a contraction but it is insufficient to move the joint.
3 = A contraction sufficient to move the joint against gravity.

4 = A contraction sufficient to move the joint against gravity and some resistance.
5 = Full power of contraction.

Grade 3 is the only accurate test as the others are subjective. When testing, it is often better to test for grade 3 and then work down or up as appropriate.

Assisted active movement – If free active movement cannot be achieved then an assessment can be made to see whether any movements are possible with the assistance of the operator. Careful consideration must be given to the position of the patient and the handling skills used to achieve the optimal results with the least discomfort to the patient.

Passive movement – As with the assisted movements the patient must be positioned carefully and the correct handling skills used. If there is no active movement or it is limited the passive movements will test whether there is any limitation to a full-range movement caused by adhesions, contractures, spasticity, rigidity or for any other reason.

Sensory mechanisms – Various tests can be carried out and these will depend on the disorder. Pain may be a problem and, if it is present, the physiotherapist should try to localize the area and indicate this on a drawing of the body image together with other areas of sensory dysfunction. Pain is a very subjective feature and it may be useful to record the impression of the patient about his pain on a visual analogue scale. Tests may include those for touch and pressure, thermal sensation, and proprioception. When there is an area of anaesthesia the testing should start in this area and move towards parts where the sensation may be normal. If the testing is started over a normal area the patient may imagine he can still feel it when the anaesthetic area is reached. Tests for perception and stereognosis should be included if appropriate.

Auditory and visual function – Although these tests will not be carried out by the physiotherapist they may be relevant to the assessment.

Reflex testing – This will depend on the specific neurological disorder. It may be necessary to assess superficial and tendon reflexes. In patients presenting with spasicity the examiner must look for evidence of the release of the primitive reflexes (tonic postural reflexes).

Function – Patients may be able to perform some movements but this will not necessarily mean that they can perform a functional activity. For example, a patient may be able to move his legs in all the actions necessary for walking but if balance in standing is not possible then this will be of no use functionally. Thus it is important to make a list of the functional activities that the patient can carry out.

Recording – The physiotherapist must keep a careful record of the examination so that changes can be noted following treatment.

Other aspects of assessment

Before making plans for the patient (or with the patient) the physiotherapist may need to liaise with other members of the team so that the plans are coordinated. It may be necessary to visit the patient's home and meet his relatives and friends, but this will depend on the particular case.

Planning

The physiotherapist will make an assessment of the examination, noting the problems as seen by the patient and as found by the examination. This will enable the physiotherapist to decide on the priorities for treatment and to set short- and long-term goals. Long-term goals may be difficult to set in some neurological disorders because of the difficulty in predicting the final outcome. It may thus be necessary to change goals as the effects of the disease and treatment become apparent.

Principles of treatment

Once the goals have been set the plan of treatment can be made. The selection of techniques for treatment and the order of use will depend on the specific disorder, the condition of the patient at the treatment session, and the physiotherapist. Plans that have been made following the assessment may need to be changed if the condition of the patient has altered.

Some of the techniques that can be used are given in Appendix 1, whereas others are mentioned under the specific conditions.

Cooperation of the patient

However good the chosen techniques are, and however well they are carried out by the physiotherapist, they will not be successful without the cooperation of the patient. Therefore, the first technique that the physiotherapist requires is the ability to communicate to gain the confidence and thus the cooperation of the patient. The treatment must be a joint operation between therapist and patient. In this way the patient will achieve the goals aided by the physiotherapist.

Techniques

In selecting the appropriate techniques the physiotherapist must have made the correct assessment of the problems and those that have priority in the treatment plan. For example, spasticity may prevent normal movement and function and this must be reduced before the next stage can be carried out. This will require correct positioning and choice of suitable techniques to reduce the spasticity. Following this it will be necessary to try to build a normal or better pattern of movement. In building a normal pattern the developmental sequence of movement may be followed. A paraplegic with no hope of recovering any movement must be taught to compensate for this loss. This may include teaching the patient to be mobile in a wheelchair and to carry out activities from the wheelchair. If a patient is unable to balance in sitting, he will be unable to carry out any useful activities with the arms. Therefore, the priority is to enable the patient to balance in sitting.

Evaluation

Evaluation of treatment is an ongoing process to assess the effectiveness of the techniques and the goals that have been set. The physiotherapist will consider at the start of a treatment session whether there has been any change since the previous session. Then, during the treatment, changes in the patient may become apparent which will indicate the

need for further alteration of techniques. Finally, at the end of the session the physiotherapist must evaluate the effects of the treatment and make plans for the next session. It is important that the changes are not made too quickly before there is time to assess their effectiveness, but it is equally important that techniques that are ineffective are changed. The physiotherapist must constantly be asking the question 'What must the patient be able to do in order to become functionally independent, and what matters most to the patient and the family?'

Recording

Careful records of treatment and the results must be kept so that progress or regression can be noted and reported to the team. Records are important in evaluating treatments and gaining information about the use of different techniques. Future research and evaluation depends on the keeping of adequate and accurate records.

Chapter 20

Diseases of the brain and spinal cord

Classification

In the past, diseases and injuries have tended to be classified according to the predominant symptoms, for example lesions that affect either the upper or the lower motor neurons, or those affecting the sensory tracts. However, this can lead to some confusion as many of the diseases can show both motor and sensory, and possibly other, symptoms. The lesion may extend over more than one area or there may be multiple lesions as in the case of multiple sclerosis (disseminated sclerosis). Therefore, the diseases and injuries given in this chapter are listed alphabetically and are those in which physiotherapy may play a significant part in the management.

Hemiplegia/stroke

These two terms can both be used although the meaning and interpretation differ.

Hemiplegia

This term implies a paralysis of one side of the body and usually affects the arm, leg and trunk. The degree of involvement of the limbs and trunk will depend on the position and extent of the lesion, and the face may also be affected. As the lesion affects the upper motor neuron there is usually some spasticity but this will depend on the position of the lesion and on the management of the patient. The problem with this definition is that it relates to one particular feature of the condition, the paralysis, and most cases present with one or more other clinical features. There may be disturbance of sensation, speech, neglect of one side, apraxia and emotional disturbance. Each patient will differ and therefore it is very important that the physiotherapist appreciates the possible impairments when making an assessment.

Stroke

This term usually refers to patients who have had a cerebrovascular accident as the result of circulatory defects in which the symptoms have continued for more than 24 hours (terminology recognized by WHO). An attack that lasts for less than the 24 hours is known as a transient ischaemic attack (TIA).

A hemiplegia or stroke is due to a lesion affecting the opposite side of the cerebrum. Thus a right cerebrovascular accident causes a left hemiplegia/stroke or vice versa.

Aetiology

The majority of cases of stroke are due to a cerebrovascular accident occurring as the result of atheromatous changes in the blood vessels supplying the cerebrum (Figure 20.1). Consequently the risk of having a stroke increases with age and in those people who have marked atheromatous changes in the blood vessels. The actual lesion causing the cerebrovascular accident may occur in a number of different ways.

1. *Ischaemia* – There may be a gradual occlusion of a vessel or vessels which will give a slow onset of symptoms. The patient may not lose consciousness and there may be an initial weakness of muscles followed by a paralysis.

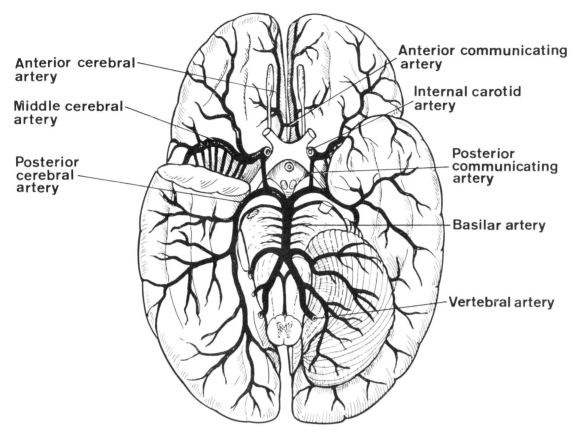

Figure 20.1 Arterial circle at the base of the brain (the circle of Willis)

2. *Cerebral haemorrhage* – The patient is often hypertensive and this combined with the weakening of the vessel walls may lead to a haemorrhage.
3. *Subarachnoid haemorrhage* – This usually arises from a berry aneurysm with a haemorrhage into the subarachnoid space. The clinical features will depend on the position of the lesion.
4. *Cerebral embolism.*

There are other causes of hemiplegia/stroke, head injuries, tumours and cerebral palsy, but these are much less common than those mentioned above.

Clinical features

These will refer to strokes resulting from circulatory problems as they form the majority of cases.

The onset will depend on whether there is a slowly developing occlusion of blood vessels or a sudden incident, as with a haemorrhage.

Occlusion of blood vessels

This occurs in approximately two-thirds of patients suffering a stroke. The patient may complain of a headache and weakness of one side of the body, and there may be a dysphasia. Loss of consciousness is uncommon in this type of stroke although the patient may be drowsy. The weakness is followed by a flaccid paralysis and later spasticity may develop, unless it is a transient attack.

Haemorrhage

This is the result of weakening of the arterial walls, and if a rupture occurs the escaping blood forms a haematoma. In these cases the onset is sudden and the patient may present with a severe headache, possibly vomiting, and most patients lose consciousness. The damage caused by the haemorrhage may prove fatal in a short space of time and in many of those who do survive the initial lesion the prognosis is not good. As with the patients suffering an occlusion there is a flaccid paralysis and later spasticity may develop. Some patients may improve dramatically if the haematoma is reabsorbed.

The following are some of the other features that may occur in addition to the one-sided paralysis.

Sensory loss – particularly if the middle cerebral artery is occluded and the post central gyrus is affected. Depending on the area damaged various sensory modalities may be affected: superficial sensation, proprioception, stereognosis or perception.

Visual defects – Visual field defects can occur particularly when the posterior cerebral arteries are affected. Visuospatial disturbances may be related to damage in the parietal lobe. It is important to realize that as most patients are elderly they may have had visual defects prior to the stroke.

Communication defects – There may be aphasia as the result of damage to the inferior gyrus in the frontal lobe in the left or dominant hemisphere. Sometimes the loss of speech may not be total but it may be abnormal. Damage to other areas in the cerebrum may make it difficult for the patient to understand what is said to him, or he may be confused. It is necessary to find out whether the patient has had any difficulty with hearing prior to the stroke which may make communication difficult.

Behavioural problems – The memory may be affected by posterior cerebral artery occlusion. Emotional disturbances may be present if there is damage to the frontal lobe.

Management

Medical

Once a stroke has occurred management will usually be conservative. However, in a small number of cases surgery may be indicated, for example in some patients, following a sub-arachnoid haemorrhage, it may be possible to clip an aneurysm to prevent further damage, or it may occasionally be possible to drain a haematoma before it has caused irreparable damage.

Conservative treatment

Patients who are unconscious after a stroke may be treated in the intensive care unit so that they can be carefully monitored and receive the necessary respiratory care. Otherwise patients may be admitted to a stroke unit, or if this is not available a general medical ward. If the stroke is mild and there is adequate domiciliary back-up the patient may be treated at home, particularly if there are relatives who are able to cope with the problems. Apart from the clinical examination of the patient it may be necessary to carry out various other investigations, which may include CT scans, possibly angiography, and blood tests.

For patients who are recovering the management will include efforts to try to prevent further strokes by treating the underlying condition when appropriate, for example hypertension or diabetes mellitus. Other factors that may be considered as precipitating causes – smoking, diet and stress – should be investigated, and advice should be given to the patient.

Physiotherapy

Physiotherapy should start at once whether the patient is in intensive care, in a ward or at home.

Assessment

The initial assessment will vary depending on the state of the patient. If the patient is unconscious and in the intensive care unit the physiotherapist will take note of the medical history, charts and monitors. There will be discussion with the medical and nursing staff on the management of the patient. The physiotherapist will carry out an objective examination of the chest and the range of movement in the limbs.

Patients who are conscious may be confused and if in hospital may not realize where they are or what has happened. Others will quickly be aware that they have had a stroke and initially be frightened and anxious. Subsequently many patients may become depressed, and those with emotional problems may very easily be upset. The physiotherapist must be able to assess these problems as they will make a difference to the way in which she approaches the patient.

Some patients will have communication problems which may be overcome in some instances but not in others. These may vary from aphasia to dysphasia, inability to express what they want to say, inability to understand what is said to them or they may previously have had a hearing difficulty.

Examination of the conscious patient

It may not be possible to carry out a complete examination on the first visit to a patient and this may have to be built up in conjunction with the treatment.

Subjective examination

This will depend on the state of the patient and his ability to communicate with the therapist. It is important to gain the confidence of the patient and not to worry him with questions that upset him or he cannot answer. Some information may be gained from the medical notes and possibly from relatives. Otherwise further information may be gained from the patient as treatment progresses. During both the subjective and the objective examination it is important for the therapist to observe the behaviour of the patient.

Objective examination

1. *Observation* – The physiotherapist must observe the patient throughout both the subjective and objective examination and note some of the following points: the resting position of the patient, any abnormalities of facial expression, any activity (normal or abnormal), general posture and ability to balance in sitting.

2. *Extent of the paralysis* – At the initial assessment it is important to ascertain the amount of paralysis in the arm, leg and trunk. At first there is hypotonia but this can change to increased tone (hypertonia) in a few days or over a longer period. A continuous record must be kept to note any changes in the degree of paralysis and any alterations in tone.

3. *Activity* – Any normal activity on the affected side must be observed and recorded. Sometimes the patient may be able to perform gross movements but not isolated activity. There may be abnormal activity, such as associated reactions. Alterations of position may increase or decrease the hypertonicity when it is present, and if a decrease occurs this may allow some active movement.

4. *Sensory mechanisms* – All sensory modalities should be tested if the patient is able to cooperate: superficial and deep sensation, proprioception, stereognosis, perception, vision and hearing.

5. *Speech* – The patient may be aphasic or have some other abnormality of speech. It is important to assess whether the patient can understand what is said to him and cannot answer, or whether it is a more complex problem with the patient not understanding what is said, or being confused. In the first instance it is very important to establish an alternative form of communication because the patient can become very frustrated and depressed if he is unable to talk or make people understand. Speech problems will affect the ability of the physiotherapist to make an accurate assessment of motor and sensory problems.

6. *Functional activity* – Some patients may be able to carry out some activities of daily living and the extent of these should be noted.

Following the examination the physiotherapist will be able to formulate goals and a plan of treatment. These must take into account the overall management of the patient.

Treatment

The aim of treatment is to minimize the effects of the stroke and to regain as much functional independence as possible. The results will vary for many reasons, for example degree of permanent neurological damage, which parts of the nervous system are affected, the age and previous ability of the patient, the mental state and motivation of the patient, and associated conditions.

Early stage treatment

Intensive care unit – The physiotherapist will be concerned with three particular aspects of care at this stage:

1. *Respiratory care* – This will be similar to that given in Chapter 13.
2. *Positioning* – The patient must be positioned correctly each time he is turned. All staff in the unit should be aware of the required positions.
3. *Passive movements* – These should be carried out to maintain the range of movement in all joints and to maintain muscle length.

Stroke unit or general ward – In this situation the patient will usually be conscious and so will require careful explanation about the treatment. The method will depend on the ability of the patient to communicate and understand, and on his reaction to the stroke. The treatment will be similar to that given in the intensive care unit although respiratory care may not be necessary. If possible the patient should be made aware of the correct position and try to maintain it. The emphasis will be on a symmetrical position and movements (Figure 20.2). The physiotherapist will try to facilitate movements, and particularly those pertaining to function such as rolling, bridging, sitting up and progressing as the patient shows any sign of recovering movement.

Department/home – If the patient is treated at home and not in hospital then similar treatment to that described above should be given. The physiotherapist cannot give the same intensity of treatment and so the relatives should be taught the importance of correct positioning and how to do the passive movements. This may not always be possible or appropriate, and other courses of management must be considered.

Later stage treatment

Progression of treatment – Once the patient is able to sit out of bed a more active programme can be started and may include some of the following. The order of treatment, the progression and intensity will depend on the response of the individual patient.

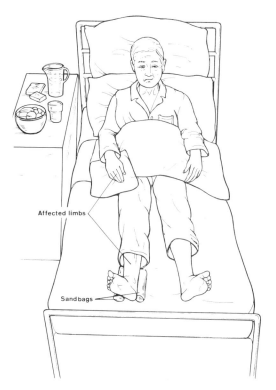

Figure 20.2 Symmetrical position in bed

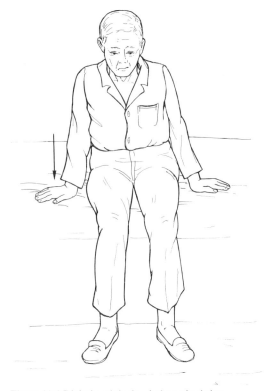

Figure 20.3 Right hemiplegia – balance in sitting

Correct positioning will continue to be emphasized, progressing through sitting and standing. The patient must learn to make his own adjustments. Passive movements should be continued as long as is necessary and the patient should be taught to do his own if possible, particularly of the upper limb. If movement returns facilitatory techniques should be used to strengthen weak muscles and encourage normal movement patterns.

It is important that the patient should be able to move around as soon as he can, and if it is not possible for a patient to walk then he may be taught to use a wheelchair.

Once a patient is able to sit unaided and adjust his position without falling (Figure 20.3) he can learn to perform other movements in the sitting position, progressing to transferring up and down a plinth. Gradually activities will be carried out in standing (Figure 20.4) and progress to walking and stairs.

It is important for the whole team to consider the preparation for the patient to return home, if this is realistic, or if not to prepare the patient for an alternative.

Once the patient has returned home the physiotherapist should visit regularly to assess the patient and give further advice if necessary.

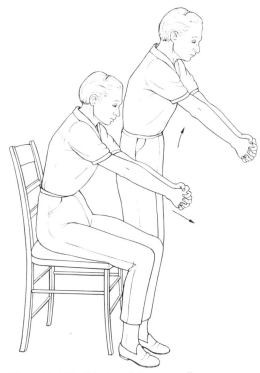

Figure 20.4 Hemiplegia – sitting to standing

Multiple sclerosis (disseminated sclerosis)

As the name implies this condition causes multiple lesions which can occur in various parts of the central nervous system. It is a disease characterized by exacerbations and remissions which may continue over many years.

Aetiology

The cause of this condition is still unknown although many causes have been suggested. There is a high incidence in temperate climates and this would tend to suggest an environmental factor. Interestingly, consumption of polyunsaturated fats is low in these areas although dietary treatment does not seem to have had any marked effect on the disease. Other possible causes may be a viral infection, an auto-immune reaction, or a genetic abnormality. There are a number of factors that seem to predispose to an exacerbation of the disease: trauma, emotional disturbance, surgery and pregnancy are among them.

The condition usually affects adults between the ages of 20 and 40 although occasionally it occurs in children or in an older age group. The incidence is slightly higher in females, particularly those aged 20–30 years.

Pathology

This disease affects the white matter of the brain and spinal cord. Active lesions include areas of demyelination called plaques which are accompanied by oedema and proliferation of cells. Nerve transmission may be affected by the demyelination and also by pressure from the oedema. Sometimes the axis cylinders may degenerate, possibly owing to the loss of the myelin sheath. After the active phase there is a gliosis, and the plaque becomes sclerotic. This scarring may cause further damage and loss of nerve transmission. Sometimes after the active stage has passed and the oedema has subsided there may be an improvement in the condition of the patient. Occasionally remyelination of the nerve fibres may occur which may result in a complete recovery of functions which had been lost during an exacerbation. However, more often the disease is progressive and there are further active phases leaving more sclerotic areas and further loss of function. This pathology explains the varying course of the disease with its exacerbations and remissions which may occur frequently or with fairly long intervals between the exacerbations.

In some patients the disease progresses very slowly and with minimal disability. An exacerbation can be followed by a remission lasting for several years. However, in other patients the disease can progress rapidly and the patient can become severely disabled, sometimes in a matter of months rather than years.

Clinical features

These are highly variable as it depends on the position and extent of the lesions. The disease may have an acute or a sub-acute onset. It may start with one focal lesion or sometimes several occurring close together.

The first symptoms vary. There may be an optic neuritis, often there is numbness of upper or lower limbs (or both), or numbness of the face. There may be weakness which is particularly noticeable in the lower limbs with possibly a dragging of one foot, or there may be a frequency of micturition. Following the initial lesion(s) there may appear to be little or no abnormality depending on whether or not there is any permanent damage.

Other early signs that may occur are nystagmus, slight intention tremor, altered reflexes, diminished or lost abdominal reflex, exaggerated tendon reflexes and an extensor plantar response.

Later – If the pyramidal tracts are affected the patient may develop a spastic paraplegia. Initially this may be a paraplegia in extension but as further damage occurs this may change to a paraplegia in flexion.

Sensory impairment may include loss of cutaneous sensation, posture and vibration sense leading to the development of ataxia.

Some patients may have a combination of a spasticity and ataxia in the lower limbs and ataxia in the upper limbs.

Speech – This may be affected and the patient may have a staccato or scanning speech.

Emotional changes can also occur and may present as euphoria, depression or irritability.

The complexity of these features, particularly in the early stages of the disease, may make it difficult for the doctor to make a diagnosis. Obviously it is important to exclude other conditions that may present with similar features.

Management

As the cause is unknown there is no specific treatment available. However, based on the possible causes a number of treatments have been tried which may appear to help in some individual cases, but when controlled trials have been carried out there has been no evidence of any benefit:

1. Based on the theory that a virus may be the causative factor some antiviral drugs such as interferon and amantadine have been tried.

2. Immunosuppressant drugs such as azathioprine have been tried but the side-effects, and a tendency to an increase in the relapse rate when the drugs are stopped, has limited their use.

3. Steroids have been used in an acute phase because of their anti-inflammatory action and their use in reducing oedema. But they cannot be used on a longer term basis because of other adverse effects.

4. On the basis of multiple sclerosis developing in areas where there is a decreased intake of polyunsaturated fats certain diets have been tried. For example, sunflower seed containing linoleic acid added to polyunsaturated fats has been given in conjunction with a decrease of animal fat.

5. Injections of vitamin B have been used because it is required for myelination. However, they have given no useful results.

Symptomatic relief can be given for some of the problems that occur in this disease. For example, catheterization may be used for urinary incontinence, drugs such as baclofen can be given for the relief of spasticity, and drugs may help to relieve depression.

Prolonged bed rest should be avoided as this tends to lead to stiffness and further weakness of muscles and it may be very difficult to regain any lost function.

Counselling

Once a diagnosis has been made counselling is an essential part of the management. The patient will require help and support to cope with his worries about the future. If the patient is married the couple may be concerned about whether their children will inherit the disease. The patient may be concerned about his ability to work, or whether he will be able to continue driving a car. It is important for members of the team to know when they can undertake the counselling role and when a professional counsellor is required.

Physiotherapy

Assessment

The findings of an examination may change quite quickly with this condition or they may remain static for a period of time. The numbness and weakness of muscles that is apparent one week may recover completely during a remission and no further treatment may be required at that time. However, it is more likley that there is some residual weakness following an exacerbation, and the physiotherapist must help the patient to achieve optimum function. After this there could be a period of months or years before the next relapse. It is very important that a careful record is kept because over the years that treatment may be required the physiotherapist and other professionals may change several times.

Gradually over the months and years more symptoms are likely to appear, increasing loss of muscle power, spasticity, ataxia, other sensory changes, nystagmus or other eye symptoms, altered speech and loss of sphincter control.

Behavioural changes must also be noted as these will make a difference to the method of management. Behavioural changes may be those normally associated with progressive disability – depression, irritability, anxiety – or they may be partly due to the position of the lesions. Euphoria is a symptom that may occur in patients with this condition but its incidence is not as common as was originally indicated.

The clinical features found at an examination must be related to the problems of the patient in deciding on a programme of treatment. The problems are those perceived both by the patient and by the physiotherapist. They may or may not be the same and they may be placed in a different order of priority by the patient and the therapist. Thus it is important for the physiotherapist to make a correct assessment of the situation in order to give the appropriate treatment.

Treatment

The overall aim of the management programme is to keep the patient functionally independent as long as possible. As can be understood from the varied course of the disease this may be many years or only months.

It is important that the physiotherapist realizes the complexity of the condition as only then can she formulate a rational and intelligent plan of treatment. Because of the exacerbations and remissions there is a constant need to reassess and possibly change the plan of management in the light of new findings. Two patients may have exacerbations which leave them unable to walk: in one case there will be a recovery with the remission but the other patient may have little or no recovery with the remission and be confined to a wheelchair. It is the unpredictable nature of this condition that makes it very difficult to manage. It is not easy to maintain the motivation of a patient who can see a rapid deterioration in his condition, or even when it is slower. In planning the physiotherapist must consider possible outcomes and prepare the patient both physically and psychologically for possible change.

Specific symptoms may require certain treatment techniques, but these must be related to the overall management and cannot be taken in isolation.

Weak muscles – Attempts can be made to strengthen weak muscles and regain functional movement. If the muscle strength returns to normal during a remission then a return to normal function may be achieved. If the loss of muscle power in the legs makes it difficult for the patient to walk then the use of an appropriate walking aid should be considered. When this occurs, strengthening exercises for the arms should be included as the patient will need this power to use the walking aid but also because the patient will probably need it later if they have to use a wheelchair, and also for transfers.

Spasticity – If hypertonicity is one of the clinical features then this will probably increase either rapidly or slowly depending on the course of the disease. It may start in one leg and then both with the spasticity being extensor in the early stages and possibly changing to flexor with increased neurological damage. Passive movements will help to prevent contractures developing and make it easier for the patient to move, or if this is not possible it will be easier for the carers to move the patient. The physiotherapist must note which movements increase the spasticity and teach the patient to try to avoid them. Pressure sores will increase spasticity and the patient and carers must be taught how to prevent them and also to watch carefully for any signs of pressure. Careful management of urinary and bowel problems are important as they may increase spasticity, particularly if there is infection. Standing and walking are important factors in inhibiting spasticity and should be continued as long as is practicable. Other techniques that inhibit spasticity may be used, such as cold, warmth, relaxation and inhibitory postures.

Ataxia – Treatment will depend on which parts of the nervous system are damaged and whether it is combined with other clinical features such as spasticity. The physiotherapist must ascertain whether the uncontrolled movement is ataxia or some other form of involuntary movement so that the appropriate techniques can be used to try to gain some control. Repeated active movements carried out at the speed that will allow the patient most control may help, perhaps with assisted movement to start with and then free active to see whether the patient can gain more control. These may be helped by the use of the eyes (Frenkel type exercises) or the use of the voice to try to assist control. It is very important to consider the position of the patient in order to give adequate stability for the movement to occur.

Self-care – The patient must be taught the importance of self-care, particularly in relation to prevention of contractures, prevention of pressure sores, care of the bladder and bowel if there are problems. There will be periods of time when the patient is not on treatment or is only monitored intermittently, and this is when trouble can very quickly occur if the patient is not aware of the dangers.

Community physiotherapy

Many patients with multiple sclerosis are living at home with varying degrees of disability and handicap. Some need to attend a physiotherapy department for special treatment periodically and may be able to manage at other times. Others may be able to manage on their own or with the help of relatives and other carers in the community. It is important for the patient at home that a physiotherapist working in the community monitors their physical activity at regular intervals, the frequency depending on the individual patient and their particular problems. Thus any deterioration can be seen and treatment commenced if necessary. It also ensures that the patient is managing a self-care programme and that it is altered or modified as appropriate.

Apart from the actual assessment these visits can have a considerable psychological effect as the patient knows that someone will be coming and they will be able to discuss any problems and gain further help when required. This often helps to allay unnecessary fears and give the patient more confidence in their ability to manage at home.

Parkinson's disease (paralysis agitans)

This condition was first described by James Parkinson in 1817. It is a slowly progressive disease which produces gradual weakening of voluntary movement, muscular rigidity and possibly tremor.

Aetiology

This condition usually starts in the 50–60 year age group, with men being affected a little more often than women.

The cause of the disease is unknown but it affects parts of the basal ganglia (corpus striatum) and pathways from the substantia nigra. The gradual deterioration may take place over 10 or more years.

There are other conditions that can produce similar clinical features to Parkinson's disease, for example Alzheimer's disease or some types of head injury, and this is known as a parkinsonian syndrome.

Pathology

There is a degeneration in some of the neurons of the basal ganglia which results in a reduction of a neurotransmitter substance called dopamine. The level of this substance is normally higher in the basal ganglia than elsewhere in the brain. Some of the synaptic terminals have stores of dopamine and others have stores of acetylcholine – the former is inhibitory in its action and the latter is excitatory. Thus the activities of these two normally counterbalance each other.

Clinical features

Disorders of movement – akinesia

All movements become much slower and are difficult to initiate. This leads to clumsiness with hand function, particularly writing and similar activities, although other functions may be unaffected. Walking is difficult partly because of the difficulty in starting the movement and partly because of the loss of ability to make quick adjustments of muscle action which are necessary to maintain balance. The gait is described as 'festinant' because the patient leans forward in order to initiate movement and then has to take short quick steps to try to maintain his balance. The normal swinging movement of the arms is absent.

Posture – The patient usually stands in a slightly flexed position.

Muscle weakness

This is also a feature of the disease, not only because of the rigidity but because the facilitatory pathways from the lentiform nucleus to the motor areas are interfered with. Fine movements are most affected and there is a lack of precision as the weakness affects the normal coordination.

Rigidity

There is a hypertonus in all muscle groups resulting in a diffuse rigidity. This gives resistance to passive movement throughout the range which is unlike that seen in diseases affecting the upper motor neuron. The rigidity may be described as 'lead pipe' when the resistance to movement is similar throughout the range, or it may be the 'cog wheel' when the resistance is intermittent.

The rigidity affects activities, giving slow delayed movement and a characteristic facial expression. This consists of the 'parkinsonian mask', rigidity causing the face to become immobile and expressionless. The blinking reflex occurs less often than usual, hence the patient appears to have a fixed stare. Because of the mask-like appearance it is easy to underrate the intelligence and mental capabilities of the patient. Since changes of facial expression are few and infrequent, the inexperienced tend to assume that the mind is equally 'vacant'. This is not so; the mental powers remain normal throughout the disease, unless dissociated degeneration occurs elsewhere in the brain.

Pain

This quite often occurs as the result of the rigidity and may present as cramps, aches or more acute pain.

Tremor

This may be unilateral or bilateral, but it often begins in one hand and is very characteristic. The fingers are alternatively flexed and extended, especially at the metacarpophalangeal joints while the thumb rests against the index finger. The movements are quick, varying between 2 and 6 cycles per second, and produce the so-called 'pill rolling' movement. The tremor may spread to the legs but the trunk and head are rarely affected and the eyes never. The tremor is usually absent during voluntary movement but continues when the limb is at rest and particularly when it is unsupported. The tremor is aggravated by emotional stress or when the patient is conscious of being observed. It ceases during sleep. Approximately half the patients with this condition have no tremor.

Speech

As the disease progresses the voice tends to become weaker and there is less variation in tone.

Cough

The patient is usually unable to cough effectively, which can cause serious problems if a respiratory infection develops.

Swallowing

Automatic swallowing is affected and the patient may tend to dribble which can be very embarrassing in company.

Reflexes

These are usually normal but occasionally may be increased.

Sensory changes

Pain has already been mentioned. The patient often suffers sensations of great heat, with sweating and rise of local temperature.

Reactions of the patient to the disease

He is likely to become very depressed because of the loss of function, pain and lack of facial expression. He may become self-conscious and unwilling to attend any social occasions.

Management

Some patients may not seek medical help for some time as they think the increasing stiffness is to be expected as they grow older. Once a diagnosis has been made treatment can be started and it is important that the drug therapy is accompanied by physiotherapy to gain optimum function. The patient will need advice about coping with the condition and possibly help from the community services to enable him to remain independent as long as possible.

Medical advances in the last 30 years have made a considerable difference to the management of this condition. In the 1950s it was discovered that a surgical procedure – stereotaxis – which consisted of the coagulation of areas in the globus pallidus and the thalamus reduced tremor and rigidity. It was particulary effective in the reduction of tremor. Then it was found that a drug called Levodopa stimulated the production of dopamine and, provided that it was given in conjunction with an anticholinergic drug, it reduced the rigidity and to some extent the tremor. This has replaced the surgical treatment as it is more effective and avoids the risk of a surgical procedure in the elderly. The Levodopa and anticholinergic drugs can be given in combination and are marketed as Madopar and Sinemet.

Physiotherapy

Assessment

It is necessary for the physiotherapist to know the medical history because there may be accompanying conditions of ageing such as cervical spondylosis or osteoarthritis of the hips or knees. The patient may have other conditions that will affect the treatment given, such as heart failure or respiratory disease. It is also important to have a knowledge of the social conditions as this can affect the management plans. What is the housing situation? Has the patient any relatives who can help? Sometimes the spouse is equally or more disabled and so help at home is very limited.

Subjective examination

It is important to gain the confidence of the patient and to try to discover the problems as he sees them. It is not always easy to do this because the patient feels depressed and anxious – he feels that it is a problem of old age and that he is not going to be able to cope with his ordinary everyday activities. Thus it may take some time to make an accurate assessment of the situation.

Objective examination

It is necessary to assess the functional activities and not to rely on the patient saying he can or cannot do them. Observation will indicate the time taken to perform an activity, which movements are limited and therefore inhibit function. Rigidity may prevent the patient turning over in bed, or sitting up easily. Walking may be difficult with a festinant gait. It is important to realize that the ability to perform functions may vary from day to day and at different times during the day.

Pain may be a problem and may prevent the patient from performing some movements. It may keep the patient awake at night and affect his general health.

Tremor may not upset functional activities, as it is worse at rest, but the patient may be very upset by the tremor and not want to take part in social activities where it will be noticed.

An examination will be carried out to assess the range, muscle strength and coordination of all movements.

The physiotherapist should keep a record of functional activities so that any improvements or deteriorations can be noted.

The ability of the patient to learn and to understand instructions must be tested so that a realistic programme of treatment can be planned.

Treatment

The drugs may allow some relaxation of rigidity and it is important to take advantage of this in building up the level of activity and function. The aims of treatment are to enable the patient to relax, to initiate and perform smoother movements and to gain as much functional independence as possible.

Positioning

The patient should be encouraged to sit in a well-supported position so that he can relax. Similarly, a comfortable lying position should be found. It is important that the positions should avoid the development of deformities if possible.

Passive movements

Smooth repetitive movements performed slowly will encourage relaxation, help to maintain the range of movement and the length of muscles.

Assisted active movement

There can be a gradual change from passive to assisted and then to free active movement. This overcomes the difficulty of initiating movement and as the patient improves he can try to initiate the movement.

Free active movements – It is easier for the patient to start with pendular type movements and then progress to coordinated *functional* movements. Walking is a problem and much of the difficulty lies in initiating the first step. It may help some patients to try marking time on the spot and then when they are moving easily start moving forward.

Music – Exercise to music is helpful to those who have a good sense of rhythm provided the music is chosen carefully to allow for the speed and range of the patient's movements.

Advice – The patient will need advice and encouragement to manage at home. If there are relatives willing and able to help they should be shown what the patient can do and when they need to help. Many relatives tend to give too much help unless the situation is explained to them and they are shown what the patient can do. It is important for the patient to do his exercises at home to maintain and improve any function that he has gained.

Community physiotherapy – A physiotherapist should visit the patient regularly to assess the situation and give further advice and help if necessary.

Spinal cord lesions

A lesion may occur in any part of the spinal cord – cervical, thoracic or lumbar – and the resulting disability may be temporary or permanent depending on the cause and extent of the damage. A complete transection of the cord in the thoracic or lumbar region would result in a paraplegia, which is a paralysis of both lower limbs. Depending on the level of the lesion in the thoracic region there may be some paralysis of the trunk muscles as well. Lesions transecting the cord in the cervical region will result in a tetraplegia with arms, trunk and legs paralysed. Patients with a high cervical lesion do not usually live because of the paralysis of all the respiratory muscles, although some may survive on a life-support machine.

In the early stage of development the spinal cord is approximately the same length as the vertebral canal and the spinal nerves pass out horizontally through the intervertebral foramina. During development *in utero* the vertebral column and the spinal cord grow at different rates and eventually the cord finishes at the lower border of the second lumbar vertebra. The upper spinal nerves still emerge horizontally but lower down the nerves become more vertical and do not emerge at the level of the corresponding vertebra. For example, a fracture dislocation of the 9th and 10th thoracic vertebrae will give a paraplegia which is effective from the 11th thoracic segment.

Lesions of the cord may be complete or incomplete.

Aetiology

Lesions of the spinal cord may be congenital or acquired, although the majority are acquired. Because of the diverse causes this can affect any age group.

Causes

1. *Trauma* – Lesions can be due to road traffic injuries, industrial injuries, accidents in the home or sports injuries. The last occur particularly in the young and can be caused by diving into shallow water (fracture dislocation of the cervical spine), some contact sports such as rugby, or riding accidents.
2. *Inflammatory lesions* – The post-viral infections are the most common of the inflammatory lesions, for example the Guillain–Barré syndrome described in Chapter 21. Other diseases such as anterior poliomyelitis and tuberculosis were fairly common causes of spinal cord lesions but with the advent of vaccines and modern drug therapy these are rarely seen in this country.
3. *Degenerative conditions of the vertebral column* – In severe cases this may cause partial or complete disruption of the spinal cord. This is more likely to occur with cervical spondylosis than lumbar spondylosis.
4. *Degenerative conditions of the spinal cord* – For example sub-acute combined degeneration of the cord.
5. *Developmental abnormalities* – Cerebral palsy, spina bifida.
6. *Neoplasms*.
7. *Other diseases* such as multiple sclerosis may progress to a paraplegia.

This chapter will deal with traumatic spinal cord lesions as they are the commonest cause of paraplegia and tetraplegia, accounting for approximately 70% of cases.

Clinical features

Complete transection of the cord

Several segments of the spinal cord may be damaged, which will affect the grey matter in these segments and the tracts passing up and down the cord.

Initially there is a period of spinal shock with a flaccid paralysis below the level of the lesion and then there is a tendency for flexor spasms to develop as reflex activity below the lesion recovers. The descending tracts carry impulses relating to motor activity, and if they are interrupted this releases the lower motor neuron from central control and so all activity is reflex. The paralysis of muscles below the level of the lesion will be permanent. The level of the lesion will determine the extent of the paralysis and some of the other problems that may emerge.

Sensory information is carried to the brain in the ascending tracts and so all sensation will be lost below the level of the lesion.

Peripheral nerves with cells in the damaged segments will be affected. Loss of the anterior horn cells will result in a flaccid paralysis of the muscles supplied by that nerve. Sometimes only a few of the fibres in a nerve are affected and this may give a muscle weakness rather than a paralysis. There may also be a loss of sensation in the areas supplied by the peripheral nerves because of destruction of cells in the posterior root ganglion.

In the thoracic region there are cells of the sympathetic system in the lateral horns, and loss of these may affect blood pressure, temperature control and other visceral activities.

The lower lumbar and sacral segments have cells of the parasympathetic system with nerves passing to the pelvic viscera. Interruption of these nerves will lead to bladder and bowel problems.

Even with a complete lesion the clinical features will vary depending on the number of segments involved.

Complete transection of the cervical cord below C5

1. *Tetraplegia* – There will be a paralysis of both arms, trunk and legs. There may be some muscle power in the arms, depending on the exact level of the lesion.
2. *Respiratory problems* – The diaphragm will still be innervated but the intercostal muscles are paralysed and so respiratory movements are decreased. Great care is needed to prevent additional problems such as retention of secretions and infection.
3. *Vasomotor control* – Loss of vasomotor control, and this leads to postural hypotension.
4. *Temperature control* – The normal regulating control is upset.
5. *Sensation* – This is lost below the level of the lesion and affects all sensory modalities.
6. *Bladder and bowel problems* – These can vary depending on the neurological damage. There may be incontinence or retention of urine and/or faeces.
7. *Psychological reactions* – These can vary enormously depending on the ability of the patient to cope with such a devastating disability. The reaction of the patient can be affected by the reaction of those around him, relatives, friends and health care professionals.

Complete lesions of thoracolumbar segments

If the lesion is at T12 then the muscles of the legs will be paralysed but the intercostal muscles and the abdominals will be innervated. There will be a complete loss of sensation in the legs and urinary incontinence.

Cauda equina lesions

The spinal cord ends at the lower border of the 2nd lumbar vertebra, and so lesions below this level will affect the peripheral nerves to the legs resulting in a flaccid paraplegia and a loss of sensation. These nerves may regenerate and there may be some recovery if the conditions are favourable, as discussed in Chapter 21. However, full recovery is unlikely.

Incomplete lesions

Some lesions may appear to be complete immediately after the injury but once the inflammatory reaction has subsided and the patient has recovered from spinal shock some activity may become apparent. This has to be carefully assessed in order to formulate management plans.

The psychological reactions of the patients with incomplete lesions will vary and are not necessarily related to the severity of the injury.

Complications

There are many complications that can occur, and all those caring for the patient and the patient himself must try to avoid them. The most serious of these are pressure sores, contractures and urinary infection. The high lesions may have the problem of developing respiratory complications.

Management

Immediate

The patient must be handled with extreme care following an injury to the vertebral column to avoid damage or any further damage to the spinal cord.

Ideally the patient should be admitted to a special unit dealing with spinal injuries as soon as possible. The work of the late Sir Ludwig Guttman in the treatment of these patients has reduced the mortality rate and improved the quality of life dramatically.

Once the patient has been admitted to a unit a decision has to be made concerning the need for conservative treatment or surgical intervention. Generally, the former is the choice as the damage has already occurred. The surgeon tries to gain as normal a position of the spine as possible to prevent any further damage. This position is usually maintained for 8–12 weeks to gain a stable spine. Surgical intervention may be required when the relief of pressure on the spinal cord may allow some recovery. Cervical lesions may require reduction by traction with skull calipers.

If the paraplegia is the result of an accident there may be other injuries that will require treatment and they may complicate the general treatment of the spinal cord lesion.

General management in hospital

A team approach is very important from the beginning, and ideally the members specialize in the treatment of spinal cord lesions.

Neurological assessment

This must be done as soon as possible in order to ascertain the level of the lesion and the extent of the paralysis and loss of sensation. It may not be possible to gain a true picture until the spinal shock has worn off and any inflammatory reaction has subsided.

Treatment

The patient is going to require treatment for a long period, and it is essential that he is a member of the team. In some cases the reaction of the patient to the injury can make it very difficult for him to work with those around him, which will need very careful handling by the other members of the team. The patient and relatives need careful counselling about the problems that have to be faced at the various stages of the rehabilitation programme. Initially the patient may be very depressed and unwilling to make any effort to help himself. Later patients may react in a variety of ways, depending on their particular situation, how they view the future and their ability to come to terms with the disability. Some are aggressive and take out their frustrations on those around them, others come to terms with the problem and set out to make the best of it. Amongst the most difficult to help are patients who will not express their fears and anxieties and thus make it very difficult to understand and help them.

There are a number of important aspects of care in the early stages which everyone in the team should know about, including the patient:

1. *Positioning and relief of pressure*:
   (a) Position of the vertebral column – the spine must be kept in the required position of reduction, which will depend on the level of the lesion. In the lumbar region pillows are used to keep the lumbar lordosis whereas some cervical lesions may require traction as

mentioned above and sandbags to prevent movement.
   (b) Position to avoid pressure on bony prominences – pressure may be prevented by the use of a sectioned mattress and pillows in conjunction with frequent turning, or by the use of electrically controlled turning beds.
   (c) Prevention of circulatory problems – pressure on veins in the leg can lead to a deep vein thrombosis and general inactivity can result in a slowing of the circulation. Prolonged pressure on the veins in the leg will be prevented by frequent turning and by passive movements. Active movements where possible will help the circulation.
   (d) Prevention of deformity – again positioning is important as one of the measures to prevent contractures developing. Also passive movements will help to maintain joint range and the functional length of soft tissues.
2. *Chest care* – This is particularly important for the tetraplegic patient because of the paralysis of the intercostal muscles. However, all patients who are recumbent are at risk of developing chest infections because of poor respiratory movement and decreased speed of blood flow. Some patients may be at special risk because they have been heavy smokers or they may previously have had a respiratory disease such as chronic bronchitis or asthma.
3. *Urinary bladder and bowels* – As the neurological supply to the bladder is mainly from the lumbar and sacral nerves most lesions will have bladder dysfunction. The initial treatment is usually intermittent catheterization. Depending on the level and type of lesion some patients will develop an automatic (reflex) bladder (for lesions above T10/11), whereas others will develop an autonomous bladder. In both types the patients may be trained to empty the bladder at regular intervals.

Later management

Once weight bearing through the spine is permitted the team must carry out a careful assessment to try to determine the level of independence that the patient is likely to achieve. This will depend partly on the motivation and realistic aims of the patient. At this stage there will be a gradual decrease in medical and nursing care and an increase in the level of physiotherapy and occupational therapy. Planning for a return to the community must be approached with great care as there are many points to consider:

1. The aims and needs of the patient – the preparation may be for the patient to live alone, with spouse and children, or with parents.

2. The type of accommodation that is required and the adaptations that will have to be made.
3. The amount of support that will be required from relatives or carers in the community.
4. What forms of assistance to mobility will be required – wheelchairs (self-propelled or electric), adapted car?
5. Will the patient be able to work? If so will he be able to return to his former work or will he have to be retrained? Sometimes patients cannot return to their former work because of lack of access for a wheelchair or travel problems rather than inability to do the work.
6. Leisure activities – it is important to help and encourage the patient to take part in some leisure activities.

Physiotherapy

The physiotherapist as a member of the team is involved in most of the above aspects of management and if not directly concerned must understand the rationale and the procedures used.

Assessment

A neurological assessment was mentioned under general management. The physiotherapist will undertake an assessment of muscle power and chart which muscles are paralysed, which are weak, and which are normal. This may take some time depending on the condition of the patient and whether further recovery may take place. Similarly, a chart of the areas of sensory loss will be made. The findings of the examination, both subjective and objective, will lead the physiotherapist to defining the aims and objectives of the short-term and possibly long-term management. This will be discussed with the team (including the patient) so that it may be related to the overall management and be altered or modified if necessary. There is a continuous evaluation and resetting of goals as treatment continues.

Early-stage treatment

This links very closely with the points made under general management.

Positioning

If the patient is turned manually the physiotherapist may be one of the team undertaking the turning. She plays an important part in positioning the limbs to prevent deformity and in observing pressure areas for any signs of abnormality.

Passive movements

These must be carried out daily to all joints of the lower limbs with a paraplegic and include the upper limbs with a tetraplegic. Care must be taken with lesions in the lumbar and lower dorsal areas that hip movements do not cause movement of the spine. Similar care may be required with the upper limbs in relation to the cervical spine.

Chest care

Paraplegics may not require physiotherapy for the chest unless there is a chronic chest condition but the therapist must watch for any signs of respiratory problems. The tetraplegic patient will require physiotherapy because of the paralysis of the intercostal muscles. The patient may have a tracheostomy and be on a respirator.

Exercises

Paraplegics – Strengthening exercises should be started for the upper limbs as soon as this is permitted.

Tetraplegics – Any active movement in the upper limbs should be encouraged provided that they are not likely to upset the positioning of the cervical spine.

Physiotherapist/patient interaction

One of the most essential aspects of treatment in the early stages is to establish a good rapport with the patient. This can be very difficult depending on the reaction of the patient to the condition. The physiotherapist must understand the reaction of the patient and use all her skill to develop the cooperation and motivation of the patient.

Later stage

Once weight bearing through the spine is permitted intensive physiotherapy must be given to develop maximum independence.

Paraplegics

Goals

1. *To achieve a sitting balance* – Despite the loss of sensation in the lower part of the body this can be attained. The patient can learn to use sensation in the upper part of the body and make more use of vision. Any suitable methods of balance training can be used.
2. *To enable the patient to be mobile in a wheelchair* – This may be a hand-propelled chair or in the case of a tetraplegic an electric wheelchair may be required. This is very important as it allows

the patient to move around and develop some independence. Patients using hand-propelled wheelchairs can be taught to go up and down slopes, and up and down kerbs.

3. *To teach the patient to transfer* – The patient will previously have been taught to roll over and sit up in bed. Now the patient is taught how to transfer from bed to wheelchair and back, and from a plinth to the wheelchair. Once these can be carried out safely the patient can transfer to a lavatory seat and into a car seat.

4. *To teach self-care* – The importance of this must be instilled in patients from the start of treatment. The patient must be taught to relieve pressure on his seat every 10–15 minutes so that it becomes an automatic reaction. The patient must be taught to observe pressure areas, or if he cannot do so to see that someone else can look at them. The patient must see that the skin is not damaged by knocks or orthoses. The patient is taught to do his own passive movements and report if there is any loss of movement. The patient is taught how to do as many functional activities as possible – dressing, washing. He should be able to look after his own urinal and report any problems.

5. *To strengthen the upper limbs* – This may be carried out on a mat and in a wheelchair. The physiotherapist can use manual resistance to start with and then the patient can become more independent using weights and body weight. Sporting activities that develop the upper limb strength – such as archery, volley ball and swimming – can be encouraged if appropriate.

6. *To teach standing and walking if this is appropriate* – As with sitting the patient must learn to compensate for the loss of sensation in the lower part of the body. The patient will require some form of orthoses and will need to use crutches. The choice of these will depend on the level of the lesion and the individual patient.

7. *To encourage independence* – A young well-motivated paraplegic will probably be able to live independently and work. Employment retraining may be necessary if his previous occupation is unsuitable. It is important that the preparations for a return to independent living are considered early enough in the rehabilitation programme.

Tetraplegic

Although some of the goals are similar they are more difficult for the tetraplegic to accomplish and take longer. One of the particular problems with high lesions is postural hypotension resulting from loss of vasomotor control. Patients can learn to adapt to this with changes of position but they must be watched carefully in the early stages as they are likely to faint.

The wheelchair will require adaptations, such as a higher back rest and the position of controls. Patients with low cervical lesions may be able to transfer unaided but those with higher lesions will require assistance.

Self-care is not so easy for a tetraplegic but he must be responsible for knowing what is required and for seeing that relatives or carers can help when necessary.

The degree of independence reached will not be as high as for the paraplegic and each patient must be carefully assessed.

Motor neuron disease

There are several diseases that come under this heading: progressive muscular atrophy, amyotrophic lateral sclerosis, bulbar palsy and peroneal muscular atrophy. In the first two diseases there is an underlying pathology of progressive degeneration which either starts in the upper motor neuron and continues down to the lower motor neuron or it may be confined to the lower motor neuron. In some cases motor neuclei in the brain stem may be affected, leading to a progressive bulbar palsy which may either precede or follow degeneration of the upper and/or lower motor neurons. There is no known cause for these motor neuron diseases which tend to occur in people between the ages of 50 and 70 years, with more men being affected than women. Peroneal muscular atrophy occurs in childhood or adolescence and is due to an autosomal dominant or recessive gene.

Progressive muscular atrophy

Pathological changes

This disease is due to degeneration of the anterior horn cells of the spinal cord and is therefore a typical lower motor neuron lesion. It is progressive and incurable, although it occasionally becomes arrested at a late stage. Degeneration of the motor nuclei of the cranial nerves may occur, and if the features of a bulbar palsy predominate the patient may only survive for 2–3 years. The prognosis is usually better if the atrophy and weakness is mainly in the limbs and trunk, and the patient may survive for 15 years or more when death may be due to an intercurrent infection.

Clinical features

The initial problem is atrophy and weakness of the small muscles of the hands. This gradually spreads to the forearm, shoulder and back muscles. Later the lower limbs and trunk muscles are similarly affected. Dyspnoea may occur if the diaphragm and intercostal muscles become weak. Similarly, other functions of the body may be affected, for example weakness of the abdominal muscles may lead to urinary retention. There is no sensory loss but pain is often a feature of this disease and occurs because of the musculoskeletal problems. Fasciculation of muscle is a common feature.

Amyotrophic lateral sclerosis

Pathological changes

This is really a variety of the previous disease but in this case the degeneration begins in the cortico-spinal tracts and spreads downwards to the anterior horns and nerve roots. Thus it begins as an upper motor neuron disease, and ends as one of the lower motor neuron.

Clinical features

The disease begins as a spastic paralysis in the fingers and hands and spreads up the arms, the upper limb assuming an appearance like that seen in hemiplegia. At the same time the muscles of the limb atrophy very slowly as the anterior horn cells degenerate. The reflexes are increased at first, but gradually decrease and are finally lost. Ultimately, therefore, the spasticity disappears, and its place is taken by flaccidity, the symptoms due to the lesion of the lower motor neuron masking those caused by that of the upper motor neuron.

Later, the legs are attacked, spastic symptoms appearing first and then as degeneration spreads into the anterior horn cells of the lumbar enlargement atrophy and paralysis follow in the same way as in the arms. The legs, therefore, may be in the spastic stage when weakness and atrophy are well advanced in the arms. The reflexes in the legs, as in the arms, are first exaggerated, ankle clonus and the Babinski's sign being present, but these are finally lost.

As with progressive muscular atrophy the motor nuclei in the medulla may be affected. The respiratory and cardiac centres may be affected. Patients may have difficulty in swallowing and have increased salivation which may cause them to choke. Dysarthria may occur with speech becoming indistinct or impossible. Death may occur as the result of the bulbar palsy or because of an intercurrent infection.

Management

As there is no cure for these diseases, medical and health care professionals have an important role in supporting these patients and trying to maintain independence as long as possible. A number of services may be required, for example a patient with

dysarthria may need speech therapy, then as the disease progresses the occupational therapist may need to make an assessment for any special equipment that may be needed in the home, and the community nurse will probably be needed if the patient is being nursed at home. Other services such as a home help may be necessary. Counselling for the patient and relatives may be very important.

Physiotherapy

Treatment and/or advice will depend on the particular problems presented by a patient. If there is spasticity it may cause considerable discomfort to the patient as well as preventing normal function. Muscle relaxants may help in the upper limbs and active or assisted active movements should be carried out to maintain range of movement and muscle power, or if active movement is not possible passive movements should be given to maintain the range of movement. Spasticity in the legs may enable the patient to stand and so it may not be desirable to give muscle relaxants. When the muscles are weak the patient should be encouraged to use them to maintain function for as long as possible. If the patient cannot perform the movement, assisted or passive movements should be given to maintain the range. This is very important as stiff joints may make it very difficult for carers to move the patient. Also the pain can be an important feature, and maintaining joint range will help to alleviate this problem.

It is tiring for these patients to attend a physiotherapy department and so treatment sessions should be kept to a minimum provided that the patients and carers know what to do at home. In these circumstances the physiotherapist must ensure that there is regular monitoring of the physical condition of the patient and careful records are kept. The patient must know that there is support available when he needs it. If community physiotherapy is available this is preferable for the patient, rather than attending a department. Patients with respiratory problems will require breathing exercises and help with removing any secretions. It may be difficult for the patient to cough because of muscle weakness and it may be helpful to support the chest while attempting to cough, adding vibrations to loosen the secretions if necessary. Changes of position may help the patient but postural drainage positions, particularly for the lower lobes, are usually too stressful.

Patients can suffer a great deal of discomfort from poor positioning and so the physiotherapist must help them to find comfortable positions which are well supported and which do not encourage deformity.

The physiotherapist should give all the encouragement and sympathy that she can to enable the patient to maintain independence as long as possible. It is important that she never holds out false hopes to a patient as the deterioration may then be an even greater blow.

Peroneal muscular atrophy (Charcot–Marie–Tooth disease)

This genetically determined disease usually becomes apparent in late childhood or adolescence.

Pathology

The motor neurons are predominantly affected although there may be some sensory involvement. There is a demyelination of the peripheral nerves leading to axonal degeneration.

Clinical features

The early signs are wasting and weakness of the peroneal muscles, which gradually progresses to the other muscles in the lower legs and feet. The muscles in the upper part of the thighs are not usually affected. The weakness in the feet often leads to pes cavus and clawing of the toes. Later a similar symmetrical wasting and weakness occurs in the forearms and hands.

Management

There is no cure for this disease and so management is concerned with maintaining independence and watching for the development of any deformities, particularly in the feet. If deformities occur orthopaedic surgery may be necessary.

Physiotherapy

Treatment is aimed at maintaining as much independence as possible and giving advice on any aids or adaptations that may be required in the home.

Neurosurgery

Patients requiring neurosurgery are normally cared for in a special unit. At one time the majority of these surgical procedures were carried out for brain or spinal tumours but the changing pattern of modern civilization has increased the incidence of trauma affecting the brain and spinal cord.

In some cases the patients are admitted for emergency surgery whereas in others the surgery may be a planned procedure following careful clinical assessment and the use of special tests.

Surgery for intracranial lesions

Tumours

These may be benign or malignant and as they are space-occupying lesions there is a gradual increase in intracranial pressure as the tumour grows. The presenting symptoms of increased pressure are headaches, nausea, vomiting and later the patient may become drowsy and show signs of mental deterioration and eventually go into a coma. There may be pressure on a specific area of the brain which will cause clinical features linked to the function of that area. For example, patients with cerebellar lesions may develop ataxia, hypotonia, and nystagmus, or in those with lesions of the parietal area of the cerebrum the features may be motor, a hemiparesis or hemiplegia, with or without sensory features.

Benign tumours may be more easily removed as they tend to be more localized and less likely to invade the brain tissues, but they are very vascular and there is always the risk of haemorrhage or a blood clot. The decision about operating on patients with malignant tumours is more difficult and may not be feasible if there is an extensive infiltration of other tissues.

Metastic tumours are secondary to a primary growth elsewhere in the body and usually occur as the result of spread through the vascular or lymphatic system. A single metastic tumour causing specific problems may be successfully removed but if there is a wider spread of the metastases then surgery may not be helpful. Also treatment will depend on the general health of the patient and the success of treatment for the primary tumour.

Prior to surgery the surgeon will carry out a full examination to assist him in making a diagnosis and an indication of the extent of the lesion.

Tests to aid diagnosis

It may not be easy to establish a diagnosis by clinical examination only and various tests may be used to assist this process such as lumbar puncture, electroencephalography, ventriculography and brain scans.

Surgery

Some patients will not be suitable for surgery because the tumour is too extensive or it has infiltrated too far into the brain tissue. Sometimes radiotherapy, chemotherapy or both may be used as an alternative, and they may also be used after surgery.

The type of procedure used will depend on the position and the extent of the lesion. Exploratory burr holes may be used to give a more accurate assessment of the position of the lesion. Following this a bone flap will be partially or completely removed to give access to the lesion – a craniotomy. Special care has to be taken in the use of anaesthesia for neurosurgery, as intracranial pressure should not be increased and cerebral oxygenation must be maintained. Also the patient must regain consciousness before leaving the theatre as this allows the surgeon to test the level of responses, such as speech and the movements of the limbs. This will enable members of the team to judge whether there is subsequent improvement or a deterioration which may indicate the development of complications. The use of modern anaesthetics and hypothermia to reduce metabolic activity allows these conditions to be met.

Postoperative management

Great care must be taken by all members of the team during the immediate post-operative period to observe any changes, particularly those that may indicate a deterioration in the condition of the patient. Any change must be reported immediately as emergency treatment may be required. The advantage of the neurosurgical unit is that the members of the team are immediately available or on call.

The type of care post-operatively will depend on the condition of the patient. Usually the patient is nursed in side-lying as this decreases the risk of the aspiration of vomit or secretions. The patient may have a tracheostomy and be on a respirator.

A nasogastric tube may be necessary if the patient is unable to swallow. If the patient is unable to carry out active movements of the limbs and trunk it is important that care is taken to avoid pressure sores, by frequent turning and observation of pressure points.

Further management will depend on the progress of the patient. Once the patient is out of bed and becoming more active the level of nursing care may be reduced but the active rehabilitation may need to be intensified.

The team must observe the behaviour of the patient both from the point of view of recording any changes and because it may affect the management of the patient. The tumour could have exerted pressure on areas of the brain which might have resulted in mental abnormalities prior to the operation, and if the operation is successful there may be an improvement or even full recovery. Alternatively these symptoms may appear after surgery as the result of damage to the tissues in removing the tumour or because of postoperative complications. Both before and after the operation the patient may suffer from psychological symptoms such as anxiety, depression and frustration.

Possible complications

The following are some of the complications that may occur after surgery, and the team must know what signs and symptoms to watch for during this period:

1. Intracranial haemorrhage/clot.
2. Infection.
3. Respiratory problems.
4. Meningitis
5. Epilepsy.

Physiotherapy

Preoperative

If surgery is not an emergency the physiotherapist will assess the patient. Careful examination of the chest is required, particularly if the patient is at risk of developing pulmonary complications because of an existing chest problem. A neurological examination will determine the extent of any loss of physical function that has occurred as a result of the tumour.

Preoperative treatment will include breathing exercises, simple active exercises or, if active movement is not possible, passive movements. As always this is an important time to try to establish a good rapport with the patient.

Postoperative treatment

This will depend on the condition of the patient, and the physiotherapist will work very closely with the other members of the team. If the patient is on a respirator the physiotherapist will carry out treatment for the chest including suction to remove excess secretions. This must be closely correlated with the nursing care as the nurses will carry out suction at other times and quite often the nurse and physiotherapist may carry out the procedure together.

If the patient is conscious and able to cooperate the physiotherapist will give breathing exercises to encourage full expansion of the lungs and assisted coughing if there are any secretions. Sometimes postural drainage may be necessary, and the physiotherapist must check with the medical staff that there is no contraindication to altering the position of the patient, particularly for the basal lobes.

The patient will be encouraged to do active movements for all the limbs. The physiotherapist will have found out whether the patient was able to carry out active movements immediately after surgery and the level of that response and then she will be able to watch for any improvements or deterioration during the early post-operative period. If the patient is unable to carry out active movements postoperatively then passive movements will be performed through full range. A loss of movement may have occurred preoperatively because of the pressure of the tumour in which case the release of pressure after surgical removal may allow movements to recover. However, if there has been infiltration of the tumour that has caused permanent damage recovery cannot be expected, although sometimes there has been a mixture of permanent damage and pressure and some movements may recover. On occasions loss of movement may follow surgery as it may not be possible to remove the tumour without some damage to the surrounding brain tissue. If tissue is damaged then the loss of movement will be permanent, but sometimes oedema occurs and as this gradually subsides partial or total recovery may occur. The physiotherapist must observe and keep careful records in order to note progress, or any deterioration that could indicate complications.

Rehabilitation of physical function may include stimulation of muscle contraction, strengthening of muscles, developing balance reactions and regaining coordination of movement. This must go hand in hand with regaining the optimum independence of the patient within the home and community and, if appropriate, at work and leisure activities. Sometimes a patient may be able to work but not in his previous occupation, and this may require discussion with the resettlement officer with a view to retraining or a change of occupation.

Treatment may have to be modified if there is any mental deterioration or change of behaviour. Some patients may suffer from a loss of memory immediately after surgery and usually this recovers after a few days. Other patients lack the ability to concentrate and therefore treatment has to be little and often. The physiotherapist must appreciate the emotional problems that are likely to occur and help the patient with psychological as well as physical adjustment. Any of the above problems may hinder the process of rehabilitation.

Vascular lesions

Aneurysms are the most common vascular lesions and may be congenital or the result of arteriosclerotic changes. In some cases there may be no obvious clinical features until a haemorrhage occurs whereas in others the aneurysm may cause pressure on surrounding structures and there may be signs and symptoms. An extensive haemorrhage may be fatal but if the patient survives the initial incident the recovery rate is higher now than it used to be as the result of improved medical and nursing care followed by a good programme of rehabilitation. However, there is always the risk of a recurrent haemorrhage and so angiography is usually carried out to discover the extent of the lesion or lesions. It

is carried out where there is a suspected lesion unless the patient is unfit for surgery. Other investigations such as a lumbar puncture or a CAT scan may be necessary.

Surgery may be considered necessary to deal with the aneurysm and usually a ligature or clip is placed on the vessel. Post-operative management is similar to that for other cranial surgery.

Head injury

The seriousness of a head injury is not always indicated by the degree of external damage. Some scalp lacerations with a fractured skull and damage to brain tissue may have very localized neurological damage, and recovery may be good, whereas some head injuries with no laceration or skull fracture may cause severe brain damage. This type of closed injury may give a contrecoup lesion where the damage is on the opposite side to the blow. Because of the mobile nature of the brain tissue within the skull, blows can lead to shearing strains with resultant damage to brain tissue and/or blood vessels. Many head injuries are complicated by injuries to other parts of the body such as fractures, dislocations and lacerations.

Management

First aid

When the patient is unconscious the immediate treatment is to maintain an airway as many patients could die from asphyxia rather than brain damage if this is not carried out.

Hospital

Observation is the keyword following admission. If the patient is conscious he must be watched carefully for any of the following signs:

1. Alteration in the level of consciousness.
2. Altered respiratory rate.
3. A rise in blood pressure and fall in pulse rate.
4. Any alteration in the pupils – dilation of one or both.

With a closed injury one of the most likely complications is a haematoma, and as this may occur in some relatively trivial injuries it could be missed without very careful examination and observation by all members of the team. The development of an intracranial haematoma is one of the occasions when emergency surgery may be the only way of saving life.

Many head injury patients may suffer from mental disorders, disorientation, confusion, loss of memory (post-traumatic amnesia, PTA), or behavioural changes. Some of these may be transitory or there may be permanent damage. The patient may not be able to function at the same level intellectually and will be unable to work or lead a normal life. If this is associated with a marked physical handicap then the patient will need long-term care and support.

Surgery

Apart from the instance cited at the end of the last paragraph, surgery is not generally necessary for the treatment of head injuries. A patient with an open injury who has sustained a depressed fracture of the skull will require surgery with the main emphasis on removing any dead tissue, foreign bodies and cleaning the wound. The depressed piece of bone may be elevated to allow drainage if there is a haematoma or to relieve pressure. Surgery for a haematoma requires location of the clot so that it can be removed. Usually an exploratory burr hole is made to locate the lesion and then a small bone flap may be lifted in order to expose the clot.

Physiotherapy

If the patient has a tracheostomy and is on a respirator the physiotherapist will give chest care and suction to remove the secretions as mentioned under intracranial surgery.

An unconscious patient will require passive movements to all limbs. The physiotherapist on the neurosurgical unit can plan this to fit in with the nursing care and when the patient is turned. All members of the team must observe the pressure points for any signs of pressure sores as these can occur very quickly, particularly if the patient is very restless.

A careful watch must be kept for any increase of tone in muscles as this may give some indication of the position of the lesion or it may indicate some deterioration in the condition of the patient. Patients may go through a stage of hyperactivity while still unconscious which may make handling very difficult.

As an unconscious patient begins to recover the level of response rises, and the physiotherapist should talk to the patient during treatment in order to give further stimulation. Patients may be helped to respond by various stimuli. Some patients respond to the voice of a close relative or friend, while others may respond to music or some other familiar noise. The following responses should be observed during treatment: eye opening, talking and whether it is coherent, movement to a command or to a painful stimulus (use of the Glasgow coma scale). These responses must be related to the more general reactions of the patient, whether he is aware of his surroundings and his general behaviour.

Surgery for spinal lesions

Traumatic lesions resulting from fractures or fracture dislocations of the vertebral column have been dealt with earlier in this chapter. There are other spinal problems that may require surgery such as neoplasms, vascular lesions, or intervertebral disc lesions that do not respond to conservative treatment. Congenital abnormalities such as spina bifida will be described in Chapter 22.

Spinal tumours

There are various types of tumours, of which some are extradural and a larger proportion intradural. The latter may be either extramedullary or intramedullary. Some tumours, such as the malignant extradural, grow very quickly and compression of the cord can occur within hours or days resulting in paraplegia, whilst other tumours are very slow growing and the patient may complain of back pain for a number of years before he begins to develop any neurological signs and symptoms.

Management

Surgery is usually indicated for tumours in order to relieve the pressure on the spinal cord. This involves a laminectomy to expose the tumour; the number of laminae removed will depend on the extent of the tumour. A large part of an extramedullary tumour may be removed, particularly if it is benign, but it is less likely that the surgeon will be able to remove much of an intramedullary tumour as it may cause further damage and loss of function.

After surgery the patient is nursed in side-lying and turned frequently to prevent the development of pressure sores. The patient may be allowed out of bed once the sutures are removed as a laminectomy has little effect on the stability of the back unless there has been destruction of other parts of the vetebrae. If the pressure on the cord has been relieved by the surgery, considerable or even complete recovery may occur. However, if there is permanent damage to the cord this may result in paralysis of some muscles or even paraplegia.

Physiotherapy
Preoperative

Unless surgery is performed as an emergency the physiotherapist will be able to assess the patient preoperatively. The aim is to assess whether there is any risk of respiratory or circulatory problems and to assess any loss of physical function due to neurological damage.

Postoperative

Treatment will depend on the condition of the individual patient. If there is any risk of a chest problem or secretions have been produced in the lungs after surgery, breathing exercises and assisted coughing will be given until there is no further risk or the problem is resolved. If the patient is able to move the limbs normally then general exercises will be given to prevent slowing of the circulation and to maintain mobility while the patient is in bed. Gentle static exercises for the back extensors and the abdominals can be given once the surgeon gives permission and then they may be progressed to active movements within the pain-free range. Once the patient is allowed up the physiotherapist will make a careful assessment to determine the short- and long-term management. If there is normal activity in the legs treatment may not need to be prolonged but the patient will require gradual mobilizing and strengthening for the trunk until he has regained normal function. Also advice will be given on general care of the back.

Some patients may have had a temporary paralysis of muscles because of the tumour and these will recover with graded strengthening exercises and re-education of function. Others may have a permanent paralysis of certain muscles or even a complete paraplegia. Assessment of the individual will determine whether he needs an appliance and/or crutches to enable him to walk. A paraplegic will need training in the use of a wheelchair and rehabilitation as described earlier in this chapter.

Intervertebral disc lesions

Herniation of discs occurs most commonly in the lumbar region and more rarely in the cervical region. The lumbar lesions tend to occur between the 4th and 5th vertebrae or the 5th lumbar and 1st sacral vertebrae. The majority of these patients are treated conservatively but if treatment is unsuccessful and particularly if there is nerve root involvement then surgery may be necessary. In some instances the disc protrusion presses on the spinal cord, and the patient begins to develop signs of a cauda equina lesion and possible involvement of the bladder. These cases require surgery before permanent damage occurs.

Management

The operative technique used will depend on the extent and position of the lesion. In some instances it may be sufficient to perform a partial laminectomy on the side of the lesion, whereas in other patients it may be necessary to remove the spinous processes and the laminae on both sides.

Postoperatively the patient is nursed in side-lying and turned frequently. Usually the patient is allowed up in 2 or 3 days and allowed to mobilize gradually. The length of the rehabilitation period will depend on the individual patient and his needs.

Physiotherapy

Preoperative

This will be similar to that given for a patient with a spinal tumour.

Postoperative

As with all postoperative patients the physiotherapist will try to prevent any respiratory or circulatory complications by assessment and treatment as necessary.

Gentle active movements for the lower limbs can be started in the side-lying position with care being taken to avoid taking the hip movements too far and causing back pain during the first day or two.

As soon as possible static work for the back extensors and the abdominals should be started, followed by gradual mobilizing and strengthening exercises. It is important in the early stages to watch for any loss of movement or recovery if movement had been lost. Loss of movement may be temporary owing to oedema after surgery, and as this subsides the movement will recover.

Surgeons vary about methods of postoperative care, some advocating vigorous mobilizing of the back to regain as full a range of movement as possible and to prevent the formation of adhesions which could lead to further problems. Other surgeons prefer to allow the patient to mobilize gently on his own and, in some cases, to avoid flexion of the spine. Thus the physiotherapist will need to discuss the postoperative management with the surgeon before planning a treatment programme.

The needs of the patient will vary according to his occupation, home and lesiure activities. A patient who has had a job demanding heavy manual work may be advised to seek alternative employment and will need the help of a resettlement officer and possible retraining. If a patient is to be allowed to return to heavy manual work he will need an intensive programme of mobilizing and strengthening with special attention to lifting and general care of the back. For a patient returning to office work such an intensive programme may not be necessary but the physiotherapist will need to assess the requirements of the patient for leisure activities as well as work. Patients returning to office work require advice about sitting, height of chair and desk and position of equipment, and must be taught correct lifting techniques.

Chapter 21

Peripheral nerve lesions

Anatomical structure of peripheral nerves
Types of nerve injury

Specific lesions of nerves
Polyneuropathies

The first part of this chapter is concerned with nerve lesions due to injury and the second part gives a brief description of the polyneuropathies.

Anatomical structure of peripheral nerves

A spinal nerve is formed by the union of a ventral nerve root and a dorsal nerve root and then, after emerging from the intervertebral foramen, it divides into a dorsal ramus and a ventral ramus (Figure 21.1). The dorsal rami are generally smaller than the ventral rami and supply the muscles and skin of the posterior region of the neck and trunk. Because of their position and the manner in which they supply structures they are not as often damaged as the ventral rami. So the lesions discussed in this chapter concern peripheral nerves formed by the ventral rami. The ventral rami form nerves passing to the upper and lower limbs and the anterolateral aspects of the trunk. Those in the upper cervical region unite to form the cervical plexus and those in the lower cervical region plus the first thoracic ramus unite to form the brachial plexus. The plexuses then divide into nerves which supply the head, neck and upper limbs. In the lumbar and sacral regions the rami form the lumbar and sacral plexuses which then supply the lower part of the trunk and the lower limbs. The rami in the thoracic region run separately and are segmentally arranged in their supply to the upper and lateral aspects of the thorax.

The fibres forming a peripheral nerve are derived from the somatic and autonomic nervous systems. They are divided into three classes according to their

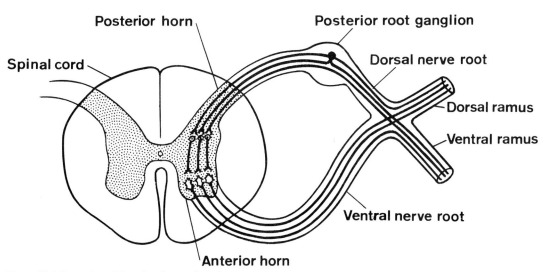

Figure 21.1 Formation of dorsal and ventral rami

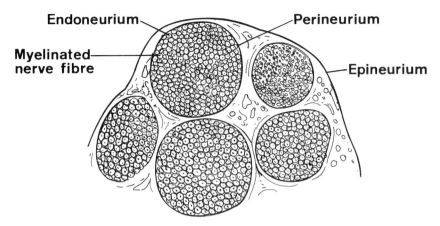

Figure 21.2 Transverse section of a peripheral nerve to show the connective tissue sheaths

size and rate of conduction. Class A are the largest, fastest conducting and are comprised of somatic efferent and afferent fibres. Class B are myelinated preganglionic autonomic fibres. Class C are non-myelinated slow-conducting autonomic and sensory fibres.

A peripheral nerve comprises nerve fibres arranged in bundles called fasciculi. Each fasciculus may contain anything from a few fibres to hundreds depending on the size of the nerve and the structures that it supplies. Likewise the number of fasciculi forming a nerve vary in size and number. Each fasciculus is surrounded by a connective tissue sheath of perineurium, and extending between the nerve fibres is a rather more delicate connective tissue called endoneurium. Binding the fasciculi together is a more fibrous connective tissue called the epineurium (Figure 21.2).

In both myelinated and non-myelinated fibres there are a large number of Schwann cells which surround the axon, or in some instances a number of axons may be invaginated in the Schwann cells. In the myelinated fibres there is an extension of the Schwann cell cytoplasm – the myelin sheath – which wraps itself round the axon. The nodes of Ranvier are gaps between adjacent Schwann cells and these occur at regular intervals along the fibre (Figures 21.3 and 21.4). The axolemma is exposed at the nodes of Ranvier and it is this arrangement that allows the fast conduction that occurs as the impulse leaps from node to node by saltatory conduction (Figure 21.5).

Types of nerve injury

These will depend on the nature and degree of the initial trauma.

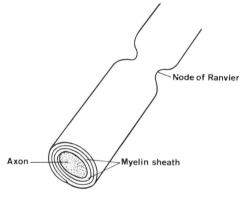

Figure 21.3 Structure of the myelin sheath of a nerve fibre

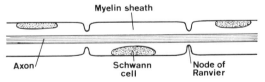

Figure 21.4 Schematic structure of a myelinated nerve to show the Schwann cells

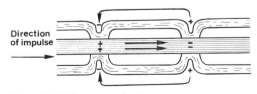

Figure 21.5 Saltatory conduction

Compression injury of a nerve

The pressure on a nerve can be brief, prolonged or intermittent and may be classified as a neuropraxia or an axonotmesis.

Neuropraxia – This is due to a brief intermittent or possibly longer pressure which causes minimal or no structural damage and recovery should occur within a few weeks.

Axonotmesis – Prolonged or chronic recurrent pressure may cause degeneration of the nerve. Recovery will take considerably longer as the nerve fibre (or fibres) has to grow from just above the lesion to its destination. Sometimes stretching of a nerve causes disruption of the axon and consequent degeneration. The chances of recovery are much greater with an axonotmesis than with a severed nerve because the nerve sheath is intact.

Severance of a nerve – neurotmesis

This occurs when the axon, Schwann cell and myelin sheath are severed, and degeneration takes place.

Mixed lesions

As a nerve consists of many fibres damage can consist of a mixture of the above types of lesions, which may make diagnosis and treatment more difficult.

Pathological changes

Brief pressure on a nerve resulting in a loss of conduction is due to ischaemia and is rapidly reversible. For example, sitting with one leg crossed over the other for a short period may result in a temporary loss of conduction in the common peroneal nerve.

A longer term compression injury may result in a mechanical displacement of the nodes of Ranvier with stretching of the paranodal myelin. Provided that the pressure is released before any structural changes have taken place recovery will occur in a few weeks.

Sometimes pressure may be intermittent and result in a mixed segmental demyelination and remyelination. This type of lesion can affect the ulnar nerve at the elbow, or the median nerve as it passes through the carpal tunnel.

Severance of a nerve may be partial or complete. In either case those nerve fibres that are severed will undergo Wallerian degeneration.

Wallerian degeneration (Figure 21.6)

The changes take place in the nerve fibres from the point of severance distally to the effector or receptor organ and proximally to the node of Ranvier above the incision. Although the initial degeneration starts at the site of the lesion subsequent changes occur simultaneously down the length of the nerve fibre. Recent studies have shown that the sequence of events occurs more quickly than was previously described. Originally it was thought that there was biochemical stability for at least a week after the disruption of the fibres. Now it has been shown that there is an increase in the concentration of hydrolytic enzymes within 12 hours of the injury which is associated with the loss of the basic protein from the sheath.

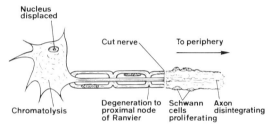

Figure 21.6 Wallerian degeneration

The myelin sheath breaks down into fatty droplets within the Schwann cell cytoplasm. These droplets are subsequently extruded into the endoneurial space and phagocytosed by macrophages. As this process occurs the Schwann cells begin to proliferate, especially around the gap produced when there is severance of the nerve. The axon breaks down and the debris is removed. These changes take place within 14–21 days after the injury, and the end result is an empty endoneurial tube with the proliferating Schwann cells.

Changes occur in the cell body of the neuron and can be seen as a reduction in the number of Nissl granules and a movement of the nucleoli towards the periphery of the nucleus. However, provided that the cell is not destroyed these changes are reversible and are linked with the subsequent regrowth of the axon.

Regeneration

Regrowth of the axon will take place down the endoneurial tube provided that it is intact. However, when there is severance of the nerve, and consequently a gap in the tube at the site of the lesion, regeneration is unlikely to be successful unless the nerve is sutured. The proliferation of the Schwann cells, which occurs down the length of the tube and particularly at the point of severance, helps to guide the axon down the tube and they may bridge the gap if the disruption is not too severe. The stump of the axon develops a swelling and from this a number of fibres grow into the surrounding tissue. One of these may enter and grow down the empty neural tube, if there is good apposition, whilst the others will eventually disappear. Thus it can be seen why an axonotmesis has a good chance of recovery. But the chance of obtaining good apposition of the fibre relative to an empty neural tube following severance of the nerve is not good, although recent advances in microsurgery have improved the level of recovery. Also the degree of recovery will depend on the type of neurons in the nerve fibre. Mixed nerves, containing afferent and efferent fibres, are a greater problem than those containing only one type of fibre. For example, a fibre from a sensory neuron could grow down an endoneurial tube which terminates on an effector organ and so be useless, and similarly a fibre from a motor neuron would be useless in growing to a receptor organ. Another factor that could stop regeneration is the presence of scar tissue which could block the pathway of the growing axon. If the nerve is severed a long way from some of the muscles that it innervates then degeneration of the muscle fibres may take place before the regenerating nerve reaches the end organ. This could occur with a lesion of the sciatic nerve when the motor fibres that supply the intrinsic muscles of the foot are severed. Lesions of a nerve fibre close to the cell body may result in irreversible damage to the cell, and then regeneration will not occur.

During regeneration the axon will grow at the rate of 1–2 mm a day, although the rate will tend to be a little slower as it extends further away from the cell body. Thus it is possible to measure the length of the nerve from the lesion and estimate the time that it will take for the fibre to grow down the tube and when some recovery might be expected. Before function can recur the myelin sheath and nodes of Ranvier must be re-formed. Also the axon and myelin sheath need to recover sufficient diameter for transmission to take place. So any calculations of recovery time must take all of these factors into account.

Clinical features

The severity of these will depend on the extent of the neurological damage and upon the type of lesion.

Somatic motor function

Paralysis

The extent of the paralysis will depend on which nerves have been damaged. A lesion of the median

nerve in the axilla would result in paralysis of all the muscles supplied by the median below the level of the lesion. However, it would be less if the median nerve were severed at the wrist or only a branch of the nerve affected. The paralysis may be partial, as for example when some of the fibres to a muscle are intact but others are damaged, resulting in muscle weakness. Paralysis of muscles will result in the loss of tendon reflexes.

Weak muscles

A neuropraxia may sometimes cause a weakness of muscles rather than a paralysis. When some muscles which work as part of a group are paralysed then the other muscles may become weak because they are unable to function normally. This may apply to movements of a whole limb when activity is impossible because of the paralysis of one or more groups of muscles.

As regeneration of a nerve occurs and contraction of a muscle becomes possible there will be a period of muscle weakness until it can be strengthened to full power again.

Somatic sensory function

If somatic afferent nerve fibres are damaged then the modalities of pain, touch, pressure and temperature may be affected. There is a considerable overlap in the sensory distribution of nerves and so the area of sensory loss may not be as large as anticipated.

Anaesthesia – This is a loss of sensation in the area affected which can cause considerable disturbance of function depending on the area affected and the extent of the anaesthesia. The hand is a particular problem and may suffer further injury if the patient is not made fully aware of the difficulties arising from the sensory loss.

Dysaesthesia – Incomplete lesions may lead to a disturbance in sensation, resulting in numbness and tingling. During re-innervation there is initially a hypersensitivity (hyperaesthesia) which gradually returns to a more normal sensation.

Analgesia – Complete lesions affecting fibres giving sensations of pain may result in analgesia.

Hyperpathia – Pain is a feature in some lesions, especially if it is an incomplete lesion. Sometimes pain can be very acute, particularly if sympathetic fibres are involved (causalgia).

Autonomic disturbances

These result in the loss of the normal function of sweating, and the skin becomes dry and scaly. The local circulation is affected partly by interference with the sympathetic innervation of blood vessels and partly because of the loss of normal movement.

These disturbances may result in the development of trophic lesions although these may also develop as the result of damage to an anaesthetic area.

Contractures

Contractures of muscle may occur as the result of an imbalance between normal and paralysed groups. Muscles that are paralysed for a prolonged period may undergo fibrous degeneration. Contractures can occur because of damage to soft-tissue structures or because adhesions develop in tendon sheaths or around joints.

Prognosis

The outlook following a neuropraxia is good, and there should be full recovery, which is usually within a few weeks but occasionally may take longer. The prognosis for an axonotmesis is also quite good although full function is not always achieved. A neurotmesis is quite a different problem, and the prognosis depends on many factors; for example:

1. There may be associated injuries, and treating the nerve lesion may not be the first priority.
2. There may be infection.
3. If the nerve ends are clean and in good apposition then the results of surgery are likely to be better.
4. The results after a mixed nerve lesion are not as good as with an unmixed nerve.
5. If the lesion is close to the effector and/or receptor organs the result is likely to be better.
6. The age and general health of the patient.

Even if all the factors are favourable to recovery it is unusual to obtain better than a 60% recovery.

Management

This will depend on the cause of the injury and the type of the lesion. Often there are associated injuries of bones, joints, and/or soft tissues, so the surgeon may have to deal with a complex situation in which the nerve injury is only one of a number of injuries. This chapter is dealing with peripheral nerve lesions, and so other injuries will be alluded to only when they are the cause of the lesion or they have a specific effect on the total management.

Diagnosis

If paralysis of muscles supplied by a particular nerve has occurred it is important to ascertain the type of nerve lesion so that suitable treatment may be arranged. In some cases where there is a wound or surgical intervention is required, because of a fracture or other damage, the surgeon will be able to see whether there is an neurotmesis. Otherwise electromyographic tests can be used to find out whether the nerve is conducting. Sensory testing will be carried out to discover the degree of sensory impairment.

Treatment

Once the type of lesion has been confirmed then treatment can be arranged. Neither a neuropraxia nor an axonotmesis will require surgical intervention unless there is a need to relieve pressure on the nerve. A neurotmesis will need to be sutured if there is to be any chance of recovery.

There must be an integrated plan of treatment and all the health care professionals in the team must have regular discussions so that progress is carefully monitored. Whenever possible and appropriate the patient should be involved as a member of the team, or if not one of the members of the team should have a counselling role.

Physiotherapy management
Neuropraxia

This may not require any treatment as recovery is likely to occur with in a few weeks. However, a patient may need advice on carrying out as much movement of the limb as possible and reassurance about the gradual recovery of normal function. Occasionally with an apparent neuropraxia a few fibres may be more extensively damaged (axonotmesis) with resulting degeneration, and then more treatment may be required.

Axonotmesis and neurotmesis
Assessment

The initial assessment is very important in determining management. The physiotherapist needs to know the history, the likely prognosis, the proposed medical or surgical management, and how much detail has been explained to the patient. If the nerve has been sutured, following a neurotmesis, it must not be stretched for 2–3 weeks and so it may not be possible to carry out a full assessment.

During the subjective examination the physiotherapist can assess the reaction of the patient to the injury and their motivation towards recovery. An assessment will be made of the problems as seen by the patient in relation to the activities of daily living, their occupation and leisure activities. This will be linked with the problems as seen by the physiotherapist following the physical examination and taken into account in formulating the treatment programme.

The objective examination will give details of paralysis and muscle weakness. This can be charted using the Medical Research Council grades 0–5 as described in Chapter 19.

If only some of the muscles in a group action are paralysed then the movement may be produced but with reduced power. Some patients adapt quickly to a loss of movement and may perform trick movements, whilst others may have more disability than the loss of muscle power would seem to indicate. The latter may be due to sensory loss, and it is important to check the extent of this very carefully.

An examination of the sensory modalities will reveal which modalities are altered by the lesion. Areas of anaesthesia can be shown on a diagram of the limb or body (Figure 21.7). When an area of anaesthesia is present the test should start in this area and move towards the normal part (Tinel's test), otherwise once the patient has felt touch in a normal area they may imagine that they can feel it in the anaesthetized part. There may be areas of

hyperaesthesia, particularly if the lesion is incomplete.

The examiner should note alterations in the colour and texture of the skin, loss of muscle bulk and any deformities.

Functional loss will depend on the extent of the lesion and the particular muscle groups affected. For example, a lesion of the radial nerve will allow very little use of the hand even though the flexors and intrinsic muscles are still innervated.

Electrical tests

The use of electromyographic tests for diagnosis has already been mentioned. The physiotherapist may also use forms of modified direct current to test nerve/muscle reactions. If there is a normal nerve conduction to a muscle then the electric impulse will stimulate the nerve directly. A strength–duration curve may be plotted on a graph by starting with a long duration pulse and using the minimum intensity of current to produce a response (rheobase) and then gradually decreasing the duration of the pulse until a response can no longer be obtained. A chronaxie is the minimum duration of impulse that will produce a response with a current of double the rheobase. If the reaction is normal a graph will be produced as shown in Figure 21.8(a). The scale is logarithmic which gives more detail for small numbers than a linear one.

Denervated muscle can be stimulated directly but the shorter the pulse the greater is the intensity needed to produce a contraction. Eventually the pulse is too short to produce a response regardless of the intensity of the current and the graph shows complete reaction of degeneration (Figure 21.8(b)). Sometimes a variable number of nerve fibres supplying a muscle have escaped damage whilst others have been severed. When this happens the strength–duration curve shows a combination of a normal curve and that of degeneration (Figure 21.8(c)). If more nerve fibres become degenerated the 'kink' in the curve will move to the left. As the nerve starts to regenerate and some nerve fibres are remyelinated a similar curve showing partial innervation will develop, and the 'kink' in the curve will move to the right.

If the muscle tissue degenerates to fibrous tissue there will be no response to any type of electrical stimulation, which is known as the absolute reaction of degeneration.

Electrical tests are not carried out for the first week or two as the changes of degeneration may not be complete and the tests could give a false picture of the changes.

Once the examination has been carried out and the findings have been considered, a plan of treatment can be arranged. The goals must be realistic and take into account the future needs of

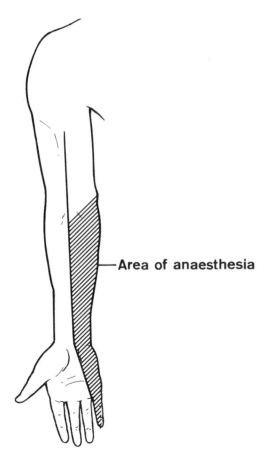

Figure 21.7 Outline of the arm to show an area of anaesthesia

Area of anaesthesia

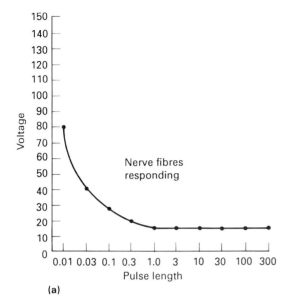

(a)

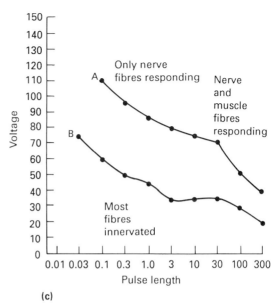

(c)

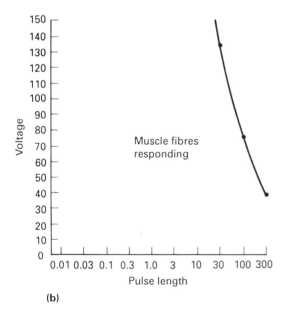

(b)

Figure 21.8 Strength–duration graph. (*a*) Normal curve (rheobase, 15 V; chronaxie, 0.1 ms). (*b*) Complete reaction of degeneration (rheobase, 40 V; chronaxie, 100 mv). (*c*) Partial reaction of denervation (rheobase A, 40 V; rheobase B, 20 V; chronaxie, 1–10 ms)

the patient. For example, paralysis of the muscles in the dominant hand might mean the loss of livelihood to a patient unless a good recovery is achieved. The level of recovery needed will vary according to the occupation, as some patients may undertake their type of work with an incomplete recovery whereas others such as concert pianists could not continue to play to the standard required. The problem of waiting several months to know how much recovery they will achieve may be very difficult for a patient

to cope with and the therapist will have to consider this aspect in management.

Principles of treatment

Initial care during stage of paralysis

There are certain basic aims of treatment and these can be modified or altered depending on the specific lesion and the assessment of the individual patient.

To prevent or reduce oedema

The patient must be shown how to position the limb, particularly when at rest, and be given general advice on preventing oedema. There may be a problem if there are other associated injuries that prevent suitable positioning and movement.

Movement is very important because of the pumping action of the muscles on the vessels and the active movement of joints which stretches and compresses vessels thus maintaining an adequate circulation. If this is not possible passive movements will help to maintain the circulation. Massage may be given to reduce the oedema, ideally with the limb in the elevated position.

To maintain the circulation in the affected area

A slowing of the circulation will reduce the effective supply of nutrition to the tissues and removal of waste products. Active movements are the best means of preventing this slowing but passive movements and massage will help if there is paralysis.

To prevent contractures

It is essential to prevent the development of any contractures which would impede recovery. Passive movements must be carried out to maintain the full range of joint movements and to maintain the full length of muscles. The latter is particularly important when muscles work over more than one joint as the muscles must be stretched over both joints at the same time. Passive movements must be carried out daily as stiffness can develop very quickly. A patient may be able to carry out their own passive movements, or they may be performed by a relative, but the physiotherapist must ensure that full movements and full stretch of muscles is being maintained.

To maintain activity and power of unaffected muscles

The patient must be encouraged to use the unaffected muscles in the limb. If this is not possible because of the paralysis the physiotherapist may be able to facilitate movement by supporting the limb, or functional splinting may allow movements to occur.

At one time electrical stimulation in the form of interrupted direct current was used to try to prevent muscle fibrosis and maintain contractility. However, recovery seemed to be as good using the other techniques described and so this was no longer used. Recent research has shown that there may be some value in using some of the new current forms, such as pulsed electromagnetic energy, and some authorities advocate the use of this.

To maintain function

As indicated above the patient must be encouraged to use the limb as much as possible. The use of well-designed and well-applied lively splints (functional splints) may allow some functional activity.

To look after areas where there is any sensory disturbance

The patient must be told how to care for areas of anaesthesia. If a lesion of the skin and soft tissues occurs it may be difficult to heal and will impede recovery.

Stage of recovery

In a mixed nerve the recovery programme will include both motor and sensory re-education. Depending on the particular nerve and the extent of the sensory and motor loss the re-education can be equally important, especially in the case of the hand.

Muscle re-education

During the performance of passive movements before any recovery occurs it is useful for the patient to think about the movement provided that it does not cause too much anxiety. It is difficult to predict the recovery time exactly for the reasons given above, but as the anticipated time approaches it is useful to start using methods of initiating a contraction. When a successful outcome is doubtful the physiotherapist must be careful not to raise the hopes of the patient too high.

Initiation of a contraction

There are many techniques that can be used to try to stimulate a contraction. As some of these depend on sensory stimulation this may be part of the sensory re-education.

A muscle works in a number of ways – as an agonist, or fixator, or synergist – and attempts should be made to use it in all of these actions. During recovery a muscle may work as a fixator or synergist before it will work as an agonist. A muscle may work with one group of muscles to produce one movement and with another group to produce a different action. For example, the extensor carpi ulnaris will work with the flexor carpi ulnaris to produce ulnar deviation and with the extensor carpi radialis longus and brevis to produce wrist extension. Thus all actions should be attempted when trying to initiate a contraction. It is also important to try to irradiate impulses to the affected muscles by demanding maximal effort from normal muscles that work with them. For example, to stimulate the finger flexors using the eating pattern maximal resistance could be given to the elbow and shoulder components (flexor adduction lateral rotation pattern – proprioceptive neuromuscular facilitation (PNF) technique).

Other methods of initiating a contraction include a quick stretch, tendon tapping, brief ice or quick brushing.

Muscle strengthening

Once there is a flicker of contraction recorded as grade 1 on the MRC scale then the muscles can be strengthened through the grades of this scale (see Chapter 19). Once there is a perceptible contraction the number of these must be counted and gradually progressed. As free movement becomes possible the number of movements, firstly with gravity and later against gravity, must be recorded and progressed. Maximal effort must be demanded if an effective programme of recovery is to be achieved. The muscles should be worked in all their actions.

Once external resistance to movement can be used a form of progressive resistance exercise can be used either by manual resistance (PNF) or by the use of weights. If weights are used there is some controversy as to the most suitable programme. Some authorities recommend one maximum contraction per treatment as being the most effective whereas others advocate a 10-repetition maximum.

It is necessary to remember that endurance is an important part of functional activity, and re-education of this factor demands a high-repetition, low-resistance scheme.

The strength and endurance required will differ from one patient to another depending on their occupation, leisure activities and age. Usually younger patients will rehabilitate more quickly than older patients.

Muscle coordination

Movement must be smooth and well coordinated to allow normal function.

Sensory re-education

Some of this is integrally linked with motor re-education, as mentioned above. However, specific attempts can be made to stimulate sensation particularly in lesions affecting the hand. The techniques will depend on the modality that is being re-educated. For example, the patient may try to identify different objects by shape and texture with their eyes closed. If proprioception is affected the patient can try to identify the position of the limb or part of the limb, again with the eyes closed.

Functional activities

The level of normal functional activitiy regained will depend on the extent of the recovery. When this is full the patient should be able to resume their normal occupation and leisure activities. However, if recovery is limited a careful asessment must be made to see whether the patient is capable of their original employment and other activities. If their previous employment is not possible then the patient must be counselled and an assessment made for a change of occupation if this is practical.

Following suture of the nerve

The rehabilitation programme will have to be modified for the first 2–3 weeks following the suture as the nerve must not be stretched. In some instances a splint may be applied to prevent movement.

Minimal or no recovery after the lesion

The physiotherapist must try to achieve optimum function. Sometimes functional splinting may help to give a reasonable level of activity. However, a number of patients do not like appliances and would prefer to manage without. The surgeon may consider further surgery to try to improve function.

Specific lesions of nerves

Upper extremity

Axillary nerve lesion

This is not a common lesion but it can occur associated with injuries around the shoulder, in particular a dislocated shoulder or a fracture of the surgical neck of the humerus. Usually the type of lesion is a neuropraxia or axonotmesis rather than a neurotmesis, as the nerve is likely to be stretched or compressed by the lesion rather than severed.

Clinical features

The main functional disability due to the nerve lesion is the inability to abduct the arm because of paralysis of the deltoid. A number of patients will develop a trick movement, enabling them to lift the arm up.

The muscle will waste. This can be observed by the loss of contour over the shoulder which is normally provided by the bulk of the deltoid. The sensory loss is minimal because of the overlap of sensory supply, but there is a small area of anaesthesia over the lower part of the muscle.

Specific points of management

The orthopaedic surgeon will reduce the dislocation as mentioned in Chapter 5; or if the associated injury is a fracture of the surgical neck this will be managed as described in Chapter 4. Usually these injuries do not require open surgery and so the nerve will not be examined, but intervention will probably not be required if the lesion is a neuropraxia or an axonotmesis.

Physiotherapy

Passive abduction of the shoulder should be carried out with care, because of the associated injury, as soon as the surgeon permits it. The physiotherapist must ascertain that there is a full range of other movements, particularly lateral rotation.

If the lesion is a neuropraxia recovery should occur within a few weeks although progress may be a little slower than following an uncomplicated dislocation. Following an axonotmesis progress will be much slower because of the nerve degeneration. It is essential to keep full passive movements until the nerve regenerates and the muscle can be strengthened.

It should be remembered that many of the patients with these injuries are older and so there is a greater danger of a stiff shoulder developing.

Ulnar nerve lesion

The nerve may be injured in the axilla by pressure such as that caused by falling asleep with the arm over the back of a chair or, in patients using axillary crutches, by the pressure of the crutch. Occasionally there could be injury due to a wound. At the elbow the nerve could be stretched or torn when a fracture or dislocation takes place. Later, following these injuries the nerve could be compressed by scar tissue or callus formation. Injury at the wrist usually occurs as the result of direct trauma caused by a cut or wound.

Clinical features

Lesion in the forearm or above – This will cause paralysis of the flexor carpi ulnaris and the medial half of the flexor profundus digitorum. This will result in weakening of ulnar deviation and the loss of flexion of the terminal phalanges of the third and fourth fingers. In the hand there will be paralysis of the following small muscles: abductor digiti minimi, flexor digiti minimi, opponens digiti minimi, the interossei, the third and fourth lumbricals, adductor pollicis and usually flexor pollicis brevis. This results in a loss of the ability to abduct and adduct the fingers, and to flex the third and fourth fingers at the metacarpophalangeal joints while the interphalan-

geal joints are extended. This disability severely limits the use of the hand, particularly in a power grip. The loss of the adductor pollicis and flexor pollicis brevis will weaken the pinch grip.

The sensory loss will depend on the level of the lesion: if it is at the elbow the palmar cutaneous, the dorsal cutaneous and the superficial terminal branches will all be affected. This will give an area of anaesthesia on the ulnar side of the hand, on both palmar and dorsal aspects, and on the little, ring and part of the middle fingers.

If the lesion is at the wrist the paralysis will affect only the muscles in the hand, and the sensory loss may affect only the fingers unless the injury has also severed the dorsal and palmar cutaneous nerves.

Specific points of management

If scar tissue or callus formation is causing pressure at the elbow this will be dealt with by the surgeon and there should be a full recovery unless the pressure has been prolonged.

Lesions resulting in a neurotmesis will need to be sutured. When degeneration of the nerve has caused paralysis of the muscles in the hand a functional splint may be given to the patient. This comprises a light padded bar across the dorsal aspect of the proximal phalanges of the third and fourth fingers and a similar one over the upper end of the metacarpals. These are attached to another padded bar in the palm of the hand by a small spring which pulls the metacarpophalangeal joints into flexion but allows the patient to extend the joints (Figure 21.9).

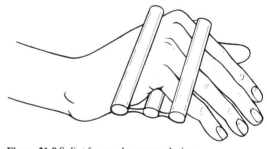

Figure 21.9 Splint for an ulnar nerve lesion

Physiotherapy

The paralysis will impede most activities of the hand, which will be particularly incapacitating if it is the dominant hand. The functional splint described above may allow reasonable use of the hand if the patient is encouraged and taught how to use it.

The sensory loss can cause problems and the patient must be warned to be careful of activities using the ulnar side of the hand, for example taking something out of the oven.

If the nerve has to be sutured at the elbow this will not normally interfere with treatment to the hand. However, a lesion at the wrist may require a modified treatment in the early stage to avoid stretching the nerve. There will probably be damage to other structures, possibly the median nerve and/or flexor tendons, which will complicate the rehabilitation.

Median nerve

The median nerve can be damaged in any part of its course but the commonest lesions are in the region of the wrist. Lacerations in this area that cause a lesion of the nerve are often combined with a lesion of the ulnar nerve and damage to the flexor tendons. The other type of lesion is a compression of median nerve in the carpal tunnel.

Laceration at the wrist causing a neurotmesis

Clinical features

The muscles paralysed are those of the thenar eminence, abductor pollicis brevis and opponens pollicis (the flexor pollicis brevis is usually supplied by the ulnar nerve), and the first two lumbricals. As a result of this the thumb lies back on the same plane as the fingers, producing the deformity known as the monkey hand (main en singe).

The sensory loss gives anaesthesia of the lateral side of the palm of the hand and the palmar surface of the thumb, index, middle and half the ring fingers. Sometimes there is a disturbance rather than a loss of sensation which may cause hyperaesthesia and pain.

Trophic changes are often apparent in this lesion which may be due to the large number of vasomotor fibres in the nerve and in part may be due to damage to the area because of the lack of sensation.

Specific points of management

The nerve will be sutured and the wrist maintained in flexion for approximately 3 weeks. Following this the patient will be supplied with a lively splint to keep the thumb in partial opposition which should enable the patient to use the hand. The splint consists of a strap round the wrist and another round the proximal part of the thumb. The two bands are connected by an elastic band which pulls the thumb into partial opposition and yet allows the patient to extend and abduct the thumb.

Physiotherapy

Passive movements must be given to all movements of the thumb. The patient may be taught to do the movements but care must be taken that they are properly carried out.

The patient must be given instructions about the care of areas of anaesthesia. When a lively splint is fitted the patient can be encouraged to use the hand as much as possible. Motor and sensory re-education must be given to try to regain normal function.

Carpal tunnel compression

This may occur in women in the fourth or fifth decade and may be the result of soft-tissue changes, particularly swelling of synovial sheaths. It is also a complication that occurs with rheumatoid arthritis.

Clinical feature

The early problems may be largely sensory, with pain and tingling in the area of sensory supply. Later there may be an area of anaesthesia and paralysis of the muscles mentioned under laceration at the wrist.

Management

Surgical division of the flexor retinaculum will give relief of compression. This is usually followed by complete recovery of sensation and almost full function.

Radial nerve

Lesions in the axilla may be due to compression or, more rarely, a wound. Pressure can be caused by falling asleep with the arm over the back of a chair, or in the case of patients using axillary crutches it may be due to incorrect use of the crutches.

Fractures of the mid-shaft of the humerus may cause a lesion of the nerve because of its position in the humeral sulcus. This could be a neurotmesis, axonotmesis or neuropraxia. A neuropraxia is sometimes a late complication following this fracture if there is a lot of callus formation.

Supracondylar fractures of the humerus or fracture dislocations of the elbow may injure the radial nerve.

Clinical features

A lesion of the nerve below the axilla will result in paralysis of the following muscles: brachioradialis, extensors carpi radialis longus and brevis, supinator, extensor digitorum, extensor digiti minimi, extensor carpi ulnaris, extensor pollicis longus, extensor indicis, abductor pollicis longus and extensor pollicis brevis. The main problem is the inability to extend the wrist and fingers. The loss of the synergistic action of the wrist extensors prevents the patient using the finger flexors adequately to grip. If the lesion is in the axilla there may be a slight weakness of the triceps.

The sensory loss causes minimal disability in this lesion as the area of anaesthesia would be on the dorsal aspect of the hand apart from a tiny area on the anterolateral side of the thenar eminence.

Specific points of management

If the injury results in a neurotmesis the nerve will have to be sutured. A lively splint will be fitted when possible to allow functional use of the hand. This comprises a leather (or other suitable material) support for the forearm incorporating a metal bar on the lateral side. This has a spring hinge at the wrist and a horizontal bar which goes across the palm to keep the wrist in extension. Thus the patient can use the finger flexors but also can actively flex the wrist.

Physiotherapy

Passive movements are very important in this lesion both to maintain joint range and muscle length. A number of the muscles work over more than one joint and must be fully stretched otherwise it may be difficult to gain good function even if regeneration of the nerve occurs. If the patient is going to do their own passive movements these points must be emphasized, and the physiotherapist must see that they are being carried out properly.

Re-education will be related mainly to motor function.

The above lesions are those that are most commonly seen. Any others will demand basic principles of management and any specific points depending on the lesion. It is worth mentioning three other lesions, but details of management will not be given here:

1. *Brachial plexus lesion* – These are usually traction injuries or may be caused by a wound. There may be damage to all the roots of the plexus: C5, C6, C7, C8, and T1.
2. *Erb's palsy* – Usually this is the result of a birth injury and damages the fibres of the 5th and 6th cervical nerves.
3. *Klumpke's paralysis* – This may be caused by sudden traction or possibly a birth injury and damages fibres from C8 and T1. Birth injuries are not as common now with better obstetric care.

Lower extremity

Sciatic nerve

It is fortunate that the whole nerve is seldom injured, as the resulting functional loss is so considerable. Occasionally it may be damaged as the result of a traumatic posterior dislocation of the hip joint. If the whole nerve is damaged the paralysis will affect the hamstrings and all the muscles of the lower leg and foot. There will be a sensory loss of the whole of the lower leg and foot except for the medial side.

Femoral nerve

This nerve is seldom damaged but if it were, the result would be a paralysis of the quadriceps and anaesthesia over most of the anterior aspect of the thigh and the medial side of the lower leg and foot.

Management

Details will not be given for the above two lesions as they are relatively uncommon.

Common peroneal nerve

This is the most commonly injured of the nerves in the leg and usually occurs as the result of injury round the neck of the fibula. The lesion may occur as a complication of fractures of the neck of the fibula or lateral tibial condyle, or there may be compression by splints or plaster of Paris. The injury may affect the common peroneal or one of the two branches. The deep peroneal nerve is the most likely to be damaged.

Clinical features

If the common peroneal nerve is damaged there will be paralysis of the tibialis anterior, extensor hallucis longus, extensor digitorum, peroneus longus, peroneus brevis and peroneus tertius. This will give a loss of dorsiflexion, extension of the toes and eversion. Inversion will be weak because of the paralysis of the tibialis anterior. Hence the patient will tend to drag the foot when walking and to avoid this usually flexes the hip and knee, thus giving a high-stepping gait. The sensory loss is over the lateral side of the lower leg and the dorsum of the foot, but this does not cause any functional disability.

When only the deep peroneal nerve is damaged the peroneus longus and brevis are not paralysed and so eversion can occur in the plantar flexed position. The functional disability in walking will be the same as with the common peroneal lesion. The sensory loss is much less, only affecting the web between the big toe and second toe.

Specific points of management

It is important that a patient is carefully watched after the application of a splint or plaster so that any loss of toe extension can be seen or any altered sensation on the dorsal aspect of the toes noted. If any loss is observed then the pressure can be relieved and there should be full recovery. If the trauma has caused a neurotmesis then this will be sutured. Following this the patient may be supplied with a light-weight plastic splint which prevents the foot dropping into plantar flexion. This can be worn inside the shoe, the splint passing from the sole of the foot under the heel and up the back of the calf where it may be kept in place with straps and Velcro fastenings. A splint may be necessary at night to stop the foot falling into plantar flexion for a prolonged period which could result in a contracture of the calf muscles.

Physiotherapy

A neuropraxia may not require any treatment, but when there is degeneration of the nerve it is important to keep full-range passive movements especially of dorsiflexion. If the patient is able to walk this will help to keep a stretch on the tendo-calcaneum.

During the stage of paralysis the physiotherapist must ensure that the patient walks as well as the disability allows, particularly when the patient is wearing a splint to keep the foot in dorsiflexion.

As regeneration occurs the muscles must be strengthened and normal function regained. The extent of re-education will depend on the needs of the patient both at work and for leisure activities.

Polyneuropathies (polyneuritis)

As the name implies this disorder results in a widespread dysfunction of the peripheral nerves and affects both somatic and visceral systems. There are a number of known causes but some causal agents are unknown particularly in the neuropathies produced by metabolic defects. Direct infection is rare but indirect infection such as occurs in the Landry–Guillain–Barré syndrome is relatively common. This is a post-infective polyneuropathy and seems to be the result of an autoimmune response following a viral infection or an allergen. Metabolic causes include toxic substances, such as some of the heavy metals; one of the side-effects of some drugs can be a polyneuropathy; lack of certain vitamins such as B_1 and B_{12}; and some endocrine disorders, the most common of which is diabetes. Vascular disorders such as atheroma can lead to a polyneuropathy because of the upset in blood supply to the nerve fibres. Collagen disorders, for example rheumatoid arthritis and polyarteritis nodosa, can develop a polyneuropathy. There are also genetic disorders, for example peroneal muscular dystrophy.

The method of onset will vary depending on the cause, and so an infective or post-infective polyneuropathy will have an acute or subacute onset. Some metabolic disorders may give an acute or subacute onset although endocrine disturbances such as diabetes tend to be more chronic. Vascular and collagen diseases usually have an insidious development.

Pathology

Depending on the cause of the condition there are two different pathological processes that can take place:

1. *Axonal degeneration* – The nerve cell body and the axon are affected, and the process is similar to Wallerian degeneration. If regeneration occurs it is not complete and recovery is slow. Axonal degeneration tends to occur in neuropathies with the following causes: poisons, nutritional deficiencies, ischaemia.
2. *Segmental demyelination* – This affects the Schwann cell, resulting in a demyelination. Recovery is more likely to occur in this type of lesion and if it does it happens quickly and is usually complete. This type of process may occur with a diabetic neuropathy and the Guillain–Barré syndrome.

Clinical features

An early feature is often sensory with the patient complaining of pain, tingling, and numbness, which usually occur in the hands and feet. Muscle weakness and/or paralysis occurs mainly in the limbs, and the lower more than the upper limbs. It is more marked distally than proximally and often results in a foot drop or wrist drop.

Contractures develop early and there may be fibrous adhesions. Loss of proprioception gives an ataxia which can be observed if the patient has some active movement, and is particularly marked in the lower limbs giving the patient a high-stepping gait.

The tendon reflexes will be decreased or lost. Trophic changes may lead to the skin appearing red and shiny, and there may be increased sweating and oedema. Sometimes there can be cardiac involvement resulting in cardiac arrhythmia.

Some of the cranial nerves can be affected in certain neuropathies.

Guillain–Barré syndrome

Usually this has an acute onset although sometimes it is subacute, and the patient may have a fever. The paralysis starts distally and moves proximally. Also it may affect the trunk and head muscles. Respiratory and bulbar paralysis may be a complication of this condition.

Sensory changes are variable and may be severe, with hyperalgia and hyperaesthesia, or there may be some cases with no sensory disturbance.

Management

This will depend on the cause of the neuropathy. Improved safety precautions in industry have decreased the incidence of cases due to heavy metals or chemicals. Careful testing of drugs should reduce side-effects such as polyneuropathy. Polyneuropathies resulting from vitamin deficiencies may recover or the progress be halted if the deficiency is remedied. Polyneuropathies from vascular or collagen diseases are unlikely to recover although drug therapy may slow the progress of the disease. Patients with the Guillain–Barré syndrome will usually recover fully although the rate of recovery may be slow. Nevertheless there can be fatalities with this syndrome particularly when there is an epidemic. Some of these patients with respiratory and bulbar problems will have to be treated in an intensive care unit.

Physiotherapy

In cases where there is little chance of recovery the main objective is to retain as much function as possible. It is important to prevent the development of contractures, and so passive movements to maintain joint range and muscle length must be given regularly. These are necessary to assist the circulation as deep vein thrombosis can be a complication particularly with loss of movement and the effect of the muscle pump. The patient probably cannot perform his own passive movements and if not it may be possible to teach a relative to do them.

The patient must be taught correct positioning and support for sitting and lying and the importance of moving to prevent any pressure sores. The patient (or relatives) must be taught to look for any evidence of pressure causing reddening of the skin.

Light-weight splints may be given to keep the correct position of joints, and in some cases to assist function, but these must be padded and care must be taken to see that that they do not cause pressure sores.

Pain and hyperaesthesia may present a problem in performing passive movements; consequently techniques and positioning may have to be modified. If analgesics are given to relieve pain, treatment should be carried out when relief of pain has occurred, if possible.

When recovery is occurring re-education of sensory and motor function should be carried out using the appropriate techniques. Coordination exercises may be given if the patient is ataxic. Patients must be helped to gain their maximum potential, both psychologically and physically.

Physiotherapy in the intensive therapy unit

Physiotherapy in the intensive therapy unit will be similar to that described elsewhere. Apart from respiratory care particular attention must be given to passive movements and maintaining a good functional position of the joints. Pain and hyperaesthesia may be a problem as mentioned above in treatment for general polyneuropathies. Both nursing and physiotherapy staff will be concerned in the prevention of pressure sores.

Once the patient recovers sufficiently to leave the intensive therapy unit recovery may begin, and the physiotherapist will be concerned with motor and sensory (if needed) re-education. This progress is likely to be slow, and it is important that the patient is aware of this as he is likely to become depressed and frustrated unless sufficient counselling and support is given by the professionals concerned. Improvements must be carefully charted so that the patient and therapist are aware of the points of recovery.

Acknowledgement

We thank Mrs Ann Reed for her help and for the use of the strength–duration curve (Figure 21.8).

Chapter 22

Neurological conditions affecting children

Cerebral palsy *Spina bifida*

The two conditions that form the majority of cases requiring physiotherapy management in the UK are cerebral palsy and spina bifida. Anterior poliomyelitis was a common disease affecting children until the advent of the Salk vaccine, and it is still common in countries that do not have an adequate inoculation programme. Other neurological conditions – some of which have already been described, such as peripheral nerve lesions and post-viral polyneuropathies – may affect children as well as adults. In these cases the management must be related to the age and needs of the child.

Cerebral palsy

In the past many children with severe cerebral palsy did not survive infancy, but now with improved medical and surgical care a greater number of these children survive, and present considerable problems for management. It is often difficult for families to cope with severely handicapped children and to try to integrate them into society.

Causes

There are a number of known causes as given below, but there are also cases in which the cause is unknown. Modern research has shown that some cases are the result of genetic abnormalities which may explain a number of those previously listed as unknown:

1. *In utero* – There may be a failure in development or maldevelopment of the brain. This may be due to the mother having a viral infection such as rubella, although the incidence of this has

decreased with the use of vaccination. Vascular insufficiency can occur *in utero*, and if the carotid or middle cerebral artery is occluded it may cause a hemiplegia.
2. Injury during birth may cause damage to the brain, particularly when there is a breech or forceps delivery. Injury may result in asphyxia and consequent brain damage. Preterm babies are especially at risk from injury at birth, or after birth because of immature development of some systems.

   An assessment of the baby may be carried out by the APGAR scale (Table 22.1) and resuscitation will be required if the score is under 7. If the scale is 7 or over then this may be regarded as normal. If the score is between 5 and 7 simple measures such as clearing the airway and administering oxygen may evoke an adequate response. Resuscitation of a baby when the score is under 5 is more difficult and depends on maintaining an adequate airway and gaining sufficient oxygenation.
3. Recent research has indicated that genetic abnormalities may be a cause of cerebral palsy.
4. Jaundice as a result of rhesus incompatability can lead to brain damage but this is less common now with better medical care.

Clinical features

These cover a wide range of problems depending on the specific areas affected and the extent of the damage. Some infants may have signs and symptoms similar to a hemiplegia, diplegia or monoplegia but on a detailed assessment less obvious abnormalities may be discerned elsewhere. Features can occur

Table 22.1 The Apgar scoring method

Sign	0	1	2	Score	
				1 min	*5 min*
Heart rate	Absent	Slow (below 100)	Over 100		
Respiratory effort	Absent	Weak cry; hypoventilation	Good; strong cry		
Muscle tone	Limp	Some flexion of extremities	Active movement, extremities well flexed		
Reflex irritability, (response to stimulation of sole of foot)	No response	Grimace	Cry		
Colour	Blue, pale	Body pink, extremities blue	Completely pink		

singly or in various combinations, for example one child may have a mild monoplegia, another may be a quadriplegic with the legs more affected than the arms whereas another may be a severe diplegic, mentally retarded and with visual and hearing defects. The following are some of the features that can occur:

1. Impaired movement.
2. Sensory defects.
3. Deformities.
4. Mental retardation.
5. Emotional disturbance.
6. Epilepsy.

Impaired movement

Spasticity

This is one of the commonest features presenting in cerebral palsy. There is increased tone in the affected muscles, with the degree of spasticity varying and being greater in some muscle groups than others. Sometimes reciprocal hypotonicity can be seen in opposing muscle groups. The degree of spasticity is also dependent on other factors. For example, if the child is frustrated, anxious, or frightened of moving because of pain the spasticity could be increased. External factors can increase or decrease the tone depending on the stimulus and which part of the body is affected. Poor handling, splints and chairs can all affect the level of spasticity. Skin irritation such as may be caused by incontinence can increase the hypertonicity.

Spasticity will impair the use of normal movement patterns, in some instances totally whereas in others abnormal patterns are created. Lack of use of normal muscles will lead to weakness which can further exacerbate the problem of trying to obtain effective movement.

Reflexes

Depending on the area and level of damage in the central nervous system there may be abnormalities of reflex action. Spinal reflexes may be affected with increased sensitivity to stretch of muscle or tendon. There may be a release of primitive reflexes: tonic neck symmetrical or asymmetrical reflexes, tonic labyrinthine reflexes, Moro and grasp reflex.

Athetoid and choreiform movements (dyskinesias)

These abnormalities occur as the result of damage to parts of the corpus striatum, the associated nuclei and pathways. Athetoid and choreiform types of abnormalities both give unwanted, uncontrolled movements. In the case of athetosis the movements are slow, large and writhing in character and are made worse by attempts at voluntary movement. If both sides of the body are affected then there are usually marked facial movements, grimacing, protrusion and withdrawal of the tongue. Choreiform movements are quicker and purposeless, or may appear to be part of a purposeful movement which is then changed. Thus there are a series of disorderly movements which again are exacerbated by attempts at voluntary movement. Facial movements are bilateral and as with the body movements they are quick-changing and disorderly resulting in bizarre grimaces. Athetoid movements cease during sleep but choreiform activity continues.

Ataxia

This is a rare feature in cerebral palsy. If it occurs it is usually the result of cerebellar damage resulting in hypotonia, incoordination, intention tremor and possibly dysarthria.

Incoordination of movement

This will occur with all the above abnormalities of movement. However, in some children with cerebral plasy a mild incoordination resulting in the child being labelled as 'clumsy' may be the only apparent problem and the underlying cause may only be revealed as the result of a detailed assessment.

Flaccidity

In the first year or two after birth the child may appear 'floppy' with a hypotonia which may later change to hypertonia, or become athetoid.

Speech defects

Movement disorders can affect speech giving dysarthria, or speech may be affected by deafness or mental retardation.

Chewing and swallowing may be a problem in some of the severely handicapped children.

Sensory defects

Defects may occur because of damage in the cerebral sensory areas or pathways. The child may have a sensory agnosia and be unable to recognize objects by feeling them. Perceptual defects may result in the child being unaware of the limb and so they may ignore the affected arm or leg.

Vision

This can vary from normal to severe visual handicap or blindness. Squints occur fairly commonly in these children.

Hearing

If the damage has affected the auditory centre or pathways the child may have impaired hearing or even be deaf.

Deformities

These are very likely to occur as the result of abnormal movement or lack of movement. The child tends to adopt certain postures for a number of reasons. Spasticity may produce abnormal postures or the child may only be comfortable in a certain position. The child may need to hold an abnormal position in order to produce an effective movement. Athetoid and choreiform movements will give distorted postures. Initially these deformities will be postural, but if they are not corrected they will become structural which will lead to increased problems in obtaining any useful movement and also difficulties in handling.

Mental retardation

It is very difficult to assess the degree of intelligence of a severely spastic or athetoid child as the usual intelligence tests rely on the possession of normal faculties. This is made even more difficult in children who in addition may have visual, speech and hearing defects. A high proportion of children with cerebral palsy do suffer from true mental retardation which will decrease their ability to respond to treatment. It is important to realize that a child who suffers from a combination of severe physical defects may appear to be mentally retarded because of his inability to explore the world around him. A normal toddler of 18 months is continually exploring his environment and so is learning all the time. However, this experience is denied to the child with cerebral palsy, who is relatively immobile.

Emotional disturbance

This may accompany mental retardation as a result of the brain damage. However, children with severe physical defects and normal intelligence may develop emotional disturbances as a result of their frustration at their inability to move, or difficulty in communicating, inability to participate with other children in education or play, and sometimes because of lack of love and care from the family.

Epilepsy

This is quite a common complication occurring with some children with cerebral palsy and may complicate the management of the child both at home and at school. It may lead to further brain damage and a gradual deterioration of the condition.

Management

The damage causing the various problems of physical and/or mental disability is not progressive. However, the disabilities may become worse or more apparent as the child grows. Contractures may lead to the development of fixed deformities which will increase the difficulty in positioning, and the ability of the child to move. The child may have difficulty in coping with the increasing demands involved with passing from infancy to childhood to adolescence and finally into adult life which may lead to emotional disturbance as mentioned in the previous section.

Any young baby who appears to have abnormalities of muscle tone, posture and movement should attend a specialist unit for assessment as soon as possible. The medical history of the mother, particularly during pregnancy, and details of the birth might indicate the possibility of a neurological problem. It may be impossible to arrive at a definite conclusion with regard to any neurological abnormality in the early months after birth, but nevertheless there are two good reasons for seeing the child at this stage. Firstly the parents can be shown how to handle their baby and be asked to report any progress or adverse changes. Secondly the assessment will give an indication of the need for further assessments.

An assessment of the level of intelligence may be very difficult to make in a young child, particularly when there is difficulty with speech. An educational psychologist will be an important member of the team in assessing the mental ability of the child.

The management will depend on the number of problems and will also differ with each child. It is essential to know whether the parents are fully committed to helping the child, and their ability to cope as this will make a difference to the amount of specialist help required. In mild cases the parents may be able to manage the child with help and advice from specialists when required. Severely handicapped children may need to be managed by a team of specialists, perhaps within a specialist unit.

The child may require treatment from a number of specialists and it is important that this is carefully discussed by the management team to ascertain which members are essential to the treatment programme. Too many professionals dealing with the child and parents can be detrimental to progress as well as being confusing. There must be careful coordination between the members of the team and each must understand the role of the others in the programme.

School age

This may present a dilemma between the priorities of medical care and the education of the child.

This subject cannot be discussed in detail in this book but it is important that the physiotherapist is aware of the problems and that the team consisting of parents (and child if possible), educationists and health care professionals can look at all the issues involved before deciding on the management. The aim of all concerned is to allow the child to have as normal a development as possible, in all respects.

If the child is able to benefit from a normal education it is preferable for this to be in a normal school. However, in the case of severe physical disability and handicap this may present problems because of the amount of assistance needed for any physical activity and special requirements for toileting, sitting, use of wheelchairs, and not least the requirements for treatment by health care professionals. Up to the present the majority of these children have attended special schools where all the specialist facilities are available, but this removes them from the stimulus of mainstream

and from the opportunity to be accepted in the normal school community. Sometimes the problems can be overcome if there is a specialist unit within a school so that the child can mix socially. This still leaves some children who will require special schooling because of their physical disability and consequent learning problems. In the case of the child with severe mental retardation care may be needed in a special unit.

Surgery

This may be necessary to correct a deformity such as talipes equinovarus, or adducted thighs, or flexed knees. Unfortunately the deformity may tend to recur following surgical correction as the muscle imbalance that caused it is still present. However, it may be worth taking this risk if it is likely to allow the child to walk.

Paradoxically the correction of a deformity may occasionally make it more difficult to walk as he may have become accustomed to the abnormal gait, and to the balance of the trunk that is required to achieve it.

The use of drugs

Epilepsy, which is relatively common in these children, may be controlled by the regular use of drugs.

Some children with severe spasticity may benefit from the administration of anti-spasmodic drugs, such as baclofen, but they may have unpleasant side-effects and should not be used when there is epilepsy.

Counselling

Whenever possible the parents must be included in the management team. They need to be able to discuss their problems in managing the child and how he relates to family life and their social environment. Then the professionals must explain their plans based on their assessment and taking into account the problems and prospects as seen by the family. The parents will not always accept that the goals they set for the child may be considered to be over-optimistic by the professionals. Sometimes the parents may be right and the child may achieve more than was anticipated, particularly when the child is intelligent, well motivated and in a family where there is help, encouragement and love. Sometimes parents are not satisfied with the treatment offered and look for other methods of treatment. They have every right to do this but it can lead to enormous cost, sometimes disappointment when no more is achieved, and it can cause a great strain on family relationships.

There are other aspects of counselling, which cannot be discussed here, but the management team should be aware of the need for counselling and should arrange for the appropriate person to do this, whether it is one of the team or a professional counsellor.

Physiotherapy

Assessment

An assessment should be carried out as soon as any abnormality of movement or lack of movement is detected. This may be prior to a firm diagnosis of cerebral palsy as this may be difficult to establish, particularly in children with a mild disability or where the severity of the disability is not apparent immediately after birth. The physiotherapist will be able to keep a record of the stage the baby has reached in the developmental sequence of movement and to note whether this is normal for the age of the baby. It is important to remember that the stages of development vary considerably in normal children which may make assessment difficult. If abnormality is suspected then the child must be assessed regularly, and some treatment and advice to the parents may be required.

When an assessment has been made of a child with cerebral palsy this will be discussed with the team so that a coordinated management programme can be arranged.

Treatment

There are a number of special methods of physical treatment which have been developed to facilitate movement and function in the child with cerebral palsy. It is beyond the scope of this book to give details of any of the methods that need to be studied at post-registration level by those physiotherapists wishing to specialize in this field.

The physiotherapist must be flexible in her approach to the child and the family and must adapt the treatment plan to suit the particular child, possibly making use of a selection of methods. The earlier any physical treatment is started the better, before deformities and stereotyped patterns of movement have become fixed.

The physiotherapist should encourage the development of skills such as head control, rolling, balance in sitting, kneeling and later in standing, and movements such as creeping, crawling and walking. She should try to inhibit abnormal reflexes and patterns of movement, and to prevent deformity. The goal must be to achieve as much independence with regard to normal function as possible, taking account of the individual disabilities, particularly in the multiply-handicapped child.

Mobility – It is very important to enable the child to move around as this enables him to explore a wider area, to have a measure of independence and to mix with other children. If the child is not able to walk he may be able to use a wheelchair. A number of children cannot manage a wheelchair and nowadays there are a variety of powered chairs which can enable a severely disabled child to move around with some freedom.

Special methods of treatment

Neuro-developmental treatment

Dr and Mrs Bobath stress the use of the developmental sequence of movement patterns together with inhibition of abnormal patterns, which are present because of the persistence of tonic reflexes. Correct handling of the child with the use of key points of control and various sensory stimuli is used by the physiotherapist and is taught to the parents.

Facilitation of normal postural control is stressed as the child is unable to perform functional activities, which involve limb movements, if he is unable to maintain and control his posture. The parents must be shown how to handle their child at home for feeding, bathing, dressing and other activities.

Sensory stimulation for activation and inhibition of movement

This approach has been developed by Margaret Rood, who is a physiotherapist and occupational therapist.

Miss Rood makes use of different types of stimulation, both cutaneous, such as stroking, and deep, such as muscle stretching, in order to activate or inhibit motor activity. She classifies muscles according to their use for light or heavy work and has indicated the appropriate stimuli in each case. The developmental sequence of movement suggested by Temple Fay is used to try to activate normal patterns. This is based on primitive patterning which start with reptilian and amphibious types of symmetrical movements of the arm and leg on the same side and then the other side, followed later by asymmetrical movements as in human movements.

Miss Rood makes use of some reflexes to reduce spasticity and encourage movement.

Proprioceptive neuromuscular facilitation (PNF)

This method was developed in America by Dr Kabat and two physiotherapists, Margaret Knott and Dorothy Voss. It makes use of functional patterns of movement rather than individual muscles or groups. These patterns all include rotatory and diagonal components. Sensory stimulation is used to facilitate the movements, touch, quick stretch of muscle, traction or compression of joints, pressure and the use of voice.

These techniques were not primarily developed for the treatment of children with cerebral palsy and they are probably of most value in children with muscle weakness.

Doman delecato

This is based on the work of Temple Fay and uses repeated passive patterning. It is claimed that if these patterns are repeated often enough and are accompanied by reverse hanging and the developmental sequence of movement it may facilitate the use of dormant pathways in the nervous system and even development of the brain.

The insistence upon repeated patterning throughout the day with the assistance of friends and neighbours places a considerable strain upon the family and can affect the home life of other children.

Conductive education

This method was devised by Dr A. Peto in Hungary and concentrates on all aspects of the life of the child. A 'conductor' supervises the child from when he wakes up until bedtime, and is concerned with all the activities of the child throughout the day. Speech is used to reinforce movements firstly by the conductor and then the child states the movement while attempting to perform it. As with the Doman delecato method it is very intensive and requires dedication from the 'conductor' and considerable effort from the child and parents.

Other techniques

There are many other techniques or methods of treatment available to the physiotherapist. For example, biofeedback which indicates to the child his position in space and the activity of muscles, which may enable some children to gain more control over their movements.

Spina bifida

This is one of the most common of the major congenital abnormalities, occurring in between 1 and 2 per 1000 births.

There is a developmental defect in the vertebral column (Figure 22.1) resulting in a lack of fusion of the vertebral arches and so the vertebral canal is not closed. The bony defect may or may not be accompanied by defects of the spinal cord and meninges. Usually the lesion occurs in the lumbosacral region but in a few cases it may be found in another area of the spine. The vertebral defect occurs early in embryonic life and may be associated with other developmental abnormalities giving deformities such as talipes equino varus.

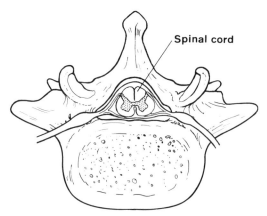

Figure 22.1 View of superior aspect of normal lumbar vertebra to show position of the spinal cord

Cause

The cause is not clear but it would appear that there may be a genetic link or it may be due to something that affects the neural tube *in utero*.

Pathology

There are two main types of this abnormality, spina bifida occulta and spina bifida cystica.

Spina bifida occulta (Figure 22.2)

This is the mildest form of the defect and is supposed to occur in only a small percentage of children with spina bifida. The actual number may be larger because there may not be any obvious defect or abnormality. There is a defect in the fusion of the laminal arch but this may only be evident on X-ray. Quite often there is a band of fibrous tissue

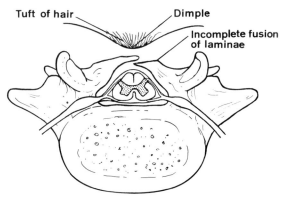

Figure 22.2 Spina bifida occulta

between the skin and the bone which results in an indentation (dimple) in the skin over the vertebrae, and sometimes there may be a small tuft of hair over the area. The nervous tissue may be unaffected in some children but in others neurological symptoms may appear as growth occurs and if so are usually apparent in adolescence. A common feature of this type of lesion is abnormality of bladder control with either an enuresis or urine retention.

Spina bifida cystica

Menigocele

The vertebral arch is not fused and a sac protrudes containing meninges and cerebrospinal fluid. The spinal cord lies in the vertebral canal and is normal, so there are no signs of neurological abnormality (Figure 22.3).

Myelomeningocele (Figure 22.4)

This is the most severe form of spina bifida and there is inevitably neurological damage. In this instance the protruding sac contains part of the spinal cord or the cauda equina, depending on the

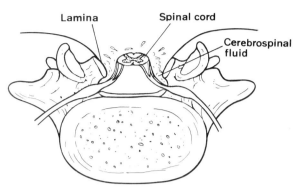

Figure 22.5 Rachischisis

level of the lesion. The spinal cord or cauda equina are abnormal, being dysplasic or underdeveloped. There may be a thin fragile skin covering over the sac or it may only be covered by arachnoid mater. Breakdown of this covering leads to infection which may cause further neurological damage. In the most severe type of myelomeningocele called rachischisis (Figure 22.5) there is no protruding sac or skin covering and a flattened spinal cord lies on the surface.

Hydrocephalus

Over 80% of children with myelomeningocele have an associated hydrocephalus due to obstruction of the flow of cerebrospinal fluid. The obstruction usually occurs between the 4th ventricle and the subarachnoid space. Absorption of cerebrospinal fluid from the subarachnoid space to the veins is also impaired. The resultant rise of pressure within the lateral ventricles leads to distension of the ventricles. In the baby this distension causes expansion of the skull which is possible because of the flexibility of the sutures and fontanelles at this age. As the head becomes enlarged there are signs of compression of the cerebral hemispheres. These signs may include mental retardation and sometimes optic atrophy.

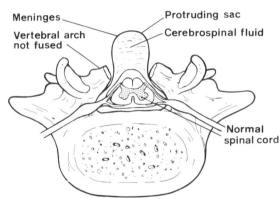

Figure 22.3 Meningocele

Clinical features of a myelomeningocele

1. There is an obvious lesion over the vertebral defect on the back. This may appear as a mass with a thin covering of skin which can easily break down and become infected. Alternatively in rachischisis the neurological tissue is outside the vertebral canal and is uncovered.
2. *Muscle paralysis and/or weakness* – This will depend on the level and the extent of the lesion. If the upper motor neurons are affected there may be a spastic paraplegia with no voluntary

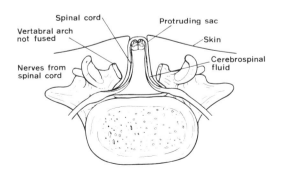

Figure 22.4 Myelomeningocele

movement below the level of the lesion. However, in some cases the cord is only partially damaged and there may be some voluntary movement. When the cauda equina is damaged there will be a flaccid paralysis which again can be partial or complete depending on the extent of the lesion.

3. *Sensory impairment* – As with the motor loss this can be variable depending on the extent and level of the lesion. A complete loss of cutaneous sensation in the lower limbs presents considerable problems in management.

4. *Rectal and/or bladder incontinence* – The majority of these children will have a neurogenic bladder and loss of sphincter control.

5. *Hydrocephalus* – Enlargement of the head will be an obvious indication of this condition.

6. *Other congenital abnormalities* – As spina bifida is a defect in development it is quite likely that there may be other abnormalities particularly of the lower limbs or spine.

7. *Mental retardation* – This is particularly likely to be a problem in children with hydrocephalus.

Management

Surgery may be necessary to repair the spinal defect and prevent further damage but this will depend on the severity of the lesion and the likely prognosis. If there is a hydrocephalus then the child is usually fitted with a shunt to drain the cerebrospinal fluid from the ventricles in the brain to a vein in the neck, or the right atrium in the heart (Spitz–Holster), or the peritoneum. However, there is a danger of infection, or the shunt may become blocked, and so the child must be watched carefully.

When spina bifida is diagnosed a detailed assessment may be carried out by the paediatrician and if necessary a neurosurgeon. Then plans will be drawn up for the short- and, if possible, the long-term management. Initially it may be difficult to decide on long-term management until the extent of the neurological damage is clear, and also whether there is any mental retardation.

Urinary incontinence may be dealt with by catheterization and sometimes in girls by ureteroileostomy, although the latter is less commonly used now because of the problem of back-pressure.

Various deformities can develop in the spine, hips, knees or feet. Some cases of spina bifida, and particularly those with a higher lesion, can be complicated by spinal curves such as a kyphosis, scoliosis or kyphoscoliosis. These may be the result of structural abnormalities of the vertebrae or because of muscle paralysis. Braces may help mild structural curves or those due to paralysis but are of no use for the severe structural curves which may require surgery. There may be subluxation or dislocation of the hip(s) which can be left if the child is unlikely to walk. However, if there is a likelihood of the child being able to walk the dislocation may be reduced and in some instances surgery may be required. Foot deformities such as talipes equino varus may require passive stretching and strapping.

Depending on the level of the lesion and the extent of the paralysis, braces may be supplied to enable the child to stand and walk. However, these have to be considered very carefully as many children will not wear them and gain better independence in a wheelchair, tricycle or other form of wheeled frame.

Counselling of parents

Counselling and support for the family is an important aspect of management.

Education

The problems are similar to those mentioned under the management of children with cerebral palsy. Integration into a normal school is the goal whenever possible, but it must be after a careful assessment of the child to see whether he will be able to cope with the various aspects of school life. Sometimes although the child can manage, the school is not a suitable environment because it is not able or prepared to deal with physically handicapped children. It may be difficult to find a suitable school within travelling distance for the child, so there are many problems to be overcome in giving the child both the best education and a normal school environment.

Physiotherapy

Assessment

As soon as the diagnosis of spina bifida is made the physiotherapist will make an assessment. The findings and proposed management will be discussed in conjunction with the other members of the team so that an overall plan can be made. The techniques for assessing posture and movement follow the normal developmental patterns and will depend on the age of the child. An assessment to determine the extent of any sensory impairment is important partly because of the problem of anaesthesia and partly because it will affect motor development. The areas of anaesthesia must be carefully noted because of the danger of developing pressure sores.

The physiotherapist will notice the reactions of the baby or child to the assessment, and with a child this may give an indication of his ability to understand and cooperate with the treatment. This in turn will affect the objectives and methods of treatment that can be chosen.

It is important that the physiotherapist asks the parents, or other health care professionals, to report any activity or reactions so that as much useful information as possible is gained.

Treatment

The plans formulated as a result of the examination must aim to develop the full potential of the child, but they must be realistic. It may be some time before an estimate can be made of the level of physical and mental ability that the child will attain. Thus it is very important that there is a continuous evaluation in order to keep a record of any changes that may indicate progression or regression.

The following are some of the problems that the physiotherapist may have to deal with:

1. Lack of movement or abnormal movement patterns.
2. Deformities.
3. Anaesthesia.
4. Psychological problems.
5. Functional activities.

Lack of movement or abnormal movement patterns

These will depend on the extent of the paralysis and weakness of muscles. The physiotherapist will give maximal stimulation to encourage and develop any active movement that can be potentially useful. The parents and other carers will be made aware of the programme and goals so that they can assist and encourage the child. If there are weak muscles the physiotherapist will try to strengthen them using techniques suitable for the age of the child. When there is sufficient normal activity in the lower limbs and the trunk the physiotherapist will try to develop the normal sequence of movement through rolling, sitting, crawling and eventually to standing. However, not all children go through the same sequence; for example not all children crawl, as some go from sitting to standing and then walking.

If the child has sufficient activity in the legs and trunk to stand and walk they may need some form of support. There are various forms of orthoses available or they may have to be specially made for the child with a particular problem. As well as giving adequate support these should be light so that the child can move. Many children prefer to use a wheelchair, tricycle or other form of aid to mobility which will give them greater freedom to move around, particularly if the orthosis is cumbersome and does not allow them the same mobility.

Deformities

The physiotherapist will try to prevent deformities occurring by correct positioning and by teaching parents and other health care workers how to handle the child. Passive movements will be carried out to try to prevent contractures and it is particularly important to maintain full extension as flexion deformities are most likely to occur. Maintaining full range in the joints will allow the child the opportunity to develop any active movement if it is present. It also helps those who are caring for the child to handle and position him more easily. If deformities are present the treatment will depend on how much structural change has occurred. For example, a talipes equinovarus can be treated with passive movements and strapping before structural changes have developed, and this is very important if the child is likely to be able to walk. Later the child may wear specially made shoes. Physiotherapy cannot alter structural deformities but their presence may affect the ability of the child to achieve physical activity and function. The physiotherapist may help by advising on positioning and handling in order to allow optimum function, and also comfort.

As the child grows there is a need to look at seating, particularly if the child is restricted to a sitting position. A chair must give correct support and be adequately padded as well as allowing the child to use the upper limbs as fully as possible. A specially made chair may be required to give adequate support, and when there is a deformity of the spine a plastic mould may be made which is then fitted to the chair and padded. If the chair is used at school the teacher should be consulted as adjustment of other apparatus may be required, such as a writing surface or work-top.

Anaesthesia

This is a difficult problem and everyone looking after the child must be taught how to prevent pressure sores and avoid knocks or friction on anaesthetic areas. Once the child is old enough and can appreciate the problem he must be taught how to avoid pressure and friction. Everyone must watch for any signs of pressure and report it at once so that it can be dealt with before the skin breaks down and becomes infected. The physiotherapist is a key person in dealing with this as she is concerned with positioning and movement. She must look at pressure areas and be careful when treating the child, as well as teaching others to do the same.

Psychological problems

These children are very likely to have a variety of reactions to their disabilities and handicaps. There may be frustration at their inability to do something, depression, irritability or anger. The intelligent child may show some of these reactions, but so may the mentally retarded child who is unable to communicate. The physiotherapist requires sufficient knowledge to understand and cope with these problems. If the reactions are severe the child may need help from a clinical psychologist, or from an educational psychologist if there are learning problems.

Functional activities

All treatment is designed to gain as much functional activity as possible. The physiotherapist must work with other members of the team, the child and the parents to achieve this. Problems with access to buildings often make it difficult for these children to take part in normal activities, and health professionals must work to make others aware of the facilities required.

Chapter 23

Principles of surgery and physiotherapy management

Reasons for surgery
Preoperative treatment
Types of anaesthetic
Types of incision

Clips, ligatures and sutures
Postoperative treatment
Physiotherapy management

Reasons for surgery

Certain specialist surgical procedures have been described elsewhere in this book and so this chapter deals with the procedures that may be seen in a general surgical unit.

Surgery is undertaken for the following reasons:

1. *To remove diseased tissue* – In the case of an organ or a gland the operation is referred to by the suffix -ectomy. For example, haemorrhoidectomy is the removeal of haemorrhoids, a pneumonectomy is the removal of a lung, a mastectomy is the removal of the mammary gland. The removal may be complete or it may be partial, as with a partial gastrectomy. The removal of a limb is known as an amputation.

2. *For purposes of repair* – In these cases the suffix -orraphy is applied, and so the repair of a hernia is a herniorraphy, the repair of a lacerated perineum is colporrhaphy. Sometimes a repair has the suffix -plasty; for example, re-shaping a joint may be called an arthroplasty.

3. *To produce an artificial opening* – In such cases the suffix ·-otomy or -ostomy is applied. An opening made in the stomach for the purpose of feeding, or evacuating the stomach is a gastrostomy or gastrotomy. An opening made in the transverse or sigmoid colon for the evacuation of contents is called a colostomy, and an opening made in the trachea to assist breathing is termed a tracheostomy.

4. *For inspection* – If a speculum or some type of viewing apparatus is passed the suffix -oscopy is applied. A cystoscopy is the inspection of the bladder, gastroscopy the inspection of the stomach, sigmoidoscopy the inspection of the sigmoid colon. If an area is opened up for

inspection the term -otomy is again used; for example, a laparotomy is performed to inspect the abdominal contents.

Surgery may be planned or be carried out as an emergency life-saving procedure.

Preoperative treatment

Ideally the patient is admitted to hospital 24 hours or more before the operation. This allows the patient to settle in and to meet those who will be responsible for his treatment. Any necessary checks on the condition of the patient will be carried out, the operation site can be prepared, premedication given, and sedatives administered if required.

If any specialized treatment, tests, or investigations are considered necessary the patient will be admitted several days, or even weeks, before the operation.

Types of anaesthetic

Many of the former operative risks and complications arose from the methods of anaesthesia used. Today both the method and type of anaesthesia given have changed and this enables patients who would formerly have been unsuitable for operation to undergo and withstand surgery. It also enables surgeons to perform operations that were previously impossible.

The following methods are commonly used:

1. *General anaesthetic* – This is used for most major operations when it is necessary to render the patient unconscious. The anaesthetic may be

administered by inhalation or intravenously. Unlike chloroform and ether which were used in the past, modern drugs, such as pentothal, are easily broken down and excreted from the body. This avoids much of the nausea and vomiting common in former days, together with many postoperative risks.

2. *Local anaesthesia* – This is often used for minor surgery and has the advantage of reducing the post-operative risk of chest complications which can follow inhalation anaesthesia.

3. *Spinal anaesthesia* – The anaesthetic is injected in to the subarachnoid space surrounding the cauda equina. Anaesthesia of the perineal region and the legs can be achieved and this may be used for certain surgical procedures to the pelvis and legs.

4. *Regional anaesthesia* – Anaesthesia of a limb may be achieved by injecting an anaesthetic into the nerve plexus. This method may be used if the patient is not fit enough to tolerate general anaesthesia.

Types of incision

There have been many advances in the techniques of surgery which allow operations to be performed more speedily and so again reduce the risks to the patient that can occur with prolonged anaesthesia. The incisions shown in Figure 23.1 are those commonly used for abdominal surgery. The choice of incision will depend on a number of factors – such as the site of the organ or tissue to be operated on or whether it is necessary to inspect other parts of the abdominal cavity – and surgeons may have minor variations on the incisions that they will use.

Clips, ligatures and sutures

Materials used to hold the edges of a surgical incision in close apposition vary according to the operation and which method of closure a particular surgeon wishes to use. It is important to reduce the risk of infection as much as possible and this makes a difference to the materials that can be used. Catgut is still used as it is absorbed by tissue digestion and although it may act as a tissue irritant this only occurs for a few days. There are different types of catgut but chromic catgut is used for suturing the abdominal wall. It is strong and retains its strength for about 2 weeks and is usually absorbed after this time. Other materials used are lined thread, silk, nylon and stainless steel (or tantalum wire). More recently strips of micropore are being used, particularly for superficial wounds. These materials can be used as sutures when a surgical needle is used to stitch the tissue edges together, or for ligatures when the material is tied round a blood vessel or piece of tissue.

Clips may be used when it is important to gain a good cosmetic effect, as on the throat following a thyroidectomy. Clips are usually removed after 4–5 days and then the subcutaneous stitches protect the wound from any stretching.

Dressings are used to protect the incision from infection, make the patient more comfortable and to absorb any exudation. It is important to keep the wound as dry as possible. Gauze and adhesive strapping have been used to cover the incision but more recently some surgeons prefer to use an adherent seal.

Postoperative treatment

The patient may be moved to a recovery room where staff are specially trained to deal with

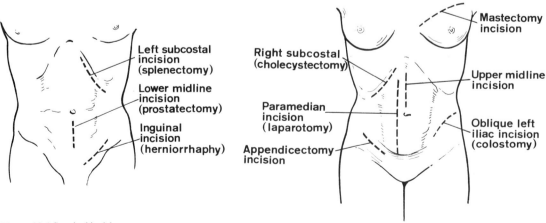

Figure 23.1 Surgical incisions

immediate postoperative complications and there is apparatus to deal with resuscitation, or he may be returned to the surgical ward depending on the particular circumstances.

Postoperatively, the trachea must be kept patent and free from obstruction until the patient regains consciousness, and for this purpose an air tube is used. The patient is nursed flat in bed in a side-lying position until he regains consciousness. If the patient is shocked, he may have a saline drip. Sedatives will be given to relieve pain but care must be taken in the type and amount used as they can depress respiratory activity and increase the risk of pulmonary complications. Normal micturition must be established as soon as possible, a catheter being passed if necessary to prevent retention and the possibility of bladder infection. After certain abdominal operations it will be necessary to rest the stomach and the gastrointestinal tract. The diet will be a fluid one administered intravenously, and the contents of the stomach will be evacuated by means of suction apparatus. The suction apparatus will have been inserted in the theatre, as will any drainage apparatus that may be required. In cases other than abdominal operations it is better to re-establish bowel action as soon as possible, and even if a fluid diet is required it will be given for as short a time as necessary. It is essential to keep a careful watch on the patient's chart as any alteration in temperature, pulse rate or respiration may herald post-operative collapse, haemorrhage, infection or embolism.

Post-operative complications

Respiratory

Despite modern advances in anaesthetics, certain complications do still arise which can, in part, be attributed to anaesthesia. One of its effects is to dry and thicken the mucus secretions in the respiratory tract. The mucus then becomes difficult to dislodge and tends to remain in the air passages. Plugs of mucus may form, and the bronchi and bronchioles are in danger of becoming blocked. Normally the cough reflex would be stimulated but this could be depressed by the administration of analgesics or the patient may try to stop coughing because it is painful.

Several chest conditions may arise:

1. *Post-operative atelectasis* – This is due to the blockage of a bronchus or bronchiole causing an absorption collapse of a segment or lobe of the lung. The basal lobes are the most commonly affected as the patient is nursed in the half-lying position once he has regained consciousness. If the main bronchus is occluded the whole lung collapses but this is a rare occurrence. High abdominal, thoracic, and mediastinal operations carry a higher risk of atelectasis than do lower abdominal or pelvic operations because of the proximity of the lung tissue to these regions. Atelectasis usually occurs between the first and third day after operation.

2. *Pneumonia or bronchopneumonia* – If the mucus secretions are not removed there is a danger of infection with the development of one of these conditions, particularly in the elderly. Aspiration pneumonia can occur due to the inhalation of vomit although this is much less frequent with modern anaesthesia.

To prevent or reduce the risk of the above complications it is essential to clear the secretions and to maintain full ventilation postoperatively.

Deep vein thrombosis

There are a number of factors that may predispose to the development of a deep vein thrombosis. There may be a slowing of the blood flow due to pressure on the calves during surgery and post-operatively if the patient is lying in bed, and also if the patient is inactive during the early stage after operation. There is a rise in the number of platelets and the concentration of fibrinogen after surgery which will predispose to coagulation. The risk is higher in low abdominal and pelvic operations when there may be handling of abdominal or pelvic viscera. The patient may have another condition, such as varicose veins, which could increase the risk of a thrombosis following surgery.

It may indeed be a combinaiton of some of these factors that causes a thrombosis.

Pulmonary embolus

The great danger following a deep vein thrombosis lies in the fact that a small fragment (embolus) may break off the clot and travel in the bloodstream until it lodges in a smaller vessel. The most likely destination is the pulmonary circulation as the blood passes back to the right atrium and then from the right ventricle into the pulmonary circulation. The point at which the embolus lodges depends on its size. If it occludes a large artery then there may be a rapid collapse and the patient will die, whereas if it occludes a small vessel there may be pain and dyspnoea and there may be time to treat the patient.

Post-operatively the patient must be active as soon as possible to reduce the risk of a deep vein thrombosis and the further danger of a pulmonary embolism.

General muscle weakness and loss of mobility

Early mobilization following surgery has decreased the incidence of muscle weakness and loss of mobility. However, elderly patients may already be weak either because they have been confined to bed waiting for surgery or because of other conditions such as osteoarthritis of the hips or knees. Some younger patients may be weak if their illness has prevented them moving about freely for a period of time before surgery.

Other complications

Pressure sores should be prevented but they can occur very quickly in anyone who is very ill and immobile for any length of time, and again the elderly are particularly at risk.

Wound infection is always a risk although modern theatres and surgical techniques along with improved postoperative care in the wards has reduced this risk.

Haemorrhage can be a postoperative complication although the risk is greater with some surgical procedures than others.

There are other complications that can occur but most of these are linked with the particular operation.

Physiotherapy management

Preoperative care

The physiotherapist has an important role to play in assessing which patients being prepared for surgery are at risk of developing complications that she may help to prevent. As a member of the surgical team in the surgical ward she may be alerted about any problems, or potential problems, by the medical or nursing staff. The medical history of any patient must be checked for any respiratory or circulatory problems that could place the patient at risk, or any other factors such as smoking, obesity, inactivity because of another disease or injury, or age, that could predispose to post-operative complications.

Examination

Any patient considered to be at risk should be examined. If any problems, particularly those relating to the chest, should become apparent these should be discussed with the surgeon, or appropriate member of the medical staff. When surgery is essential in a patient with a respiratory problem the surgeon may admit him some days before surgery so that the physiotherapist may clear secretions and ensure that the respiratory movements are as good as possible before surgery.

Treatment

The physiotherapist will explain to the patient why treatment is necessary and teach the patient the exercises that he will be required to perform post-operatively. Respiratory movements will concentrate on lower costal and posterior basal movements. The patient will be taught how to cough effectively and how to support the wound site. Instruction will be given on the leg exercises that the patient will be expected to do postoperatively and any other exercises or postural correction that may be related to specific surgical procedures.

The patient should practise the exercises so that they become familiar and are performed correctly. If the preoperative treatment is taught carefully it will be much easier for the patient to respond to instructions postoperatively. It is very important that whenever possible the same physiotherapist should treat the patient both preoperatively and postoperatively.

Postoperative care

Assessment

The physiotherapist must take careful note of the surgery that has been performed as sometimes this may differ from the preoperative plans. It is important to discuss the condition of the patient with the nursing or medical staff so that the physiotherapist is aware of the post-operative management particularly related to drips and drains and also of any problems that may affect the physiotherapy. Next the physiotherapist must look at the chart of the patient to see whether there is any abnormality of temperature, pulse rate, blood pressure or respiration. She must also know when the patient is receiving analgesics as treatment will be most effective when there is less pain.

Careful observation of the patient may indicate whether he has pain, the amount and rate of respiratory movement and the general posture. The physiotherapist will need to assess the ability of the patient to communicate coherently, his general degree of alertness and ability to follow instructions.

The objective examination will depend on the condition of the patient and may form part of the treatment. Each treatment will involve an evaluation of the patient and subsequent treatments will be changed in the light of this. Treatment will be altered, modified, progressed or stopped as judged to be necessary by the physiotherapist.

Treatment

It is important to start treatment as soon as possible after surgery, whether the patient is in the recovery unit or on the surgical ward.

Prevention of chest complications

The physiotherapist must take other factors into consideration besides the effects of the anaesthetic on secretions in the respiratory tract. One is that pain causes reflex inhibition of the diaphragm and therefore breathing is difficult. Another is that in any operation affecting the abdominal muscles the patient tends to avoid using them because of pain or fear of pain and this again hampers respiratory movements. Administration of too much analgesic may inhibit the cough reflex and lead to the accumulation of secretions.

Breathing exercises should be given to all parts of the chest but particularly the lower costal and posterior basal areas as mentioned previously. Breathing should be as deep as possible with emphasis on the expiratory movements as this helps to loosen the secretions and stimulate the cough reflex. It is important not to make the patient take too many deep breaths at one time as this may make the patient feel faint.

The patient must be encouraged to cough and try to clear any secretions. It is important to give as much support as possible when the patient attempts to cough. It is easier to cough if the patient sits forward and the physiotherapist supports him in this position. It helps if the patient places his hands over or around the wound as the pressure helps to prevent stretching of the wound as the patient coughs. In abdominal surgery it may help if the patient can bend his knees up as this relaxes the abdominal wall and decreases the stretch on it as the patient coughs. If the secretions are very sticky the patient may need an inhalation to loosen them.

If secretions cannot be removed it may be necesssary to use other techniques such as postural drainage and vibrations. These may have to be modified depending on the condition of the patient and the particular surgical procedure.

The frequency and length of treatment will depend on the individual case. Chest complications are most likely to occur in the first 48 hours after surgery and so treatment should be given frequently during this time and the patient should be encouraged to do them on his own if he can. The physiotherapist can stop treatment when there appears to be no further risk and the patient has good respiratory movement and no secretions. If a complication does occur then the treament must be frequent and intensive until the problem is solved.

Prevention of thrombosis

Adequate movement post-operatively is essential. While the patient is in bed he must be encouraged to move about and be as independent as he can. Leg exercises should be given until the patient is up and moving around the ward. It is particularly important to give full-range dorsi- and plantar flexion as this improves venous return from the lower limbs by the use of the muscle pump. Hip and knee exercise and quadriceps contractions should also be included.

The exercises may have to be modified if the patient has an intravenous drip in the leg, or if there is any form of pelvic drainage. Once the patient is up the physiotherapist should see that he is moving around as it is not sufficient for the patient just to sit in a chair.

It is important that these exercises are done properly. Initially the physiotherapist should supervise them but the patient must practise them on his own. So the physiotherapist must try to set up a realistic schedule, such as before or after each meal. They must be practised frequently if they are to be effective.

Prevention of pressure sores

These should not occur in patients who have early mobilization after surgery. However, for patients who have to remain in bed for some days or longer and particularly for the elderly there is a risk. Care must be taken in positioning the patient and he must be encouraged to move around in bed. All members of the team must watch and report any signs of pressure.

Prevention of muscle wasting and joint immobility

Muscle weakness and joint stiffness are particularly likely to occur in the elderly if they remain in bed for any length of time before or after surgery. The physiotherapist may need to give general mobilizing and strengthening exercises to enable the patient to regain independence.

Danger signals

A very careful watch must always be kept on the patient's chart. The physiotherapist must know what she is looking for. A rise in temperature may presage any of the post-operative complications. A swinging temperature usually indicates sepsis.

Alterations in pulse rate and/or respiratory rate and depth may indicate respiratory or circulatory complications, shock or haemorrhage.

Specific clinical features

It is important that the physiotherapist is aware of the significance of any abnormalities and that they are reported immediately.

Post-operative atelectasis – The chart will indicate a rise in temperature, pulse rate and respiratory rate. In addition the patient is usually flushed and feverish and may complain of a feeling of tightness and discomfort on the affected side. There is poor chest expansion on the affected side, the percussion sounds are flat and there are adventitious sounds. An X-ray reveals the collapse.

Thrombosis – If there is a deep thrombosis the chart may reveal a rise in temperature, and the calf may become swollen and tender. Passive dorsiflexion may cause pain in the calf muscles – Homans' sign. If the thrombus is superficial the site is painful and swollen and the skin is red and shiny.

Pulmonary embolism – In serious cases the chart reveals a rapid rise in temperature, pulse and respiration. The patient's colour is poor and he complains of severe pain in the chest. Death may ensue within a few minutes. If he survives he will be very ill for some time. In less serious cases the chart reveals a rise in temperature, pulse and respiration. The patient complains of a sharp stabbing pain in the side of the chest. To all intents and purposes he has pleurisy. In 2–3 days the sputum becomes blood stained, and the condition begins to subside.

Chapter 24

Common operations

It is not proposed to deal at length with any specific operations but to give a brief résumé of operations commonly encountered by the physiotherapist, together with particular points that should be noted. The basic principles of preoperative and post-operative physiotherapy care should be applied to patients undergoing surgical procedures not mentioned here if the patient is at risk of developing pulmonary or circulatory complications. If the patient is elderly he may require further physiotherapy in order to gain optimum independence following surgery.

Cholecystectomy (Figure 24.1)

This operation may be performed following the development of stones in the gall-bladder and cystic duct (cholelithiasis). The stones cause attacks of colic and jaundice and may obstruct the bile duct. If there is an acute attack of cholecystitis the surgeon may treat the condition conservatively until the inflammation has subsided and then operate. The pain experienced by the patient may be very acute and cause considerable distress.

The surgeon may use a Kocher's incision, a right paramedian or midline incision. Following the removal of the gall-bladder a T-tube is inserted and left for approximately 48 hours, or longer if necessary, to allow drainage of any bile or blood into a bag. The amount of bile is measured to ascertain whether any leakage is occurring. Provided that there are no postoperative complications the patient usually makes a good recovery. Removal of the gall-bladder does not require any special diet once the patient has recovered from the operation. Complications that may occur after this operation are: pulmonary, haemorrhage, or leakage of bile.

Physiotherapy

The problem that is most likely to concern the physiotherapist is the risk of pulmonary complications. Provided that the patient is not admitted for emergency surgery it should be possible to assess the patient and decide on the treatment required. The patient may be taught breathing exercises and how to cough effectively. A careful explanation must be given to the patient about the reasons for treatment and what will be expected of him after surgery.

There are a number of factors that increase the likelihood of chest problems after surgery. The actual surgical procedure is very close to the diaphragm, and the irritation may cause the production of increased mucus secretions in the

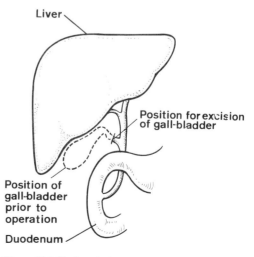

Figure 24.1 Cholecystectomy

Liver

Position for excision
of gall-bladder

Position of
gall-bladder
prior to
operation

Duodenum

lung. Postoperatively, deep breathing will be painful because of the position of the incision and the presence of a drainage tube. Initially the patient will have a Ryle's tube which will make coughing difficult. Atelectasis is most likely to occur in the lower lobe of the right lung because of the position of the gall-bladder on the right side of the upper part of the abdominal cavity. Analgesics given to relieve pain before treatment will enable the physiotherapist to be more effective, although care must be exercised in the amount of analgesic given as too much can depress the cough reflex. Emphasis must be placed on gaining good expansion of the right lung and getting rid of any secretions. As stressed in the last chapter, the first 48 hours postoperatively are important in trying to prevent pulmonary complications.

The physiotherapist should give the patient leg exercises and advice about the amount of activity to try to prevent any circulatory problems. There is a tendency for these patients to be overweight and if so they may not have been very active before the operation which further increases the risk of pulmonary and circulatory complications.

Colostomy

This is an artificial opening in the large bowel to divert the faeces to the exterior where they are collected in a disposable, adhesive plastic bag. Usually this procedure is carried out because of obstruction or disease of the large intestine caused by diverticulitis, Crohn's disease or carcinoma. The colostomy may be temporary or permanent. A temporary colostomy is often placed in relation to the transverse colon whereas a permanent one is usually placed as far distally as possible.

There are a number of problems for a patient with a permanent colostomy. Firstly, there is the worry about the success of the operation if it has been carried out to remove a malignant tumour. Secondly, the patient will probably be concerned about his ability to manage a colostomy, particularly if he is elderly. Thirdly, the patient will be concerned about whether he can lead a normal life, and once out of hospital may tend to shun social activities. The patient must be helped to overcome these problems by all the members of the team. In some hospitals there are nurses who have had special training in dealing with colostomies, and they are known as stoma nurses or therapists.

Physiotherapy

As this operation involves the lower part of the abdominal cavity and pelvis there is an increased risk of a deep vein thrombosis developing postoper-

atively. The physiotherapist must teach the patient leg exercises preoperatively and they should be continued for a couple of weeks postoperatively. It may be considered that the patient is active enough when he is up and walking but this activity may be minimal and it is wise to encourage the patient to do a series of leg exercises before getting out of bed and at regular intervals when sitting in a chair. It may be necessary to give breathing exercises pre- and postoperatively if the physiotherapist has assessed that the patient is at risk because of a chest condition, or because he smokes, or because he is elderly and relatively inactive. Before the patient leaves hospital he should be taught how to lift correctly and avoid excessive strain on the abdominal muscles. The physiotherapist must help the patient to appreciate that he will be able to undertake normal activities, both physically and socially after he has recovered.

Ileostomy

This is similar to a colostomy except that the opening is in the right side of the lower abdominal cavity. Usually it follows a more extensive resection of the colon than a colostomy.

Gastrectomy

A partial gastrectomy for the treatment of gastric ulceration is a common operation if healing does not occur following medical treatment. The formation of ulcers usually occurs along the lesser curvature of the stomach and if they do not heal they may undergo malignant changes. There are a number of operations that may be used although the most common are the Billroth 1 (Figure 24.2) and the Polya type (Figure 24.3). If there is a carcinoma of the stomach this may be treated by a total gastrectomy, and sometimes splenectomy, provided the disease is localized.

Duodenal ulcers are usually treated by a vagotomy, but if there is duodenal and gastric ulceration the surgeon may perform a partial gastrectomy and vagotomy.

Complications – Immediate postoperative complications may be a gastric or duodenal fistula, gastric retention, haemorrhage or pulmonary problems.

Physiotherapy

As the operation is closely related to the diaphragm there is likely to be irritation of adjacent tissues which could cause increased production of mucus, particularly in the lower lobe of the left lung. The patient will be reluctant to breathe deeply because of pain. Similarly, coughing will be inhibited by pain and the presence of a Ryle's tube. So it is very important that the physiotherapist pays special attention to the chest. Generally the patient may be treated preoperatively with emphasis on deep breathing, particularly lower costal, and taught how to cough effectively. Postoperatively the patient must be encouraged to do the deep breathing with emphasis on the left lower costal area. Before attempting to cough the patient should be helped to sit up in bed and lean slightly forward as this makes it easier for him to cough. The patient places his hands over the incision while the physiotherapist supports him in sitting and places one hand over the patient's hands and the other round his back to give pressure on the left lower costal area. Treatment to the chest should be intensive, particularly if there is the slightest indication of a problem. The patient is likely to tire quickly and so the treatment should be given for a short duration and frequently. The nurses can remind the patient to do the deep breathing after carrying out nursing procedures, and the patient must be taught to practise on his own. The patient should do leg exercises to reduce the risk of developing circulatory problems.

If the patient has been ill for some time before the operation the physiotherapist may need to give general mobilizing and strengthening exercises.

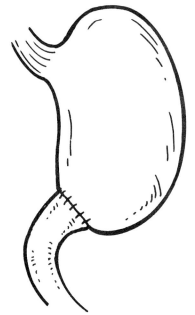

Figure 24.2 Partial gastrectomy. Billroth I operation

Hernias

A hernia is a protrusion of a viscus or part of a viscus through an abnormal opening in the wall of the containing cavity.

Hiatal hernia

In this condition there is a weakness in the oesophageal opening of the diaphragm and part of the stomach may pass upward into the thoracic cavity. Treatment may be conservative but if this fails, surgery may be required. The surgeon may use a thoracic or abdominal route, although the latter is preferable as it may be necessary to investigate for other causes of dyspepsia. There are various surgical procedures that can be used but the main aim is to repair the hiatus.

Physiotherapy

This is similar to the treatment described for a gastrectomy as there is a risk of pulmonary complications with operations in the upper abdominal cavity.

Inguinal hernia

This may be indirect or direct and is a protrusion of a sac of peritoneum containing omentum and possibly intestine through the inguinal canal. The indirect hernia is usually congenital and passes through the length of the canal whereas the direct hernia is medial and projects through a weakness in the posterior wall of the canal. The latter usually

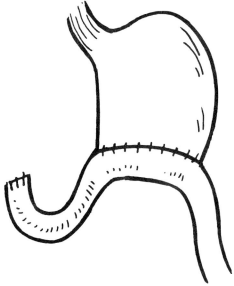

Figure 24.3 Partial gastrectomy. Polya-type operation

occurs in middle-aged to elderly men and often is associated with stress on the abdominal wall caused by a chronic cough or strain on lifting. In infants with a congenital abnormality a herniotomy with removal of the sac may be adequate. However, in the adult more extensive surgery is preferable, unless the risk of operation is too great because there are pulmonary or circulatory problems. The operation performed is a herniorraphy which reduces the herniation and repairs the weakness of the posterior wall.

Femoral hernia

These are more common in women and are a protrusion of the peritoneal sac through the femoral ring. The increase of intra-abdominal pressure that occurs in pregnancy may be a precipitating cause. Surgery is usually the treatment of choice because of the risk of strangulation.

Strangulated hernia

This may require emergency surgery with resection of the gangrenous section of the bowel.

Physiotherapy

For patients undergoing surgery for an inguinal hernia, pulmonary complications may be a risk when there is a chronic chest condition, in which case pre- and postoperative breathing exercises are important. The surgeon may sometimes request physiotherapy to improve the condition of the chest before he will operate.

A deep vein thrombosis is a possible complication after herniorraphy and so exercises for the legs should be given before and after surgery.

These patients are likely to have weak abdominal muscles which should be strengthened after surgery. A progressive scheme of exercises starting with static contractions in the middle to inner range and following with free active exercises should be implemented. Care should be taken not to go beyond the ability of the individual patient and exercises in the outer range of the abdominal muscles should be avoided. Patients should be instructed in correct lifting techniques especially when the history indicates that lifting might have been a precipitating cause in producing a rupture.

Patients undergoing surgery for a femoral hernia should have similar physiotherapy. The risk of pulmonary complications is smaller but there may be a greater risk of developing a deep vein thrombosis. Correct lifting techniques should be taught so that the intra-abdominal pressure is not abnormally high during lifting.

Umbilical hernias

These are more common in children although they can occur in older, obese patients with weak abdominal muscles and possible weakness of tissues in the umbilical region.

Incisional hernias

These may occur through previous operation scars, usually because of infection at the site of operation, or poor healing which weakens the incisional area. Surgery may be necessary if the hernia cannot be controlled with a pad and abdominal belt as there may be a risk of strangulation.

Mastectomy

This entails removal of part or the whole of one breast for a malignant, or sometimes benign, growth. This is the commonest site of carcinoma in women, and if treatment is to be successful it is important to have early diagnosis. Thus health education should aim to teach women to report any lump in the breast to their doctor. Tests can then be carried out and if treatment is required there is a greater chance of success before the disease has spread. Some benign growths can be removed without removing the whole breast and may not cause any disfiguration. Malignant tumours will require more extensive surgery to remove the diseased tissue and there are a number of operations that can be carried out. A simple mastectomy removes the breast and if necessary may remove the axillary lymph nodes, whereas a radical mastectomy removes breast, lymph nodes and pectoral muscles. The latter is performed less often now as it did not give a greater success rate than the less radical procedures and there was the problem of the patient developing an oedematous arm and stiff shoulder. Radiotherapy or chemotherapy may be given after surgery.

This operation may cause severe emotional upset and the patient may be very concerned about the disfigurement. All members of the surgical team must be aware of these problems and try to help the patient through a difficult time with understanding and advice. Good prosthetic devices are available, and arrangements must be made for patients to be fitted with suitable prostheses for their individual needs.

Physiotherapy

General pre- and postoperative care should be given to patients who are at risk of developing complications. As the chest will be painful after surgery the patient may be reluctant to breathe deeply or cough and if there is a history of a chest problem or if the patient smokes she may require treatment.

There is a danger of a stiff shoulder developing particularly with the more extensive surgical procedures. The physiotherapist will discuss the management with the surgeon as some surgeons prefer the arm not to be abducted for the first few days because of the risk of developing a haematoma. Hand and wrist movements should be carried out from the beginning with shoulder shrugging and static contractions of deltoid. If a radical mastectomy has been performed the physiotherapist may be concerned with trying to prevent or treating oedema and mobilizing the shoulder.

Nephrectomy

The kidney may be removed because of a malignant tumour or infection, provided the remaining kidney is normal. The kidney lies in close proximity to the diaphragm and so pulmonary complications following surgery are a risk.

Physiotherapy

The emphasis should be on posterior basal and lower costal breathing, concentrating on the side of the nephrectomy.

Prostatectomy

This is usually carried out for benign growths of the prostate which commonly occur in elderly men. It is less commonly performed for carcinoma because early diagnosis is difficult and the growth may have spread too far. However, surgery may be required to relieve urinary obstruction.

Physiotherapy

Pulmonary complications may occur because these patients are elderly and may be relatively inactive. Also a number are likely to suffer from chronic chest disease and so are at risk. In view of this, these patients should be carefully assessed and treated if necessary. They are generally up within a day or two after surgery but it is important to see they are sufficiently active otherwise there is the risk of developing pulmonary complications.

Chapter 25

Obstetrics

The physiotherapist studying obstetrics needs a knowledge, *inter alia*, of the basic anatomy and physiology of human reproduction. A brief résumé of pregnancy and childbirth follows.

Anatomy and physiology

Bones and joints (Figure 25.1)

The bones of the pelvis comprising hips, sacrum and coccyx, form a cavity through which the fetus passes during labour. The two large hip bones meet together in the midline anteriorly, forming the symphysis pubis, and the sacrum posteriorly, forming two sacroiliac joints. These joints allow a small amount of movement during birth, giving the fetus an easier fit. The hormone 'relaxin' increases ligament laxity (Calguneri *et al.*, 1982). It is liberated from the corpus luteum during pregnancy (under the influence of the anterior pituitary) causing hypermobility of all joints, not just the pubis, to which it is specific.

The pelvic brim (arcuate line) divides the pelvis into the 'false' pelvis above and the 'true' pelvis below. The brim is known as the 'pelvic inlet', and in the female it is wider and deeper than in the male, being described as 'apple shaped'. The 'pelvic outlet' at the base of the true pelvis comprises the following points: the tip of the coccyx, posteriorly; the ischial spines and tuberosities laterally, and the pubic arch anteriorly. Its outline is diamond shaped. At mid-cavity the true pelvis assumes a circular shape. It is this shape of the bony pelvis that allows the fetus accommodation during the process of birth. There is, of course, a variety of positions the fetus may adopt. The fetus' head changes its positions through the cavity of the true pelvis, its

nose turning towards the maternal sacrum as it descends and escapes under the pubic arch at vaginal delivery.

Muscles (Figure 25.2)

Although there are many muscle groups on which demands are made and met, the physiotherapist's understanding of the stretch made on the abdominal and pelvic floor muscles in pregnancy and labour respectively is important, for there is no other area of physiotherapy where it is necessary to exercise stretched muscle tissue. The abdominal muscles form a 'four-way stretch' elastic support for the abdominal contents. They are the rectus abdominis, transversus abdominis, internal oblique and external oblique. Superficially, the recti abdomini stretch either side of the linea alba ligament attaching to it in midline, running from the pubic arch below to the ribs and the xiphoid process above. Their function is to flex the spine, as well as give support. The growing pregnant uterus not only stretches the abdominal muscles but, due to the laxity of the linea alba caused by relaxin, the recti separate, leaving a gap of some 1–3 cm between the two muscles by the end of pregnancy. The transversalis consists of horizontal fibres and the two pairs of oblique muscles interlace diagonally deep to the recti, not only taking part in trunk rotation and side flexion but, together with the pelvic floor muscles, helping to maintain intra-abdominal pressure.

The pelvic floor muscles form a sling of elastic support for pelvic and abdominal contents. The pelvic floor is also known by other names: the perineum, perineal area, urogenital diaphragm, pelvic diaphragm, or muscle names such as levatores ani, or pubococcygeus. These many descriptive

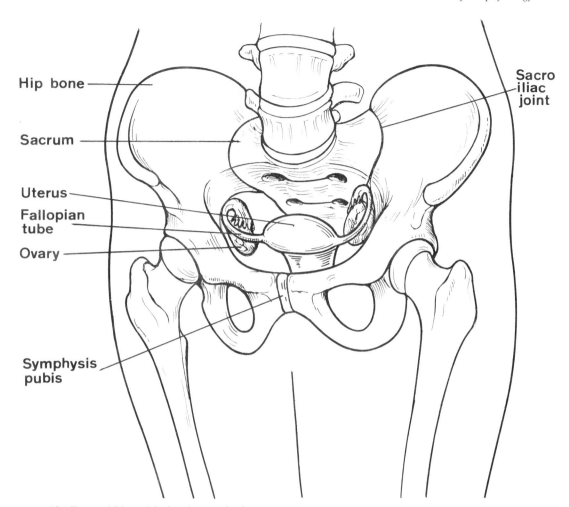

Hip bone

Sacrum

Uterus

Fallopian tube

Ovary

Symphysis pubis

Sacro iliac joint

Figure 25.1 True and false pelvis: female reproductive organs

terms indicate the obstetric and therapeutic import- ance of this muscle group and may help in the understanding of its anatomy and function, for by its position it cannot easily be seen or felt to contract as can other muscles. Body awareness of this muscle group needs careful teaching by an experienced physiotherapist. The pelvic floor consists of a superficial and a deep layer of muscle tissue. Three openings penetrate the floor in the female, the urethra and vagina anteriorly and the anus post- eriorly. The superficial muscles form two loops which meet at the central perineal body, the anterior loop enclosing the urethra and vagina and the posterior loop enclosing the anus. Their action is to close these openings.

The deep levators ani form the main part of the pelvic floor, which on contraction compress the anterior walls of the urethra, vagina and anus

against their posterior walls, thus maintaining continence. The deep layer is formed of two powerful muscles lying on each side of midline, many of the fibres crossing between the vagina and the anal canal to form the strong perineal body. Each levator ani is composed of three bands of fibres: pubococcygeus, ischiococcygeus and ileococ- cygeus, named from their attachment on the hip bone and the coccyx. The anatomical outlet is flexible; the coccyx behaves like a spring after the elastic stretch on it is released during defaecation and parturition. The bands of fibres interlace and sweep from pubis to coccyx enclosing the whole pelvic outlet and forming a firm undercarriage of muscular support. The nerve supply is the 4th and 5th sacral nerves and a branch of the pudendal nerve.

Although the superficial and deep layers of the

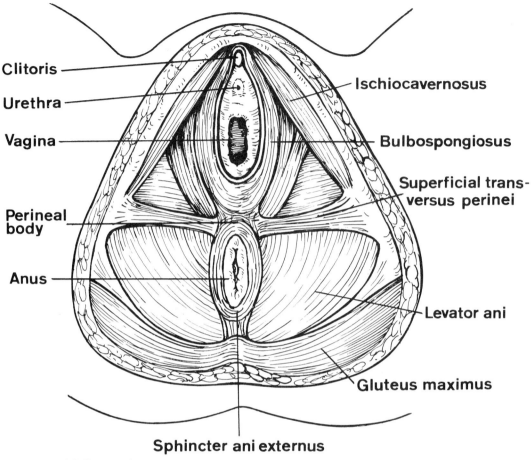

Clitoris

Urethra

Vagina

Perineal body

Anus

Ischiocavernosus

Bulbospongiosus

Superficial trans- versus perinei

Levator ani

Gluteus maximus

Sphincter ani externus

Figure 25.2 Pelvic floor muscles

pelvic floor muscles and their action have been described separately, it should be understood that in health, the muscles contract as a harmonious whole, which is the physiotherapist's objective in treating muscle weakness.

Organs of reproduction

Female (Figure 25.3)

The contractile uterus and two ovaries lie suspended in connective tissue and peritoneum in the true pelvis (see Figure 25.1). The broad ligament surrounds the uterus and divides the pelvic cavity into two compartments: the anterior, containing the bladder; and the posterior, containing the rectum. The ovaries, the size and shape of almonds, are situated in the broad ligament on either side of the uterus. Just behind and slightly below are the soft, trumpet-shaped open ends of the contractile Fallopian tubes. Their openings have anemone-like fringes (fimbriae) which catch the ovum when it

erupts from the ovary at ovulation. The free ovum is attached to the Fallopian tube and is able to travel along it to the uterus by the beating sweep of the tiny cilia lining the tube walls. If it is fertilized, the ovum is embedded in the endometrium, the receptive lining of the uterus. The uterus is remarkable for its growth capacity: from a flattened, pear-shaped hollow muscular organ (approximately the size of the heart) it becomes a large container in 10 lunar months, to accommodate a 3 kg (7 lb) baby, 0.75 kg (1.5 lb) of placenta and 1 litre of fluid, all enclosed in a membranous sac.

The uterus comprises a body (the main part), the fundus (the upper part) and the cervix (the lower part). The cervix opens into the vagina. At the lower end of the vagina is the vulva which comprises the mons pubis (a pad of fat), the labia major and minor (folds of skin) and the clitoris. The uterus is directed forwards and upwards and the vagina forwards and downwards and they are therefore at right angles to each other. The pelvic floor muscles guard and close the distal end of the vagina.

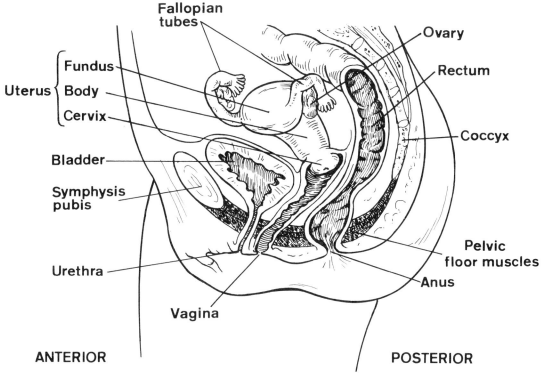

Figure 25.3 Female pelvic organs

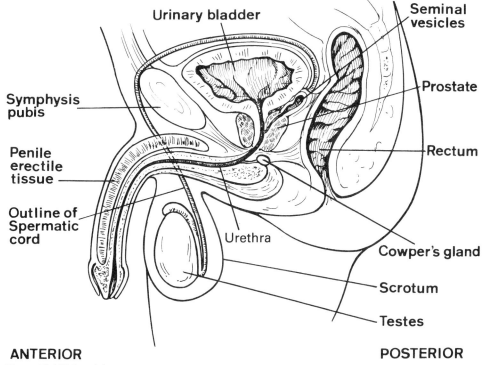

Figure 25.4 Male pelvic organs

Male (Figure 25.4)

The external genitalia in the male consists of two testes which produce spermatozoa, suspended in the scrotum by spermatic cords. These ducts lead from the testes through the true pelvis, joining the urinary tract from the bladder, to descend to the outside through the penis. The epididymis in the testes stores the manufactured sperm. Inside the pelvis the fine seminal tubules are thickened to form the vas deferens, powerful muscle tissue for contraction and ejaculation of seminal fluid. Two small sacs, the seminal vesicles, open into the ejaculatory duct. They and the prostate gland produce and store a volume of seminal fluid. The 3.5 ml of semen at ejaculation contains 20 million microscopic sperm. Sperm (having a head which contains the nucleus and a mobile tail) are the smallest cells in the human body whilst ova are the largest (the size of a pin-head).

Reproduction

Menstruation

Menstruation is the monthly period of bleeding from the vagina when the lining (endometrium) of the uterus, apart from the basal layer, is shed. It begins at puberty, and follows ovulation.

Terms associated with menstruation

Amenorrhoea – Bleeding does not occur as ovulation is suppressed.
Menorrhagia – Excessive bleeding at menstruation.
Dysmenorrhoea – Pain or difficulty accompanying periods.
Climacteric – When ovulation and menstruation cease, between the ages of 35 and 55.

The menstrual cycle (Figure 25.5)

The menstrual cycle is a cyclic release of gonadotrophic hormones from the anterior pituitary which stimulate the events and levels of hormones of the ovarian cycle, which in turn govern a cycle of endometrial events of the uterus. There are three phases:

1. *Menstrual phase* – When fertilization of the ovum does not occur, the corpus luteum degenerates and the output of oestrogen and progesterone falls. The endometrium, apart from its basal layer, disintegrates and sheds, accompanied by bleeding from the many blood vessels. This phase varies from 3 to 6 days.

2. *Proliferative phase* – Following menstruation the growth of a graafian follicle in one ovary occurs, stimulated by follicle-stimulating hormone (FSH) from the anterior pituitary gland. This governs the rise of circulating oestrogens and the endometrium repairs and proliferates under this influence. At this stage the cells of the endometrium are narrow and straight. This phase also varies, taking 7–10 days.

3. *Secretory phase* – Ovulation occurs through the rupture of an ovum through the tense ovary wall, due to the ever-increasing growth of the graafian follicle near its edge. The reorganization of the ovary occurs under the influence of luteinizing hormone (LH) from the anterior pituitary. The follicle now secretes progesterone. This influences further growth of the endometrium, the cells becoming longer, dilated and more tortuous in shape. This phase is constant and lasts precisely 14 days.

   During the last 7 days of secretion the endometrium becomes more vascular, congested and thicker, awaiting the embedding of a fertilized ovum. There is general fluid retention; some women notice discomfort ranging from tingling breasts to headache. The term pre-menstrual tension (PMT) has been used to describe these symptoms.

Conception and fertilization

Gamete formation

During the process of maturation of gametes the parent cells undergo a reduction by half of their original complement of 46 chromosomes, a process known as meiosis. This process is finalized just before the release of each ovum at ovulation and during the formation of spermatozoa in the testes. This preparation allows for the full complement of chromosomes (46) to be restored when they come together at fertilization. The mature sperm, with its thrashing, motile tail, is able to make its way from the vagina into the Fallopian tube where it meets the much larger shed ovum, about a third of the way along.

Zygote formation

The fertilized ovum or zygote now contains 22 pairs of autosomes and one pair of sex chromosomes, which under the microscope resemble an X and a Y form. The pair of sex chromosomes in female cells form XX and in male cells form XY. Thus at meiosis, when each chromosome pair is reduced to a half in each gamete formed, every ovum will contain an X chromosome, whilst the sperms may contain an X or a Y. The sex of the baby is determined by the male component at the union of the gametes.

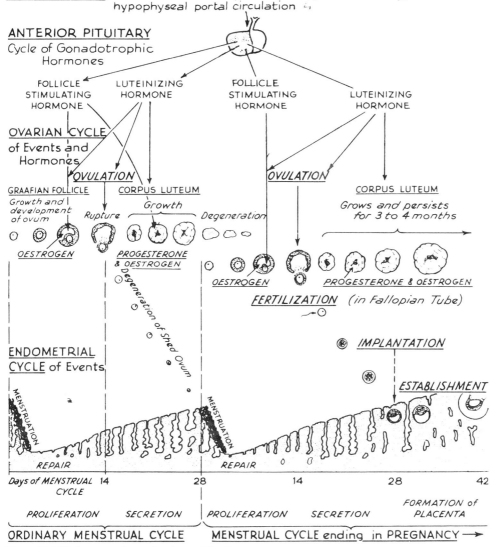

HYPOTHALAMUS *secretes Gonadotrophin Releasing Factor into hypothalamic-hypophyseal portal circulation*

ANTERIOR PITUITARY
Cycle of Gonadotrophic Hormones

FOLLICLE STIMULATING HORMONE   LUTEINIZING HORMONE   FOLLICLE STIMULATING HORMONE   LUTEINIZING HORMONE

OVARIAN CYCLE
of Events and Hormones

OVULATION   *OVULATION*

GRAAFIAN FOLLICLE   CORPUS LUTEUM   CORPUS LUTEUM
Growth and development of ovum   *Rupture*   *Growth*   *Degeneration*   *Grows and persists for 3 to 4 months*

OESTROGEN   *PROGESTERONE & OESTROGEN*   *Degeneration of Shed Ovum*   *OESTROGEN*   *PROGESTERONE & OESTROGEN*

FERTILIZATION (in Fallopian Tube)

IMPLANTATION

ENDOMETRIAL CYCLE *of Events*

ESTABLISHMENT

MENSTRUATION   MENSTRUATION

REPAIR   *REPAIR*

Days of MENSTRUAL CYCLE 14   28   14   28   42

PROLIFERATION   SECRETION   *PROLIFERATION   SECRETION*   *FORMATION of PLACENTA*

ORDINARY MENSTRUAL CYCLE   MENSTRUAL CYCLE ending in PREGNANCY →

Figure 25.5 Pituitary, ovarian and endometrial cycles
(From McNaught and Callender, 1983, with permission.)

Morula formation

Cell division (cleavage) results in a cluster of cells forming a ball called the morula (because it resembles a mulberry). Cleavage continues whilst the morula continues to be moved gently towards the uterus.

Blastocyst formation

The growing cluster of cells reorganize to form an outer layer of trophoblast cells that will form the placenta and an inner cell mass that becomes the embryo, the process being known as gastrulation. The blastocyst formed enters the uterine cavity on approximately the seventh day. These trophoblastic cells secrete an enzyme which digests the endometrial wall of the uterus, leaving a small indentation into which the blastocyst sinks, becoming completely embedded (invagination or implantation). This usually occurs within 10 days of fertilization, during the secretory phase of the menstrual cycle. Now the corpus luteum keeps the progesterone level high and becomes the corpus luteum of pregnancy. Implanting should be in the upper segment of the uterus and occurs at different sites with each pregnancy. If the placental growth takes place in the lower segment of the uterus, placenta praevia can occur, blocking the fetus' vaginal exit. As the blastocyst embeds, slight bleeding from the vagina may be seen in some women as a scanty period.

Embryo formation

Differentiation of three primary cell layers takes place, each developing into several tissue types as follows:

1. *Endoderm* – Alimentary tract, respiratory tract, gonads.
2. *Mesoderm* – Heart, blood vessels, bones, connective tissue, mucous and serous membranes, urinary system.
3. *Ectoderm* – Nervous system, epithelial structures including skin, nails and hair, endocrine and exocrine glands.

There is rudimentary circulation. By the fifth week, bones begin to ossify and by the eighth week a recognizable head, trunk and limbs can be seen although the fetus is only the size of the thumb-nail.

The amniotic cavity gradually enlarges and surrounds the embryo, yolk sac and body stalk. Most of the yolk sac is enclosed with the embryo and goes to form the alimentary tract. The body stalk becomes the umbilical cord.

Fetal membranes

The fetus, placenta, cord and liquor amnii are enclosed in a double layer of membrane, the amnion. This lines the uterine cavity and is adherent to the chorion. It is smooth and transparent, tougher than the chorion and secretes liquor amnii which fills the amniotic cavity. The chorion is the outer layer attached to the endometrium. It is more opaque than the amnion and is more likely to be retained at delivery, so the placenta is always examined very carefully.

Liquor amnii

This is a clear straw-coloured fluid with an alkaline reaction, composed of 99% water with a small percentage of protein, glucose, urea and various mineral salts. Also to be found are lanugo (fetal hairs), vernix caseosa (white creamy substance secreted by the fetus' sebaceous glands to protect the skin) and desquamated cells of the fetus and amnion. The contents can be examined by amniocentesis – a procedure to investigate fetal abnormality by drawing off liquor containing fetal cells, through the abdomen. At full term the uterus contains approximately 1 litre of fluid, the total volume being irrigated about every 3 hours as the fetus continually swallows, absorbs and excretes it

via the placenta and hence by the maternal skin and kidneys. Its constant production allows for free movement of the fetus and acts as a shock absorber to protect the fetus from jarring. A constant temperature of the fetus is maintained by the warmth of the fluid, and during labour the liquor assists in equalizing the pressure on the fetus during strong uterine contractions and marked interference of placental circulation.

Umbilical cord

A large umbilical vein and two smaller arteries form a twisted rope-like structure 50 cm long and 2 cm in diameter. It arises from the fetal surface of the placenta at its centre and passes oxygen and nutrients to the fetus through its navel and reabsorbs fetal waste products back through the placenta to be excreted by the mother's kidneys, lungs and skin.

Placenta

The placenta is round and flat and by full term weighs approximately 100 g, about one-sixth of the fetal weight. It is made up of twenty lobes or cotyledons, each containing numerous chorionic villi. The maternal surface is tough, reddish and may appear gritty, as fibrin deposits become calcified. Its fetal surface is smooth, shiny and bluish, covered by the inner layer of the amnion. The two arteries branch and radiate from the fetus throughout the placenta, dividing into smaller branches, each supplying a cotyledon, and then into yet smaller branches into a capillary network to each tiny villus. The network re-forms as a venous network to form the umbilical vein.

Functions of the placenta

The placenta does the work of a number of fetal organs which cannot function during intrauterine life. It is a highly complex organ, comparable in many ways to the liver. Its biochemical activities and pathways appear to model very closely the complete animal, with the exception of neural, skeletal and muscular systems; therefore it is a good tool for research. Hence the placenta has:

1. A respiratory function, the fetus obtaining oxygen and excreting carbon dioxide through it.
2. A nutritive function, the placenta selecting the necessary amino acids, monosaccharides, lipids, fat-soluble vitamins, minerals and water. Some pass by simple diffusion, others are broken down by enzymes in the placenta into lower molecular weight items for fetal absorption.
3. A glycogenic function, storing glycogen and supplying it in the form of glucose on demand.

4. An excretory function, the fetal waste products diffusing through the placenta to the maternal circulation.
5. A barrier function, preventing many harmful substances from passing through. This latter function is not complete and care has to be taken in administering drugs during pregnancy. The thalidomide disaster is an example of the harm that can be done. Certain viruses can also harm the fetus in early pregnancy, before the placenta is fully formed, German measles (rubella) being the most feared.
6. The endocrine function is of prime importance to maintain the pregnancy. From the twelfth week the oestrogen and progesterone levels are kept high by production from the placenta. Human chorionic gonadotrophin (HCG) is produced by the placenta's basic trophoblast cells and helps maintain the corpus luteum through the necessary progesterone levels. Human placental lactogen (HPL) affects carbohydrate metabolism concerned with fetal growth and the levels of HPL in maternal blood is one method of assessing placental function. It normally rises as pregnancy advances. A measure of oestrogen found in maternal urine is a guide to fetal well-being. It is low for anencephalic babies, for instance.

Pregnancy

Physiological changes

The uterus grows from a weight of 50 g to 950 g at term. The myometrium (muscle tissue) increases in number and length of fibres which grow to fifteen times their pre-pregnant length. The endometrium (lining) thickens as the blood supply increases and the lymphatic drainage is greater with the increased fluid volume; the liquor bathing the fetus reaching a peak of 1000 ml at 35 weeks of pregnancy. The cervix and vagina are more vascular and softer with increased secretions of mucus. At ovulation the mucous secretions become more fluid and pour down into the vagina to aid sperm mobility. During pregnancy, however, ovulation is inhibited and the secretions remain thick, resulting in a tenacious mucous plug which fills the cervical canal aiding the prevention of infection of the fetus. The breasts and nipples enlarge and the veins distend as the individual cells of these glands multiply.

Apart from these effects on the reproductive system pregnancy has an effect on the following systems of the body. The abdominal muscle fibres lengthen and as the linea alba separates (diastasis) the abdomen protrudes from 20 weeks to accommodate the growing fetus. Skin stretch may cause stretch marks (striae gravida) in the fairer, dryer skin type, as the elastic tissue tears. Skin pigmentation causes the nipples and areolae to darken and

a fine brown line, the linea nigra, appears between the navel and pubis. Sometimes a butterfly freckled effect (chloasma) appears around the eyes. The rib cage widens to accommodate the uterus.

The hormone relaxin has an effect not only on the ligaments but also on blood vessels and the alimentary tract. Veins appear distended and peristalsis changes slightly; the stomach and gut empty more slowly, accounting for the common problems of heartburn and constipation. Although venous return slows there is little change in blood pressure. There is also a 50% increase in blood plasma volume by the 34th week. The red cell production and volume are adjusted to, and regulated by, the increased demand for oxygen transport. (The concentration of red cells falls because of the increased plasma volume; the total haemoglobin is raised.) The white cell count is proportionally high to give protection potentially against infection. The blood flow through the skin and mucous membranes increases 70% by 36 weeks and accounts for increased sweating, heat sensitivity and nasal congestion.

The kidneys are required to cope with an increased blood flow. This, together with the pressure of the growing uterus on the bladder, causes frequency of micturition. Urinary tract infections sometimes occur due to the effect of relaxin which relaxes the bladder and ureters, encouraging urinary stasis. The thyroid, suprarenal and pituitary endocrine glands enlarge to improve their metabolic function.

Posture and gait change as the weight increases in the abdomen and the pelvic joints relax. The centre of gravity shifts forwards resulting in strain on the lumbar spine as the abdominal muscles lengthen.

Psychological/emotional changes

Emotions are more labile. Obviously the impending birth, with its responsibilities, dramatically changes life styles but the basic emotional type does not change. Pregnancy induces vulnerability, and the first trimester (3 months) is coloured by whether or not this baby is wanted. By mid-term, second trimester, the emotional high or low becomes stable. Anticipation, often mixed with anxiety or fear, predominates in the last 3 months (third trimester).

Signs

The presumptive signs of pregnancy are amenorrhoea and abnormal fullness of the breasts which may be the earliest indication even before the first missed period. During the first 12 weeks bladder irritability causes frequency of micturition. Nausea and vomiting occur in 50% of women which may be related to blood sugar assimilation. From about the sixteenth week the first faint fluttering movements of fetal activity (quickening) can be felt. The movements increase in strength as the pregnancy proceeds.

The earliest positive sign (7 days after the missed period even) can be achieved by the result of a simple immunological test. Human chorionic gonadotrophin (HCG) is released into the circulation with the development of trophoblast cells. The woman's urine is first exposed to anti-HCG serum which will neutralize HCG in it if it is present. When a serum containing HCG is added no agglutination (clumping of cells) occurs. However, if the urine contains no HCG (not pregnant) agglutination will occur. This agglutination-inhibition is the principle of the positive result.

Ultrasound can be used to visualize the fetus as early as 6 weeks. Reflected at any interface (boundary between tissues), ultrasound screens the uterus to see detail of the fetal heart and spinal cord and therefore detect certain malformations. Women are often examined routinely between the 10th and 20th weeks and again at the 34th week to provide diagnostic help in assessing fetal growth. Although the fetal heartbeat can be observed from the 6th week, its sound cannot be heard with accuracy using an ultrasonic detector until the 16th week. A Pinards fetal stethoscope can only detect the heartbeat from the 20th week. The rate varies from 120 to 160 beats per minute. The fetus can be directly palpated after the 25th week, and with skill its position and presentation can be defined.

From the 12th week the fundus of the uterus becomes palpable. Its height gives some estimation of pregnancy duration; reaching the level of the pelvic brim at 12 weeks, the umbilicus at 20 weeks and the diaphragm at 32 weeks. In the last 4 weeks or so the fetus moves down into the pelvic brim (engaged), the woman feeling less pressure (lightening) under her rib cage. To achieve this objective uterine contractions (Braxton–Hicks) become frequent and stronger after the 30th week. These are palpable and may cause discomfort.

Complications

Pregnancy does not always take an uncomplicated course and indeed sometimes does not even proceed to fruition. The following account will indicate the importance of antenatal screening. 'Abortion' means the expulsion of a fetus before it reaches viability (the gestation period of more than 22 weeks recommended by the World Health Organisation). Once pregnancy is confirmed, the sign of vaginal bleeding is presumed to be a 'threatened abortion', which fortunately resolves itself in 80% of pregnancies. Bleeding can be a sign of local cervical lesions such as polyps or cervicitis. However, should bleeding continue, accompanied by rhythmical pains, then the term 'inevitable abortion' describes the condition. This leads to either a 'complete abortion' or to an 'incomplete abortion' where the uterus does not empty its contents completely. If the entire products of conception are not expelled rapidly, active medical intervention to evacuate the uterus is needed. Very occasionally, 'missed abortion' occurs when the dead embryo and placenta are not expelled spontaneously. The threatened abortion settles down but the uterus fails to enlarge and the signs of pregnancy cease. The diagnosis of 'carneous mole' is established by ultrasound and treated by careful curettage to remove it.

In 0.6% of pregnancies 'ectopic pregnancy' occurs. This describes the implanting of the fertilized ovum in the Fallopian tube when it has failed to reach the uterine cavity. The attempt to abort may rupture the tube wall, known as a 'ruptured tubal pregnancy', but in any case will result in bleeding with severe pain. This serious condition needs treatment instantly and a laparotomy examination is followed by a partial or total salpingectomy, a removal of the tube, depending on the severity of the damage to the tube.

'Cervical incompetence' accounts for 20% of recurrent abortions. Ultrasound detects it and the dilated internal os is held closed by a soft unabsorbable suture placed around the cervix. The pregnancy usually progresses normally and the suture is left until 7 days before term, permitting the woman to deliver vaginally.

'Antepartum haemorrhage' refers to bleeding from the birth canal after 22 weeks when the fetus is viable. Occurring in 3% of pregnancies, it has two main causes, accidental haemorrhage and placenta praevia. 'Accidental haemorrhage' is so called because the separation of the placenta was thought to be produced by some sort of trauma like a blow or fall. It is more likely that the bleeding is induced by vascular dysfunction between the placenta and the uterus lining from hypertensive disease or pregnancy-induced hypertension. Vaginal bleeding is accompanied by abdominal tenderness and pain and, depending on its severity, the baby may be delivered by caesarean section as an obstetric emergency. In 'placenta praevia' the placenta lies before the presenting fetus when the ovum has implanted abnormally in the lower uterine segment, instead of in the upper segment. The growing placenta then either completely or partially covers the internal os (except in marginal cases), preventing the baby from delivering vaginally. The sign of bleeding is recurrent but painless and when the diagnosis is confirmed by ultrasound the patient is admitted under observation. Having had blood loss replaced if necessary, she is treated by bed rest, with the objective of prolonging the pregnancy to the 37th week. The baby is delivered by caesarian section.

The uteroplacental blood supply is crucial to fetal growth and to its survival. 'Placental insufficiency', when the placenta fails to transport adequate supplies of nutrients and oxygen, can lead to a 'small for dates' baby at best, or to intrauterine death at worst. Screening to evaluate fetal well-being and placental function can pick up the 'at risk' fetus. Serial ultrasound examinations can estimate fetal growth; and cardiotachography (CTG) records fetal heart rate. Blood and urine tests measure the related qualities of oestriol and human placental lactogen (HPL) to the normal range of weekly gestation. Studies have shown that rest, a maternal diet rich in protein, and correcting anaemia can improve uteroplacental blood flow. Higher risk pregnancies, including multiple pregnancies, are monitored from the 28th week to detect when the risk to the fetus becomes critical, and then the mother can be delivered immediately.

Pregnancy is achieved by a compensation of metabolism, but imbalance can result in 'pregnancy induced hypertension' (PIH) known as 'pre-eclampsia'. This normally occurs after the 30th week of pregnancy, and 5% of pregnancies are complicated by hypertension. If this is not diagnosed and treated it can lead to the extremely serious condition of 'eclampsia', producing convulsions and coma, with possible loss of life to mother and baby. Because PIH is insidious, the woman feeling well until eclampsia is imminent, the health care team should be vigilant to detect potential pre-eclampsia and to recognize the three signs that indicate it:

1. Oedema present in the ankles after a night's rest, or in the hands and face.
2. Raised diastolic blood pressure, to 90 mmHg or more than ten points above the level recorded in early pregnancy.
3. Proteinuria, which is usually the last and most serious symptom to appear.

A combination of any two of these three signs is significant and requires treatment. The effect of bed rest improves renal blood flow, and the management will be able to control blood pressure and monitor the well-being of the fetus. Labour is induced at 38 weeks or before, if the mother and baby are at risk, and the hypertension usually resolves within 72 hours of delivery. Blood pressure can change quite suddenly and develop into 'eclampsia' in a few days. If this dangerous condition, which should be prevented, occurs, then hypotensive drugs, diuretics and adequate sedation are used to control blood pressure, and the baby is delivered by caesarian section.

There are some maternal conditions that may affect the baby but not the placenta. 'Infectious diseases', particularly virus infections, can cross the placenta. 'Rubella' (German measles), endemic in most countries, has very serious effects on the fetus, especially when the virus is contracted in the first 14 weeks of pregnancy. It causes congenital malforma-

tions to the fetal organs that are forming at the time, which can result in sight, hearing and heart defects as well as other systemic problems related to widespread cellular growth retardation. Preventative measures include vaccinating girls between the ages of 11 and 14 years; testing for rubella immunity immediately after childbirth and offering women appropriate vaccination; and offering therapeutic abortion to all women who develop rubella in the first weeks of pregnancy.

'Hepatitus B' virus is carried by up to 30% of migrants from parts of Africa and Asia and it may be transmitted to the baby at birth. Health care workers are potentially at risk for they may be infected by contact with blood and body secretions. Precautionary hospital protocol has been developed in caring for carriers of hepatitis B in childbirth and for vaccinating their babies at birth and again at 1 and 6 months. Sexually transmitted diseases, for example 'active genital herpes' or women who are HIV positive (human immuno-deficiency virus – the AIDS virus) can pass these conditions to their children. Vaginal delivery makes the transmission of the virus more likely, and consequently these high-risk women are delivered by caesarean section.

Great care is necessary in administering therapeutic drugs during pregnancy as these can pass through the placenta and damage the fetus. We all need to remember the deformities of people affected by thalidomide, which was prescribed to control nausea and sickness in the mid-1960s. Babies are also affected by 'drug addiction'. Not only 'hard' drugs, but even smoking can cause underweight babies.

'Iso-immunization' complicates 0.5% of pregnancies. Rhesus incompatibility occurs when maternal and paternal genes have differing rhesus blood groups, for then a rhesus-negative mother may carry a rhesus-positive baby. If sufficient fetal cells enter the maternal circulation, antibodies are produced. This means that in the next pregnancy these antibodies, now present in the maternal blood, cross the placenta and can cause haemolytic disease in the second child. This risk increases with each subsequent pregnancy. In about 98% of cases this can be prevented by giving an injection of rhesus anti-D gamma globulin to every rhesus-negative woman giving birth to a rhesus-positive baby. A similar treatment is given to this group of women when the fetal blood group incompatability is detected by amniocentesis and after abortion. Every rhesus-negative woman is screened for rhesus antibodies from early pregnancy so that the appropriate treatment can be given.

The full range of medical disorders may affect the mother and not the fetus. For example, cardiac and respiratory disease, neurological and orthopaedic conditions, etc. They will all invite attention in pregnancy with the stresses placed on maternal metabolism, but diabetes needs special mention because impaired glucose tolerance may be induced by, and disappear between, pregnancies, and established diabetes is made worse due to its effect on metabolism. A healthy outcome for the baby depends on good management of the diabetic condition. With good control, most diabetics are permitted to continue the pregnancy to approximately the 37th week if possible, and then labour is induced because after that the diabetes may directly affect the baby.

Labour (childbirth; parturition)

Full-term labour takes place at 40 weeks of pregnancy, but normal limits are within 2 weeks either side of this estimated delivery date (EDD).

Physiology

The myometrium of the uterus is composed of a thick middle layer of interdigitating spiral fibres and two much thinner layers, an outer layer of mainly longitudinal fibres and an inner layer of largely circular fibres. The thick muscle tissue is especially marked in the upper pole, decreasing in the lower pole to no more than 10% at the cervix, compared with 90% at the fundus.

Labour is insidious. The trigger is still not fully understood, since research into this finely tuned event has not given a precise picture. For its occurrence, however, the cervix 'ripens', that is, the collagen tissue becomes softer, and the myometrial contractions are coordinated. Current evidence suggests that cervical ripening is due to prostaglandins which are inhibited by progesterone. Labour contractions are influenced by a rising level of oxytocin (a hypothalamic hormone released from the posterior pituitary) whilst the placental progesterone is gradually reduced. The involuntary muscular activity is established by the neuromuscular control of the autonomic nervous system. The parasympathetic sensory nerve fibres innervating the uterus pass through the juxtacervical plexus lying adjacent to the cervix, reaching the spinal cord at T11, T12, and L1. The motor nerve supply leaves the spinal cord at the level of T7 and T8, passing through the plexus to reach and spread through the uterus. This higher level of the emergence of the motor nerves permits the sensory nerve supply to be blocked by epidural anaesthesia, if required, without affecting uterine activity. The vulva is innervated by branches of the pudendal nerve, derived from S2, S3 and S4, allowing perineal analgesic infiltration to be used when assisting delivery.

Established labour contractions cause retraction at the fundal upper pole of the uterus and allow progressive dilatation at the cervical lower pole.

This polarity of contraction is a special property of uterine muscle causing the fetus to descend into the pelvis. Once the cervix has dilated, contractions of the diaphragm and abdominal muscles assist the uterus in its expulsive efforts until the child is expelled through the elastic, muscular perineum.

Signs

The signs of labour are variable and therefore the onset of labour is difficult to define; bearing in mind that labour is established when the cervix is dilated to more than 2 cm and contractions are strong, regular and frequent. During the effacement and early dilatation of the cervix the tenacious mucous plug named 'the show' is discharged. It is often streaked with blood from the vascular cervical mucosa and it may be broken up so that there may be indications occurring over several days. Natural rupture of the amniotic membranes, termed 'waters breaking', usually occurs much later in labour, but if it should be one of the early signs it requires management because of the risk to the fetus from infection or prolapsed cord.

Labour is divided into three stages.

First stage – cervical dilatation

This takes an average of 12 hours in the primigravida and 7½ hours in multigravida. The contractions increase variably in intensity and frequency until the cervix is fully dilated. The first stage is further divided into a longer 'latent' phase of approximately 8 hours leading to a shorter 'active' phase of 3–5 hours on average. Here the contractions increase from 1 to 1½ minutes in duration and occur at a frequency of 3 minutes or less, causing distressing pain which may require analgesia. Each contraction produces a wave of sensation, starting with a feeling of tightening in the abdomen and reaching a peak of intensity before dying away. During the active phase the pain feels constant but increasing with contractions and decreasing in between them. The pain is referred from the dilating cervix and the deep pressure of the fetus descending into the pelvis, and it is felt in the abdomen, lumbar region, pubic area and often the thighs.

Second stage – the birth (Figure 25.6 (a)–(c))

This takes an average of 1 hour in the primigravida and 15 minutes in multigravida. Bearing down (pushing, straining) of the diaphragm and abdominal muscles reflexly assist the uterus to expel the baby through the curved birth canal. Each contraction advances the fetal head but it is protected by a short retreat between contractions until eventually the child's head is 'crowned' by the perineum. It slips through, escaping under the pelvic brim and after a short pause, while the head rotates, the shoulders enter the antero-posterior diameter of the lower pelvis between the ischial spines. One expulsive effort delivers the anterior shoulder first from under the pubis and then the posterior shoulder, trunk and legs. The baby is born.

Third stage – afterbirth (Figure 25.6 (d))

The cord is divided near the baby's abdomen and within 5 minutes or so of the birth the placenta has separated from the uterus, causing some retro-placental bleeding. However, the lattice arrange-ment of the muscle fibres virtually blocks the blood vessels supplying the placental bed, stemming the blood loss. This natural process is encouraged by an intramuscular injection of Syntometrine (oxytocin and ergometrine). This oxytocic drug combines the rapid effect of oxytocin with the sustained, contrac-tile effect of ergometrine to minimize haemorrhage, and the placenta is expelled with the cord and membranes. This completes the labour.

The baby at birth

Although many babies gasp for air and cry immediately, using their lungs for the exchange of air for the very first time, most will need suction to prevent their gagging on mucus and some will need oxygen from a tiny oxygen mask. The baby's extremities may appear bluish at first. The Apgar scale (see Table 22.1) gives a measure of fetal well-being at birth. A score out of 10 is given at 1 minute and 5 minutes. A maximum of two points each are scored for five signs: colour, respiration, heart rate, muscle tone and reflex irritability.

Assisted delivery

There are some women who need a varying degree of assistance during the birth, by methods such as:

1. *Episiotomy* – A relatively small incision in the perineum will make a much larger space for the baby to emerge. An episiotomy is used:
   (a) To speed up delivery.
   (b) With forceps to allow easy delivery.
   (c) To prevent tearing of the tissues that are not stretching easily. A repair using soluble perineal sutures is required in the third stage of labour.
2. *Forceps/vacuum extraction* – The blades of the forceps fit the sides of the baby's head and smooth gentle movements are used with the uterine contractions to lift the baby out and may assist in rotation as well as traction. Vacuum extraction is achieved by attaching a small

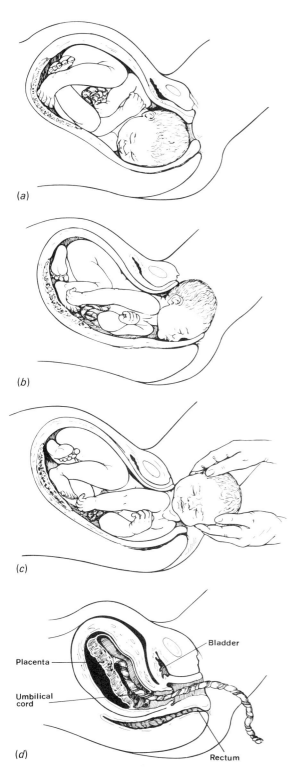

(a)

(b)

(c)

Bladder

Placenta

Umbilical cord

(d)

Rectum

Figure 25.6 The stages of labour. (*a*) Beginning of second stage. (*b*) Second stage continues. (*c*) Delivery of head and shoulders. (*d*) Third stage

vacuum cup to the baby's head to exert gentle traction as before.

3. *Caesarean section (lower section caesarean section, LSCS)* – A transverse incision is made though the skin and muscles of the lower abdomen known as a bikini incision so that baby and placenta may be removed. There are five indications for an LSCS:

   (a) Poor fit between pelvis and fetus.
   (b) Malpresentation including breach.
   (c) Fetal distress and failure of labour to progress, with poor uterine contractions.
   (d) Placenta praevia and ante-partum haemorrhage.
   (e) Some maternal disorders, e.g. pregnancy-induced hypertension.

Pain relief in labour

1. *Psychophysical preparation* gives a knowledge of the physiological events of labour and teaches relaxation through tension control. It instils confidence in attendants and induces a willingness in the patient to cooperate and participate in giving birth, therefore raising the pain threshold.
2. *Analgesics* – Pethidine is a muscle relaxant and induces drowsiness which takes effect within 20 minutes and lasts 2–3 hours. It may be passed to the fetus and therefore timing is important and an antidote must be used if the baby is affected.
3. *Nitrous oxide and oxygen* – Inhalation of a mixture of 70% N_2O and 30% O_2 is self-administered at the end of the first stage and through the second stage of labour. Its effect is immediate.
4. *Epidural analgesia* – This is an anaesthestic agent introduced into the dural space between the dura mater and the periosteum, blocking upwards to the level of the 10th dorsal segment of the spine. The difficulty of correlating expulsive effort with painless uterine contractions may result in increased length of second stage and higher incidence of forceps delivery.
5. *Perineal infiltration* – This anaesthetizes the perineum, permitting the painless repair of episiotomy wounds, and allowing outlet forceps to be used with little discomfort.

Puerperium

This is defined as the period following completion of labour during which the reproductive organs return to their non-pregnant state and in which lactation is established. It lasts 6–8 weeks.

Physiology of the puerperium

The retrogressive changes of the uterus are termed involution. At the end of the labour the contracted uterus is approximately the size of a 20-week pregnancy and lies above the pelvic brim below the umbilicus. Involution reduces the size by approximately a finger breadth a day and by the 12th day its level is below the pelvic brim. By the 7th week the uterus is only slightly larger than its pre-pregnant size.

Involution of the placental site

After expulsion of the placenta, the placental bed contracts in size rapidly. New epthelial tissue covers the inner area of the uterus within 10 days except for the placental site which takes approximately 6 weeks to heal. A discharge is seen during this time.

Lochia

This discharge from the vagina lasts approximately 4 weeks. It resembles a heavy period and is mainly blood in the first 4 days. The colour changes from red to reddish brown and after 12 days will be yellowish until it finally ceases.

Endocrine changes

Blood levels of oestrogen and progesterone fall significantly by the third day after childbirth and will reach basal levels by the 7th day. While breast feeding continues the levels remain low because of the high prolactin concentrations in the blood. If the woman decides not to breast feed, the oestrogen and progesterone levels begin to rise between 14 and 21 days after delivery. This indicates return of ovarian follicular development and ovulation.

Breasts

In the first 3 days the baby is nourished by the secretion called colostrum which is rich in protein and more easily digested than milk, secretion of which is established around 3–5 days. The breasts become firm, large and heavy. Milk production is controlled by the release of prolactin, stimulated by the anterior pituitary. Milk expression is stimulated by the baby's sucking, through the release of oxytocin controlled by the posterior pituitary. While breast feeding, ovulation and therefore menstruation is delayed. However, when considering contraception it should be realized that ovulation takes place before the visible menstrual bleeding occurs.

Abdominal muscles

In pregnancy these not only lengthen but the two recti abdomini separate (diastasis). The connective tissue between them (the linea alba) widens from 2 cm to at least 4 cm. By 6 weeks after birth the gap should narrow so that normally only the tip of one finger can be inserted between the muscle bellies at the level of the umbilicus. The abdominal muscles are severed by caesarean section.

Pelvic floor muscles

These are stretched at childbirth by the presenting part of the fetus. They also recover their pre-pregnant firmness by 6 weeks. These muscles are cut and sutured when an episiotomy is necessary.

Postnatal complications

The following complications are not common but when they occur either physiotherapy may be contraindicated or the condition may limit the normal progression of postnatal exercise.

Puerperal infection

A local infection can be caused by the bacteria *Escherichia coli*, staphylococci or anaerobic strepto-cocci. The infection delays the healing of the placental site and the patient shows signs of general malaise, a raised temperature and offensive lochia. Investigations of urine, blood and a cervical swab examination are made to determine the bacterial type. Immediate treatment with antibiotics prevents spread from the primary site causing a more serious pelvic infection.

Breast infection is caused by the organism *Straphylococcus aureus* entering a crack in the nipple. Early treatment of mastitis with breast care, antibiotics and analgesics prevents the occurrence of breast abscess. This rare condition is indicated by a painful, red, wedge-shaped area of inflammation and enlarged axillary lymph glands. The patient has a raised temperature and feels generally ill. Antibio-tics are prescribed. Incision and drainage under anaesthetic may be necessary – the drainage tube is required for 48 hours.

Venous complications

Thrombophlebitis is a superficial venous throm-bosis. It occurs in 1% of patients. Inflammation usually affects an existing varicosed superficial vein. There is local tenderness, and the vein is visibly distended. Re-absorption of the clot usually occurs and the condition resolves with a support bandage or elasticated stocking and encouraged activity.

Phlebothrombosis is a venous thrombosis occur-ring in the deep veins of the legs or pelvis and occurring in 0.02% of puerperal women. The signs are a raised temperature, leg pain and tenderness. Anticoagulants and analgesics are prescribed. The patient is nursed in bed (with the foot of the bed elevated and a cradle to take the weight of the bedclothes off the leg) until all the pain and tenderness has subsided. When the deep pelvic veins are affected there is a serious risk of the patient developing a pulmonary embolism. Prevention of deep vein thrombosis is therefore very important. Early mobilization and activity are encouraged following delivery, especially after caesarean sec-tion.

Physiotherapy in obstetrics

Antenatal care

In early pregnancy, women are referred by the general practitioner (GP) to antenatal clinics at district hospitals which have the resources to carry out screening and monitoring. It is usual to be seen at monthly intervals up to the 24th week, then fortnightly until 32 weeks and then weekly during the last 8 weeks.

Women may choose to use the domiciliary service, visiting their GP throughout the pregnancy. The GP will use the hospital resources, referring the patient to the obstetrician for routine screening once during each trimester. Most babies are born in hospital, the mother and baby returning home often within 48 hours to the care of the domiciliary midwife.

Antenatal education

This takes the form of a programmed course in the third trimester. Pregnancy provides for health promotion because prospective parents are keen to learn how best to cope with the experience of childbirth and a new baby. This health education should meet both physical and emotional needs. Midwives, health visitors, and obstetric physio-therapists work together as a team and are termed antenatal educators. Also included are obstetri-cians, paediatricians, dietitians and dental hygien-ists. Each team member reinforces the role of the others and this requires good communication with regular contact to operate an effective referral system.

Programme aims, content and plan

Aims

1. Prepare the prospective parents for the birth and care of the baby and for parenthood.

2. Give confidence to the woman in her own abilities through an understanding of how her body functions and the various changes occurring during pregnancy and birth.
3. Introduce each member of the team and ensure that the woman knows who to go to for advice.
4. Provide a forum for the prospective parents to meet each other and discuss aspects of hopes, fears, problems and expectations.

Content

1. Outline of the anatomy of the reproductive system.
2. Outline of the physiology of pregnancy, birth and after the birth.
3. Components of labour.
4. Self-care.
5. Baby care.

Plan

If possible, two or three classes should be attended by the woman at around 6–8 weeks pregnancy for early physiotherapy advice and instruction.

Then there is usually a course of six classes of 2 hours each, once per week during the third trimester. The physiotherapist takes 1 hour of each class and the other hour is taken by various members of the team, e.g. the midwife, health visitor or dental hygienist.

Time of classes – It is important to have different times of the day on offer, and an evening session should be available so that fathers may attend.

Role of the physiotherapist

1. Complement instructions from other members of the team, relating to policies of the hospital and community care.
2. Assess physical health and identify any musculoskeletal or neuromusclar problems that could be aggravated by pregnancy. Teach leg, abdominal and pelvic floor muscle exercises.
3. Advise on continued sport or work, and how to recognize fatigue as an important sign of overactivity.
4. Advise on back care and lifting.
5. Treat any problems with appropriate physiotherapy skills.
6. Teach methods for controlling neuromuscular tension.
7. Teach positions that may be used for labour.
8. Teach postnatal exercises.

Items (2), (3), (4) and (6) particularly should be covered in the early classes.

Complementing instructions from other team members

The approach to the running of the programme varies but the principle of each member of the team explaining his or her role is common to all. The midwife is sometimes the main coordinator and instructor whereas in others it is the physiotherapist. The ideal situation is to have compatible personalities who work together for the benefit of the parents and are not concerned about professional identities which can create artificial barriers.

Generally, the midwife looks after the mother and baby until 10 days after the baby is born, then the health visitor cares for the baby and the physiotherapist teaches and advises the mother throughout antenatal and postnatal care.

The teaching of the anatomy and physiology of labour is covered by a physiotherapist or midwife depending on local policy.

Assessment of physical health

The physiotherapist should identify and try to prevent problems. For example, a woman who has a history of backache needs special attention to perhaps strengthen weak muscles or mobilize stiff joints. Leg exercises are taught, to keep circulation moving and to prevent varicose veins. Lying, move feet up, down, in, out and circle, twice daily with the legs in elevation on one occasion. Standing, heels raising and lowering – this should be performed every quarter of an hour 10 times if the lifestyle involves standing for long periods. Abdominal contractions are taught to be practised in sitting, lying and standing. Pelvic tilting and posture awareness are also taught in these positions. Pelvic floor contractions are taught in stride sitting with the elbows resting on the knees.

Continued activities

General exercises of walking, swimming and cycling are beneficial. Bicycling is an excellent form of non-weight bearing activity but it is often abandoned because roads are dangerous, in which case a static cycle is useful. Group aqua-exercises are becoming popular at leisure centres. (They have followed the 'mother and baby splash' courses of the late 1970s.) Heavy forms of exercise and unaccustomed activities (e.g. moving heavy furniture) are unwise in pregnancy because of the extra stress on top of the increased weight already present, altered centre of gravity and altered blood distribution. Particular note must be taken of the ligament laxity (due to relaxin). Hypermobility occurs in all joints, which then become vulnerable to strain and so competitive sport is not recommended. Also the level of fatigue rises more rapidly in pregnancy owing to the metabolic needs of the fetus.

Back care and lifting

Back strain is minimized when the spine is held in its normal curves but spinal posture has to change with pregnancy. The centre of gravity moves forwards and there is a tendency to an increased lumbar curve with consequent stress on the posterior muscles and ligaments. There are also compensating changes in the thoracic and cervical spines which cause discomfort in these areas. It is important to teach the woman how to adopt positions which minimize stress and to change position regularly (Figure 25.7). Posture advice is given in different positions. Attention to good posture has been shown to reduce the incidence of backache in pregnancy (Mantle *et al.*, 1981).

Standing (Figure 25.7) – Stretch head up out of shoulders. Feel baby sit in the pelvis, pull in abdominal muscles, tighten buttocks. Feel poised, release tension without sagging. Avoid transferring the weight through one leg for long periods of time. Lean back against a wall or chair back for support if standing is essential and try to go up and down on the toes several times to keep the circulation moving and ease muscle tension.

Sitting – Practise sitting back into the chair so that it feels as if the weight of the baby is taken on the seat, and try to have the feet well supported – on a little stool if necessary. If sitting for a long time pelvic tilting should be practised regularly. A small cushion should be placed in the back to preserve a slight lumbar curve and reduce the stretch on the posterior spinal structures. It is also important when resting in sitting to have the legs supported in slight elevation or at least horizontal.

Whether sitting or standing it is important to remember that if the arms are in use in front of the body the spinal extensors are working hard and need to be eased by placing the hands on the pelvis along the iliac crest and extending backwards. It is important to avoid twisting with the knees or feet apart because this causes stress on the sacroiliac joints, as does stepping on to high stools or going up two stairs at a time.

Sleeping positions – In pregnancy, sleeping positions may have to be altered because of the body's weight gain and altered shape (lying prone is not possible). For most women, quarter-turn from prone (recovery position) is acceptable as the weight of the baby is taken on the bed. With a pillow under the abdomen and another under the top knee the position can be very comfortable. Sleeping supine should be avoided but, if necessary, a pillow under the thighs and another under the head and shoulders (perhaps two under the head) will ensure flattening and support of the lumbar spine. When changing position in bed, e.g. turning, keeping the flexed knees together reduces the strain in the sacroiliac joints. Getting in and out of bed, the woman should go into side-lying and avoid abdominal strain from sitting up or lying straight down.

Lifting advice – This involves lifting from a height and carrying as well as lifting from the ground level. The principles to follow are: never stoop, feet should be apart to increase the base and any object to be lifted must be held close to the body (if held at arm's length the leverage on the spine causes high loading of the spinal extensors). When lifting from the floor, it is important to ensure that the weight is light enough to be lifted comfortably. It may be advisable to lift in stages such as floor to chair and then chair to upright. When lifting from a height, it is important to hold the object close to the body and to make sure that the height is within easy reach. Later in the pregnancy, it is inadvisable to stand on high stools or to climb step-ladders because balance is less secure with the centre of gravity moved forward.

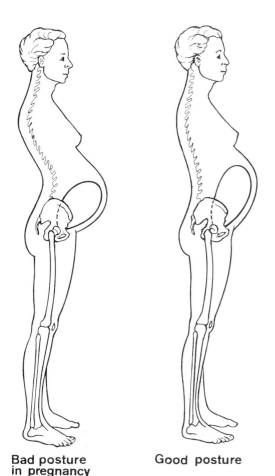

Bad posture in pregnancy may cause backache   **Good posture**

Figure 25.7 Posture during pregnancy

Activities and back care – Low-down activities should be performed from kneeling positions, for example cleaning the bath, making beds or playing with small children. Standing at work surfaces is more comfortable for the back with one foot forward and possibly on a low stool. When hoovering, hanging out washing or ironing it is important to ensure that the body weight is over a base with the feet apart and one in front of the other. At intervals during these activities and others involving flexion it is important to ease the spinal extensor muscle tension by placing the hands on the iliac crests and easing the spine into extension.

Treatment of neuromuscular and musculoskeletal problems

Sacroiliac pain, due to immobility, is treated with low-grade mobilizations. For example, with the patient lying, the knee of the affected side is flexed towards the opposite shoulder and then an oscillatory force is applied along the long axis of the femur. At home, it helps if the woman lies on her back and pulls the knee and foot of the affected side up to her chest, holds and rests a few times to ease the pain (ankle towards groin and knee towards shoulder).

Pubic pain is often related to diastasis of the rectus abdominis muscles, especially following many pregnancies. This pain is treated by pelvic support, for example from a Fembrace – a firm elasticated corset, modified in design to fit under the main bulk of the baby. Abdominal contractions must continue as a daily routine.

Lumbar pain may be eased by soft-tissue kneading and mobilizations such as transverse vertebral pressure to the spinous processes with the patient in side-lying or lumbar rotation.

Hip pain often responds to longitudinal oscillations.

All these treatments are followed by reinforcing education on posture, back care and lifting plus any exercise specific to the patient's requirements.

Rib-cage pressure – If the patient supports the arms above the shoulder height this feeling of pressure can be reduced.

Pelvic pressure – Some patients find kneeling, with knees shoulder width apart and leaning forward on to the forearms is helpful. It is important to instruct the woman to keep her feet together.

Cramp – This occurs most commonly in the calf muscles often at night or after a period of rest. It can be relieved by slow sustained stretch on the muscles pushing the foot and ankle into dorsiflexion. Some people find that it is possible to prevent cramp by performing foot exercises just after getting into bed and when turning in bed to keep the feet in dorsiflexion.

Stitch – This is a sharp pain in the side brought on by fast activity, particularly fast walking. Therefore activities should be performed at an even, steady pace and become slower as the pregnancy proceeds.

Bladder control – Strong pelvic floor muscles are needed to support the ever-increasing weight. If these muscles are weak a slight dribble of urine can occur when the abdominal pressure is increased, for example in coughing, sneezing, laughing or lifting. Previous pregnancies make the woman more likely to have this problem. The treatment is pelvic floor exercises. The woman is instructed to tighten and pull up muscles between the legs plus tightening the abdominal muscles, hold for a count of 4 and rest; repeat six times. This should be practised during pregnancy so that the woman understands how to do the exercise during the difficult postnatal time when the area is numb. Since these muscles fatigue easily with voluntary exercise only 4–6 isometric contractions should be performed at any one time, but frequent practice throughout the day is essential. Once mastered, the exercise can be performed with the woman in any position; but to start with sitting on a hard chair with knees apart, leaning forwards so that the perineum is in contact with the chair seat, assists learning through awareness and proprioception.

Neuromuscular tension control

Relaxation techniques

Relaxation techniques are taught as 'coping strategies' for measuring pain tolerance in labour and also as a means of reducing stress in all life situations. The method used is physiological relaxation based on the Laura Mitchell method. The principle underlying this approach is to make a group of muscles contract isometrically so that there is a relaxation and lengthening effect of the antagonists. The general position of tension is flexion with hunched shoulders, arms held in, elbows flexed, hands clenched, legs flexed, chin held down and forward, and teeth gritted. Other signs of tension are a dry mouth, sweating, tachycardia and breath holding. The physiotherapist must teach the woman how to recognize tension and how to deal with it. At first it is helpful to practise relaxation in lying. The woman is taught to tighten the muscles opposing the tension position:

1. Push the legs into the supporting surface, feel the support, now stop pushing and register the comfort.
2. Stretch the hands and elbows, push the arms into the floor, feel the support and then stop pushing.
3. Push the shoulders down, feel that they are comfortable and stop pushing.

4. Push the head down into the pillow, stretch the head out of the neck (feel that this is comfortable) and then stop pushing and stretching.
5. Face and jaw. Feel smoothness over the face and up over the head. Open mouth like a yawn and rest, to release clenching of the teeth.

These principles, once they are understood, can be applied in any position and in several everyday situations. The value of this method is that it is simple to practise stretching into the positions opposite to those of tension thereby gaining relaxation of the tight muscles. With practice the woman can learn to register quickly when a part of the body is tense, and take appropriate action. There is then a better balance between muscles and joint receptors which register comfort and a feeling of well-being which eases mental stress. During labour, an ability to apply relaxation principles can help to reduce the severity of the pain.

Breathing awareness

The respiratory centre in the medulla is sensitive to carbon dioxide excess so that breathing rate and depth change to meet the oxygen debt. Care is therefore necessary in explaining the use of conscious breathing so that hyperventilation does not occur. Keeping to the natural breathing rhythm, the woman is taught to sigh out slowly during the expiratory phase of respiration and fill up comfortably. This can help with relaxation during the painful contractions of labour.

Touch and massage

Touch is known to release the body's own opiates that help to block sensory pain; it is a natural reaction to rub an intact area that hurts. Firm holding of the lower back or deep, slow massage by the partner or midwife can reduce the pain of labour. Also self-stroking, or holding of the abdomen or pubis can help to reduce pain and release tension.

Rocking movements

Rocking in a rocking-chair can induce comfort, again – it is thought – by releasing the body's own opiates. This principle can therefore be incorporated into gaining relaxation during labour, e.g. rocking the pelvis backwards, forwards and sideways in different positions.

Teaching positions for labour

First stage (waiting for cervical dilatation)

Remaining upright and mobile with gravity assisting fetal descent can make contractions more effective and possibly less painful. The following may be helpful:

1. Walking about, changing to leaning forwards on a support during contractions when necessary.
2. Sitting comfortably, leaning on a table or using the chair back and sitting astride the chair seat or use a rocking-chair.
3. Kneeling leaning forward with the forearms and trunk on a bank of pillows, big bean pillow or bed backrest.

As labour progresses fatigue sets in and rest is essential in side-lying, quarter-turn from prone or tailor position. Relaxation techniques can then be used as already described to preserve energy between contractions. It is helpful to imagine a contraction coming on and to practise breathing, rocking or touch and massage techniques already described.

Second stage (expulsive effort of giving birth)

Midwife and physiotherapist together describe the sensations of the expulsive effort and of giving birth. Most women sit supported in bed in a modified squat position, but some use side-lying and a few use kneeling or a childbirth chair. The midwife explains the various types of obstetric assistance available (episiotomy, caesarean section, forceps delivery) as well as the forms of pain relief (pethidine injection, nitrous oxide plus oxygen inhalation, spinal epidural). This enables the woman to understand the effects and implications of these procedures and to participate in the choice when the time comes. The physiotherapist may teach the woman how transcutaneous electrical nerve stimulation (TENS) may be used to relieve pain during the birth.

Third stage (expulsion of the placenta, cord and membranes)

The midwife explains this stage. Relaxation and breathing awareness are again useful.

Teaching postnatal exercises

The physiotherapist explains the importance of postnatal exercises in regaining fitness and preventing long-term problems such as abdominal weakness, backache and stress incontinence.

Postnatal care

Postnatal support groups are organized at Community Health Clinics and exercise sessions are arranged by the physiotherapist. Most mothers are home within 48 hours, and a physiotherapy session should be attended within the first 6 weeks.

The time taken to return to fitness after childbirth will vary according to the lifestyle beforehand and the type of delivery. It takes longer to recover from a caesarean section than from an uncomplicated delivery and the fitter the woman beforehand the quicker is the return to normality. Emotionally the woman is affected by the bodily changes and by her new responsibility. Parenthood creates a new dimension which is difficult to imagine and the feeling of responsibility can be almost overwhelming. Protective maternal instinct is strong but feelings of love for the new-born may take some time to develop. Elation at the time of the birth may be replaced by mild depression due mainly to fatigue and perhaps discomfort. A new mother is very sensitive to the attitudes of members of staff and it is important to temper a positive approach with compassion and sympathy. It is very important to listen to any problems as they are perceived by the mother especially in relation to uncertainty in caring for the new baby.

Aims of physiotherapy

These are to:

1. Re-educate and strengthen pelvic floor muscles.
2. Instruct in the care of the perineum.
3. Relieve pain in the perineum.
4. Strengthen abdominal muscles.
5. Give postoperative care following a caesarean section.
6. Advise on posture and prevention of backstrain with activities related to the baby.
7. Give instructions in a long-term exercise (6 weeks to 6 months).

Pelvic floor muscles

It is important to start pelvic floor exercises within 6 hours of the delivery to regain the strength of these stretched muscles as soon as possible. The contraction may be felt only around the anus because the perineum is numb but antenatal practice helps as the mother knows what to aim for. The physiotherapist needs to encourage the mother to practise the contractions four or five times at frequent intervals throughout the day. The mother may be afraid to try because of the postdelivery discharge (lochia) or because of stitches or pain. It helps, therefore, to explain that the exercises will increase the circulation, promoting healing and removing inflammatory exudate which will in turn relieve pain. Because the muscles have been stretched it is important to tighten and relax slowly. As feeling returns, the mother can gauge the recovery of strength by trying to arrest urine mid-flow. The number of contractions should be increased to 50 per day in small groups of five at a time and linked to a daily activity,

e.g. when washing hands, getting out of a chair, or feeding the baby. At the 6-week postnatal appointment the obstetrician will check the perineum for healing, the vaginal opening for size, the cervix for erosion and the muscles for strength. If, on testing at 12–16 weeks for stress incontinence there is a problem, the mother is referred for out-patient physiotherapy. Interferential therapy is very useful in re-educating the pelvic floor muscles (see stress incontinence). Pelvic floor exercises should be continued indefinitely to reduce the likelihood of stress incontinence in later life. The suggested ultimate test for incontinence is to try jumping up and down (2–3 hours after passing urine) and coughing at the same time to raise the intra-abdominal pressure.

Care of the perineum

Frequent bathing and changing of sanitary pads is important. The area should be kept dry and during a bowel movement supported with a clean folded sanitary towel.

Relief of perineal pain

Sitting is more comfortable on a ring cushion or between folded pillows so that pressure on the perineum is relieved. Side-sitting or side-lying may be tried for breast feeding. Prone lying with pillows under the lower legs and the abdomen to relieve pressure on the breasts may be restful. Mild sedation may be prescribed. The sooner the bruising is absorbed the quicker healing takes place and the pain is relieved. Ice may be applied as a pack for 4–5 minutes or as an ice cube wrapped in a wet swab moved gently over the area for 2–3 minutes twice a day. Both these methods can be carried on at home by the mother herself. Pulsed electromagnetic energy can be applied to the area at a low intensity for 5–10 minutes to promote healing. Ultrasound may be applied under water with the mother in a bath if, at a later stage, there is dyspareunia (pain on sexual intercourse) because scar tissue around the vagina can be softened by the effects of ultrasound.

Strengthening the abdominal muscles

Immediately after the birth, the muscles are slack, and intra-abdominal pressure is reduced. At first the uterus remains above the pelvic rim and the woman is concerned about looking 5 months pregnant. Involution of the uterus is generally complete in about 14 days but the abdominal muscles may take 6 weeks to return to the pre-pregnant state and it can be 6 months before full strength is returned.

Care of the back must be explained, e.g. rolling onto the side to get in and out of bed, avoiding straight sit-ups, lifting as already taught, because the normal support of the abdominals for the lumbar spine is diminished and the ligamentous laxity still present renders the spinal structures more vulnerable to strain.

Diastasis of the rectus abdominis, i.e. separation of the two muscles, should be monitored. The women lies in crook lying with the lumbar spine flattened and the head is lifted to produce an abdominal contraction. The gap is felt with the fingers just below the umbilicus between the internal borders of the two muscles. At first the muscles are two finger breadths apart but by 6 weeks the gap should be reduced so that only the tip of one finger may be inserted. If the gap is greater, e.g. 3–4 finger breadths, then rotation and side-flexion should be avoided, and straight abdominal muscle work only is recommended until the gap is narrowed to two finger breadths. Diastasis is more common in women who have had several pregnancies, are obese and prone to bronchitis. Suitable strengthening exercises are:

1. Crook lying, pelvic tilting.
2. Crook lying, back flattening, hold to count of 4 and rest – progress to holding for 10.
3. Crook lying, back flattening and, keeping the back flat, slide the heels slowly down the bed and slide slowly back.
4. Crook lying, tighten abdominal muscles, lift head and shoulders and lower slowly. (There may be a couple of pillows under the head to start with which are removed as the muscles become stronger.)
5. Half crook lying, hip hitching on the side of the straight leg.
6. Sitting, trunk bending side to side.
7. Crook lying, knees rolling from side to side.
8. Sitting, trunk turning from side to side.
9. To work the hip extensors which help to maintain the backward/forward pelvic tilt.
10. Prone lying, alternate leg raising and lowering.
11. Prone lying, tighten buttocks, hold for count 10 and rest.

It is important to remember that the abdominal muscles should be contracted and released slowly at first and jerking must be avoided.

Physiotherapy following caesarean section

First day

1. Breathing exercises.
2. Huffing with a pillow held over the wound.
3. Foot and leg exercises are performed to assist circulation.
4. Teach mother how to move about and to roll on to the side for getting in and out of bed.
5. Feeding the baby in bed – have a pillow under the thighs to prevent sliding down and an extra pillow under the knee on the side of feeding.

Second day

1. Add pelvic floor exercises.
2. Straight abdominal exercises.
3. Pelvic tilting.
4. Continue deep breathing exercises.
5. Standing, stretch tall, tighten buttocks.
6. Walk tall to prevent backache.

Subsequent days

1. Progress exercises along the same lines as for vaginal delivery.
2. Stitches are generally out by 7 days.
3. Abdominal contractions are very important to maintain mobility of the healing tissues as well as increasing circulation to promote healing.

Involution of the uterus is slower following a section. The mother may attend classes after discharge from hospital.

Advice on activities related to the baby

Feeding the baby

A variety of positions can be tried:

1. Sitting in bed, back supported, bend the hip and knee on the side the baby is feeding. Side-sitting can be tried.
2. Sitting on chair back supported, support one foot on a stool – on the side the baby is feeding.
3. Sitting tailor position may be used with the back supported.
4. Side-lying in bed can be used but is not easy for first-time mothers.
5. Checking suitable heights. When bathing or changing the baby arrange an easily accessible height. Stooping must be avoided – kneel down instead.

Carrying the baby

Carrying the baby close to the body is important for security and well-being of both mother and baby. Over the shoulder is a natural position for carrying. Holding the baby on one hip for too long can cause a strain on the back.

Class two

1. Abdominal strength is assessed.
2. Diastasis of the rectus abdominis muscles is checked.
3. Exercises are progressed.
4. Pelvic floor muscle function is considered in relation to stopping urine flow mid-stream.
5. Ability to relax is ascertained so that the mother can regain energy when the baby is asleep – this is especially useful for the mother whose baby is keeping her awake for large parts of the night.

Class three

Posture, back care and lifting are checked and the importance of these emphasized in the long term to reduce the incidence of sacroiliac and spinal joint strain. If there is pain of musculoskeletal origin, the appropriate treatment must be implemented to prevent the disorder becoming chronic.

Continuation classes

The exercise regimen should be continued and progressed to enable the mother to return to her normal activities, including yoga and sport, in a fit condition and with safety.

Leisure centres

Postnatal sessions and aqua-exercise groups are becoming increasingly available under the auspices of local councils or private enterprise. Mothers pay a small fee for a series of about six sessions. These contribute to the overall fitness of the mothers and as such constitute an important aspect of health care. The exercises are similar to those quoted above plus general trunk, leg and arm movements, often to music. Hydrotherapy is of special value in providing a medium of weight relief for strengthening abdominal and pelvic floor muscles, as well as swimming for general fitness. Generally exercises in water should not be started until 6 weeks after the birth when the placenta site has healed. It is important that the group leaders are qualified to teach exercises, have an understanding of the physiological changes of childbearing, have a knowledge of the advantages, precautions and dangers of hydrotherapy, and experience in dealing with the psychology of parenthood. Physiotherapists are well suited to develop expertise in this field.

Lifting

Antenatal education on back care and lifting must be reinforced.

Practising physiological relaxation is also very beneficial.

Postnatal exercises from 6 weeks to 6 months

It is important that the mother can fit exercise into a busy day and that she can combine her own programme with baby play.

For exercises in crook lying the baby can lie prone on the mother's tummy and chest. During exercise in prone kneeling the baby can lie between the mother's arms. Suitable exercises are back humping and hollowing, pelvis swinging from side to side and alternate leg stretching backwards with abdominal contractions. In standing, the baby can be held in the arms and the mother bends and stretches the knees and hips with her back against a wall. Abdominal and pelvic floor contractions and pelvic tilting can be performed during activities such as washing dishes or queueing at a supermarket.

Suggested plan of postnatal management

Three classes are the necessary minimum to cover all the important points. Class one should be about 6 weeks after discharge from hospital, and the other two at 2- or 3-week intervals.

Class outline

1. Exercises are checked for timing and quality of movement re-taught as necessary, and progressed.
2. Posture advice is reinforced.
3. Questions are answered.
4. Group discussion is encouraged to provide mutual support.

References

Calguneri, C., Bird, H. and Wright, V. (1982) Changes in joint laxity occurring during pregnancy. *Annals of Rheumatic Disease,* **41**, 126

McNaught, A. and Callendar, R. (1983) *Illustrated Physiology,* 4th edn, Churchill Livingstone, London, p. 201

Mantle, M. J., Holmes, J. and Curry, H. L. F. (1981) Backache in pregnancy II: prophylactic influence of back care classes. *Rheumatology and Rehabilitation,* **20**, 227

Chapter 26

Gynaecology

Anatomy and function of the female bladder
Medical conditions

Surgical conditions

Gynaecology is the study of the disorders of the female genital organs. Obstetrics forms part of and overlaps the gynaecological field. In the treatment of these disorders it is important to realize that the control and function of the reproductive system is influenced by the endocrine system. Effective treatment requires a sensitive approach which considers the whole woman, not just her pelvic organs. The physiotherapist needs an awareness of the social and emotional aspects of femininity as well as a sound knowledge of anatomy and physiology.

Anatomy and function of the female bladder (Figure 26.1)

The female bladder is a hollow organ positioned behind the symphysis pubis. Posteriorly it is related to the cervix and anterior wall of the vagina, laterally and inferiorly to the pelvic floor. Two ureters enter the bladder near its base at the trigone. This is a triangular shaped part of the bladder with three orifices – two for the ureters and one for the urethra. The bladder has a wall with three layers: an inner mucous membrane, an outer layer of connec-

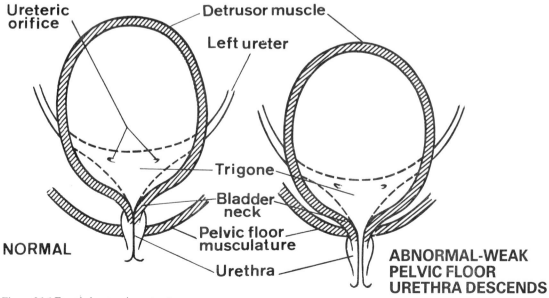

Figure 26.1 Female lower urinary tract

tive tissue and a middle layer of muscle tissue – the detrusor muscle. This muscle has an interlacing arrangement of smooth fibres which run in all directions. The female urethra is 3–4 cm in length passing from the bladder neck through the pelvic floor muscles to its orifice in the perineum. The muscle fibres of the urethra are striated and of the slow twitch variety, enabling the sphincter to maintain a closure pressure and hence continence of urine over prolonged periods without fatigue. The musculature of the bladder has both reflex autonomic and higher centre control. In the normal bladder a mild desire to void is experienced at 200 ml capacity. This can be postponed by voluntary inhibition until micturition is allowed by relaxation of the urethral and pelvic floor muscles with contraction of the detrusor muscle. The pubococcygeus of the levator ani muscle group exerts a closing force on the urethral opening (see Figure 25.2). These pelvic floor muscles contain both fast and slow twitch types of fibre, pubococcygeus making an important contribution to continence during increases of intra-abdominal pressure such as coughing, sneezing and jumping.

The description and treatment of gynaecological conditions will be limited largely to those benefiting from the particular skills of the physiotherapist. The student should note that physiotherapy treatments will include invasive techniques.

The conditions studied are divided into medical and surgical categories.

Medical conditions

Incontinence is defined as the passage of urine at any time that is not both personally desired and socially acceptable.

Three types are described:

1. *Genuine stress incontinence* is the involuntary small leak of urine occurring when intra-abdominal pressure is raised. If high intra-abdominal pressure exceeds the urethral pressure and the outlet mechanisms are incompetent, urine is voided.
2. *Frequency incontinence* is defined, as its name suggests, when the patient needs to void frequently through the day and more than twice at night. It is due to loss of higher centre control over the detrusor muscle which is then described as unstable.
3. *Urge incontinence* occurs when the desire to micturate overcomes the voluntary control of bladder function. It is a sensory or motor disorder. Sensory dysfunction is treated by antibiotics or surgery since it is related to infection, urinary calculi or bladder tumour.

Motor dysfunction is due to detrusor muscle instability and is seen more commonly in the elderly patient.

Some patients have mixed stress and urge or frequency incontinence.

Genuine stress incontinence

Although the degree of dysfunction may require surgery, muscular re-education of the pelvic floor can often restore continence. Like any other muscle in the body these muscles may be damaged, disused, or merely fatigued, leading to atrophy.

Causes

1. Over-stretching or damage of the pelvic floor muscles and fascia during childbirth, leading to inhibition of muscular tone which diminishes function.
2. Loss of elasticity of musculature due to hormonal changes after menopause.
3. Atrophy of the pelvic floor muscles in the elderly sedentary person.

Assessment of muscle strength and function

Digital evaluation of the vagina

This is an invasive technique of a sensitive area and requires great skill. The patient is comfortably supported in half-lying with knees crooked and apart. The physiotherapist, wearing disposable gloves and using a lubricant jelly, gently and slowly inserts the index and middle fingers into the vagina. The therapist palpates the posterior vaginal wall with the distal two phalanges, then judges the strength of the muscles by withdrawing the fingers gently while the patient is asked to hold the fingers there. Strong muscles will squeeze the fingers firmly, thus a graded assessment may be made: 0 nil, 1 poor, 2 fair, 3 good, 4 very good condition.

Perionometer

A vaginal pressure gauge or perionometer may be used to assess the progress of muscle strength and it is often encouraging because it is visual. The gauge needs some experience to be used properly since a gluteal or abdominal contraction can give a misleading reading.

Pad test

This is an objective test of improved function. It is used in urodynamic studies. First the patient voids, then wears a pre-weighed sanitary pad. After drinking 1000 ml of fluid, she rests for 45 min, then exercises for 30 min (which includes walking, climbing stairs, coughing, jumping and hand washing under running water). The pad is then re-weighed; the resulting measurement is given in grams of urine lost.

Physiotherapy

Sensitivity to the patient's condition and attention to comfort and privacy are essential.

A recording of the patient's history is charted. Stresses to which the pelvic floor muscles are subjected are noted; obesity or persistent cough may require referral. The patient needs to participate fully in her recovery and for this an understanding of her condition is necessary. A simple explanation of the anatomy of the pelvis is given and the action of the pelvic floor muscles is demonstrated. (The cupped hands, palms uppermost, gives a model of the approximate size of this group.)

Most patients with genuine stress incontinence will improve with the practice of carefully taught pelvic floor exercises and electrotherapy.

Exercise – For this to be effective the patient should understand that a definite routine of exercise must be followed. Pelvic floor contractions may be performed in all positions (sitting, standing, lying, for example). The legs should be slightly apart, the therapist guarding against the patient breath-holding or contracting the abdominal or gluteal muscles whilst learning the exercise. Some proprioception of muscle contraction can be achieved by the patient leaning forward in stride sitting; the perineum will be in contact with the chair seat. The contractions should be repeated a few times only because of fatigue. Patients are instructed to perform exercise frequently and are encouraged to do so during daily activities. Laycock (1987) described the different demands of fast and slow twitch muscle fibres; some contractions should last 4–10 seconds and some should last 1 second. Stress exercises that raise intra-abdominal pressure (jumping, bending) should include active pelvic floor contraction before attempting the activity. When this is taught the patient's confidence is increased.

Electrotherapy – When the contraction of pelvic floor muscles is graded as poor, the weak muscles may be re-educated by electrotherapy as an adjunct to exercises. Faradism: external electrodes can be used to stimulate pelvic floor muscle contraction. The active pad is on the perineum and the larger indifferent pad is on the lumbar spine or sacral area. However, it is accepted that the use of an internal vaginal electrode is the most effective way to stimulate the pubococcygeus of the levatores ani group in the female. This method of using faradism is both invasive and very uncomfortable, so it is being replaced by interferential therapy. Interferential: Laycock (1988) described different electrical parameters which should be selected for different types of incontinence. A frequency sweep of 10–50 Hz is used for genuine stress incontinence and 5–10 Hz for urge incontinence. A bipolar technique of electrode placement is recommended, the posterior pad placed under the ischial tuberosities and the anterior pad on the perineum just below the symphysis pubis.

Urge and frequency incontinence

When these conditions are the result of an unstable bladder they are treated by bladder training. The physiotherapist teaches re-education of the pelvic floor muscles by encouraging the patient to delay micturition for a few minutes. This can inhibit detrusor muscle activity and lessen the urge to micturate. (Interferential therapy is also used – see above.) Progression is achieved by encouraging the patient to hold on for longer periods.

Surgical conditions

These are divided into minor and major surgery.

Minor surgery

The obstetric conditions requiring short-term hospital treatment are: threatened and inevitable abortion, vaginal termination of pregnancy, ectopic pregnancy and cervical incompetence. Other conditions are hysterosalpingography, dilatation and curettage, laparascopy and colposcopy.

1. *Hysterosalpingography* – This is one of the many investigations that are systematically carried out for infertility (childlessness). A water-soluble radio-opaque medium is passed through the uterus and Fallopian tubes and monitored by an image-intensified screen to determine the patency and function of the tubes.
2. *Dilatation and curettage (D&C)* – This is used as a diagnostic tool to determine the cause of abnormal uterine bleeding. The curettage provides samples of endometrium for histological examination (endometrial biopsy). Dilatation and curettage is also used following abortion to complete the evacuation of the products of conception.
3. *Laparoscopy* – This is a direct inspection of the pelvic organs through a tiny sub-umbilical incision. The laparoscope can detect abnormalities of the ovaries and the uterus. Operative procedures may be performed such as:
   (a) Ovarian biopsy – differentiating ovarian

endometrial cysts from chronic pelvic infection.

(b) Sterilization – performed through the laparoscopic removal of a segment of the Fallopian tubes, ligating each cut end or using metal clips to occlude the tubes.

4. *Colposcopy* – This uses a system of lenses to examine the tissues of the cervix visually and is a means of diagnosing cervical intraepithelial neoplasia and of differentiating mild to severe dysplasia and carcinoma *in situ*. Cyto-diagnosis (smear test) begins with routine examinations of cervical cells. Smears of cells obtained from the lateral wall of the vagina are used to detect a woman's hormonal state and examination of a cervical smear detects or excludes the presence of pre-clinical malignancy of the cervix. Early detection can be followed by successful treatment and since cervical cancer accounts for 11% of all cancer (Llewellyn Jones, 1986), cervical screening should be available to women throughout life. Positive smear tests are indications for inspection and magnification of the cervix with a colposcope. Dysplasia requires further investigation and treatment. Multiple punch biopsy is performed in the region of the suspicious areas and the lesions may be treated by electrocautery or cryosurgery under anaesthetic. Should the lesion extend beyond the cervix then a radical cone biopsy to remove the cervix or a hysterectomy (major surgery) is the appropriate treatment, depending on the lesion and the woman's reproductive age.

Major surgery

The major surgical procedures that will be described briefly are hysterectomy and repair operations.

Hysterectomy

Total hysterectomy refers to the removal of the uterus, and one or both tubes and ovaries may be included depending on the condition. Wertheim's hysterectomy is an extended operation removing uterus, tubes and ovaries and includes lymphadenectomy.

Hysterectomy is used in the treatment of organic pelvic disease for the following conditions:

1. Dysfunctional uterine bleeding after failure of hormone treatment.
2. Endometrial carcinoma and carcinoma of the cervix.
3. Severe uterine or ovarian endometrioma type cysts.
4. Myomatal – benign tumours that develop in the myometrium of the uterus.

The hysterectomy is performed through either an abdominal or a vaginal incision. The abdominal incision most commonly used is the lower midline incision (referred to colloquially as the bikini incision). Vertical median and paramedian incisions are used occasionally.

Repair operations

The range covers corrective surgery relating to prolapse. Prolapse is a form of hernia and occurs through failure of some of the supporting tissues of the muscular vagina and transverse cervical ligaments of the uterus. Depending on the degree of strain there is often enough tone in the supporting tissues to prevent prolapse until the climacteric (menopause). Then muscular atrophy occurs and prolapse may become evident. For this reason operative repair procedures are more common after the age of 45 years.

Vaginal prolapse – When the anterior wall of the vagina is damaged it may cause herniation of the bladder (cystocele) and damage to the posterior wall may affect the rectum (rectocele).

Utero-vaginal prolapse – Descent of the uterus is accompanied by the upper vagina and is also associated with rectocele and cystocele.

Operations used

1. Anterior and posterior colporrhaphy – repair of vaginal tissue and fascia.
2. Manchester repair which combines colporrhaphy with amputation of the cervix and shortening of the transverse cervical ligaments.

Preoperative care and advice

The physiotherapist teaches the patient the value of postoperative physiotherapy and the main exercises are taught.

Post-operative care and advice

The aims of the physiotherapist will be to:

1. Assist in the prevention of circulatory and respiratory complications.
2. Strengthen pelvic floor, abdominal and back muscles.
3. Teach postural correction.
4. Advise on back care.
5. Advise on progression of activities to full function.

Method of treatment

1. Deep breathing and frequent foot and leg movements practised slowly in full-range assist

general circulation, aiding venous return in the first 48 hours.

2. The patient is taught to remove secretions by coughing, supporting the abdominal or perineal incision, with forearms supporting the abdominal wall over a pillow to prevent the pain of the abdominal movement; supporting the perineum, one hand placed on a sanitary pad with gentle pressure upwards prevents pain after vaginal surgery. Long, slow breaths emphasizing the breath out and repeated 'huffs' will help project mucus into the mouth with minimum discomfort.

3. *Exercises:* Pelvic tilting is performed slowly and smoothly. This helps to relieve pain by preventing protective muscle spasm in abdominal and back muscles. Abdominal muscle contractions can help to relieve flatulence and the discomfort of this. Pelvic floor exercise: It is common following hysterectomy and some repair operations that catheterization is used to drain the bladder and rest repaired tissues. The catheter is usually removed within 48 hours. Some surgeons prefer pelvic floor exercises to be delayed until after the catheter is removed.

4. *Posture* – Once drainage tubes are out the patient is encouraged to ease herself out of bed comfortably with knees together and to stand and walk tall. It is very tempting to stoop to guard against pain of the abdominal wound but if the advice is followed pain is lessened because standing tall corrects the spinal curves, and muscle balance, removing the protective tension that adds to pain.

5. Advice on level of activity until returning to normal function from hospital discharge:

(a) Rest and activity should be balanced; lying on the bed for an extra rest daily for 3–4 weeks.

(b) Reduce standing. Sit on a stool or chair for light household tasks.

(c) Graduated exercises will help to strengthen abdomen and back muscles: (i) crook lying knee rolling; (ii) crook lying sit up; (iii) crook lying hip hitching; (iv) 2–3 weeks, prone lying buttocks tightening, alternate leg raising.

(d) Avoid pushing or pulling objects forcefully.

(e) Avoid lifting and carrying for 6 weeks. When lifting, hold objects close in to the body, feet apart. Use leg muscles by bending knees – never stoop.

(f) Return to work will be advised by the surgeon. Depending on the type of work it will vary between 6 and 12 weeks.

Generally, after 12 weeks, the patient may return to a full lifestyle – normal for her. It is important, however, that for at least a year she pays attention to warm-up and stretching before sport or heavy household tasks such as furniture removing.

References

Laycock, J. (1987) Graded exercises for the pelvic floor muscles in the treatment of urinary incontinence. *Physiotherapy,* **73**, 371

Laycock, J. (1988) Interferential therapy in the treatment of incontinence. *Physiotherapy,* **74**, 171

Llewellyn-Jones, D. (1986) *Fundamentals of Obstetrics and Gynaecology,* 4th edn, Vol. II, Faber & Faber, London

Chapter 27

Care of the elderly

During the twentieth century there has been a dramatic increase in the number of elderly people in Western society. Theoretically, people are classified as elderly on reaching retirement age (65 for men and 60 for women). In health terms, most patients who require the services of an elderly-care team are aged over 75 years. Changes in medical, social and economic factors have resulted in people being fitter for longer, and the final period of illness is tending to be shorter. This trend is likely to continue so that more people will live to old age with men having a life expectancy of 69 years and women of 75 years.

Physiotherapy in care of the elderly

Physiotherapy is directed at the early rehabilitation of elderly patients. Prevention of the problems of old age should also be an important theme for all physiotherapists. The main diseases and disorders that affect the elderly and require a very positive physiotherapy input may be considered under headings as follows:

1. Orthopaedics and trauma.
2. Rheumatology.
3. Respiratory.
4. Cardiovascular.
5. Neurology.

Physiotherapy principles are outlined in the chapters indicated.

Orthopaedics and trauma (Chapters 3–7)

Joint replacement surgery is directed at restoring movement and function in patients with degener-

ative or inflammatory arthropathies. Patients undergoing this surgery may not necessarily be elderly but rehabilitation is essential to restore fitness and encourage independence, which helps to reduce disability in later years. Fractures of the neck of femur and surgical neck of humerus are injuries of the elderly. Soft-tissue injuries may be spontaneous rupture of a tendon (often the long head of biceps). Capsulitis of the shoulder can also occur.

Deformities – particularly of the feet (hammer toe, hallux rigidus, hallux valgus) – can be very disabling in the elderly.

Rheumatology (Chapters 8–11)

Degenerative, inflammatory and metabolic arthropathies give rise to problems in the elderly. Osteoarthrosis of the hips, knees and hands can be very disabling. The patient suffers from both pain and slowness of movement.

Respiratory (Chapter 13)

Chronic obstructive airways disease and late-onset asthma are features in any elderly group. Physiotherapy has often been instituted before the patient is elderly and should be aimed at prevention of disability by encouraging patients to have a daily exercise programme and regular checks – especially as winter sets in each year. During an exacerbation of bronchitis or asthma, physiotherapy can be life-saving and often has to be fairly aggressive to regain mobility before the patient succumbs to the problems of bed rest.

Cardiovascular (Chapters 15 and 16)

Cardiovascular disease is the commonest cause of death in elderly patients. Coronary artery disease, congestive cardiac failure, heart valve disorder, cardiac arrhythmias, heart block and infective endocarditis are conditions that affect the elderly. A myocardial infarction (due to coronary artery disease) can be 'silent' in the old, and infective endocarditis is easily missed.

Venous leg ulcers can be present, causing great pain and distress. Often they are dressed by a visiting nurse without any active treatment. Peripheral vascular disease may lead to leg amputation in the elderly.

Neurology (Chapters 19–22)

Cerebrovascular accident producing hemiplegia causes disability in the elderly. Transient ischaemic attacks (TIA) often precede an episode of paralysis. Gradual onset of paralysis can be due to a cerebral tumour. Parkinson's disease causes slowness of voluntary movement and particular distress in relation to loss of emotional response, facial expression and communication.

In addition to treating patients with specific disease-related problems, the physiotherapist should have a broad understanding of the other age-related problems and the importance of health promotion for the elderly. Also, the multiple-pathology nature of disease complicates the picture, e.g. chronic obstructive airway disease and osteo-arthritic hips. These may be considered under the following headings:

1. The biology of ageing.
2. Health promotion including body maintenance.
3. Social problems.
4. Handicaps within daily living.
5. Effects of immobilization.
6. Psychiatry in the elderly.
7. Assessment of the elderly.
8. Services available.
9. Role of physiotherapy.

Biology of ageing

With age there is a decline in energy, faculties and tissues. Different systems change at different rates in different people. Chronological age does not necessarily correlate with biological age. An 85 year old may be active and independent (Figure 27.1) whereas a 70 year old may have many problems. Visible signs of ageing include greying and coarseness of hair, loss of elasticity and dryness of the skin

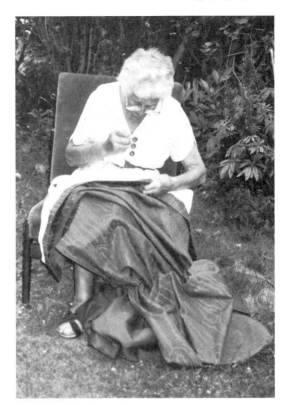

Figure 27.1 85-year-old woman sewing curtains

Hearing may be impaired – often by accumulation of wax which should be treated by a GP. Stiffening of the ossicles causes loss of high frequency sound and it is frustrating for an elderly person who can hear quite well – but not in the presence of background noise (as in a ward or day-room). A hearing aid is of great benefit and can be cosmetically acceptable. It is important for communication to sit on the 'good' side, to talk slowly, clearly and in short sentences. Shouting should be avoided and touching the patient's hand to attract attention before asking a question is helpful.

Eyesight may be diminished and dark adaptation is a problem. Therefore good lighting is important. Glasses can take care of some sight problems but rugs on floors, uneven paving stones and unmarked steps are hazards to the elderly who cannot see.

Speech becomes restricted and it may be helpful for the patient to have a bell to call attention because the voice is not strong enough. Reluctance to speak is often associated with depression.

The musculoskeletal system deteriorates. Bones may become osteoporotic especially in the immobile patient. This is a hazard to active exercise and manipulative procedures. Soft tissues lose elasticity. Height is lost owing to narrowing of intervertebral discs. Articular cartilage is less elastic and joints are less able to absorb stress – there is stiffness after prolonged sitting or lying. Muscle power diminishes leading to slowness of movement and loss of coordination.

Balance difficulties can develop. The causative factors are loss of proprioception from tissues on weight-bearing surfaces, muscle weakness and degenerative changes in the semicircular canals. Hence falls are a problem in the elderly.

Nervous system deterioration leads to impairment of homeostasis, for example abnormal temperature regulation leads to hypothermia.

Learning and short-term memory are impaired. Repetition of instructions and patience in waiting for the patient to remember are important.

Pain thresholds are often higher or sensitivity to pain decreases which sometimes leads to trauma (pressure sores, fractures) being missed.

The cardiovascular system diminishes in efficiency. The cardiac output is decreased and sudden stress should be avoided.

The respiratory system is less efficient. Loss of elasticity of the costal cartilages leads to diminished thoracic mobility and reduced vital capacity.

Cognitive abilities – Memory and personality do not diminish much until the middle eighties.

Health promotion and body maintenance

The measures that can be taken to promote health in the elderly include:

1. Weight control by diet and exercises.
2. Mental stimulation with preservation of self-esteem by hobbies and activities involving meeting people.
3. Stop cigarette smoking.
4. Caring for the body by regular visits to the dentist, optician, or general practitioner (for blood pressure, hearing and skin care).
5. Joint replacements also maintain mobility in the elderly.

Social problems

The main social problems of the elderly are related to:

1. Poverty.
2. Lack of heating.
3. Poor housing.
4. Loneliness – loss of partner and distance of family.

These factors interact to produce a downward spiral (Figure 27.2).

Handicaps within daily living

Pain, stiffness, muscle weakness and neurological deficit can lead to inability or profound difficulty with dressing, washing (personal hygiene), toileting, eating, moving around the house, using transport. Incontinence may be a problem because of weak pelvic floor muscles or stiff fingers and shoulders making it difficult to remove clothing quickly, or slowness in getting to the toilet. This can be helped by encouraging the patient to 'go' every 2 hours – or at regular intervals when it suits the individual's time-scale.

Effects of immobilization

These may be considered as:

1. Musculoskeletal.
2. Circulatory.
3. Skin.
4. Postural hypotension.
5. Respiratory.
6. Urinary and bowel problems.
7. Apathy and depression.

Musculoskeletal

Bones become osteoporotic. Joints become stiff and contractures may arise, e.g. hamstrings (knee flexors), gastrocnemius (tendo Achillis), biceps brachii, finger flexors, and sternomastoid muscles rapidly lose power and bulk – after 6 weeks' bed rest, power loss can be up to 20%. A normal adult takes 6 weeks to recover muscle power after 6 weeks' bed rest. This period is longer with increasing age.

Circulatory

Deep vein thrombosis in the legs can lead to pulmonary embolism which is often fatal.

Skin

Pressure sores arise due to muscle and soft-tissue loss, shearing stresses between tissue planes and loss of blood supply due to pressure on bony prominences. Aggravating factors are contamination with sweat, urine or faeces.

Postural hypotension

This may occur after prolonged bed rest. As a result, there is faintness and giddiness on standing up.

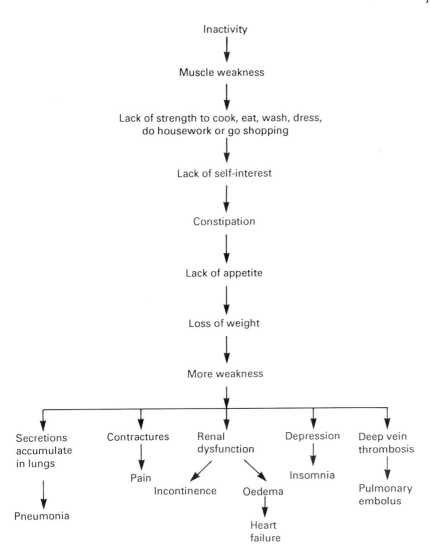

Figure 27.2 The downward spiral of problems in the elderly

Respiratory

Hypostatic pneumonia. Accumulation of secretions provides a medium for development of bacteria, e.g. *Streptococcus pneumoniae*. In the elderly the clinical features are often lethargy, loss of appetite and dry, irritating cough.

Urinary and bowel problems

Calculi can form in kidneys and incontinence develops of both urine and faeces.

Apathy and depression

Even in a young person, prolonged immobility can cause apathy, then depression. Age accelerates the onset of these.

Psychiatry in the elderly

One of the most important aspects of psychiatry in the elderly is that the various disorders or diseases are recognized and treated, otherwise patients can be simply classified as 'old' or labelled 'difficult'.

Psychiatric illnesses include:

1. Depression.
2. Hypomania.
3. Paranoid psychoses.
4. Neuroses.
5. Dementia.
6. Confusion.

Depression

This is common in the elderly – especially those admitted to hospital. It is related to physical ill health, bereavement, deafness, blindness, or social isolation. It may lead to withdrawal, apathy, or refusal to eat or drink.

Hypomania

This results in loss of concentration, non-stop talking, restlessness and swings of mood. Patience and firmness are essential in dealing with the manic patient.

Paranoid psychoses

These may be the schizophrenic type and may manifest as delusions of being persecuted, poisoned or harassed. Alcohol can be a related factor. This can be very trying for carers, particularly family, as the patient will probably tell professionals that the family do not help and 'never do anything'.

Neuroses

Anxiety is one of the commonest states. The patient tends to be irritable, forgetful and agitated. Sometimes phobias, e.g. agoraphobia, develop.

Dementia

This is impairment of memory, intellect and personality. The patient is conscious but cannot perform everyday activities. Alzheimer's disease is a form of dementia which can start in younger people (50 years). There are tangles of filaments in the cells of the cerebral cortex and hippocampus, together with neuritic plaques and lack of acetylcholine. Dementia of Alzheimer type can occur in older people.

Confusion

Acute confusion is often a main feature of underlying serious pathology – e.g. pneumonia, gastrointestinal bleeding, or pulmonary embolus. Disorientation, hallucinations and loss of awareness of environment are features.

Treatment of these conditions varies according to the underlying pathology. Tranquillizers or anti-depressants, lithium (a mood stabilizer) and anti-biotics may be appropriate. A review of the patient's drugs is often wise because these can cause confusion (iatrogenic disease).

Assessment of the elderly

This is complex and requires time because often there is multiple pathology. Team work is generally necessary to produce a real picture. Relatives, friends, neighbours, home helps, policemen, social workers, nurses, occupational therapists, physio-therapists as well as doctors of varying specialities need to make a contribution and a true assessment of a patient admitted to an acute unit may take 2–3 days.

History

1. Patient's problems/complaints.
2. Precipitating events.
3. Personality.
4. Lifestyle, degree of independence.
5. Home, family, carer situation.
6. Use of drugs, alcohol.
7. Previous physical illness.
8. Previous occupations.
9. Hobbies.

Mental state

1. Appearance and behaviour.
2. Speech and communication.
3. Mood.
4. Orientation.
5. Concentration.
6. Self-esteem.

Observation

1. State of skin, hands, nails, teeth.
2. Tension, posture, relaxation.
3. Clothing.
4. Shoes.

Investigations

1. Urine tests.
2. Blood – cell count, ESR, electrolytes, calcium, glucose.
3. X-rays.
4. CT scans.

Physical examination

Physiotherapists must identify functional restrictions and relate these to the causes.

Principles to follow are:

1. Self-care:
   (a) Dressing.
   (b) Bathing.
   (c) Washing.
   (d) Toileting.
   (e) Eating and drinking.
2. Transfers:
   (a) Moving about in bed.
   (b) Bed–chair.
   (c) Use of wheelchair.
   (d) Standing up and sitting down.
   (e) Floor–chair.
3. Mobility:
   (a) Walking with or without aids.
   (b) Stairs.
   (c) Balance.
   (d) Confidence in moving around.
   (e) Desire to move around.
   (f) Shopping.
   (g) Transport.
4. Special tests:
   (a) Joint range.
   (b) Muscle strength.
   (c) Coordination.
   (d) Cardiovascular functions (see Chapter 15).
   (e) Respiratory examination (see Chapter 12).
   (f) Neurological tests: (i) sensation, (ii) muscle tone.

Assessment continues throughout the patient's progress from initial contact to final discharge. A home visit and functional assessments are essential. Patients must be seen to actually perform tasks, as many say they can when in reality they cannot, e.g. cook, dress, wash. Team conference is essential to draw together all the findings so that problems are identified and goals set. Progress must be monitored and generally the patient should be seen to progress from medical and nursing care to rehabilitation and social care.

Services for the elderly

The elderly are cared for in:

1. Own home.
2. Family home.
3. Private residential homes.
4. Private nursing homes.
5. Sheltered housing.
6. Part III accommodation.
7. Day centre.
8. Day hospital.
9. Long-stay hospital.
10. Acute hospital.
11. About 90% of elderly people live at home – on their own or with the family.

Own home

Theoretically this is ideal for the persons' self-esteem and independence. Home help, meals on wheels, community youth visiting, dial-a-ride (taxi service), health visitor, church, home nurse, neighbours, friends, telephone help and some societies can help maintain an elderly person at home.

Family home

A 'granny flat' attached to the house of a son or daughter can work extremely well because the elderly person's independence plus security can be maintained. An elderly parent occupying a room in the family house can work most of the time but can cause stress, for example in division of loyalties. Progressive deterioration in an elderly parent puts increasing demand on the son or daughter and it is at this stage that help is needed from the services outlined above plus a regular check-up from the general practitioner. Intervention at this stage could possibly prevent some of the disability which develops and the stress on the carer could be reduced.

Private residential homes

These can be pleasant but expensive, although some welfare financial assistance can be arranged. When the person takes up residence there can be feelings of rejection on the part of the elderly person and feelings of guilt on the part of the family. On the other hand, there can be total relief to all parties, and strained relationships can change to happy mutual trust and respect.

Private nursing homes

These offer more nursing than residential homes and are highly variable in standards. Again they can be expensive although financial assistance can be arranged from local authority funds.

Sheltered housing

This varies, but an elderly person can live in sheltered housing with carers providing the support to keep the person at home.

Part III accommodation

Under the National Assistance Act (1948) Part III, Section 21, local authorities provide residential accommodation for people who need care and attention because of age. Hence 'Part III' refers to local authority residential homes.

Day centres

An elderly person may travel to a centre by social service transport or with a relative or friend. A day centre provides support in terms of group activities, meals, chiropody, hair dressing, occupational therapy and possibly physiotherapy. A meal is provided and daily programmes are varied to give interest. Activities may be chess, carpentry, cookery, painting and marquetry, for example.

Day hospital

This may have similar facilities to those in a day centre but the essential difference is that medical attention is available. There are doctors, nurses, physiotherapists and occupational therapists who develop a programme of treatment and rehabilitation according to individual needs. A patient, therefore, has the benefits of hospital treatment as well as living at home.

Other forms of day care may be in:

1. Lunch clubs.
2. Residential homes.
3. Work centres.
4. Social centres.

Long-stay hospital

This provides 24 hour nursing care for the severely disabled (both physically and mentally). Decor of the rooms, bedspreads and furniture are homely rather than clinical. The corridors and doorways are wide enough for people with walking aids or wheelchairs. Baths and toilets are adapted for easy use. Physiotherapy input is dependent on staffing levels and how much occupational therapy is available. Group activities as in the day centre, maintenance of mobility, prevention of pressure sores and contractures are all important.

Acute hospital

This includes general medical wards in a district general hospital as well as special elderly care wards or hospitals. Patients may be admitted for assessment because of 'failure to thrive'. This can be caused by the following:

1. Minor cardiovascular accidents, Parkinson's disease.
2. Masked depression.
3. Chronic infection – lungs, kidney, bladder.
4. Iatrogenic disorders – too many drugs.
5. Malignancy – lung, bowel, prostate.
6. Endocrine disorders, e.g. thyroid insufficiency.
7. Metabolic disorders, e.g. diabetes.

It is essential to diagnose and treat these disorders, otherwise the patient can be incorrectly labelled 'old' or 'demented'.

Falls and accidents (e.g. fractured femur, burns) often lead to admission. Sometimes neighbours alert the police, who enter the home of a patient who has had a black-out and been lying on the floor for several hours. The management follows the themes of:

1. Medical diagnosis and treatment.
2. Assessment of problems related to:
   (a) Patient.
   (b) Environment.
   (c) Family.
   (d) Social.
3. Development of strategy to solve or cope with these problems.
4. Early mobility and discharge so that the patient does not become dependent.

Some people who look after the elderly

Bath attendant.
Chiropodists.
Church personnel.
Continence advisor.
Dentist.
Doctors.
Hairdresser.
Home help.
Health visitors.
Neighbours.
Nurses.
Occupational therapists.
Optician.
Orthotist.
Physiotherapist.
Police.
Social workers.
Speech therapists.
Stomach advisor.
Voluntary services – WRVS, hospital friends.
Welfare rights officer.

Associations and societies

Alzheimer's Disease Society.
Chest, Heart and Stroke Association.
Parkinson's Disease Society.

Useful addresses

Age Concern,
Bernard Sunley House,
60 Pitcairn Road,
Mitcham,
Surrey CR4 3LL.

Association of Carers,
Medway Homes,
Balfour Road,
Rochester,
Kent.

Help the Aged,
St. James Walk,
London EC1R 0BE.

The Disabled Living Foundation,
380–384 Harrow Road,
London W9 2HU.

Role of physiotherapy in care of the elderly

Physiotherapy in elderly care is broad spectrum, challenging and rewarding. The environment may be acute unit (district general hospital), long-stay unit, private or council home for the elderly, sheltered housing, part III accommodation, day hospital, day centre or within the patient's own home. It demands an insight into the role of many health care professionals and others.

Technical expertise in a wide variety of physiotherapy skills is necessary in order to maximize function. Analytical skills are necessary to determine that individual goals are being achieved. Humanitarian skills are essential to enable the physiotherapist to decide when to treat, chat, listen, cajole, or leave in peace.

Care of the dying requires an understanding of how human comfort is obtained. For example, passive movements, including trunk turning, positioning in bed or chair, warmth, attention, and eye-to-eye contact are important for the patient's sense of well-being. Communication may be by touch. Nasopharyngeal suction is unpleasant but helpful to clear a 'bubbling chest' and should be given after sedation.

Improving mobility at home requires common sense and some determination to maximize the benefits of other professionals, e.g. the patient who cannot walk because of pain from ingrowing toe nails requires a chiropodist urgently.

Elderly fitness groups can be run by physiotherapists so that people are fitter longer and less dependent on family, friends or state.

There is a need for interprofessional skill development so that the patient's needs can be met by, for example, nurses, occupational therapists or physiotherapists.

Carers also need attention and physiotherapists should teach lifting, handling and therapeutic procedures appropriate to the individual patient. Courses (2–3 days) for carers are necessary to practise these skills, identify common problems and ascertain sources of help.

Carers need to be cared for in terms of shopping breaks and respite holidays. Someone needs to ensure that this takes place before the carer is ill and it may well have to be the physiotherapist.

Group therapy, music therapy, and orientation therapy (identifying time of day, weather conditions) are important activities in day centres or day hospitals. Horticulture therapy may be encouraged by the physiotherapist, and there are some units where the physiotherapist takes her dog to work and this gives enormous pleasure to elderly people (some people in elderly care homes have had to get rid of their pets before taking up residence). Anything that brings a smile to the face is important and laughter is one of the best forms of exercise.

The greatest fears of growing old, expressed by those who see the disabled elderly are loss of independence, self-esteem and dignity. It is very hard for the 'head of the household', former managing director, head of college, 'one of the boys', to lose position in life. This is a feature of western culture where families tend to live separately and retirement means little, if any, involvement in being productive or achieving. Eastern cultures have a different approach where the elderly are treated with reverence as master of the household and are cared for accordingly.

Therefore, it is important for physiotherapists to take this into account by according respect and ensuring dignity. Patients should be addressed by the name they wish (e.g. Mrs X, not necessarily the first name). They should be dressed preferably in their own clothes and cared for with courtesy and consideration. Elderly care physiotherapy is, therefore, for the imaginative, caring physiotherapist.

Examples of activities for group or individual work

Sitting

1. Sit up straight.
2. Turn head from side to side.

3. Identify five objects at different distances – two to right, one centre, two to left. Look at these as the number is called out, e.g. door knob 1, window handle 2.
4. Place hands on shoulders, stretch arms up and bend.
5. Place hands on neck – push elbows back.
6. Place hands on shoulders, circle elbows back.
7. Swing arms backwards and forwards.
8. Hold rope, push up towards ceiling, place behind neck – up to ceiling and back to lap.
9. Pass rope from right hand to left behind back (over shoulder or behind waist).
10. Touch right little toe with left thumb or touch right knee outside with left thumb and vice versa.
11. Turn to touch chair back with both hands.
12. Alternate knee straightening and bending.
13. Alternate heel and toe raising.
14. Stand up; sit down.
15. Stand up, turn round, sit down.
16. One knee straighten – circle the foot – bend the knee – repeat with other leg.
17. Deep breath in – feel air filling around waist – hold – let all air out, × 3.
18. Pass ball over head, hand to hand and behind back.
19. Pass ball hand–hand.
20. Pass bean bag round left foot:
    (a) With right hand.
    (b) With right foot.
21. Repeat with other leg.
22. Pass ball with feet around the group or to different members of the group.
23. Pass ball by hand round group.

Standing

1. Feet apart:
   (a) Bend trunk side to side.
   (b) Stretch up tall – stretch arms backwards and turning thumbs to point backwards.
   (c) Weight transference foot to foot with head held high.
2. Feet in walk standing:
   (a) Weight transference foot to foot with head held high.

To music

Sitting: 'Head and shoulders, knees and toes'. 'Daisy, Daisy' – actions demonstrated by the physiotherapist.

Without music

Sitting: 'O, Grady says do this: do that'.

Useful address for exercises for the elderly and/or disabled

EXTEND,
1a North Street,
Sheringham,
Norfolk NR26 8LJ.

Appendix 1 – Physiotherapy skills

Introduction

To regain function it is necessary to assess which of the components of a movement are not working adequately and to decide whether normal actions can be achieved. This is provided that the fault lies in the musculoskeletal system and not in other physiological activities of the body. The components of a movement are: range of movement in joints, muscle power and endurance, coordination of movement and timing. Sometimes it is not possible to achieve the normal level of one or more components of a movement because of the nature of the disease or injury, and the physiotherapist has to decide on the degree of function and independence that may be gained.

Good coordination and timing are important in producing an efficient movement and reducing the mechanical and physiological stress. If these aspects can be improved during re-education it may help to prevent further injury.

When activities such as rolling over from lying, sitting from lying, sitting to standing and walking have been temporarily lost because of neurological disease, or weakness following an illness, it may be necessary to re-educate through the developmental sequence of movement using appropriate methods of facilitation.

Children with cerebral palsy or spina bifida may require similar treatment to try to encourage functional independence.

Movement techniques

These comprise: passive, assisted active, free active and resisted movements.

Fundamental starting positions

For any movement to produce the maximal effect the correct position must be chosen. Sometimes the best position must be modified because of the disability or discomfort of the patient but the physiotherapist has to make this decision after a careful examination of the patient.

There are five fundamental starting positions and others derived from these:

1. *Lying* – The body is fully supported in the supine position. Other positions derived from lying are: half lying, side lying, prone lying. Adjustments may need to be made to these to make them suitable for patients.
2. *Sitting* – The chair must be the correct height so that the person can sit with the thighs fully supported, a right angle at the knees and the feet on the ground. The back is straight and the arms are by the side of the body. This position can be modified by having a chair with the back slightly inclined and with arms to the chair so that the patient can be more fully supported. Other derived sitting positions are on the floor – cross sitting, side sitting, long sitting – and are more useful for children than adults.
3. *Kneeling* – The person is upright from the knees and the lower part of the legs is supported on the floor. This is an unstable position as the centre of gravity is towards the front of the base. Derived positions include kneel sitting – this is sitting back on the heels from the kneeling position – half kneeling, and prone kneeling.
4. *Standing* – The body is upright with the arms by the side and the feet very slightly apart. There are a number of derived positions which are gained by altering the position of the feet – high

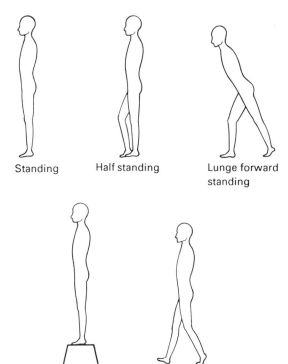

Standing   Half standing   Lunge forward
                                  standing

High standing   Walk forward standing

Figure A1.1 Derived positions gained by altering the position of the feet

standing, half standing, lunge forward standing, walk forward standing (Figure A1.1).

5. *Hanging* – The person grasps an overhead bar and allows the body to hang down. This is not a very useful position except in some advanced rehabilitation.

Apart from the above positions, further modifications can be achieved by altering the positions of the arms or legs. For example: in lying the knees may be flexed to a right angle, giving the crook lying position. The arms may be stretched above the head (stretch), stretched forward (reach) or stretched out to the side (yard). In the standing position the legs may be placed apart to give stride standing or one in front of the other to give walk standing. The arm and leg positions can be used in lying, sitting or standing.

Passive movements

These are movements produced on a person by an external force. The external force can be an inanimate object such as a chair or any object that produces a force acting on the body. Passive movements of this type can be harmless and part of

any normal activity – for example, as a person sits down in a chair and relaxes against the back of the chair, or against a cushion, this may produce a passive extension or flexion of the spine depending on the direction of the force. If the passive movement causes discomfort then the person will move to a more comfortable position. Alternatively if a person has a painful back, a cushion may be placed to produce a movement that may relieve the pain.

There are many other examples of passive movements produced during normal activity – for example, passive movements are produced in some joints in the foot when walking on an uneven surface. A violent external force may produce passive movement that causes injury, as for example a whiplash injury to the neck.

Another type of passive movement is by one person moving a part of the body of the other, passive, person. A physiotherapist uses this type of passive movement in several different ways.

Relaxed passive movements

The physiotherapist supports the limb and moves the joint while the patient relaxes. The patient must be placed in a well-supported position which will allow the physiotherapist to take the movement through the available free range. The technique may be restricted to one joint or it may affect several joints. In the latter case it is important to observe the movement at each of the joints. This technique is usually carried out when the patient is unable to perform the movement because the muscles are either paralysed or too weak to perform the movement. The movements used must be chosen to maintain both joint range and muscle length. It is particularly important to consider muscle length as many muscles work over more than one joint. The technique may be used to help initiate a contraction of muscle by reminding the patient of the movement that he is trying to perform. Relaxed passive movements may be used during the examination of a patient to determine the factor(s) causing limitation of movement.

Technique

Starting position

The patient must be as well supported as possible so that he can relax, and it should prevent unnecessary movements occurring elsewhere. For example: to perform abduction of one leg the patient should be in lying and the other leg should be fixed in abduction as this will prevent side flexion in the trunk when the movement is performed.

Grasp

When the movement is to be restricted to one joint the physiotherapist should grasp above and below the joint if possible. In the example given above this is not usually suitable and as the other leg is fixed in abduction, to prevent movement occurring in the spine, the physiotherapist supports the thigh and grasps the lower leg just above the ankle.

Position of the physiotherapist

This is important to enable a smooth movement to be carried out through the full or available free range. The therapist must be in a comfortable and stable position which will allow her to perform the movement without any tension and without upsetting her balance.

Traction

Gentle traction is given during the movement to allow a smooth movement at the joint.

Movement

The physiotherapist tells the patient to relax. If the muscles working over the joint are paralysed this is relatively easy but if the patient can move the joint actively it may be difficult for him to relax.

The movement should be carried out smoothly in the available free range. The number of times the movement is performed and the frequency will depend on the reason for using this technique. If it is being used to maintain joint range and muscle length each movement should be performed about three times and at least once daily. The decision to continue or discontinue the use of this technique will depend on an evaluation by the physiotherapist.

Assisted active movement

Sometimes a patient requires assistance to perform a movement because the muscles are not strong enough to perform the movement freely, or because free movement causes pain. The assistance can be given by the physiotherapist, or sometimes a carer may be taught to give the movement, or occasionally the patient may assist his own movement. Alternatively assistance can be given in other ways – for example the upthrust of water can be used to assist movement; sling suspension, pulleys and springs can also be used. If the assistance is given by the physiotherapist, the grips are the same as those used to give relaxed passive movements. The patient is encouraged to do as much of the movement as he can with the physiotherapist assisting when necessary. As the patient progresses he should gradually perform more of the movement unaided.

Sling suspension

Axial sling suspension assists movement in three ways. Firstly it supports the weight of a heavy limb and allows the patient to concentrate on the required movement. Secondly, the limb is lifted clear of the plinth and so the friction offered by the surface of the plinth and possibly that of a blanket is removed. Thirdly, the point of suspension is vertically over the joint that is to be moved and this allows a swinging movement in the horizontal plane.

Flexion and extension of the hip

The patient is placed in side lying with the underneath hip and knee flexed (if possible) to reduce movement in the spine to a minimum. The upper leg is then supported by slings at the foot and knee. The ropes from the slings are attached above the hip joint. This allows the leg to swing freely forward and backwards in a horizontal plane (Figure A1.2).

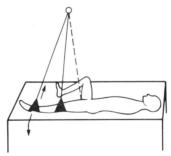

Figure A1.2 Axial sling suspension for abduction/adduction of hip

Abduction and adduction of the hip

The patient is placed in lying and the other leg is fixed in abduction to prevent movement occurring in the spine. Again, the leg is supported at the foot and knee with the axial point over the hip joint (Figures A1.3 and A1.4).

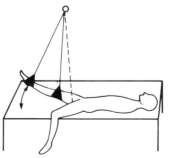

Figure A1.3 Axial sling suspension for flexion/extension of hip

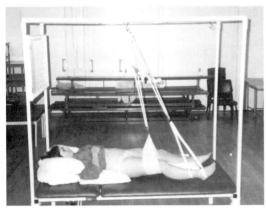

Figure A1.4 Abduction and adduction of the hip (Courtesy School of Physiotherapy, Middlesex Hospital)

Other movements

Using the same principles, sling suspension can be used for flexion/extension movements of the knee, flexion/extension, abduction/adduction of the shoulder joint, and flexion/extension of the elbow joint.

Uses

1. Movement limited by adhesions – a repetitive swinging movement with emphasis on the limited part of the range may help to stretch the adhesions.
2. Weak muscles – if a patient is starting to produce movement in a position with gravity counterbalanced, it will be easier to do this for some of the movements mentioned above if the limb is supported in axial suspension. Also it will reduce the effects of friction that occur when the patient tries to slide the limb along the plinth.
3. The physiotherapist will have her hands free to assist or resist a particular movement.
4. The patient can practise on his own for a short time provided that the instructions have been clear and the physiotherapist has seen him performing the movement correctly. The patient must know what he is trying to achieve and when to stop.

Free active exercises

These are exercises performed by the patient without external (manual or mechanical) assistance or resistance to the movement being performed. The movement may be made easier or more difficult by the position of the patient, the position of the limbs and/or trunk, the speed of the movement and the number of times the movement is performed.

Free active exercises can be used for the following purposes in a therapeutic programme:

1. To increase range of movement in joints.
2. To strengthen weak muscles.
3. To retrain balance and coordination.
4. To regain independence.

Free exercises are often used in conjunction with other techniques of movement, for example assisted or resisted exercise, and they may be used with other procedures such as manipulative, thermal or electrical therapy. The skill of the physiotherapist depends on her ability to select and use the techniques that will produce the most effective treatment.

Free exercises are particularly important for home use and so must be well taught and their performance checked regularly, both for accuracy of movement and to evaluate progress.

To increase range of movement in joints

Factors limiting movement may be due to abnormalities affecting either intra-articular or extra-articular structures. Intra-articular structures that lie within the joint capsule are the articular surfaces of the bones, articular hyaline cartilage, intra-articular discs of fibrocartilage in some joints, synovial membrane, bursae, and articular pads of fat; tendons may pass through the joint capsule (example – long head of biceps). The extra-articular structures include ligaments and tendons which pass in relation to the joint and the overlying skin and fascia. Abnormalities of muscle will limit active movement at the joint and this may be the result of disease or injury affecting the muscle directly or indirectly due to disease of the nervous system.

The following clinical features may occur as the result of the above factors and these may limit movement – pain, swelling, adhesions, abnormal contractility or coordination of muscles.

Free exercises are not always appropriate to deal with limited range of movement and this will depend on the condition, pathological changes with their consequent problems, and an assessment by the physiotherapist.

The following are a few of the techniques that may be used for particular problems.

Pain

It must be remembered that pain is a protective mechanism and may be a contraindication to active exercise. Sometimes the pain may be relieved by medical or surgical treatment but if not, and the cause of the pain is known, the physiotherapist may be able to determine whether one of the techniques available to relieve pain is appropriate – thermal, electrical, manipulative or exercise. Some indications of suitable methods for dealing with pain are discussed under the various sections in this book.

Swelling

1. The limb will be elevated to assist drainage.
2. Static contractions of muscles working over the joint.
3. Free exercises for any joints not limited by swelling.

Examples

Where there is swelling of the leg because of injury to the knee the following might be used: the patient is placed in lying on a plinth with the leg elevated on pillows and left for 10–15 minutes as some drainage of the swelling may occur by the positioning. Then exercises are given with the leg still elevated – static contractions of the quadriceps plus ankle and toe movements plus leg lifting and lowering.

Swelling of the arm as the result of injury to the hand may have similar treatment. The patient is placed in sitting with the arm elevated on pillows which have been placed on a table. The hand should be above the level of the shoulder. As with the leg the patient may be left with the arm in this position for 10–15 minutes. If movement is possible in the hand, rhythmical flexion and extension of the fingers and then wrist movements should be carried out. Following this, flexion and extension of the elbow and movements of the shoulder can be given.

Emphasis should be on teaching the patient to carry out movements rhythmically through full or the available free range, to assist the venous and lymphatic drainage.

The patient must be advised to keep the limb elevated whenever possible (certainly when at rest), and to do the exercises regularly at home. Pressure bandages may be used between treatment sessions.

Adhesions

Active exercise may be used to stretch the adhesions and improve the blood supply to the area.

Pendular movements

At certain joints such as the shoulder, hip and knee pendular-type exercises may be used. They should be rhythmical swinging movements taken to the limit of the range.

Examples

For the right shoulder to gain flexion and extension – Left walk forward standing or lunge forward

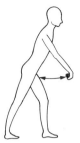

Figure A1.5 Lunge forward standing – one arm swinging forward and back

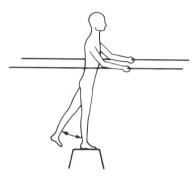

Figure A1.6 High standing – one leg swinging forward and back

standing with the right arm swinging forward and back. A small weight may be held in the hand to give a little traction (Figure A1.5). For the elderly the left hand may be placed on a support such as a table or chair.

A similar movement can be used for abduction and adduction – stride standing with the body relaxed forward so that the arms can swing across the body and out to the side.

For hip flexion and extension – Standing (between the parallel bars) with the left leg on a low platform so that the right leg can swing forward and back (Figure A1.6).

For knee flexion and extension – High sitting (on a plinth) with alternate leg swinging up and down.

Other exercises

These should be smooth rhythmical movements with emphasis at the limit of the range to stretch the adhesions.

Examples

To gain wrist flexion and extension – Sitting with the arm supported on a table and with the forearm in the mid-prone position, the wrist is flexed and extended. Alternatively the forearm may be placed prone with the hand over the edge of the table so that gravity will assist flexion. If this is used, the wrist extensors should be strong enough to lift the hand up against the pull of gravity (Figure A1.7).

To gain dorsiflexion of the ankle – Prone lying on a plinth with the foot over the end of the plinth, the movement of dorsiflexion is assisted by gravity. The main disadvantage is that the patient cannot see the movement. Another exercise is in sitting with one leg crossed over the other so that the foot may be moved freely though dorsiflexion and plantarflexion.

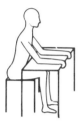

Figure A1.7 Sitting with forearms supported on table – wrist extension/flexion

Functional movements using all the joints in a movement are useful in gaining range, and in some instances may be better than isolated movements. However, the physiotherapist must observe carefully, as the patient may not gain the full available range at the restricted joint. Generally the functional movement allows the better use of muscle activity over the affected joint, particularly muscles stretching over two or more joints.

With a stiff knee – Side lying with flexion of the hip and knee will stretch the hamstrings over the hip and allow better activity of the hamstrings in flexing the knee. Similarly, with stiff finger flexion, if the wrist is extended stretching the flexors (flexor digitorum sublimis and flexor digitorum profundus) over the wrist their action will be more effective on the fingers.

When there are adhesions there is usually associated muscle weakness, and it is very important to strengthen the muscles for several reasons:

1. The muscles need to be effective at the limit of range.
2. As range of movement is gained the muscles must be able to produce the additional movement and control it.
3. The muscles must be strong enough to produce functional activities for use in the home, at work or leisure.

To strengthen muscles

The techniques used will depend on the grading of the muscles – grades 0–5. Initiation of a contraction (grade 0–1) will be dealt with separately.

Muscles must be worked maximally to gain power most effectively.

Grade 1 (flicker of contraction) to grade 2 (contraction with gravity counterbalanced)

A flicker of contraction will not be sufficient to produce movement at a joint and so at this stage the muscle activity must be increased by other techniques – for example those used to initiate a contraction. Once movement can occur the muscle can be strengthened by increasing the number of times the movement is performed. As the strength increases the range of movement will increase, and this can continue until grade 2 is achieved.

Examples

For the shoulder abductors – Lying on the plinth with the elbow flexed and the fingers touching the shoulder, moving the arm out to the side and back. Initially, movement may be prevented by the friction of a blanket and so there should be a smooth surface. Once there is approximately half the range of movement the movement may be facilitated by performing it bilaterally.

For the shoulder flexors or extensors – A similar movement can be carried out in side lying for one arm.

As soon as possible, muscles should be used in patterned movements which will lead to the return of function. Thus in the above exercise, with the patient in side lying, the shoulder should be flexed and the elbow extended as in reaching forward, and likewise the shoulder extended and the elbow flexed as in pulling back.

For the flexors of the hip – The patient is positioned in side lying with the underneath leg flexed to give a more stable position. The upper leg is then flexed at the hip and knee and then followed by extension of the hip and knee.

Grade 2 to grade 3 (movement against gravity)

Strengthening is continued by increasing the number of times the movement is performed in a position with gravity counterbalanced. Some resistance may be given in this position before trying the movement against gravity. Initially it may be possible to position the patient so that the muscle work is easier in the weaker part of the range.

Example

For weak quadriceps – If the patient cannot extend the knee fully in sitting, he may be placed in crook lying with a wedge pillow under the knee. As the patient extends the knee the maximal resistance will be in the middle range.

As in the previous grade the muscle can be strengthened by increasing the number of times it contracts, and gradually increasing the range. When possible, exercises should be given to work the muscle statically and eccentrically as well as concentrically.

Grade 3 to grade 4 (movement against gravity and some resistance)

It is more difficult to judge grade 4 as the amount of resistance is not specified. Once the muscle can perform the movement fully against gravity, resistance may be added gradually. The number of movements are increased and then the weight is increased. This is continued until the muscle is strong enough to perform the normal functions for that patient.

Grade 4 to grade 5 (normal function)

The amount of resistance required to achieve normal function will vary from one patient to another. For example an office worker who sits at a desk most of the day, and does not participate in any leisure physical activity, will not require the same strength of the quadriceps muscle as a manual worker who is involved in heavy lifting, or an office worker who is a keen amateur rugby player. Thus it is important to assess the needs of each patient.

To retrain balance and coordination

The inability to balance or to coordinate movement may be due to weak muscles as the result of inactivity or it may be due to a neurological deficit.

Balance

This is the ability to keep the body in equilibrium in either the static or dynamic positions, and should require minimal muscle activity. The point at which retraining of balance is started will depend on the particular injury or disease, and the particular problems of the individual patient.

Static positions

Balance may be started in forearm support prone lying, progressing to prone kneeling, half kneeling, sitting and standing and so follows the developmental sequence of movement (Figure A1.8).

Sitting

When a patient has been lying in bed for some time he may lose his postural sense and holding a correct

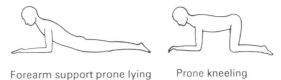

Forearm support prone lying   Prone kneeling

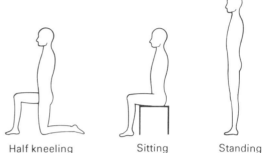

Half kneeling   Sitting   Standing

Figure A1.8 Static positions to retrain balance

sitting position may be difficult. In this instance the patient may be placed in the correct position and be supported there for increasing periods of time. This will enable him to adjust to the new position, and gradually the support may be reduced. A back support tends to encourage the patient to lean backwards and will make standing balance difficult, so unsupported sitting should be taught as soon as possible. Special facilitatory techniques may be required but the physiotherapist must teach the patient to have an awareness of the correct position and how to adjust his balance if he tends to move in a certain direction that upsets it. A mirror is sometimes helpful, particularly if the patient tends to move to one side, as he can see when he is moving out of position and correct it. If lateral balance is a problem, the patient may start by sitting on a plinth with the hands supported on either side (see Figure 20.2).

Balance may be a problem because of muscle weakness, or there may be a neurological deficit. In the case of the former, normal balance should return as the muscles are strengthened but in the latter case the patient may have to learn to compensate for some loss of sensation and/or paralysis.

Once the patient has attained a good balance in sitting he may be taught to move the arms so that an adjustment is required to maintain balance. This should be done slowly and carefully at first, but as the patient gains confidence and can maintain the position, the arm movements can be quicker. In younger or more able patients, progress can be made to throwing and catching balls.

Standing

If the patient is to walk independently without aids, a good standing balance is necessary before starting to walk. Initially the patient may require some support, such as parallel bars, to give him confidence and he may need to stand with his feet slightly apart to give him a wider base. The patient is then taught to transfer weight by bending one hip and knee up while taking weight on one leg, and then repeating it on the other side – marking time on the spot. This can then be progressed to the walk-forward position, with the patient pushing from the back leg to take the weight over the front leg. Once this can be successfully carried out with both legs, the patient can bring the back leg through to the heel strike position, following on to weight bearing and the push-off. The point at which the patient can stand and walk without any support will depend on the condition and ability of the individual patient. Once the patient is confident in the standing position he can try moving his arms to see whether he can make the adjustments required to maintain balance. To start with the therapist must stand by so that she is ready to give support if the patient begins to lose balance.

Further progress will depend on the needs of the individual patient. A balance board can be used to simulate maintaining balance on a moving object such as a train or bus.

Balance during activity

As indicated above, once the patient can balance in standing and transfer weight, walking can be started. At first the patient may need to walk with a slightly wider base but as the walking improves, this can be brought within normal limits. Progress can be made by walking more quickly, stopping suddenly and turning. Patients will also have to learn to adjust their balance to carrying objects concerned with the activities of daily living or work.

Many patients with a permanent disability may have their balance upset and have to learn to compensate. For example, the loss of an arm or leg will upset the normal balance and the patient will have to learn to adjust to this new situation, with or without a prosthesis. A patient with a hemiplegia or a paraplegia will have to learn to react to a different sensory input.

Coordination

Weak muscles – When incoordination is due to imbalance of muscle activity, strengthening exercises should redress the balance and improve coordination. It may be necessary to teach the patient some rhythmical free active exercises to help regain normal function.

Ataxia – As this is usually due to a neurological lesion, the aim of treatment is to try to improve coordination by teaching the patient to compensate for the neurological deficit.

For example, a patient with a sensory loss as the result of tabes dorsalis, which results in degeneration of the posterior columns of the spinal cord, by using his sight combined with making the fullest use of any muscle sense left as with Frenkel's exercises.

Frenkel's exercises

These consist of a carefully planned series of exercises which aim at making the patient employ what is left to him of muscle sense in an attempt to prevent its further decrease, or even effect an improvement. Frenkel considered that, despite the damaged sensory path, a tabetic patient could learn to make the fullest use of what is left in the way of muscle sense by constant repetition – much as a normal person acquires complex skills. In fact this principle is illustrated in cases where optic atrophy has supervened early, for in these the ataxia develops slowly and incompletely, since the blind man is *obliged* to depend on his muscle and joint sense, and so uses it to the utmost of his capacity. If, however, the muscle sense is practically non-existent by the time a patient comes for treatment, the object of the exercises is to teach him to replace his lost sense by the sense of sight. Treatment should begin as soon as possible. If the patient is in the pre-ataxic stage, he should perform the most complex movements possible. In the later stages the exercises should begin with very simple movements and gradually advance to more complicated ones. Certain rules must be observed at whatever stage the patient may be.

Rules for giving Frenkel's exercises

1. *Commands* should be given in an even, monotonous, sing-song voice; and the exercises should be done to counting.
2. Each exercise, or set of exercises, should have been mastered by the patient – that is, he should be able to do it accurately and smoothly – before he is allowed to proceed to a more difficult one. *Precision of performance must be attained*, but the exercises should be sufficiently varied to prevent boredom.
3. Exercises involving strong muscle work should not be given. Progression is by *complexity*, not strength.
4. Movements in *complete range* are easier than those in *small range*, therefore the former should be given before the latter, but no movement should be taken beyond its normal limit, because the hypotonia of muscles and laxity of ligaments render the patient vulnerable to dislocation or the onset of Charcot's joints.

5. The movements should first be given rather *quickly*, then *more slowly*, this being more difficult since it requires greater control.
6. The patient should practise movements first with his eyes open, and then with them shut.
7. Each patient should have individual attention, and should not be left unattended in case he should fall and injure himself.
8. *Rests* must be given between the exercises; after so many minutes' work, an equal number of minutes' rest should be taken.
9. It is necessary, when planning the treatment scheme, to take into consideration the patient's general health and mental attitude, the state of his muscles, and any complications such as Charcot's joints. A careful record should be kept of exactly what work the patient is doing from day to day.

The exercises themselves are given in *lying*, in *sitting*, or in *standing*.

Exercises in lying

The patient lies on a bed, plinth, or couch with a smooth surface along which the feet can move easily. *His head must be sufficiently raised for him to be able to watch his feet.* The exercises in this group begin with simple movements, and gradually become more difficult and complicated.

The first set are as follows (one leg moved at a time; legs moved alternately):

1. Flexion of one leg, at hip and knee, foot kept on plinth; extension.
2. Flexion as above; abduction, adduction; extension.
3. Flexion as above, but only half-way; extension.
4. Flexion as above (half-way); abduction; adduction; extension.
5. Flexion (voluntary halt made by patient during flexion); extension.
6. As (5), but halt at physiotherapist's command.

The exercises are done slowly three or four times, using each leg in turn. The foot should be kept dorsiflexed, so as not to stretch the hypotonic anterior tibial group. The physiotherapist should count four during each movement.

At a later stage both legs are moved together.

Examples of more difficult exercises in the lying series:

1. Flexion of one leg at hip and knee, with the heel raised some inches from the plinth; extension.
2. Heel of one leg placed on patella of other leg; return.
3. As above, with voluntary halt.
4. As above, with halt to command.
5. Heel is placed on the middle of the other tibia, lifted off, and put by side of leg; extension.

6. Heel placed on other knee; down on bed at side; leg extended until heel reaches middle of tibia; placed on tibia, then again on bed at side; extended to level of ankle; placed on ankle, then on bed at side; complete extension.
7. Heel placed on knee; heel slides along tibia to ankle joint; extension.
8. As above, but heel carried from ankle back to knee; extension.
9. Flexion and extension of both legs, with heels off bed.
10. As above, with halts.
11. One leg (e.g. left) flexed; left leg abducted and right leg flexed, simultaneously; left leg adducted and right leg extended; left leg extended. (Repeat with legs reversed.)
12. Left leg flexed, right leg abducted and flexed (all at the same time); right leg adducted; both legs extended, without heels touching bed till end of movement.

NB. These asymmetrical exercises are very difficult for the tabetic patient.

13. The physiotherapist places her finger on various places on the leg; the patient places his other heel on her finger.
14. As above; but as the patient reaches the finger, the physiotherapist moves it, and the patient tries to follow its course.
15. Right heel is placed on the knee of the other limb, which is in extension; with right heel in this position, the left leg is flexed and extended.
16. Right heel is placed on left knee, and slides down the tibia to the ankle; as it slides down, the left leg is flexed; as it is brought back to the knee, the left leg is extended.

These are only a few examples of the whole series of nearly 100 exercises. Frenkel's exercises may *seem* 'old-fashioned', but they are still effective, and no one has yet improved on them. It is, of course, quite possible to invent other similar exercises if desired, and to adapt them to purposeful movements, e.g. to assist the patient to dress himself more easily.

Exercises in sitting

These are not necessarily *progressions* on those in lying; they are considerably easier than some of the more advanced exercises in that series. Those given by Frenkel consist of rising from a stool or chair, and sitting down again. The patient has literally forgotten how to perform these 'stock' movements – he has lost his 'formula' for them. The rising movement, therefore, is divided into its component parts, the operator counting three. At *one*, the patient draws his knees under the stool. At *two*, he bends his trunk forward. At *three*, he rises extending hips and knees. He then sits down again, reversing the above process.

These movements may be done in the reach–grasp position, the patient sitting close to the wall-bars. Later, he rises unsupported. Later still, he attempts to do so with his eyes closed.

Other exercises may be given in sitting:

1. The patient may be directed to raise his knees and place his foot on, say, the second rail from the bottom. This is done in three movements:
   (a) Flexion of hip.
   (b) Extension of knee.
   (c) Lowering of the foot on to bar.
   He then replaces the foot on the ground.
2. He may be made to touch marked points on the floor with his foot. (Frenkel gives this type of exercise in lying; but it necessitates apparatus in that position.)

Exercises in standing

These are designed to give *re-education in walking*. They should be performed in as large a space as possible, preferably where lines can be marked out (Figures A1.9 and A1.10).

1. *Walking sideways* – The patient, accompanied by the physiotherapist, who must be prepared to support him if necessary, begins by walking sideways. Balance is easier in this way, because, except in the long step, he does not have to rise on the toes of one foot, thus decreasing his base.

   He should begin by taking *half-steps*, which are easiest, alternately to left and to right, the physiotherapist counting three for each step, e.g. for half-step to right:
   (1) he places the right foot on the ground half a step away,
   (2) he transfers his weight from the left to the right foot,
   (3) he brings the left foot up beside the right.

   He then practises *quarter-steps*, then *long-steps*, and finally combines all three lengths in one exercise. For example:
   (a) Three-quarter-step to right–one–two–three.
   (b) Quarter-step to left–one–two–three.
   (c) Half-step to right–one–two–three.
   (d) Whole step to left–one–two–three.

   The long steps are more difficult because the toes have to be put on the ground first. The heel is raised and the patient's base is therefore smaller.

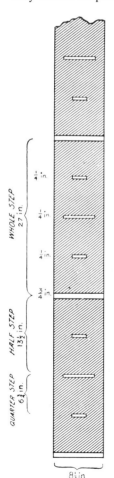

Figure A1.9 Diagram of 'steps' used in treating tabes

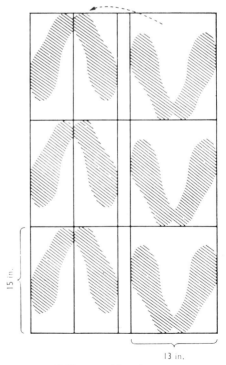

Figure A1.10 'Footsteps' for tabes treatment

2. *Walking forwards*: Whole, half- and quarter-steps forwards, beginning with each foot alternately, counting three as before. Thus, in beginning with the right foot:
   (a) Place right foot forward, heel on the ground.
   (b) Transfer weight to this foot, raising heel of left foot.
   (c) Bring left foot up beside right foot.
3. *Walking backwards*, in a similar manner.
4. *Walking heel to toe*.
5. *Walking in footsteps* painted on the floor (Figure A1.10).

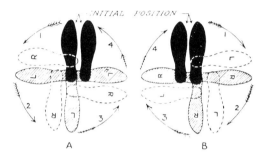

Figure A1.11 'Footmarks' for turning around in treatment of tabes. (*a*) Turning to the left. (*b*) Turning to the right

6. *Turning round*, also in footmarks on the floor (Figure A1.11), practised in three movements. For example, turning to right:
   (a) The patient turns on the right heel.
   (b) He raises the left heel and turns on the toes of this foot.
   (c) He brings the left foot up beside the right. This should be done four times, completing the full turn, and then repeated to the left.
7. *Walking up and down stairs or steps*:
   (a) The patient first goes up one step at a time. Later, he practises walking up the steps as a normal person would.
   (b) He walks up and down, with support to begin with, later without.
8. Finally, he is taught to walk while using his arms at the same time, carrying parcels, getting out of the way of obstacles, etc.

When the arms are affected

This is rare. Exercises of a similar nature are given, special attention being paid to the fine movements of hands and fingers, placing the fingers in holes in a board; inserting pegs or matches into holes; picking up small objects like marbles, and arranging them in piles or patterns. He should also practise going over diagrams with a pencil, writing, drawing, etc.

Some patients with multiple sclerosis may have a cerebellar ataxia, and in these cases the eye muscles will probably be affected, producing a nystagmus. Therefore the eyes cannot be used to assist coordination, but a modified type of Frenkel's exercises may be used, concentrating on repetitive smooth rhythmical movements to counting rather than using the eyes.

Functional movements should be carried out in a manner similar to the above methods to try to help the patient gain as much independence as possible. Sometimes a certain amount of resistance helps the patient to perform a movement more slowly. This can be applied in activities of daily living – for example the patient may find it easier to use heavier knives, forks and spoons for eating. If the patient is using a walking stick it may help to weight the stick – an adjustable tubular metal stick can be weighted with lead shot.

To regain independence

Isolated movements of joints and muscles may be necessary to achieve certain aims in the therapeutic programme, but whenever possible functional activity should be included so that the patient can become independent.

Vertigo exercises

Vertigo is defined as the consciousness of disordered orientation of the body in space. The patient's senses are deceived into feeling or seeing movement which may be up and down, side to side or whirling. It may seem that the patient's body is moving or the external world is moving. Patients describe such sensations as giddiness. dizziness or swaying. Nausea may or may not be present.

Normal spatial orientation depends on:

1. The retinas of the eyes.
2. The labyrinths of the ears.
3. Proprioceptive organs of the joints and muscles of the neck (relating to the relationship of the head to the trunk).
4. Proprioceptive organs in the joints and muscles of the trunk and limbs especially in weight-bearing surfaces.
5. Afferent impulses derived from these organs are conveyed to the cerebellum, red nucleus and vestibular nucleus, from where impulses are transmitted to the motor cortex, which in turn transmits impulses which result in adjustment of the body position. Vertigo may result from a lesion in any of these organs or the neural pathways transmitting the impulses. Dizziness or light-headedness may also arise from a disturbance of the blood supply to the brain.

Causes of vertigo

The commonest causes are:

1. Labyrinthitis.
2. Vestibular neuronitis.
3. Head injuries.
4. Cervical spondylosis.
5. Neck injury.
6. Tumours.
7. Drug toxicity.

Indications for vertigo exercises

Any patient who suffers from vertigo or loss of balance can benefit from vertigo exercises. Following medical treatment of the above conditions, therefore, vertigo exercises can form an essential component of the rehabilitation programme.

It is of particular importance to enable patients to regain confidence in moving about performing everyday activities, otherwise there is great danger that they will be afraid to move, become housebound and deteriorate into permanent invalidism or dependency on relatives and friends.

Principles of vertigo exercises

The balance mechanisms that remain intact can be educated to regain sufficient control for everyday functions.

The patient performs an exercise up to the point of dizziness, rests, then repeats the exercise. With practice, the patient finds that he can perform more complex activities without producing dizziness and that once produced, the dizziness takes a shorter time to settle.

The exercises can be performed at home daily, monitored by the patient himself. Very ill patients start the exercises in bed and gradually progress to sitting, walking, gym class and then continue as an outpatient as appropriate. Others may start as outpatients.

Education of the balance mechanism is possible, as evidence by ice-skaters, ballet dancers and astronauts who retain spatial orientation following spins, by regular training.

Anxiety is diminished and confidence restored as the patient realizes that he can perform more activities involving bending, turning or changing position until eventually he can live his normal life and forget about being unable to move without causing dizziness.

The exercises

In bed

Patient in lying or half lying with head supported:

1. Eye movements keeping the head still:
   (a) Focus on pencil end (patient and physiotherapist establish a comfortable distance between eyes and pencil).
   (b) Follow pencil end with eyes only: (i) side to side, (ii) up and down, (iii) obliquely up to the right down to the left, (iv) obliquely up to the left and down to the right.
   (c) Progress by: (i) increasing repetitions, (ii) increasing speed, (iii) altering distance.
   (d) Focusing practice. Objects at different positions and distances are identified by number then the numbers are called out in random order for the patient to focus on. Speed is slow to start with, increases and can then be varied.
2. The above exercises are progressed by the patient, moving the head as well as the eyes.
3. Eyes closed, head turning side to side, bending forward and backwards and bending side to side, turning slowly then quickly.

Sitting

Once the patient is confident, exercises may be performed in sitting. Sitting at first in an arm-chair, feet and trunk well supported, then on a chair with no arms, then on a stool:

1. The eye and head exercises are repeated.
2. Shoulder girdle raising, pushing down and resting.
3. Hands on shoulders, bend trunk side to side.
4. Pass ball from hand to hand, in front, then overhead, stretching the arms and watching the ball throughout the movement.
5. Place ball in front of feet, pick up and stretch above head, watching ball.
6. Place ball to the side, pick up and pass overhead to place down on the other side.
7. Throw ball from hand to hand.
8. Bounce ball on one side, other side and in front with alternate hands.
9. Sitting on stool place object (tall at first then small) behind stool to right and then to the left. Repeat with eyes closed.

Standing exercises

1. Standing up and sitting down.
2. Standing feet astride, eye and head movements are repeated.
3. Ball exercises are repeated.
4. Stand up, turn round, sit down.
5. Walking forwards stopping and starting to order.
6. Walking, picking up or placing objects on the floor and at different heights.

7. Walk round obstacle course with eyes open then closed.
8. Lying on floor, get up, sit on stool, stand up, step up on to stool, step down, go into prone kneeling, lie prone, turn over and rest.
9. Walk up and down stairs – repeat with eyes closed holding banister.
10. Go into darkened room – walk around feeling for objects with hands and feet.
11. Go outdoors – walk and cross street with friend or physiotherapist, then alone.

Group activities

It is helpful for these patients to join in group activities, as this further increases confidence.

Examples of activities

1. Sitting – throw and catch ball with partner.
2. Sitting in circles 'pass the parcel'.
3. Sitting in circle throw ball at random from person to person.
4. Exercises in sitting (above) may be repeated.
5. Stand in circle – walk forwards, backwards and sideways.
6. Skittles, dribbling, basketball, movement to music or other activities that involve bending and stretching.

Patients should be encouraged to join an exercise class appropriate to their age, go dancing or take up an active interest, for example rambling, hill walking, bowls, dog walking.

The number of exercises in any one treatment session should be between five and eight. The exercises are generally performed up to 20 times. If the patient feels dizzy the exercise must stop immediately but should be resumed when the dizziness has subsided.

Monitoring progress

The patient should keep a chart of the effects of the exercises. He should be asked to consider a dizziness scale of 1–4:

1. No dizziness.
2. Slight dizziness.
3. Moderate dizziness.
4. Severe dizziness.

together with a settling scale of A, B, C, D:

A   Settles quickly (as soon as exercise stops).
B   Settles in less than 5 minutes.
C   Settles in 5–10 minutes.
D   Takes longer than 10 minutes.

At first he should monitor each exercise against the two scales, but as he progresses monitoring may be of one activity only, or he may consider how he has been for a day, e.g. at 6 p.m. and record the worst he has felt that day. This is an essential component of patient management as he can see progress on his own chart, and is encouraged to increase his activities, confident that the dizziness will subside.

Relaxation, general fitness and posture training must complement this programme of rehabilitation.

Resisted exercises

Resistance can be given to facilitate activity and to strengthen muscles. It can be given manually by the physiotherapist or mechanically by means of weights, springs or weight and pulley systems.

Principles of using resistance

To strengthen a muscle most effectively it should be worked maximally. This means maximal according to the grading of the particular muscle. If a muscle can contract only through part of its range with gravity counterbalanced, it may not be able to contract at all if external resistance is applied, and so it is already working maximally, provided that it is moving through the range as many times as possible. A muscle may be able to work through part of its available free range against some resistance and in this case it should be applied in that range, but the muscle must also be worked in the rest of the range.

If a movement is being performed a number of times against resistance, the physiotherapist must check that the range of the movement does not decrease as the number of times is increased, as this means the resistance is too high.

Resistance may be given to a muscle in one part of the range with no movement occurring (isometric) or through the available range (isotonic). Isometric work may be important for a patient's work or leisure activity when he needs to hold a certain position or positions.

There are a number of different methods of applying resistance and the physiotherapist must choose a suitable one depending on her assessment and the needs of the individual patient.

The point at which this treatment is stopped depends on the requirements of each patient. A sedentary worker who does little spare-time physical activity will not require the same strength in the quadriceps as a professional footballer. An assessment of the normal limb will give a rough estimate of the requirements for the affected limb.

Methods of giving resistance

Manual resistance

The physiotherapist offers resistance to the movement made by the patient. This has the advantage that the resistance may be finely graded to allow the patient to perform a smooth movement through the available range. The disadvantage is that it is not possible to measure the amount of resistance. Movements can be resisted in a functional pattern, as with proprioceptive neuromuscular facilitation techniques (PNF), or resistance can be given to an isolated movement. PNF techniques are described separately in the next section.

The physiotherapist records the starting position for the patient, the type of movement given and the number of times the movement is performed. Each treatment is evaluated and progression made at the next treatment if appropriate. This may be carried out by increasing the resistance and/or the number of times the movement is performed. Alternatively progression may require a change of treatment, particularly when the patient is regaining normal function. Patients can become very dependent on the physiotherapist, and so it is important to make the patient more responsible for his own treatment by using mechanical resistance or body weight activities, depending on an assessment of the needs of the patient.

Self-resistance

A patient can be taught to give resistance to his own movements in some instances. This is suitable only if the patient has good kinaesthetic sense and understands what he is trying to do. For example – to strengthen the right wrist extensors, the patient sits beside a small table with the right forearm supported and the hand over the front edge of the table. He then gives resistance over the back of the hand with the left hand as the right wrist is extended.

Mechanical resistances

The type of resistance chosen will depend on the disease or injury, the stage of recovery, the part to be treated and the assessment made by the physiotherapist.

Weights

Various forms of weights are available for treatment. A boot (De Lorme or Variweight boot) which can have varying weights attached may be used for strengthening some of the leg muscles, particularly the quadriceps (Figure A1.12). Sandbags or bags containing lead weights can be strapped onto a limb to give resistance to the required movement.

There are several methods of giving weight resistance and most depend on finding the 10 RM, which is the maximum weight that the patient can lift ten times. Most of the methods involve lifting a weight a certain number of times in sets of 10 lifts

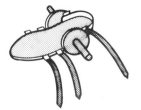

Figure A1.12 Weight-lifting boot

with a rest in between each set. The number of sets varies with the different regimes, but the usual number is 30. A modification of the original De Lorme and Watkins method starts with a lower resistance and ends with the 10 RM (for example ½ 10 RM × 10 ¾ 10 RM × 10, 10 RM × 10) which allows for warming-up. The McQueen method uses the 10 RM in three or four sets which requires a good warming-up programme prior to the weight lifting. A modification of the original Zinovieff method starts with the 10 RM for one set, decreases by 1 lb (0.45 kg) for the next 10 and another 1 lb (0.45 kg) for the next 10, and again this requires warming-up exercises before commencing the lifting. The 10 RM can be reassessed each week or more often if appropriate. The aim is to work the muscle maximally and strengthen it as quickly as possible, so the physiotherapist will choose the most suitable method for each individual patient.

Weight and pulley system

There are a number of weight and pulley systems in use, for example the Westminster pulley and the EMS Rehabilitation unit. These allow the direction of force to be altered and therefore maximal resistance can be applied at the desired angle.

Electrically operated machines giving resistance to movement

There are various machines available and some of these have an advantage over the application of weights, as the resistance can be adjusted through the range of movement according to the effort made by the patient. The Cybex (Figure A1.13) is an example of this type of machine, and as it is linked to a computer it can record the resistance at each part of the range in each session. The patient may be tested for maximum isometric resistance if required. The Cybex can be used for assessing a patient and for treatment if it is appropriate.

Spring resistance

Springs can be used to offer resistance to a movement and there are special therapeutic springs available. The extensible springs are made in

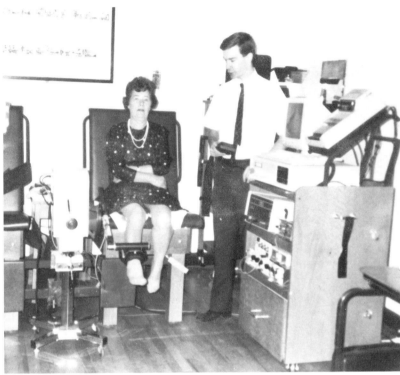

Figure A1.13 Cybex machine (Courtesy School of Physiotherapy, Middlesex Hospital)

various sizes to offer different amounts of resistance to stretch – for example a 20 lb (8 kg) spring will offer a resistance of 20 lb (18 kg) when the spring is stretched and the cord inside the spring is taut. Springs are usually made with an interval of 5 lb (2.3 kg) between one spring and the next – 10 lb, 15 lb, 20 lb. 25 lb, 30 lb, 35 lb, 40 lb (4.5 kg, 6.8 kg, 9 kg, 11.4 kg, 13.6 kg, 16 kg, 18.2 kg) – and they do not usually extend over 50 lb (23 kg). Compression or torsion springs may be used to offer resistance, and are particularly suitable for strengthening hand grip.

There are a number of problems that must be appreciated by the therapist when considering the use of spring resistance:

1. The stretch of the spring will not necessarily coincide with the range of movement, some movements being less than the full stretch of the spring and others being more than the full extension of the spring.
2. Often the maximal resistance is required in the middle range of the muscle contraction. It is relatively easy to position the patient and the spring so that it is at right angles to the bone and parallel to the line of movement at the desired range, but this does not give an accurate measurement of the amount of resistance being

given unless the spring is fully stretched at this point.
3. The patient must be taught to control the returning movement against the recoil of the spring by using eccentric muscle work, otherwise the recoil of the spring will produce an uncontrolled passive movement.
4. Springs must be attached very carefully to ensure that they do not become detached during a movement.

Springs can be used in series to give a larger range of movement, in which case two 10 lb (4.5 kg) springs would give 10 lb (4.5 kg) resistance when fully stretched. Springs can be used in parallel and then two 10 lb (4.5 kg) springs would give 20 lb (9 kg) resistance when fully stretched, which can be useful when one spring of the desired strength is not available. When using springs in series or parallel, it is important to use springs of the same poundage.

Endurance

Many activities whether at work, in the home or leisure require the ability to sustain movement for a period of time, hence endurance training is a necessary part of the rehabilitation programme. The exercises should be of low resistance and high repetition rate, and should simulate the activity. If general fitness is required, then circuit training is one method that may be used to improve endurance in a physiotherapy department.

In some instances a work situation may be more easily simulated in an occupational therapy department.

Quite a number of work places have a medical department and may have an occupational health physiotherapist who can devise a programme of retraining in relation to the normal work activity, and this is probably the most desirable way for all concerned. The physiotherapist will know when the person is ready to start work, even on a part-time basis, and can discuss this with management and the worker. The worker may not need to be off work for as long as if they were attending hospital out-patients for treatment. Management will have a better idea how to plan when they can have reports on progress from the occupational health team.

Circuit training

Circuits were developed for general fitness training and were then adapted for specific sports. Later they were modified for use in rehabilitation programmes. The circuit was designed to exercise all parts of the body, and is particularly useful for improving endurance. The circuit is made up of a number of different exercises, some or all of which may use apparatus. A person may start at any point in the circuit and therefore a number of people can participate at the same time.

The number of exercises in a circuit usually varies between 6 and 10 depending on the objectives. If all-round fitness is required for a person returning to sporting activities or heavy manual work, then 10 exercises are probably suitable. Patients who do not require such a high level of fitness may have fewer exercises, although less than six will not allow an all-round fitness programme to be carried out. In rehabilitation programmes the difficulty of the exercises may be varied, starting with a set of easy exercises and changing to more difficult ones as the patient progresses. If there are a large number of patients of different abilities, then there may be two or three circuits graded easy, intermediate and difficult.

There are several methods of carrying out circuit training but the following will indicate the basic principles of its use. Firstly each exercise must be carefully taught to ensure that it is being performed correctly. The person is then tested by asking him to perform the exercise as many times as possible in 1 minute. This may be too long for some patients, and if so, the time can be reduced to 30 s. A 2-minute rest is given before testing the next exercise and so

on until the 10 exercises are completed, giving a total time of 30 minutes (or 25 minutes if each exercise is performed for 30 s). For training purposes the number of each exercise performed for the test is reduced by half, and the circuit is performed three times, with the total time at each session being recorded. As endurance improves the total time will decrease, and once the total time for the three circuits is under 20 minutes the patient is retested and a new training schedule is set. Once the number of repetitions of an exercise in 1 minute cannot be reduced without decreasing its performance, the exercise should be changed to a more difficult one.

For a patient, the treatment is continued until he is assessed as being fit to return to work or to undertake any other activities.

Sometimes a circuit will not be suitable for all the patients, in which case alternative exercises may be inserted into the programme for a particular patient.

Circuits have a number of advantages in a rehabilitation programme:

1. The level of each exercise is tested for the ability of each patient.
2. The patient is competing against himself and so patients can work at their own level.
3. It helps the patient to become independent as he is partially responsible for his own treatment and can see his progress.
4. A number of patients can participate in a circuit at the same time, each one starting at a different exercise. This saves time in patients waiting for a particular piece of apparatus.
5. If necessary a circuit can be organized in a relatively small space.

Circuit training in rehabilitation requires very careful organization and supervision if it is to be successful. The physiotherapist must examine each patient to ensure that the needs of the individual will be met by this method of treatment. The patient must understand what he is trying to achieve. The physiotherapist must be able to observe all the patients taking part in a circuit and must keep a careful check on the progress of each patient.

Sample circuit

1. Form inclined from wall-bar. Patient starts in crouch position and lifts form as he moves to standing, and then lifts form above head. The form is then lowered until the patient is back in the starting position.
2. Cycling on a stationary bicycle – the distance is recorded for the 1 minute test and then halved for training.
3. Press-ups.
4. Running the length of the gymnasium and back.
5. Standing – lifting weighted bar to chin and lower slowly (weight determined for test).

6. Burpees.
7. Crook lying – lifting head and shoulders to touch hands on knees and lower slowly.
8. Prone lying – head and shoulder lifting and lowering.
9. Standing (by a form) – stepping up and down onto form and using alternate legs.
10. Sitting on stool with fingers on shoulders (or hands behind neck) – trunk turning to place right elbow on left knee and back, and then repeat for other side.

Group work

This can be a valuable part of the same rehabilitation programmes but it must be appropriate for the condition and stage of treatment of the individual patient.

Size of group

It is preferable for the group to be no larger than eight patients, as beyond this number the physiotherapist will have difficulty in observing and correcting the movements of the individual patient.

A larger group can be taken for general activities, provided that close supervision of movements is not required.

Uses

1. One of the main advantages of group work is to give the patient an increasing amount of independence. The patient becomes gradually more responsible for his own exercises and yet is still adequately supervised. Patients on long-term rehabilitation programmes can become very dependent on the physiotherapist and a progression to group work may help to reduce this, provided that it is appropriate.
2. A patient may require some very specific techniques for a particular part of the body, but it is essential to regain overall physical activity and function. Group work can be used for this purpose as an addition to the individual treatment. As well as being an advantage for the patient it can save valuable time for the physiotherapist by treating several patients together.
3. It gives patients an opportunity to discuss problems of common interest with the therapist and with each other. This may help to resolve problems and sometimes a patient finds that a difficulty that has assumed major proportions when viewed on his own becomes minor when discussed with others, and he is able to cope with it.
4. An element of competition can provide a stimulus for some patients, which will make them work harder and they may achieve a more effective result.
5. An important part of the rehabilitation programme is to give advice to patients on future care, and this may be usefully carried out during group work. Following injury, the physiotherapist may be able to teach the patient how to avoid a repetition of the injury. A good example of this is protection of the back by using proper lifting techniques and good positioning for work and leisure activities. The physiotherapist must have adequate knowledge of the work or sporting activity. Some physiotherapists specialize in preventing or treating patients with industrial injuries, others may specialize in the management of sports injuries. Advice is equally important for patients who have a progressive or chronic condition, such as rheumatoid arthritis or osteoarthritis, to show them correct positioning and how to protect their joints.
6. Group work can sometimes be used to advantage in helping mentally ill or mentally handicapped patients. Movement may give them another medium of expression and it may help their general physical activity and function.

Preparation for group work

Type of group

This can be specific or general depending on the aims and objectives. Specific groups may be named according to the particular area of injury or disease, for example a knee injury group, shoulder group, back group, hand and wrist group and so on. The work will include exercises for the whole limb or body, as rehabilitation must concern the function of the whole patient. If there are too many patients for a group, then the groups may be graded into easy, intermediate or advanced as appropriate. General groups may be used for advanced rehabilitation or in other cases when a general programme is required.

Selection of patient

Condition

Patients should have a similar condition and be at approximately the same stage of treatment. It is possible to take a group with patients at different stages of recovery, but this requires skilful handling from the physiotherapist – sometimes this can be achieved by using a circuit.

Age

This will depend on the type of group and the needs of the individual patients. For example it would not be suitable to take an elderly gentleman with lumbar spondylosis in a group of miners recovering from traumatic injuries to the back and being rehabilitated for work in the mines.

Sex

The same applies as for age, as the occupation and leisure needs of men and women are not necessarily the same and their physical abilities may differ.

Attitude

Some patients are not suitable for group treatment and will not benefit from it. The physiotherapist must assess the suitability of each individual patient.

Frequency

This will depend on the aims and objectives of the particular group. If group work is being used to monitor the home programme and give advice, then once or twice a week may be all that is required, provided that the patient performs the home programme adequately. Groups used for advanced rehabilitation for return to work in heavy industry or sport may be required daily, partly because of the apparatus used. In a rehabilitation centre group work may be part of a whole-day programme.

Length of time

This is usually 20–30 minutes but can vary depending on the aims and objectives and the type of group.

Space

Minimal space must allow patients to move their limbs from various starting positions without risk of hitting another patient or any fixed apparatus. Quite advanced work can be given in a relatively small space if the physiotherapist organizes appropriate exercises, but obviously it is preferable to have more than the minimal space, particularly for advanced groups. The type of exercise that can be given will depend not only on the amount of space, but also whether lights and windows are protected and if there are any radiators or other fittings projecting into the room.

Apparatus

A physiotherapy department should be equipped with small apparatus both for individual and group work, such as balls (various sizes), bean-bags, quoits, hoops, bands. If a department is large enough to have a remedial gymnasium then it may be equipped with gymnastic apparatus such as forms, wall-bars, ropes, exercise bicycles, rowing machines, weight and pulley systems, etc.

Planning group work

The physiotherapist will assess the suitability of a patient for group work. Then the individual needs of the patients within the group must be assessed in order to formulate the aims and objectives for the group.

There are certain basic principles that should be followed in organizing group work.

Before starting

Select suitable space, as the choice of exercise may depend on this. Plan exercises and decide on apparatus required.

Explanation

Every patient should have the purpose of the group work explained, and agree to take part.

Programme

Introduction

Sometimes it may be necessary to explain the aims and objectives to the group as well as the initial explanation to the individual.

Exercises

1. The number of planned exercises may vary according to the response of the group and the way in which the exercises are performed.
2. Start with easy warming-up exercises that all the group can perform. This is very important as it allows the body systems to adjust to increasing activity. It allows graduated contraction and stretching of muscle tissue before making the muscles work against resistance or be fully stretched.
3. Similarly at the end of the group work there should be some easy exercises to allow the body to adjust to normal function.
4. Progress through to the more difficult exercises.
5. Vary muscle work – for example, follow flexion/extension of shoulder by abduction/adduction or rotation and then return to another flexion/extension if required.
6. Consider starting positions carefully – keep patients in a similar position for 2–3 exercises unless there is a definite reason for moving them.
7. Apparatus must be used purposefully and not just for the sake of using it.
8. Avoid using too many pieces of apparatus in one session.

Home exercises

These must be carefully selected and taught to avoid them being performed incorrectly at home. The patients should be asked to repeat them at the end of the group work to see that they have remembered how to do them. At the beginning of the next session they should be asked to show which exercises they have been doing at home to see whether they are being correctly performed and if there is any progress.

Music

It may be helpful to perform exercises to music and this may be particularly useful with the mentally ill or handicapped. However, the music must be chosen carefully to allow the exercises to be performed properly.

Mentally ill and mentally handicapped

Planning of group work for these patients may be less structured and may develop according to the responses of the patients. This work can only be used therapeutically if the physiotherapist understands the conditions and needs of these patients and this requires specialist training.

General activity classes can be given but the therapist must still have a knowledge of the possible reactions of the patients and how to deal with the problems that may occur.

Group activities

The following are examples of some of the groups that can form part of a therapeutic programme.

General activity groups

1. *Elderly* – Activity groups in day centres and hospitals.
2. People with learning difficulties (including mental illness and handicap):
   (a) General fitness in gymnasium, hydrotherapy pool or day centre.
   (b) Relaxation.

Specific groups

For musculoskeletal disorders:

1. Ankylosing spondylitis:
   (a) Groups in hydrotherapy pool.
   (b) Posture and fitness in the gymnasium (including advice on back care).
2. Back (spinal) school to include:
   (a) Education in the care of the spine.
   (b) Biomechanics of the spine and pelvis.

(c) Exercises (mobilizing and strengthening).
(d) Posture.
(e) Diet.
(f) Self-help and pain management.
3. *Lower limb groups* – To include disorders of hip, knee, ankle and foot. Groups may be limited, i.e. foot group, but must include general leg exercises and function. Sometimes there may be a general leg group.
4. *Upper limb groups* – Similar to lower limb groups and may be general or specific, i.e. shoulder or hand group.
5. *Advanced rehabilitation* – Patients who have to return to manual work or sport after injury may require advanced rehabilitation. These groups may include patients following injury to upper or lower limbs, or back.
6. *Circuits* – Can be used for any of the above groups. (See page 432.)

Other specific groups

1. *Obstetrics*:
   (a) Antenatal.
   (b) Post-natal: (i) in hospital, (ii) in health centres, (iii) hydrotherapy pool.
2. *Cardiac rehabilitation* – Education in diet and care of the heart exercise circuits.
3. *Respiratory care* – Asthma. Childrens' classes.
4. *Cardiovascular* – Amputation groups in the gymnasium for upper limb strengthening, balance and teaching self-help.
5. *Neurological disorders* – Usually there are not sufficient numbers of patients with the same disease and in the same ability range. Group activity has been used for patients with multiple sclerosis and for patients with Parkinson's disease.

Use of small apparatus

A variety of small apparatus can be used in therapeutic programmes: balls of different sizes, quoits, bean-bags, hoops, bands, poles. If suitable apparatus is not available the physiotherapist can make use of other items – for example a sponge or an old plastic bottle filled with water for squeezing, a peg for practising pinch grip between thumb and index finger. The physiotherapist must take into account a number of factors before deciding to use a piece of apparatus.

Improving performance

The apparatus should help to improve the performance or effectiveness of an exercise:

1. A patient who has to perform an exercise a number of times in order to strengthen muscles

may find it tedious and be loath to practise. The physiotherapist may introduce a piece of apparatus and an element of competition – for example, if the exercise is arm stretching forward to strengthen the shoulder flexors ($\times 10$), this could be changed to trying to throw a quoit on to a horizontal or vertical pole for the same number of times and see how many times the patient can hook the quoit on the stick. Also this could be used to improve endurance when an exercise is practised an increasing number of times at a low resistance.

2. Apparatus may be used to increase the range of movement – for example, to encourage elevation of the arm through flexion the patient can try to tie a band on to the highest wall bar he can reach using both hands. A note can be made of this level and then the patient can see if he is making progress.

3. Small apparatus can be useful in improving the dexterity of the hands as well as strengthening the muscles – gripping, throwing and catching small balls, tying and untying knots in bands, string or rope, picking up small objects such as buttons, pins or money.

Patient motivation

The use of apparatus may motivate a patient to work harder.

Safety

This is an important factor to consider when using apparatus, both from the point of view of the patient using it, and other patients in the vicinity. As far as the patient using the apparatus is concerned safety will depend on the type of exercise and the apparatus being used. For example, when the patient is throwing and catching a ball the physiotherapist must see that he is not standing too near to any other apparatus. There must be sufficient space between patients to allow for the use of the apparatus. The patient must have the ability or the potential ability to perform the exercise. If the patient has the ability then the physiotherapist should observe the exercise to see that it is being carried out correctly and safely. Otherwise the physiotherapist will have to teach each part of the exercise, and then when the patient is proficient, allow him to carry out the full movement. The physiotherapist must be careful using apparatus if there are other people in the room, especially if it involves throwing and catching objects, as there may be a danger of another person being hit, or the object knocking another piece of apparatus over on to someone.

A remedial gymnasium will normally have protected windows and lights, but if another room is used it may not be advisable to throw balls or other objects because of the danger of breaking windows or lights.

Apparatus must not be left where it may be a hazard to other people, and it must be stored after use.

Walking re-education

Walking patterns

Walking is a complex activity involving most parts of the body. Movements of the trunk and arms facilitate the actions of the lower limbs, and the extent to which they are used will depend on the type of gait. If the length of stride is long and the person is walking fairly fast, then the arm and trunk movement is usually increased. As the left leg moves forward there will be some rotation in the trunk (to the left) to keep the person facing forward. There will be some extension in the lumbar spine to facilitate the propulsion from the right leg. The arms will also swing to assist balance and facilitate movement with the right arm swinging forward with the left leg and at the same time the left arm swinging back. In a slower walk these movements may be markedly reduced and there may be little or no swinging of the arms.

The type of gait can vary in an individual according to the activity required: for example a leisurely stroll, a fast stride or an ordinary walking pattern. Walking will also vary with age, starting with the slow, wide gait of the toddler through the confident gait of the child and adult, including the ability to run, and then to the elderly when the gait will tend to become slower. The characteristics of a person or a behavioural change may be reflected in the posture and gait pattern. The physiotherapist must be aware of these various factors when re-educating gait.

Re-education may involve teaching the patient to walk again following disease or injury, correcting an abnormal gait or keeping mobile a person who has irreversible problems affecting the walking pattern.

Assessment

The assessment will depend on whether the patient is able to walk, or if some treatment is required as a preparation for walking re-education. In the latter instance the physiotherapist must decide what objectives must be achieved before the patient can start to walk and whether he will require any walking aids.

If the patient is able to walk, the physiotherapist will observe the gait and notice any abnormality in the pattern.

Points to check:

1. Smooth transference of weight with the ability to control the position of pelvis.
2. Ability to maintain the weight on one leg while swinging the other leg forward for heel strike.
3. Swinging leg forward. Starts with flexion of hip and knee followed by extension of knee with dorsiflexion of ankle and lowering leg to heel strike.
4. Propulsion phase of back leg with extension of hip and knee, with plantar flexion of the ankle.
5. Position of body and lower limb joints in each phase of the pattern.
6. Even length of stride.

The patient is then examined to determine (or sometimes to confirm) the cause of the particular abnormality. Pain, muscle weakness and joint stiffness can all be causes of an abnormal gait. Diseases of the nervous system can lead to abnormal gait patterns. For example: spasticity occurring with cerebral palsy, or with multiple sclerosis, or as the result of a stroke; rigidity occurring with Parkinson's disease; muscle paralysis from spinal cord lesions or peripheral nerve lesions.

When the physiotherapist has analysed the problem, a decision is made as to whether treatment is appropriate or not – usually in conjunction with other members of the management team. If treatment is to be given, the physiotherapist will decide on the objectives with the patient (if possible) and a programme will be planned. This may involve trying to effect a change – relief of pain, increasing range of movement, strengthening of muscles – which will lead to an improved walking pattern. Sometimes it may not be possible to make any improvement in the factor(s) affecting gait, as for example with a permanently stiff knee joint, and then the physiotherapist will try to obtain as normal a pattern as the disability will allow. If appropriate, walking aids or an orthosis may be given to the patient, either temporarily or permanently, to assist walking.

Re-education

As in teaching any complex pattern of movement, the correct gait must be built up gradually. The patient may need to concentrate on one particular aspect of the gait, and as that improves, move on to the next stage.

For example, a patient who has had a fracture of the lower end of the tibia may have some pain and residual stiffness of the ankle (due to adhesions) after the plaster has been removed and weight bearing is started. The plan of treatment will probably include techniques for the relief of pain, increasing the range of movement and strengthening the muscles, in addition to walking re-education.

The patient may walk with a limp because of pain and will not have the range of movement in the ankle to allow the push-off phase. Initially the patient may have crutches or sticks until the pain decreases and the range of movement begins to improve, and then the amount of weight bearing will gradually be increased. To begin with the patient should be encouraged to take short steps so that the weight is not held too long on the painful ankle. Also the shorter steps will mean that the patient will not require as much propulsion to move forward. The length of stride and propulsion can be obtained as the patient improves, remembering to see that there is an even length of stride on each side.

It is important to try to keep a natural rhythm whenever possible, and concentrate on correcting one point at a time. Correcting too many points at one time and slowing the gait to an unnatural rhythm is likely to develop further problems.

When a patient presents with irreversible problems such as a permanent limitation of movement in one or more joints of the lower limbs, spasticity, or instability, it is important to help him to walk and be as mobile as possible, rather than trying to achieve a perfect pattern. The physiotherapist must recognize when walking is not going to be achieved so that alternative plans can be made.

Types of walking aids

Crutches (Figure A1.14)

Axillary crutches – These are usually wooden with a padded top and a hand rest. The padded top is pressed against the chest wall, just below the axilla, by the arm when the patient takes weight through the crutches. These crutches are made in different lengths and so the patient must be measured in order to obtain the correct length. Some of the wooden crutches are adjustable, both in length and at the hand piece, but they do not extend as far as the metal crutches and the patient will need to be measured as for the non-adjustable.

Elbow crutches – These are made of metal and are adjustable by means of a metal clip. The patient takes the weight through the hand pieces and there is a metal half-band which rests against the back of the forearm.

Forearm support crutches – These are made of metal and are adjustable in length. The weight is taken through the forearm support and there is an adjustable hand grip at the end.

There are some other types on the market but the above are those in common use.

Use

Axillary and elbow crutches can be used when the patient is unable to take weight on one leg provided

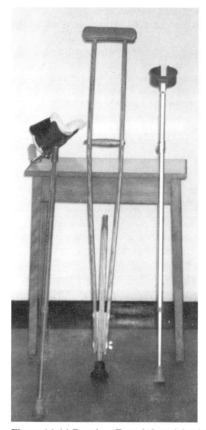

Figure A1.14 Crutches. From left to right: forearm support, axillary, elbow (Courtesy School of Physiotherapy, Middlesex Hospital)

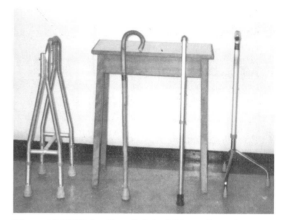

Figure A1.15 Sticks. From left to right: quadrapod, wooden, adjustable metal and tripod (Courtesy School of Physiotherapy, Middlesex Hospital)

that he has good balance, the unaffected leg is strong and his arms are strong enough to take his weight. The axillary crutches are more stable than the elbow but care has to be taken that the patient takes the pressure of the crutch against the chest wall and not through the axilla. These crutches are also used for partial weight bearing when more support is required than a stick, or as an intermediate stage before using a stick.

Forearm support crutches can only be used for partial weight bearing and are often used by patients with rheumatoid arthritis when the hands, wrists and elbows are affected by the disease.

Sticks (Figure A1.15)

There are wooden sticks, which have to be cut to the correct length for the patient, or there are adjustable metal sticks. The latter are not so commonly used because they are more expensive.

Tripod and tetrapod sticks are available and can be used if more stability is required.

Uses

Two sticks can be used for partial weight bearing as a progression from crutches or when the patient does not require the greater support offered by crutches. One stick may give sufficient support for some patients, and has the advantage of leaving one hand free. In this case the stick is used on the opposite side from the affected leg. A stick or sticks may also be used to assist balance in a patient who is a little unsteady but does not require a frame.

Frames (Figure A1.16)

There are various types of frames which are usually made of metal and most are adjustable. The majority have ferrules attached to the four struts and the frame is light in weight so that it can be lifted easily. Some frames have wheels attached but they can only be used for certain patients as there is a danger that they may run forward if not carefully used. There are some reciprocal frames which are hinged so that one side can be moved forward and then the other.

Uses

Frames are used for partial weight bearing especially with elderly patients who could not take sufficient weight through the arms to use crutches, and who may also be unsteady. They may be useful for children with cerebral palsy or spina bifida who need some support to walk but cannot use crutches or sticks. Frames may be used by patients who need some support for walking because they are unsteady.

A frame with a tray attached may be useful for a patient at home to enable him to carry items from

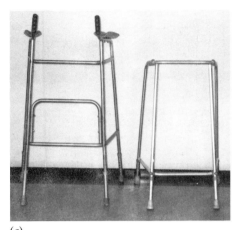

(a)

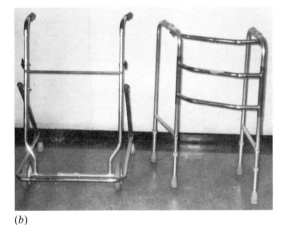

(b)

Figure A1.16 (*a*) Forearm support and hand support frames. (*b*) Rollator and reciprocal frames (Courtesy School of Physiotherapy, Middlesex Hospital)

one room to another. In this instance the frame will probably need wheels or shepherd castors.

Care of aids

The physiotherapist must check that all aids are safe to use before giving them to a patient and they must be regularly checked during use. When patients are not on treatment or are not being seen frequently, they or their relatives must be taught to inspect the aids regularly.

Points to watch:

1. Ferrules are not worn.
2. Wooden aids have no cracks or splinters.
3. Support areas are properly padded.
4. Screws and clips are not broken.

Principles of crutch walking

Preparation

Adequate preparation is required to ensure that the patient can use the crutches effectively and safely.

Measurements for axillary crutches – It is important that these are the correct height for the patient and there are two ways in which they may be measured:

1. The patient is positioned in lying with the shoes on and the measurements are taken from 5 cm below the posterior axillary fold to a point 15 cm laterally from the level of the shoe heel.
2. The patient is positioned in lying and the measurements are taken from the posterior axillary fold to the medial malleolus.

Measurements for elbow crutches – If the patient is able to stand the measurements may be taken in this position otherwise they will be taken in lying with the shoes on. The measurement is taken from the ulnar styloid with the elbow flexed to approximately 15° to a point 15 cm laterally from the level of the shoe heel.

Measurements for sticks – Similar to above measurement for elbow crutches.

Examination of patient

The patient must be able to take weight on the crutches by extending the elbow and pressing down on the hands. Additionally the shoulder adductors must be strong enough to keep the upper arm close to the body (particularly in the case of axillary crutches), the shoulder extensors to give the propulsion and the shoulder depressors to assist the downward thrust when taking the weight through the crutches.

The unaffected leg must be able to take the weight of the body and so the physiotherapist will check the strength of the hip and knee extensors, the plantar flexors, and that the abductors of the hip can control the level of the pelvis.

The patient must be able to balance in sitting and standing. Standing balance can be tested by the physiotherapist and an assistant supporting the patient or with the patient standing with the support of the crutches and the physiotherapist close enough to give additional support if necessary.

Non-weight-bearing crutch walking

The amount of assistance required in the early stages will vary from one patient to another. It may be necessary for two people to help the patient to stand and then give him the crutches, whereas another patient may be able to manage unaided. The physiotherapist must be certain that the patient is safe before leaving him to walk without any supervision.

It is helpful if the physiotherapist demonstrates crutch walking and emphasizes the important points before the patient gets up.

Stages

Standing with crutches – The physiotherapist will check that the patient can balance and that the height of the crutches is correct. The crutches should be slightly in front of the supporting foot in order to give a triangular base. The sequence is as follows:

1. Pressing down on crutches and lifting weight-bearing leg off the ground and back again.
2. The patient moves the crutches a little way forward.
3. The weight is taken forward over the crutches.
4. The patient presses the arms straight and lifts the unaffected leg forward and places it just behind the crutches.

The sequence continues in this manner. It is important for the physiotherapist to judge how far the patient can go on the first occasion and place a chair ready for him to sit.

Progression – As the patient becomes confident he may progress from a swing-to gait to a swing-through, where the unaffected leg is placed ahead of the crutches. The patient must be stable and have strong arms for a swing-through gait. Usually it is only suitable for younger patients.

Shadow walking

If possible the patient should be taught to swing the non-weight-bearing leg back as he brings the other leg forward thus making it easier to resume the normal walking pattern when he is partially or fully weight bearing.

Partial weight bearing

There are two methods that may be used:

1. The crutches and the affected leg are moved forward. The weight is then taken through the leg and the crutches while the unaffected leg is moved forward. This pattern is then repeated. Progress is made as the patient gradually takes more weight through the leg and less through the crutches (three-point gait).
2. Alternate crutch–foot gait – the right crutch is moved forward and then the left foot. This is followed by the left crutch and then the right foot (four-point gait). As the patient improves he may progress to moving the right crutch and left foot together followed by the left crutch and right foot (two-point gait).

The choice of the above methods will depend on the amount of weight that the patient can take through the affected leg. The second method gives a better walking pattern but takes more weight through the affected leg than may be possible or permissible in the first instance.

Sitting

Initially the physiotherapist may need to take the crutches and support the patient while he sits. Unless there is another helper the patient will have to use a crutch on the unsupported side or place a hand on the arm of the chair. It is important that the patient realizes where he must be positioned in relation to the chair before sitting.

If the patient is to sit and stand unaided he must know what to do with the crutches.

Axillary crutches – Hold onto hand pieces and move padded top forward away from chest wall, and then using crutches to assist balance followed by sitting in the chair. Alternatively both crutches may be held in one hand and the other hand may be placed on the arm of the chair followed by sitting.

Elbow crutches – The forearm support piece must be moved away from the arm and the hand grip held. The same methods may then be used as with the axillary crutches.

If the crutches are being held in one hand and the other hand is being placed on the arm of the chair the crutches should be on the side of the affected leg.

Stairs

Non-weight bearing – If there are no banisters the patient keeps the crutches on the ground level, takes weight through the crutches and lifts the unaffected leg onto the first step. The weight is taken through this leg and the crutches are lifted onto that step. This is repeated to progress up the stairs. The physiotherapist stands behind the patient until she is certain he is safe on his own.

When there is a banister – The patient holds the banister with one hand and the crutch with the other. Progress up the stairs is as described above. Initially the other crutch may be held by the physiotherapist but once the patient is confident he may be taught to transfer the crutch to the other hand.

Going downstairs, the patient places the crutches on the step below and takes the weight through the crutches while lowering the unaffected leg onto this step. With a banister, the patient slides one hand a little way down and then moves the crutch onto the lower step. This is followed by taking the weight through the banister and the crutch while lowering the unaffected leg onto the step. The physiotherapist goes down in front of the patient until she is certain that he is safe on his own.

Sticks

If two sticks are used, patterns similar to the partial-weight-bearing walking with crutches may be used.

When one stick is used, it is held on the opposite side from the affected leg. The stick and affected leg are moved forward together followed by the unaffected leg. In this way the weight is taken partly through the affected leg and partly through the stick. It is important to see that there is a smooth gait with equal length of stride on each side.

Frames

Adjustable light-weight frame with ferrules – The frame is moved forward and the patient walks up to it. Care must be taken that the patient does not move the frame too far forward, and that he does not move his feet too close to the frame, as either would decrease stability.

Frame with wheels – This may be required if the patient is unable to lift the frame forward or is incoordinate (as in multiple sclerosis with ataxia). The physiotherapist must ensure that the patient is safe with this type of frame, as the wheels make it less stable and liable to run forward. An alternative is the reciprocal frame, which is used by taking the weight on one side and lifting the other side forward, and then repeating to the opposite side.

Proprioceptive neuromuscular facilitation (PNF)

These are functional patterns of movement whereby the physiotherapist uses a variety of sensory stimuli to facilitate a movement. These techniques require skilful handling by the physiotherapist if they are to be effective.

The stimuli involve touch and pressure with the hands of the physiotherapist on the surface of the limb in the direction of the movement, quick stretch on the muscles to be facilitated, traction or compression as appropriate to the movement, maximal resistance to allow smooth movement through the available range (unless using resistance to a static contraction), use of voice, and the patient is encouraged to watch the movement. Good timing is essential to produce an effective result. These techniques can be used to initiate a muscle contraction, to strengthen muscles, to increase range of movement and to improve coordination.

Basic patterns

The starting positions are usually lying, although certain techniques can be carried out in other positions. The movements are named according to the movements taking place at the shoulder or hip joint, but proximal and distal joints are also involved. The degree of movement in the other joints will depend on the particular technique and the starting position used. Movement starts distally and ends proximally.

Arms

Flexion, abduction, lateral rotation/extension, adduction, medial rotation.

Flexion, adduction, lateral rotation/extension, abduction, medial rotation.

Functionally the arm is often used with elbow flexion or extension, as in eating, brushing teeth, brushing or combing the hair, pushing or pulling. The patterns may be used similarly – for example, flexion, adduction, lateral rotation with elbow flexion (eating) or flexion, abduction, lateral rotation with elbow flexion (combing hair) and so on.

Legs

Flexion, adduction, lateral rotation/extension, abduction, medial rotation.

Flexion, abduction, medial rotation/extension, adduction, lateral rotation.

As with the arm, many of the functional movements of the leg involve knee movements. For example flexion, adduction, lateral rotation with knee flexion to extension, abduction, medial rotation with knee extension (walking pattern).

Trunk

Many activities include trunk movements as well as the arm and/or leg. For example, the right arm flexion, adduction, medial rotation pattern can continue to trunk flexion and rotation to the left, and then right arm extension, abduction, lateral rotation with trunk extension and rotation to the right. Thus the arm or leg patterns can be used to facilitate trunk movements. Also trunk movements can be facilitated without including the arm or leg patterns.

It is not possible in this text to describe all the ways in which the patterns can be used and neither is it possible to describe all the techniques in detail, but the following indicates the use of some of the different techniques.

To strengthen muscles

1. Slow reversals.
2. Repeated contractions.
3. Rhythmic stabilizations.

To gain relaxation/lengthening of muscle

1. Hold–relax.
2. Contract–relax.
3. Rhythmic stabilizations.

To improve coordination

If the incoordination is due to muscle weakness then appropriate strengthening techniques can be used – slow reversals are particularly helpful.

Repetitive movement in pattern may help patients with ataxia to obtain a smoother movement.

Initiation of a contraction in a muscle or muscles

Provided that the neurons supplying a muscle have not been destroyed by injury or disease it should be possible to reactivate the muscle and then strengthen it. The time taken to recover will depend on the nature of the injury or disease and where it occurs. For example, pressure on a peripheral nerve that does not cause degeneration will recover in a few weeks, and the muscles will contract again, but when degeneration of the peripheral nerve has occurred the muscle fibre cannot contract until the nerve fibre has regrown – see Chapter 21, Peripheral Nerve Lesions.

To reactivate a muscle there must be a constant bombardment of the anterior horn cells using any sensory stimuli available – touch, pressure, traction or compression as appropriate, quick stretch of the muscle. The physiotherapist can make good use of her voice to encourge the patient to try to move and thus stimulate the muscles via the cortico-spinal pathways. Passive movements with the use of the voice will help to remind the patient of the movement which may be accompanied by some of the other stimuli mentioned above. The use of other external stimuli such as brief ice or brushings may be helpful.

As muscles work together in functional patterns rather than in isolation, increasing the activity of other groups of muscles in the pattern may encourage a contraction. For example, to initiate a contraction in the dorsiflexors of the ankle joint, strong resistance may be given to the hip flexors and knee flexors in either the flexion/adduction pattern with knee flexion, or the flexion/abduction pattern with knee flexion, as the dorsiflexors usually work with hip and knee flexion.

Sometimes normal body reactions can be useful in encouraging activity. For example, to gain a contraction of the left deltoid the patient is placed in the lying position and then strong resistance is given to the extension abduction pattern of the right arm. This will normally cause the left arm to go into extension and abduction to prevent the body rolling towards the right side.

Group action of muscles may help to initiate a contraction of the desired muscle(s) within the group. For example, the wrist extensors normally work as synergists with a grasping movement. The wrist may be supported in the degree of extension that allows the patient to grasp an object, which may encourage the synergistic activity of the wrist extensors.

It is important to try as many different ways as possible to reactivate a muscle. The physiotherapist must watch carefully for a flicker of contraction but must not be misled by trick movements. The fingers may extend if the wrist is flexed, not because the extensors are working but because of the stretch on the extensors as they pass over the wrist. Similarly with a paralysed extensor pollicis longus, if the thumb is flexed at the metacarpophalangeal and interphalangeal joints and then the flexor is relaxed there may be a small degree of extension at the interphalangeal joint, which may be due to the relaxation and not to a contraction of the extensor pollicis longus.

Once a flicker of contraction has appeared, the same methods must be continued until there is sufficient contraction to produce a little movement with gravity counterbalanced. After this the methods outlined below for strengthening muscles can be used.

Manipulative therapy

This aspect of physiotherapy involves skilful restoration of mobility to soft tissues and joints. Thorough examination, assessment of findings, formulation of a working hypothesis and identification of tests for ensuring that objectives are being achieved are essential for competent treatment of patients by manipulative therapy. Ultimately, however, it is the precision, sensitivity, care and concentration with which techniques are applied that will achieve success, and this needs dedicated practice. Complementary skills involving re-education and strengthening of muscles, coordination of movement, posture training and relaxation are essential in the overall management of the patient.

Manipulative therapy consists of:

1. Soft-tissue techniques (massage).
2. Passive mobilization of joints.
3. Passive stretching of soft tissues.
4. Autostretching of soft tissues.

Soft-tissue techniques (massage)

Soft tissues are muscles (and their fascial sheaths), ligaments, tendons, fascia (including specialized structures such as the ilio-tibial tract) and skin.

The term 'massage' has been replaced in the vocabulary of some physiotherapists by 'soft-tissue techniques' because of the bad publicity accorded to massage in the late 1960s and 1970s. The image of 'unscientific' therapy was unfortunate as it led to the reduction of practice and application of these highly effective techniques. During the 1980s the importance of treating the soft tissues in addition to the joints began to be recognized and massage in the total treatment of patients with musculoskeletal disorders is gradually being restored to its rightful place in the repertoire of the chartered physiotherapist.

The techniques are termed:

1. Stroking.
2. Effleurage.
3. Kneading.
4. Picking up.
5. Wringing.
6. Skin rolling.
7. Frictions.

Techniques for respiratory conditions – clapping, shaking and vibrations.

Stroking

This may be performed with the whole hand or fingers. It comprises the passage of the relaxed hand over the patient's skin with a rhythm and pressure that produce a relaxing, sedative effect.

Effleurage

In this technique, the hands pass over the skin with pressure and speed which is both soothing and such as to assist fluid to flow through the tissue spaces, lymph vessels and veins. The hands move in the direction of lymph and venous blood flow (distal to proximal in the limbs) and generally each stroke ends at the site of a group of superficial lymph glands.

The effects are:

1. Stretching of subcutaneous tissues.
2. Increasing of tissue fluid, lymph and venous flow.
3. Removal of oedematous fluid from tissue spaces into lymph vessels.
4. Relief of pain due to stimulation of touch and pressure receptors in the skin, removal of excess fluid and removal of metabolites from the site of injury, disease or disorder.

Kneading

In this technique, the hands are placed on the skin and allowed to mould to the part, then they move in a circular direction with pressure gradually applied over the top of the circle and released towards the bottom of the circle. The hands move the muscles and subcutaneous tissues applying alternately compression and release. On no account during the pressure phase are the hands allowed to slide over the skin. To localize the effects, the fingers or thumbs may be used, and where deep pressure is required one hand may reinforce the other. The effects are:

1. Increase in flow of circulation local to the area treated.
2. Reduction of tone in muscles which are in a state of excess tension.
3. Stretching of tight fascia and restoration of mobility of soft tissues.
4. Pain relief is obtained by releasing acute or chronic tension in muscles and by affecting pressure and touch nerve endings.
5. Where there is chronic oedema, the fibrin within the fluid can be stretched, so facilitating drainage of the fluid into lymph vessels.

Picking up

Picking up has effects similar to those of kneading but the technique involves lifting the tissues up at right angles to the underlying bone, squeezing and releasing. Tissue mobility is therefore gained in a plane at right angles to that obtained by kneading.

Wringing

Wringing involves lifting the tissues up as in picking up, and applying a twist to enhance the stretching effect.

Skin rolling

This involves lifting and stretching the skin between thumbs and fingers so that the skin and subcutaneous tissues are moved on each other and adhesions are stretched. This is particularly useful where there is a long-standing chronic problem and improvement will not be complete until the skin is moving freely.

Frictions

These are small-range movements applied with the thumb or fingers starting superficially and working deeper. They are applied in one of two ways – transverse or circular. Transverse frictions as the name implies are applied at right angles to the long axis of the structure being treated. They are used to mobilize structures on underlying tissues, e.g. supraspinatus tendon, the lateral ligament of the ankle or adhesions within hamstring muscles following a strain.

Circular frictions are used to produce localized effects on muscles which have been in a prolonged state of tension, e.g. the paravertebral muscles. They may also be applied to tissues where there is a nerve trunk which may be embedded in adhesions or consolidated oedematous fluid, e.g. the ulnar nerve on the posterior aspect of the medial epicondyle of the humerus or the sciatic nerve deep to gluteus maximus.

Contraindications to soft-tissue manipulation

These techniques in the repertoire of a competent chartered physiotherapist have few contraindications but the important ones are:

1. *Acute inflammation*, e.g. rheumatoid arthritis flare-up, tenosynovitis.
2. Weeping conditions of the skin, e.g. eczema.
3. *Infection* – This does not rule out soft-tissue manipulation but precautions are necessary to avoid cross-infection.
4. Recent fractures.
5. *Patient preference* – Some people do not like massage and their wishes must be respected.

Clinical features and conditions for which soft-tissue manipulation are indicated

1. Scar tissue – adherent and limiting movement.
2. Muscle spasm.
3. Muscle tightness.
4. Fascial tethering.
5. Oedema – particularly traumatic in origin.
6. Pain.
7. Slow healing scars or ulcers.

It is essential to see that these techniques are applied within a scientific method. For example, it is inappropriate to treat the oedema of kidney or heart failure. In fact, the underlying pathology must be considered and soft-tissue techniques must be used as an adjunct to the total patient management. That said, it can be perfectly professional to treat, for example, oedema of an arm following a mastectomy, or muscle spasm associated with spondylosis with soft-tissue techniques. The techniques may have no direct effect on the underlying pathology but the symptomatic relief and consequent improvement in the patient's quality of life justify their application. This, of course, is provided that both the patient and the physiotherapist recognize and accept the potential limitations.

Connective tissue massage (CTM)

This is a special type of stroking which pulls the skin and subcutaneous tissues away from the underlying fascia (Gifford and Gifford, 1988). The strokes are applied in a pattern starting over the sacrum and buttocks. Progression may then be up the back and out to the arms or down to the legs. The patient is usually treated in sitting but may be in lying.

The effects claimed for this treatment are related to balancing the sympathetic and parasympathetic components of the autonomic nervous system. The principal result of this is improvement of the blood supply to the target area.

Perhaps the best illustration of the value of this treatment is the story of how it started with Elizabeth Dicke (a German physiotherapist) who was in hospital awaiting an amputation of her right leg for circulation problems. She applied pulling strokes to the skin over her back to relieve pain there and found that not only did the backache disappear but the circulation to the leg became re-established such that amputation was not necessary. In these days of economic evaluation, it would clearly be attractive in terms of saving in cost (money), resources (theatre, surgeon, nurse, prosthetic training time) and patient suffering if physiotherapists were to practise this method of treatment.

Passive mobilization of joints

Movement at a joint may be lost in association with postural stress, trauma, or degenerative changes.

The restricting factors may be pain, muscle spasm, oedema, fibrous contracture of fascia, ligaments or capsule, or cartilage flake trapped between the joint surfaces.

Pain

Pain may be relieved by restoring normal movement. Treatment of the other limiting factors and regaining movement which is then maintained by exercise is often effective in pain relief or reduction.

The pain may be relieved as a direct effect of passive joint movement by the stimulation of mechanoreceptors, which in turn inhibits the transmission of pain impulses from the periphery through the spinal cord to the brain. Rhythmical passive movement of joints – which includes effects on skin, fascia, muscles, tendons and ligaments – probably moves fluid through the tissue planes and increases lymphatic and venous drainage. This results in removal of metabolites which act as an irritant to the nociceptive nerve endings in the tissues, and pain is reduced. Pain relief is a complex subject and much has been written on it.

Muscle spasm

This usually diminishes as pain is relieved, but may persist to that it hampers further improvement. Passive, rhythmical joint movement has been shown clinically to be effective in relaxing this spasm. The movement thus obtained often has to be re-educated so that the patient is able to maintain the improvement.

Oedema

Immediately after injury, oedema is in a fluid form which can readily be drained into the lymph or venous circulation. If this fluid remains in the tissues, fibrin forms within it and it becomes consolidated. This can be seen to happen in association with an injury at the ankle, knee, wrist or finger, but is not so evident at the hip, shoulder or vertebral facet joints. It is important to remember that oedema is present at these joints and will respond to passive, rhythmical joint mobilization.

Fibrous contracture

Injury of soft tissues results in formation of inelastic scar tissue which is laid down in a disorganized orientation causing loss of movement and dysfunction of muscle. This process occurs slowly as a result of postural stress and degenerative changes. Rhythmical passive joint movement together with regular exercise can help to realign and stretch this tissue. The particular value of manipulative therapy in treating scar tissue is that it can focus on an accessory movement within or at end of any range of a physiological movement. This is impossible with active exercise and it is essential that manipulative therapy precedes exercise. Otherwise, exercise can stress joint structures which are already moving freely, in an attempt to mobilize a stiff joint. The individual spinal joints, carpal and tarsal joints particularly can be mobilized only by the skilled application of passive joint mobilization techniques.

Cartilage flakes/synovial fringe entrapment

When a joint becomes suddenly 'stuck', a helpful hypothesis is to consider that a flake of articular cartilage has become impacted between the joint surfaces. Another hypothesis is that a part of the loose synovium at the joint margins becomes trapped between the joint surfaces. Separation of the joint surfaces by traction or 'gapping' technique (high velocity thrust–manipulation) releases the impacted tissue and joint movement is restored.

Indications for passive mobilization of joints

These techniques are appropriate to restore movement and relieve pain to any component of the musculoskeletal system provided that the contraindications have been ruled out.

Contraindications to passive mobilization of joints

These vary according to the degree of force being used. Absolute contraindications to all joint movement are:

1. Malignant disease.
2. Bone disease (osteomyelitis, osteoporosis).
3. Recent fractures or severe sprains.
4. Inflammatory arthropathies during acute flare-up – rheumatoid arthritis and ankylosing spondylitis.
5. Instability or hypermobility of joints.
6. Severe pain which is easily provoked and takes a long time to settle after provocation.
7. Psychological states in which the patient has an obsessional desire for manipulative therapy.
8. Rapidly worsening signs and symptoms.
9. Additional contraindications for the spine are:
   (a) Spinal cord compression.
   (b) Cauda equina compression.
   (c) Vertebro-basilar insufficiency.
   (d) Severe nerve root pain or compression.

These contraindications should be detected during examination by the physiotherapist, bearing in mind the following indications.

Malignancy

1. Grey pallor.
2. Pain worse at night, not relieved by movement or mild analgesia.
3. Previous operations.
4. 'Empty' feeling on palpation.
5. Failure to improve subjectively or objectively over 3–4 treatment sessions.

Bone disease

1. Osteomyelitis:
   (a) Deep, throbbing pain.
   (b) Recent history of infection.
2. Osteoporosis:
   (a) Prolonged steroid therapy.
   (b) Gastrectomy.
   (c) Over 50 age group.

Psychological state

Be wary of the patient who looks and moves well when not under obvious observation, smiles when the pain is described but claims severe functional restriction.

At the same time, it is important to examine meticulously and give the patient the benefit of the doubt until it is clear that manipulative therapy is inappropriate. (That is not to say that other treatment methods, e.g. posture and relaxation training, are inappropriate.)

Spinal cord compression

1. Paraesthesiae (pins and needles) in the legs – if the cervical or thoracic spines are to be treated.
2. Increased tendon reflexes.
3. Increased muscle tone in the legs or arms.
4. Patchy loss of sensation in both legs (not dermatomal in distribution).
5. Poor balance due to impaired transmission of impulses in the dorsal columns (fasciculus gracilis and fasciculus cuneatus).

Cauda equina compression

1. Straight leg raising tests on each leg separately very limited.
2. Bladder and/or bowel problems.
3. Saddle anaesthesiae.

Vertebro-basilar insufficiency

The vertebral artery arises from the subclavian artery, ascends through the foramina in the transverse processes of the upper six cervical vertebrae, passes behind the lateral mass of C1 and through the foramen magnum. The two arteries then join at the lower border of the pons to form the basilar artery. It supplies the cervical spine muscles, joints, nerve roots, spinal cord, pons, medulla and cerebellum. The basilar artery forms the circle of Willis and sends branches to the cerebellum and the visual area of the cerebral cortex.

Occlusion of the vertebral artery can, therefore, give rise to impairment of balance and vision.

The tests for insufficiency are:

1. *Patient lying* – Turn head to one side and hold 30 s. The patient is asked to report any untoward effects. Repeat to the other side. When the neck is rotated, the artery on the same side is occluded (normally). In the presence of disease, the patient may begin to feel light headed or dizzy.
2. *Patient sitting* – Hold head steady and ask patient to turn the shoulders from side to side (i.e. cervical spine rotation). Vertebral artery insuffi-

ciency is indicated if this makes the patient dizzy. If turning the head from side to side causes dizziness, this could be due to either vertebral artery or labyrinth (ear) problems.

In the presence of vertebral artery insufficiency, rotation and lateral flexion techniques should not be used, but a careful, low-force longitudinal technique may be used, as may soft-tissue manipulation.

Severe nerve root pain or compression

This is indicated by dermatomal (see Figure 11.4) loss of sensation, loss of muscle power in a myotomal (see Figure 11.5) distribution, reduced muscle tone and diminshed tendon reflexes. Traction and longitudinal oscillation may be applied with care but other techniques are contraindicated. It may not harm the patient to treat with manipulation but will not help if the compression is due to a tumour, severe disc prolapse or aneurysm.

Nerve root pain is described as stabbing or toothache in nature, and is broadly dermatomal in distribution. The pain keeps the patient awake and dominates his consciousness such that there is considerable functional restriction. Traction is indicated for this but joint mobilization is contraindicated.

Care should be taken in applying passive joint mobilization to the following:

1. Severe degenerative changes.
2. Long-standing spinal deformity.
3. Chronic inflammatory arthritis.
4. Pregnancy – low-grade oscillatory techniques are indicated for relieving backache but high-velocity thrust techniques are contraindicated.

Application of passive joint mobilization (PJM)

The physiotherapist should follow a logical procedure:

1. Meticulous examination.
2. Assessment of examination findings.
3. Decision to treat with PJM.
4. Select joint to treat.
5. Select test movement if possible.
6. Select technique.
7. Select grade.
8. Select number of oscillations.
9. Treat.
10. Test.
11. Repeat or change.
12. Treat.
13. Test.
14. Advise patient – discuss subsequent treatment.

(1), (2) and (3)

During these the physiotherapist applies examination principles, clarifies the patient's problems and relates these to the examination findings. Objectives and goals are identified, together with indications and contraindications for the techniques to be used.

(4) Selection of joint to be treated

As a general rule, the joint treated should on examination reproduce the pain, on either active or passive movement. Otherwise, there should be a lack of mobility which is likely to be contributing to the patient's problems.

NB. It is important to note that the joint to be treated may be far from the site of the pain, e.g. thoracic 4 for glove distribution of pins and needles in the hands; mid-tarsal joint, causing gait abnormality, producing backache.

(5) Selection of test movement

When manipulative therapy is applied skilfully, there should be an immediate effect. Improvement is indicated by:

1. Increased range of movement.
2. Less pain on the same range of movement.
3. Patient is more willing to move. Generally the movement chosen is the most restricted on active testing but care must be taken not to provoke a painful joint by too much testing.
4. Passive movement or testing may be chosen, e.g. straight leg raising or a quadrant of a joint may be used.
5. Sometimes the physiotherapist has to judge improvement by palpation.

As the patient improves, the test may be changed to full movement with overpressure or repeated quick and slow movements, or a sustained hold at end of range or combined movement, e.g. flexion in abduction or extension with side flexion – or maybe the patient has to try running or walking a mile or so if this is what provokes the pain.

(6) Select technique

Mobilizations are oscillatory, rhythmical, repetitive movements which may be physiological or accessory.

Physiological movements are the normal voluntary patterns, e.g. flexion, abduction, side flexion, rotation.

Accessory movements are those gliding movements that take place between joint surfaces whenever physiological movement is performed. They are essential for voluntary movement but cannot be produced separately, other than by an 'external force' as applied by a physiotherapist, e.g. when the wrist is flexed there is antero-posterior gliding of the carpal bones on the inferior surface of the radius.

Guides for technique selection are as follows.

Peripheral joints

1. Use the accessory movements necessary for the limited physiological movements, especially if the joint is very stiff, e.g. longitudinal movement of the humerus for a stiff shoulder, anteroposterior movement of the tibia for a knee with very limited flexion.
2. Use physiological movements where there are tight soft tissues or the movement is not very limited, e.g. hip extension with the patient in prone lying.
3. Combinations of techniques are sometimes important, i.e. an accessory movement performed with the joint at its limit of physiological movement, e.g. postero-anterior movement on the head of the ulna with the radio-ulnar joints in supination.

Spinal joints

Regional stiffness is best treated by regional techniques, e.g. rotation of the cervical or lumbar spine, or springing (whole hand – postero-anterior movement) for the thoracic spine.

Localized problems tend to respond to postero-anterior central vertebral pressure (on the spine of the vertebra), especially if the pain distribution is bilateral. For unilateral symptoms, rotation away from the pain or transverse vertebral pressure (on the side of the spinous process) towards the pain are often effective. Pain radiating round a rib often responds to postero-anterior movement of the rib.

In the presence of bilateral pain and tenderness (i.e. the vertebrae are very often sore to pressure), longitudinal oscillation can be useful (i.e. on the head for cervical spine problems and to the legs for lumbar spine problems).

Again, accessory movements may be performed with the spine positioned in a physiological movement, e.g. with the cervical spine in right rotation, transverse pressure from right to left on the spine of C6 or 7 is appropriate, or with the thoracic spine in flexion, central pressure on the spinous process of T7 in a cephalad direction helps thoracic spine flexion.

Technique selection should therefore be a logical process based on the palpation and active movement component of the examination.

Grade and number of oscillations

Generally, in the presence of moderate to severe pain and muscle spasm, low grades and few oscillations are indicated and in the presence of low intensity pain with fibrous stiffness higher grades and more oscillations are appropriate. Irritability is a guiding factor. An irritable joint has the following clinical features:

1. Pain at rest or which comes on early in the movement.
2. Pain takes a long time to settle after movement.
3. Muscle spasm is present.
4. Sleep is disturbed.
5. Lifestyle is curtailed – off work.

A non-irritable joint has the following characteristics:
1. No pain at rest.
2. Pain is produced only in the last one quarter of the movement.
3. Pain settles as soon as movement is stopped.
4. No muscle spasm.
5. Limiting factor is fibrous tissue/block.
6. Problem is a nuisance rather than dominating the patient's lifestyle.

Irritability must be treated with respect (grades I–II).

Non-irritable joints respond to more vigorous techniques (grades III–IV).

Grades of techniques (Maitland 1986)

Grade I is a small-amplitude oscillation performed at the beginning of available range.

Grade II is a larger amplitude oscillation performed within the available range but not going to the limit.

Grade III is the same amplitude as grade II but goes to the limit of available range.

Grade IV is a small-amplitude oscillation performed at the limit of available range.

All of these grades are within the patient's control, i.e. can be stopped by the patient.

A grade V – or manipulation – is a unidirectional, small-amplitude, high-velocity thrust performed at the limit of available range and is over before the patient can stop it.

Available range is the range the patient can perform up to the pathological limit, NOT normal anatomical range.

The procedure is to treat, e.g. L4/5 rotation right × grade II × 50 oscillations.

The test movement is then performed, the result of which may be that the patient is better, same or worse.

Better

Repeat the technique up to four times with an irritable joint or until movement is clear in a non-irritable joint.

Same

Adjustment may be made. Increase grade or number of oscillations or the direction of the movement or the patient's position (only one at a time). Then change the technique or level. Test after each change.

Worse

Leave for the session and have the patient back next day, then if worse reduce oscillations by half and grade if appropriate. Consider other treatment modalities.

Rules and safety with mobilizations

Mobilizations – passive oscillatory joint movements – are very safe procedures provided that the contraindications are excluded and there is logic in the application. The following rules are guides for safety and effectiveness:

1. Never force through spasm.
2. Examine thoroughly.
3. Listen to the patient – explain effects and make treatment like 'a partnership'.
4. Exclude contraindications.
5. Do one technique at a time and test after each one.
6. Warn the patient of treatment soreness (which wears off in 24 hours and is like post-exercise stiffness – not the original pain).
7. Start gently, increase vigour only if really necessary.
8. Concentrate on trying to achieve the effect.
   Do not chat or allow the patient to chat during a technique – but do encourage the patient to report any effects.

Spinal traction

This is a stretching force applied in a longitudinal direction of the spine. It may be applied manually but the physiotherapist can hold for only a minute or so. Therefore, mechanical apparatus is required (Figure A1.17). Electrically operated equipment allows a sustained hold or an oscillatory force (see Figure 11.10).

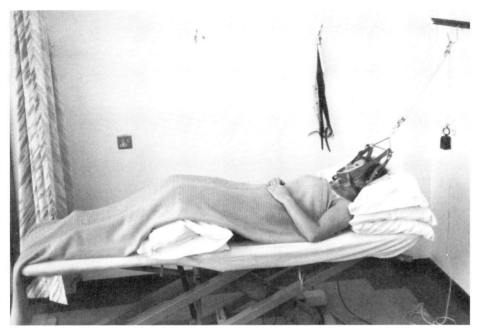

Figure A1.17 Cervical traction

Indications

1. Sustained hold is helpful for:
   (a) Tight soft tissues – not muscle spasm.
   (b) Nerve root compression.
2. Oscillatory force is helpful for general stiffness –
   to mobilize degenerative changes.

Effects

Clinical effects are relief of pain, or pins and needles
and increased mobility. How these effects are
achieved is speculative. The following are helpful
explanations for patients:

1. Separation of vertebral bodies enables fluid flow
   and therefore improved nutrition of the intervertebral discs.
2. Stretching of tight fibrous tissue for 5–20 minutes
   also allows fluid flow and increased movement –
   which is retained by exercise.
3. Stretching of tissues around the nerve root in the
   intervertebral canal enables free circulatory flow.
   This improves nutrition to the nerve and removes
   metabolites and exudate produced by low-grade
   inflammation. This may explain why root pain
   remains diminished after traction is removed.
4. Sliding (accessory movement) of the facet joints
   facilitates synovial sweep – aiding lubrication and
   nutrition.
5. Traction counteracts the effects of gravity and
   poor posture and is useful as an adjunct to
   posture training.

Contraindications

These are the same as for mobilizations but traction
is the technique of choice for nerve root pressure.
   Also, traction is contraindicated as follows:

1. Acute muscle spasm.
2. Temporomandibular joint pain – cervical traction causes compression.
3. Hiatus hernia or cardiorespiratory problems
   because the patient cannot lie down or tolerate
   the thoracic belt of lumbar traction – but it is
   possible to apply traction to the patient in an
   upright position with special equipment.

The variables to consider in the application of
traction are:

1. Position of spine.
2. Force.
3. Time
4. Sustained or oscillatory.

Position of spine

The spine is positioned to enable the force to be
effective at the target segment. Generally, the lower
the level to be treated in the cervical spine the more
the neck is positioned in flexion. Also, the lower in
the lumbar spine the level is, the more the spine is
flattened by flexing the knees and hips and tilting
the pelvis backwards. The physiotherapist should
always palpate the vertebral spines of the target
segment to check for effect.

Force

The force generally should be the smallest compatible with relief of symptoms. For nerve root pain, the patient should feel that the traction diminishes the pain by 50% – not more, otherwise the pain can be drastically increased when the traction is removed. For stiffness and degenerative changes, effective force varies from 3 kg to 7 kg.

Time

Time varies according to the condition treated. For nerve root pain, sustained traction may be left on for 20–30 minutes, released for 5–10 minutes and then re-applied for a further 20–30 minutes. Treatment is generally best on a daily basis until the overall pain reduction is 75%. For degenerative changes or regional stiffness, 10–20 minutes is the order of time used, repeated three times a week until improvement stops.

Sustained or oscillatory

Sustained traction is generally best for nerve root pain or paraesthesia or tissue tightness. Oscillatory traction is useful for degenerative joint stiffness.

Notes

1. Once a force and time are found to be effective they should not be altered until improvement rate slows. Then, as a general guide, the force may be increased where tissue tightness or nerve root compression is the problem. Time should be increased where the problem is time related, i.e. relief is obtained for 1–2 hours after traction and then returns.
2. Improvement may be reduction in pain intensity, longer pain-free spells or increased mobility.
3. Immediately after sustained traction is removed, spinal mobility is often reduced. This effect wears off in 1–2 hours. Testing movements, therefore, should be delayed until the next treatment. If after four treatments with traction there is no improvement, other modalities should be considered. A combination of passive oscillatory movements (given first) and traction is often more effective for general stiffness.
   Postural training and exercises are essential components of patient management.

Passive stretching of soft tissues

Scar tissue has an inherent property of contracture and tends to bind tissues together. This is essential in the healing of wounds and repair of the skin. However, it is a distinct disadvantge when it occurs in fascia, muscles and ligaments. Adherent tissues cannot function normally – for example muscle contraction is impaired, fluid exchange is reduced, there is pain when the scar causes traction on the surrounding tissues, and the tissues are at risk of further injury. Early movement after injury is essential to ensure that the scar tissue is laid down in the correct plane of movement, but there is still a danger of adherence of tissues particularly with chronic injuries which have excess scarring. Sometimes nerves become trapped in this scarring and may cause severe pain, for example the ulnar nerve and the deep terminal branch of the radial nerve at the elbow, and nerve roots in the intervertebral canals. Passive stretching is designed to lengthen shortened scar tissue and complement massage and joint mobilization.

The technique is to identify the 'tight tissue' and work out the position which will apply a stretch. The patient is told to report mild discomfort when the stretch is applied, the stretch is then held and the physiotherapist feels the tissues easing usually over 1–2 minutes. The slack is taken up and the tissues held again. Generally this procedure is repeated 2–3 times. Release of the stretch is often accompanied by quite severe soreness which goes off quickly. At no time is force applied as the stretch is gained by the holding and then taking up of the slack.

Following this procedure it is essential that the patient practise the active movement which will retain the flexibility gained – i.e. 2–3 movements every hour. Some range will be lost after the first treatment but 3–4 treatment sessions should suffice to achieve lengthening, maintained by auto stretching or active exercises.

Sometimes it is appropriate to apply hold–relax technique (PNF) in the same treatment session.

Passive stretching is often useful in treatment of the following:

1. Capsulitis of the gleno-humeral joint to gain elevation through flexion.
2. Tightness of the neck side flexors, for example if the left side flexors are tight the technique is to hold the head in as much right side flexion as possible and depress the left shoulder.
3. Tethered sciatic nerve – straight leg raising.
4. Stiff lumbar spine – rotation with or without straight leg raising.
5. Hip flexor tightness (e.g. in early osteoarthritis) – the patient lies prone, the pelvis is fixed and the flexed knee is lifted up to stretch the hip into extension.
6. Tight hip adductors – passive hip abduction is performed with the other leg fixed.
7. Tight gastrocnemius – the knee must be kept straight and the calcaneum pulled down while the ankle is dorsi-flexed.
8. Following 'ankle sprain' – inversion of the

subtalar joint by holding the calcaneus in a position which stretches the middle band of the lateral ligament of the ankle.

Auto-stretching of soft tissues

Prior to activity auto-stretching develops flexibility, particularly in sport but also in other activities such as gardening, decorating and even housework. The value of stretching is the subject of some debate and the evidence for its value is largely empirical. However, there is considerable belief that stretching is useful for:

1. Prevention of injury.
2. Providing flexibility and therefore a greater range of movement.
3. Promoting coordination by enabling symmetrical free movement.
4. Reduction of muscle tension or tightness.
5. Psychological preparation – makes the person feel ready for the activity to be undertaken.

The technique

The patient takes up the position with the appropriate structure or tissue on the stretch, feels the tightness and holds for 30–60 s then as the tightness reduces he takes up the slack and holds again. This is repeated 3–4 times. The procedure is then applied to the opposite side. The technique should be performed daily.

Precautions

At no time should there be a 'bouncing' or forcing. Time must be allowed to perform the stretching slowly, with care and consideration, otherwise muscles can be injured. Warmth is important and so warm-up exercises should be performed first, and clothing worn which covers the muscles during this session. When a person is starting this technique or is recently recovered from an injury, the holds should be 10–15 s and only 2–3 repetitions should be used.

Examples of stretching positions are illustrated in Figures A1.18–A1.29.

Orthoses and strapping

Orthoses

Physiotherapists should be able to:

1. Supply and make certain orthoses.
2. Recognize when a patient must be referred to another physiotherapist specializing in orthoses, or to an occupational therapist or orthotist.

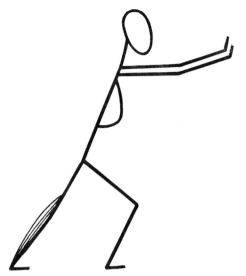

Figure A1.18 Stretching: gastrocnemius, calf muscles and tendo achillis

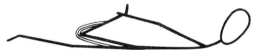

Figure A1.19 rectus femoris and quadriceps

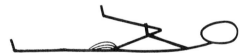

Figure A1.20 Stretching: hip flexors of the straight leg

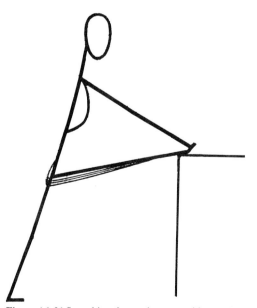

Figure A1.21 Stretching: hamstrings, one side

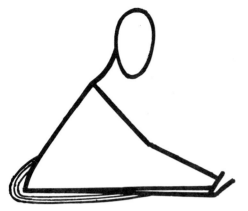

Figure A1.22 Stretching: hamstrings, both sides

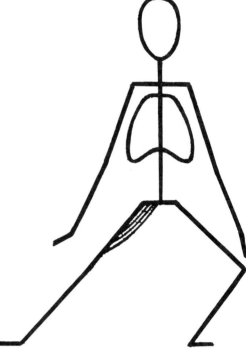

Figure A1.23 Stretching: hip adductors and groin muscles, one side

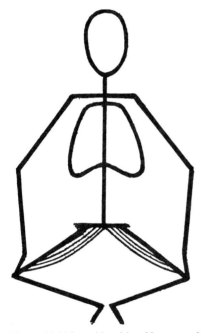

Figure A1.24 Stretching: hip adductors and groin muscles, both sides

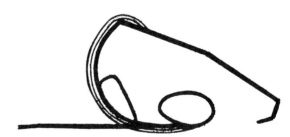

Figure A1.25 Stretching: back extensors and hip extensors

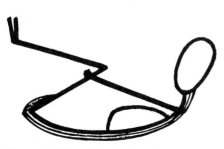

Figure A1.26 Stretching: back extensors

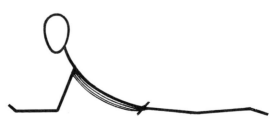

Figure A1.27 Stretching: trunk flexors, prone

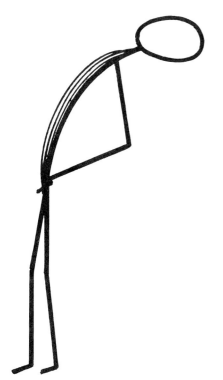

Figure A1.28 Stretching: trunk flexors, standing

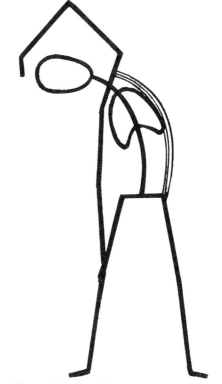

Figure A1.29 Stretching: trunk side flexors

Orthoses commonly provided by physiotherapists

These are:

1. Cervical collars.
2. Lumbar supports.
3. Sacroiliac belts.
4. Lumbo-sacral supports for pregnancy.
5. Thumb splints.
6. Wrist splints.
7. Foot pads.

Principles of use of orthoses

1. Examination findings must indicate that support or reduced mobility will benefit the patient.
2. The patient should understand that it is a temporary measure (true instability requiring permanent support is managed by a doctor referring the patient to an orthotist).
3. If the patient has a recurring problem then the support should be worn during the activity that aggravates it and then be removed.

Points to note

Cervical collars

Soft collars may be helpful in limiting movements which could cause pain and may be worn at night as well as during the day. Also they are useful for an acutely painful neck or nerve root pain in the arm, as they can reduce the jarring which aggravates the pain. The collar should not be required for longer than 1–2 weeks at a time. As the patient recovers, advice is necessary regarding the reduction in its use.

Lumbar supports

These provide a reminder to the patient to keep the lumbar spine steady and in a correct lordosis during an episode of acute pain. Belts with a broad component stretching from the thoracolumbar to lumbosacral junctions provide support for lifting and can prevent injury. According to some patients 'body warmers' are useful, and as it is important to keep the back muscles warm prior to and during exercise, there is no reason why they should not be worn.

Sacroiliac supports

Hypermobile sacroiliac joint problems respond to a support which binds the iliac bones. A broad bandage (which may be elasticated) wound round the pelvis just below the iliac crests can afford relief.

Lumbo-sacral pregnancy supports

Logic dictates that if backache or sacroiliac pain (especially in the third trimester of pregnancy) is deemed to be due to the increasing mobility of the joints, then support is the treatment. A broad elastic support which goes across the lumbosacral area, round the anterior superior iliac spines, and fixes with Velcro under the 'baby bulge' enables the patient to perform everyday functions with confidence and some pain relief.

Thumb and wrist splints

These are indicated for tenosynovitis or as a temporary measure following strain of ligaments. Materials used vary, but they should be firm and washable, so that the hand can be used for everyday activities.

Foot pads

When a patient has pain as the result of muscle weakness which causes a lowering of the arches of the foot, then pads may be indicated. These must be seen as a temporary measure whenever possible. The foot joints must be mobilized, the muscles strengthened, and posture and gait re-educated. The orthoses can then be abandoned as soon as possible. When pads are required, the most common is for the anterior arch, and a Sorbo rubber pad is placed just proximal to the metatarsal heads. Less often a pad to support the medial arch is required, and this is placed under the head of the talus.

Other orthoses

Drop foot supports, knee splints, trunk braces, and 'lively' splints are the province of the specialist. The physiotherapist treating a patient with one of these must check that it is comfortable, that the skin is not being traumatized and that the splint is in good condition. She must check that the patient understands the application, so achieving the best function.

Strapping

With the increase in sporting activities there is a greater demand for strapping, which is also known as taping. The value of strapping may be considered in three phases:

1. Immediately post-injury to reduce swelling and facilitate healing.
2. After recovery from an acute injury to enable the patient (who is often impatient) to resume sport.
3. Prevention of injury where there is an old injury or weakness.

After injury

The strapping is applied to :

1. Keep any dressings in place.
2. Give compression to the tissues and therefore reduce oedema (Figure A1.30).
3. Enable functional use of the injured part by providing support.
4. Support an injured structure in a shortened position to allow healing to occur.

After healing

A patient is generally anxious to return to sport as soon as possible. Strapping to support the healing structure not only protects it, but may enable the patient to return to activity with confidence, improving the chance of a good performance and reducing the risk of injury to other structures. It is important that the patient discards the support when there is full pain-free movement, muscle power and coordination.

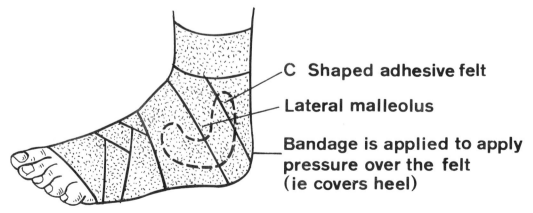

C Shaped adhesive felt

Lateral malleolus

Bandage is applied to apply pressure over the felt (ie covers heel)

Figure A1.30 Bandage with pressure pad to reduce oedema around the ankle

Chronic injuries

When a patient has had several injuries affecting the same structure, or a severe injury has inevitably left some weakness, strapping for a sporting activity is justified. An elasticated support, however, may be more appropriate as not every patient can tolerate the repeated application of adhesive tape to the skin.

Contraindications to strapping

1. Abnormal skin sensation.
2. Irritable or allergic skin reaction.
3. Skin disorders, e.g. eczema, dermatitis.
4. The absence of a meticulous examination which would have identified a real need for strapping.

Precautions and techniques

1. The skin must be prepared by being washed, dried, shaved if necessary and sprayed with an adhesive spray (e.g. benzoin tincture). An underwrap may be applied for very sensitive skin or when there is to be repeated strapping.
2. The anatomy of the part must be studied so that the injured structure is in a shortened position and joints are in a functional position.
3. Bony points that are susceptible to pressure must be padded.
4. The number and length of pieces of strapping required must be worked out and cut ready to apply. Each strip is applied to achieve its effect and, where appropriate, layers should overlap by half the width.
5. The strapping is applied smoothly, avoiding wrinkles or traction of the skin.
6. The balance between effectiveness and the strapping being too tight (causing impairment of the circulation) must be carefully considered.
7. The function of the part must be carefully checked before the patient goes home, e.g. gait pattern.

Hydrotherapy

Hydrotherapy in the strictest sense refers to the therapeutic use of water. Contrast baths and ice therapy are considered elsewhere. Pool therapy will be discussed here.

Indications

Pool therapy should be considered for patients with problems arising from muscle weakness, loss of joint mobility, poor coordination or balance, pain or lack of confidence. The particular value of pool therapy over dry-land treatment is derived from buoyancy, which counteracts gravity, provides support and relieves weight-bearing pressure on joints, for example in degenerative conditions. The warmth of the water reduces pain and can relax muscle spasm. The medium enables mobility for patients who may be wheelchair-bound or recovering from prolonged immobilization. Importantly, it also provides for enjoyment, recreation and laughter which are vital aspects of rehabilitation. Physiotherapists should consider pool therapy when treating patients with:

1. Ankylosing spondylitis.
2. Osteoarthritis.
3. Rheumatoid arthritis.
4. Juvenile chronic polyarthritis.
5. Spondylosis.
6. Capsulitis.
7. Mechanical spinal disorders.
8. Polymyalgia rheumatica.
9. Major fractures especially of the lower limbs or spine.
10. Orthopaedic surgery.
11. Neurological disorders such as hemiplegia, paraplegia, tetraplegia, polyneuropathy.
12. Children derive particular benefit from the freedom of movement afforded by the water.
13. Pool therapy is also of value for maintaining fitness and relieving backache during pregnancy and after childbirth.

Principles of treatment

Strengthening muscles

Muscles are strengthened by being worked progressively against graded resistance.

In the pool, resistance may be from buoyancy, turbulence, unstreamlining.

Buoyancy

Movements downwards in the pool are resisted by buoyancy. Floats which may be of different densities may be used to increase the effect of buoyancy.

Turbulence

This is created by movement through water and is increased if the rate of movement is increased. The patient may move as a whole through the water – this is the principle underlying muscle strengthening using Bad Ragaz techniques. Alternatively, the patient may be fixed and move one limb at a time. Walking fast through water is useful for strengthening muscles and for improving cardiovascular fitness.

Unstreamlining

If a broad surface is presented when a body is moved through water the resistance is greater than if the surface is narrow. To progress exercises with a bat, for example, the movement is first performed with the edge of the bat moving through the water and then progressed so that the broad surface is going against the water.

Manual resistance may be applied in the pool as in land treatment, but it is important that the physiotherapist ensures that the patient benefits from being in the pool.

Joint mobility

Relief of pain and muscle spasm by the warmth of the water and by support from buoyancy can restore free movement of joints. Exercises for gaining mobility are generally slow, taken to the point of limitation, held, carried a bit further and then relaxed. Full-range sweeping movements also gain range (the speed is kept to a minimum so that the muscles are not working against turbulence). Hold–relax and repeated contractions may be used to gain joint movement – generally with the patient in lying (buoyancy supporting) or positioned so that buoyancy may assist in gaining the movement.

Mobilizations – Oscillatory passive movements can be applied to joints to gain range. Fixation is a problem and it may require two physiotherapists, one fixing and one producing the movement, to localize the effect to the joint being treated. Patients report considerable relief from pain following mobilizations in the pool.

Coordination and balance

Patients can practise activities in standing, for example stride standing or walk standing, transference of weight, or arm movements. The buoyancy of the water relieves weight, for example 90% relief is obtained if the water is over the shoulders, therefore weight-bearing activities such as walking, stepping up and down, standing up and down can be practised in the pool before the patient attempts these activities on land. Components of swimming can be practised, for example the leg patterns of different swimming strokes may be performed while the patient holds the pool rail. Swimming and ball games, Bad Ragaz techniques and the Halliwick principles all help patients to regain coordination. The special value of the Halliwick approach is to teach the patient breathing control and balance in the water, thereby enabling him to be water-confident.

Pain relief

The general freedom of movement in a pool enables tissue fluid to flow through tissue planes, removing metabolites and improving nutrition. These effects, together with a feeling of well-being after physical activity, help to gain permanent reduction of pain. In some pools there is a facility for applying a high-pressure jet of water to a painful area. The patient is standing, sitting or lying and the physiotherapist directs the jet at the area to be treated and moves it either in circles or to and fro for 5–10 minutes. Patients report relief of the aching which is often associated with muscle spasm or tightness in degenerative conditions or chronic injury.

Confidence

Teaching a patient to be water-confident has particular benefit in that regular exercise can be continued at a local swimming pool. Cardiovascular, respiratory and musculoskeletal fitness can be maintained by swimming once or twice a week. Joining a club or class for exercises in water can bring social as well as fitness benefits. Some classes are run in which exercises are performed to music, and patients can be well advised to join these.

Contraindications to pool therapy

During examination of a patient the physiotherapist must rule out the following before giving hydrotherapy:

1. Infected wounds.
2. Acute skin conditions.
3. Pyrexia (temperature must be normal for 24 hours before hydrotherapy).
4. Incontinence (unless controlled).
5. Cardiac disease with resting angina.
6. Deep vein thrombosis.
7. Recent pulmonary embolus.
8. Recent CVA (within 3 weeks).
9. Gastrointestinal disorders.
10. Tracheostomy.
11. Careful consideration is essential for patients with open wounds covered with a waterproof dressing (e.g. Opsite).
12. Hypotension, hypertension.
13. Epilepsy.
14. Vertigo.
15. Low vital capacity (below 900 ml).
16. Kidney disease.
17. Diabetes.
18. Thyroid deficiency.
19. Radiotherapy in the previous 3 months.

Precautions must be taken for patients with:

1. Tinea pedis or verrucas – pool therapy must be delayed until these conditions have been cleared or special socks may be worn.
2. AIDS. Patients with this syndrome must not be treated if there are skin cuts.
3. Hydrophobia – fear of water. Breathing control must be taught.
4. Contact lenses.
5. Hearing aids.
6. Allergy to chlorine.
7. Haemophilia.
8. Severe mental retardation.

Dangers of pool treatments

1. Hazards.
2. Infections.
3. Untoward effects.

Hazards

1. Falls inside and outside the pool.
2. Burns and scalds.
3. Faulty equipment.

Infections

Contagious diseases are a problem because of the proximity of patients and staff. Waterborne diseases are typhoid, cholera, dysentry.

Untoward effects

1. Chilling.
2. Sudden changes in blood pressure.
3. Fatigue of patients or staff.

Precautions necessary to ensure patient and staff safety with pool therapy

1. Water temperature should be 34–37°C (94–98°F).
2. Chlorine levels should be 1.5–3.00 parts per million.
3. Water pH level should be 7.2–7.8.
4. Chlorine and pH levels must be tested two or three times a day.
5. There must be a complete water turnover every 4 hours.
6. Bacteriological testing must be performed regularly.
7. Backwashing must be performed regularly.
8. Results of all tests must be recorded meticulously.
9. The floor of the pool must be non-slip.
10. There must be handrails on both sides of steps for entry to the pool.
11. A cord to an emergency bell must be situated over the pool.
12. Hoists and other pool equipment must be tested and maintained regularly.
13. A footbath must be situated near the entry point to the pool.
14. The pool surround must have a non-slip floor and handrails.
15. Water must be mopped up so that it does not remain on the pool surround.
16. Air temperature should be 25°C (78°F).
17. The humidity level should be 55%.
18. Overshoes must be provided and worn by everyone within a designated area.
19. All staff must be trained and regularly tested in emergency and resuscitation procedures.
20. The maximum time for a physiotherapist to be in the water without a break is 2 hours. It is recommended that physiotherapists who are treating patients in the pool regularly should not be in the water for longer than 1.5 hours without a break.

General facilities

1. A hydrotherapy department should include rest, changing and utility areas.
2. Rest and changing areas.
3. Air temperature should be 21°–23°C (68°–74°F).
4. There must be adequate space and privacy.
5. Wheelchair accessibility is essential in all areas.
6. There must be provision for privacy for patients and security for their valuables.
7. Showers and toilets must be available both for able and for disabled people.
8. Utility area.
9. There must be a washing machine and spin dryer for cleaning swimming costumes.
10. Buckets are essential for shoes, flippers and other equipment which must be soaked in disinfectant.
11. Chemicals must be stored in a secure, cool dark place with goggles and gloves which must be worn when chemicals are being handled.
12. Storage space is essential for linen, wheelchairs, sticks and crutches.

Electrotherapy

The modalities include various methods of heating or cooling the tissues, ultrasound, electromagnetic radiations, medium-frequency currents, low-frequency currents, and iontophoresis.

Heating the tissues

The sources of heat may be:

1. Paraffin wax.
2. Infra-red radiation.
3. Heat pad.
4. Hot moist packs.
5. Short-wave diathermy.
6. Microwave diathermy.

Several factors determine the choice of modality. These include the objectives of the treatment, the part to be treated, the depth of the lesion, the state of the skin – nerve supply and nourishment – and the underlying pathology.

Paraffin wax

The wax has a low melting point and is contained in a bath thermostatically controlled between 40°C and 44°C. Owing to its low thermal conductivity, wax heats more slowly but retains its heat for a longer period than water. As the wax solidifies on the skin the energy released by the latent heat of fusion results in heating of the tissues. The advantages of wax are that it completely surrounds the part being treated and the patient does not need to remain in a fixed position. Also it is applied at a known temperature and gets cooler – therefore there is very little danger of a burn. Its disadvantages are that regular cleaning is necessary and it is difficult to apply except to the extremities. Its main use therefore is in treating hands and feet. Wax is used to relieve pain after trauma, in degenerative joint disease and in the chronic stage of inflammatory arthropathies. Skin condition can be improved following the removal of plaster of Paris. Adhesions and scars can be softened and mobilization is facilitated. It should not, however, be applied over open wounds or skin infections.

Infra-red radiation

When the radiations are absorbed the radiant energy is converted to heat. There are two types of generator:

1. Luminous, producing rays from 350 nm to 450 nm which penetrate the epidermis and dermis to the subcutaneous tissues.
2. Non-luminous, producing rays from 770 nm to 1500 nm which penetrate only as far as the superficial epidermis.

Any part of the body can be treated, but the patient must be positioned so that the rays strike the part at 90° for a maximum absorption. The tissues are heated directly on one aspect only and the patient should remain in one position throughout the treatment.

The heating effect on the area treated results in vasodilatation in the superficial tissues, thereby bringing nutrition and removing waste products. There is a sedative effect on the sensory nerve endings which aids pain relief and relaxes muscle spasm.

Owing to these effects, infra-red can be used to promote healing in uninfected wounds, relieve pain and reduce muscle spasm following trauma, and for chronic arthritic joints, when the luminous generator should be used. The sedative effect of the non-luminous generator is more suitable for recent trauma and subacute inflammatory joints. Infra-red is used to treat large superficial areas.

Heat pads

These are plastic-covered pads similar to but smaller than electric blankets. A pad has three levels of heat and is useful for treating the neck or back. The patient lies on it and heat passes to the tissues by conduction. An advantage is that the heat can be applied at the same time as traction.

Hot moist packs

These are canvas bags filled with a hydrophilic substance and stored in a thermostatically-controlled cabinet of water between 75°C and 80°C. The packs vary in size and shape and are returned to the cabinet for reheating after use. The area to be treated should be totally covered by the pack, which is moulded to the contour of the body. Layers of towelling must be placed round the pack to separate it from the patient's skin. The superficial tissues are heated by conduction, relieving pain and muscle spasm. Moist heat is conducted more uniformly than dry heat. These packs are particularly useful on uneven surfaces because they can be easily moulded to the surface, but they are heavy and may cause discomfort.

Short-wave diathermy

Short-wave diathermy is the application to the tissues of electrical fields which oscillate at a frequency of 27.12 MHz and have a wavelength of 11.06 M (condenser field method). The oscillating fields produce distortion of molecules, rotation of dipoles and vibration of ions. When the inductothermy cable is used there is a current oscillating in the cable which produces an electromagnetic field, which in turn induces eddy currents (and therefore ionic vibration) in the tissues. The movement of the molecules and ions generates heat within the tissues. The amount and distribution of heat depends on the arrangements of the fields (i.e. electrode application) and the electrical impedence of the tissues. Tissues of high impedence are bone, fat, fascia and other fibrous tissue structures. Tissues of low impedance are blood, lymph and muscle. If the oscillating electrical field is applied in parallel with the tissues, then those with low impedance will tend to be heated more, whereas the tissues of high impedance will be heated if they are in series with the field. The superficial tissues of low impedence tend to be heated when the inductothermy cable is used.

Short-wave diathermy can be used to treat both deep and superficial lesions. It produces a greater and more rapid rise in temperature than the conductive methods of heat. Large areas can be treated and it is useful for soft-tissue injuries, degenerative and inflammatory arthropathies, slow healing wounds, sinusitis and conditions of the deep-seated pelvic structures.

Short-wave diathermy may be pulsed (one form of pulsed electromagnetic energy – PEME). Pulse frequency may vary from 15 pps to 400 pps. The pulse width varies from 65 µs to 400 µs. The mean power is, therefore, considerably reduced. The therapeutic effects are similar to those produced by continuous short wave. The main difference is that during the relatively long rest period, the heat developed is dispersed by the circulation and the treatment is referred to as 'non-thermal'. Pulsed SWD is particularly useful for giving pain relief in acute soft-tissue lesions and arthropathies. In crush injuries or trauma which results in excessive swelling, pulsed SWD obtains marked reduction in local oedema. For acute lesions the recommended dosage is 65 µs at 100 pps for 15 minutes. Progression of treatment, if necessary, involves increasing pulse widths and frequencies. The possibilities of varying the treatment depend upon the machine used. In wounds treated with pulsed SWD there is increased organization of connective tissue and growth of epithelial tissue, so that healing is accelerated. Areas with metal in the field which are a contraindication to continuous short wave may be treated with pulsed SWD.

Microwave diathermy

Microwave diathermy is the application of electromagnetic radiations with a wavelength of 12.25 cm and frequency of 2450 MHz. They are produced by a magnetron, which is a special type of thermionic valve. When the microwaves are absorbed in the tissues, heat is produced. The depth of penetration is about 3 cm, which is deeper than infra-red rays but more superficial than short-wave diathermy. Microwaves are particularly absorbed by fluid tissues such as muscles, and less by fat and bone. Superficial muscular lesions will be most effectively treated, giving pain relief and resolution of inflammation. Only one aspect of a structure is heated. Localized degenerative joint disease and joint lesions can be successfully treated but widespread lesions are best avoided.

Cooling of the tissues – ice therapy

Ice therapy is the local or general application of cold for therapeutic and preventative uses. When ice is applied to the skin it melts and removes heat from the tissues – the energy required to change its state (the latent heat of fusion). The rate at which cooling occurs depends on the duration of the application, type of tissue (e.g. the thermal conductivity of muscle is greater than that of fat) and the patency of the blood vessels.

The application of cold results in alternate periods of vasoconstriction and vasodilation, reduced nerve conductivity and reduction of muscle spasm and spasticity.

Therapeutically, ice can be used to relieve pain and muscle spasm, reduce swelling, reduce spasticity, facilitate muscle contraction, increase muscle endurance, reduce haematoma formation, prevent pressure sores and promote healing of wounds.

Ice can be applied in towels, as a pack or by immersion in a bath. Damp towels dipped in an ice-and-water mixture, or containing crushed or flaked ice, can be wrapped round painful and swollen joints. Towels are applied longitudinally along muscles to reduce spasm. To reduce spasticity, towels are laid longitudinally from proximal to distal when flexor tone predominates, and from distal to proximal when extensor tone predominates. The towels are changed every few minutes. Ice baths containing 50–60% ice to water are used for painful swollen hands or feet. Spasticity can also be reduced by immersion in a bath.

In ice massage, an ice cube or ice lolly is wrapped in a towel at one end and the free end is massaged over the skin. This can act as a counter-irritant if applied for 5–7 minutes to relieve pain and muscle spasm and as a preventative measure to avoid pressure-sore breakdown. This method may be used to facilitate the following:

1. Muscle contraction, by application over the appropriate dermatome for 3–5 s.
2. Swallowing, by application over the skin just above the suprasternal notch or sipping iced water.
3. Speech, by application to the lips, tongue and inside of the cheek.

Ultrasound

This is the production of longitudinal mechanical waves above the audible range (20 kHz). The frequencies used in physiotherapy vary from 0.75 MHz to 3 MHz. These are produced by distortion of a quartz crystal by a high-frequency alternating current (reverse piezo-electric effect). The longitudinal sound waves cause to-and-fro movements of particles giving alternate areas of compression and rarefaction. With sound energy the frequency remains the same as the source but the velocity varies through different media for a given frequency. The sound waves require a medium (not air or a vacuum) for transmission, therefore a coupling medium such as oil or water is necessary to transmit ultrasound from the treatment head to the patient's tissues.

To avoid refraction of sound energy, the treatment head must be applied perpendicular to the skin surface and continually moved to ensure that the sound energy does not concentratre on one tissue area. The higher the frequency the greater the absorption and the smaller the depth of penetration. Superficial lesions should be treated with 3 MHz frequencies and deeper lesions with 0.75–1 MHz. Depending on the site of the lesion ultrasound may be applied directly using a coupling medium, immersion in a water bath or by a water cushion. Continuous ultrasound is used for chronic injuries or large areas, and pulsed ultrasound mainly for acute conditions. Empirical clinical evidence suggests that underdose is better than overdose and low intensities are very effective. For acute injuries the starting dose may be 0.25 W cm^{-2} for 5 minutes twice daily. Progression is made by increasing the time and reducing the frequency of treatment. For chronic conditions the intensity may be increased up to 1 W cm^{-2}. Ultrasound is thought to promote the release of chemical mediators, which results in the proliferation of granulation tissue and stimulates the activity of the fibroblasts. There is increased circulation, increased cellular activity of phagocytes and microphages to reduce oedema. This accelerates the healing process and results in pain relief. Because of these effects ultrasound may be used in recent soft-tissue injuries, back pain, recent and chronic scar tissue, skin grafts and venous ulcers or pressure sores.

Ultraviolet rays (UVR)

These are electromagnetic rays between the visible rays and X-rays in the electromagnetic spectrum (400–100 nm) – see Chapter 17.

Sources

The ultraviolet rays are produced by vaporization of mercury in a quartz tube. All ultraviolet burners produce visible and infra-red rays. For therapeutic sources of UVR see Chapter 17. In the Kromayer lamp water absorbs the infra-red rays and allows treatment in contact with the patient's skin. With the air-cooled source the patient is treated at a distance of 45 cm or more to avoid burning of the skin from the infra-red rays.

Laws of radiations

A larger area is irradiated but the intensity is decreased when the distance from the source to the patient's skin is increased. UVR are governed by the law of inverse squares which states that 'the intensity of rays falling on a plane surface varies inversely with the square of the distance from the point source'.

To irradiate a smaller area the source is moved nearer to the patient but the time of exposure must be altered to maintain the same intensity in accordance with the law of inverse squares:

$$\text{New time} = \frac{\text{Old time} \times (\text{new distance})^2}{(\text{Old distance})^2}$$

UVR must strike the surface at 90° to obtain maximum absorption in accordance with the cosine law, which states that 'the proportion of rays absorbed varies directly with the cosine of the angle of incidence'. This is necessary for UVR to be effective. Grotthus' law states that 'rays must be absorbed to produce an effect'.

Calculation of UVR dosages

UVR dosages are graded according to the erythema reaction (see Chapter 17) after an E1 has been determined from a skin test. The other erythema dosages can then be calculated as follows:

Suberythema 75% of E1
E2 = 2.5 × E1
E3 = 5 × E1
E4 = 10 × E1
Double E4 = 20 × E1
E4 + Double E4 are used on open wounds.

Progression of dosages

When UVR is applied to normal skin there is thickening of the epidermis therefore progression of dosage is necessary to obtain the same effective level. Doses can be progressed as follows:

1. Suberythema – previous dose plus 12.5%.
2. E1 – previous dose plus 25%.

3. E2 – previous dose plus 50%.
4. E3 – previous dose plus 75%.

Dosages used on open wounds are not progressed because there is no epidermis to thicken. Should desquamation occur the dosage is reduced to the original dose to protect the new, underexposed skin. Repetition, progression and termination must be determined by the response of the patient to treatment. Criteria for assessing success must be identified at the initial examination, e.g. ulcer tracings, acne (skin clearance), psoriasis becoming flatter.

Physiological effects of UVR

UVR are absorbed in the epidermis and superficial dermis to a depth of 2 mm. There are local effects and in addition general effects with whole-body treatments.

Local effects

1. *Erythema* – When UVR are absorbed chemical changes in the skin produce a latent erythema. The level of erythema is dependent on skin type, intensity of treatment (time and distance related to E1 of the burner). The rays irritate the epidermis with the release of a histamine-like substance causing a triple response.
2. *Desquamation (peeling)* – This occurs as a result of the shedding of cells destroyed by the rays.
3. *Pigmentation* – This follows repeated exposure of the skin to UVR. Melanin is formed by melanoblasts as a result of stimulation from the UVR.
4. *Thickening of the epidermis* – There is proliferation of the basal layer cells resulting in the thickening of the epidermis.
5. *Antibiotic effect* – The UVR destroy bacteria and infections on the skin surface.

General effects

Esophylactic effect – UVR increases the resistance of the body to infection due to stimulation of the reticuloendothelial system.

Formation of vitamin D – The UVR is absorbed by the 7-dehydrocholesterol, and vitamin D is formed which results in an increased absorption of calcium and phosphorus from the intestine into the blood.

Therapeutic effects of UVR

UVR is given primarily for its local effects, but the general effects may be useful in some conditions. UVR can be used in the treatment of:

1. Open wounds such as ulcers, pressure sores or surgical incisions. Uninfected wounds are given an E1 or E2 and infected wounds an E4 or double E4.
2. Psoriasis, acne and other skin conditions. The peeling effect of UVR improves acne and the accelerated reproduction of the epidermis in psoriasis is reduced (see Chapter 17).
3. General debility and a history of recurrent infections. The esophylactic effect of general UVR reduces the frequency of infection.
4. Calcium and phosphorous deficiency diseases, e.g. rickets, are improved by vitamin D formation.

Contraindications to UVR

1. Deep X-ray therapy during the preceding 3 months because the skin may be hypersensitive to UVR.
2. Tuberculosis or malignant disease may be exacerbated by UVR.
3. Hypersensitivity to sunlight – patients who react adversely to the sun should not be treated with UVR.
4. Dermatological conditions such as acute eczema, lupus erythematosis may be exacerbated by UVR.
5. After infra-red therapy – UVR given whilst the erythema from the infra-red is still present may result in increased effects.
6. Pyrexia – UVR may produce a further increase in temperature.

Applicators

An applicator is a small quartz tube which can vary in size and shape and is attached by an adaptor to the Kromayer. It can be used to irradiate a deeply seated wound, shelf of an ulcer, deep sinus or a small area of infection in an otherwise non-infected wound.

The dosage with an applicator is increased to compensate for the loss in intensity as the UVR passes down the quartz tube. For an E1 in contact, multiply the E1 of the burner by the coefficient of the applicator. Each applicator should be tested by the manufacturer to determine the loss of intensity. As a rough guide, the length of the applicator (in inches) is squared or the length (in mm) is divided by 25 and the total squared.

Laser

The word laser is an acronym for Light Amplification by Stimulated Emission of Radiation. It obeys the laws of radiation. Specific substances are stimulated electrically to emit radiations which produce greater energy levels. In physiotherapy laser beams are produced from a helium/neon mixture at 632.8 nm and a variety of infra-red emissions, e.g. 865 nm and 904 nm. The helium/neon mixture produces a red light and the infra-red produces no light. The probe may produce a single wavelength or a cluster of wavelengths. Laser is different from other forms of light because it is monochromatic (one wavelength only), the beam of light being narrow, parallel and uniform. The laser waves are identical, superimposing on each other and therefore giving an amplifying effect.

There are three types of laser:

1. Power laser used in surgery for destructive effect.
2. Soft laser (helium/neon) used for superficial lesions of the skin.
3. Mid-laser (galium, aluminium, arsenide). The wavelength produced depends on the ratio of each material. These are most commonly used because of their depth of penetration (30–40 nm).

Effects of laser

1. Increases collagen synthesis – useful for tissue repair.
2. Increases permeability of cell membranes with increased efficiency of sodium pump.
3. Increases number of fibroblasts and promotes granulation tissue – useful for wound healing.
4. Increases levels of prostaglandins. Causes an increase in cellular ATP, which is useful for pain relief.

The effects spread from one cell to another, and therefore to surrounding tissues.

Uses of laser

1. Open wounds – ulcers, postoperative wounds.
2. Skin conditions – psoriasis, burns.
3. Soft-tissue injuries – tendons, ligaments and muscles.
4. Degenerative and inflammatory arthropathies.
5. Pain relief over trigger or acupuncture points. The main beam is useful for localized lesions, e.g. soft-tissue injuries and trigger points.

Contraindications

1. Carcinoma.
2. Skin irritation.
3. Chest treatment in cardiac patients should be avoided, together with those who have a pacemaker.
4. The eyes.

Medium-frequency currents

Medium-frequency currents alternate at 1000–100 000 Hz. Interferential is the use of two medium-frequency currents around 4000 Hz to produce a low-frequency effect within the body without the problem of high skin resistance.

Skin impedance is much greater with low-frequency currents and much smaller with higher frequency currents:

$$Z = \frac{1}{2\pi F C}$$

where Z = skin interference (in ohms),
   F = frequency in Hz,
   C = skin capacitance in microfarads.

This gives skin resistance at 50 Hz = 3200 ohms and at 4000 Hz = 40 ohms per 100 cm^2.

Low-frequency currents, due to high skin resistance, require a high current intensity to achieve the desired effect, and this causes marked sensory stimulation to the patient.

Medium-frequency currents, due to low skin resistance, require a low current intensity to achieve the desired effects, which results in less sensory discomfort.

High-frequency currents, such as short-wave diathermy and microwave, have frequencies too high to stimulate skin or muscle and produce only thermal effects.

If two medium-frequency currents at constant intensity but different frequencies are applied to the body at the same time, the intensity of the combined current will increase and decrease rhythmically. The combined current has a frequency equal to the difference between the two medium frequencies known as the beat frequency, and this is the interference effect.

In interferential equipment one frequency is fixed at 4000 Hz (generated by one pair of electrodes) and the other is variable between 4000 Hz and 4200 Hz (second pair of electrodes). By selecting the variable frequency, a beat frequency between 0 and 200 Hz may be generated.

Vector effect

The interference field is rotated to an angle of 45° in each direction; the field thus covers a wider area. This is useful in diffuse pathology or if the site of the lesion cannot be accurately localized.

Frequency swings

Some equipment allows a variation in the speed of frequency swing. A rhythmic mode may be a continuous swing from 0 to 100 Hz in 5–10 s and back in similar time or it may hold for 1–6 s at one frequency followed by 1–6 s at another frequency with a variable time to swing between the two.

Constant frequency

Some treatments may be carried out with the interference fixed at a certain frequency, e.g. 100 Hz. Rhythmic frequency is useful if several types of tissue are to be treated at once. A variation in frequency also overcomes the problem of tissue accommodation where the response of a particular tissue decreases with time.

A constant frequency has the advantage of giving selective effects, e.g. pain relief. Some patients obtain pain relief at one frequency and others at a different frequency. Small sweeps are fairly selective, and overcome the problem of accommodation without the disadvantage of being too unselective.

Effects of interferential

These depend on:

1. Frequency:
   (a) Range selected.
   (b) Constant or rhythmical.
2. Intensity of currents.
3. Electrode placement.
4. Localization of the lesion.

Frequency

100–150 Hz constant or 90–100 Hz rhythmic

These frequencies are useful for pain relief. Interferential acts on large myelinated fibres in the dorsal horn, blocking off small pain fibres. The higher frequencies have a triggering effect on the endogenous opiates in the mid-brain which inhibit pain.

0–10 Hz rhythmic or 10–50 Hz rhythmic

These frequencies are useful for muscle stimulation. They produce stimulation of deep, normally-innervated muscle tissue with little sensory stimulation. The higher frequencies stimulate the parasympathetic and inhibit the sympathetic system. Skeletal muscle is stimulated at most frequencies but as the frequency increases the contraction changes from a twitch to a tetanic contraction.

0–100 Hz rhythmic

This range of frequencies produces vasodilatation via the autonomic nervous system. This is stimulation and relaxation of vessel walls, giving a 'sinusoidal' effect.

Intensity of current

The current is increased until the patient feels prickling. As accommodation occurs the intensity is increased up to the point of muscle stimulation if this is necessary. The duration of treatment varies between 10 and 20 minutes.

Electrode placement

With the four-electrode method the electrodes are placed equidistant from the lesion. With the two-electrode method the electrodes are placed on either side of the lesion. The electrodes may be fixed with straps or suction. There is, however, more sensory stimulation with the two-electrode method.

Indications for interferential

1. *Pain relief* – Pain of sympathetic origin such as causalgia, neuralgia, pain from herpes zoster, amputation-stump complications and recent injuries.
2. *Swelling* – Interferential aids absorption of exudate particularly for haematomas.
3. *Stress incontinence* – The muscle stimulating frequencies aid weak pelvic floor muscles.
4. *Back pain or disc lesions* – Interferential is useful for relief of acute back pain where the pain is localized to the back or referred down a lower limb.
5. *Sudeck's atrophy* – This responds to interferential when other modalities have failed but treatment may need to be prolonged.
6. *Ligamentous and muscle injuries* – Interferential can be given in acute or chronic conditions to relieve pain, promote healing and restore function. Treatment can be given with strapping in place.
7. *Rheumatic conditions* – Relief of pain arising from osteoarthritis, rheumatoid arthritis and ankylosing spondylitis may be obtained, with a resulting increase in function.

Contraindications for interferential

1. *Pacemakers* – Patients with pacemakers should avoid high- and medium-frequency currents.
2. *Malignancy* – Spread of the disease may occur.
3. *Pregnancy* – Treatment should not be given to the pelvic organs during pregnancy.
4. *Bacterial infections* – Treatment may cause spread of the infection.
5. *Thrombosis* – Interferential tends to spread the blood clot and is contraindicated in deep venous thrombosis or thrombophlebitis. The heart and stellate ganglion should also be avoided.

Combined therapy

It is possible with some machines to combine ultrasound and interferential therapy. Ultrasound has been found to enhance the effect of interferential and it is possible to use lower intensities. Two-electrode interferential using pain relief frequencies is applied with the ultrasound beam. The ultrasound head acts as one electrode and the other electrode is placed on the opposite side of the limb or lesion if this is on the trunk. This technique has been found to be useful for tennis elbow and trigger points in muscles.

Low-frequency currents

Low-frequency currents alternate at 1–1000 Hz. At this frequency currents can stimulate both motor and sensory nerves. Without modification these currents produce a tetanic contraction. Low-frequency currents used therapeutically are:

1. Faradic.
2. Direct.

Faradic current

Faradic current is an unevenly-alternating current with a frequency of 50 Hz with a pulse duration of 1 ms. The current is surged to produce a contraction similar to active muscle contraction. The length of the surges varies from 1 to 5 s and they are repeated 15 times per minute for large muscles and 30 times per minute for small muscles.

Direct current

Direct current is a unidirectional current, the intensity of which must vary to produce a muscle contraction. The current is normally interrupted. The duration of flow can vary from 0.01 ms to 600 ms and the rest period should be at least 2–3 times pulse width, e.g. 100 ms pulse width with a frequency of 1.5 Hz has a rest period of 500 ms. The pulse forms can be rectangular (quick rise and fall), triangular (gradual rise and fall) or saw-tooth (gradual rise, less gradual fall). The interrupted current produces a muscle twitch. In modern muscle stimulators the 0.1–1 ms pulse lengths with frequencies of 50–100 Hz are surged to produce a faradic current.

Uses of faradic-type currents

Muscles must be normally-innervated to respond to this current.

1. Re-education of muscle. When muscle contraction is inhibited by pain or incorrect use, faradism can be used to facilitate a muscle response. This method is particularly useful for the quadriceps and intrinsic muscles of the foot.
2. Training a new muscle action after a tendon transplant.
3. Reduction of oedema by increasing venous and lymphatic drainage. Pressure pumps have begun to supersede faradism in this function.
4. Prevention and loosening of adhesions. If active exercise is not possible electrical stimulation may stretch and loosen adhesions.

Muscle testing

The state of innervation of a muscle can be identified by plotting a strength–duration curve (see Chapter 21).

Transcutaneous (electrical) nerve stimulation (TENS)

TENS is a method of producing pain relief by the application of a pulsed biphasic rectangular wave form through electrodes on the skin. The principle of working is related to the pain gate theory (Melzavk and Wall, 1965, 1982). There is closing of the gate by stimulation of A-β fibres and activation of the descending pain suppression system. It has been suggested that 50–150 Hz achieves this effect. Low frequency (2 Hz pulsed) is said to relieve pain by increasing the body's production of endorphins.

The TENS stimulators are commonly small battery-operated machines with a current output of 0–50 mA. The pulse widths may be fixed at 200 μs or variable between 50 and 300 μs. The frequency is also variable on most machines from 2 Hz to 300 Hz, although some are fixed at 150 Hz. The low frequencies are used for chronic pain and the slightly higher (80–120 Hz) for acute pain. The wide variables of pulse width, frequency and current output allow adjustments for the individual.

The electrodes are applied with conducting gel and are self-adhesive or fixed with tape. Their position may be above and below the painful spot, over the affected nerve, nerve trunk or the affected dermatome. They should not be applied over anaesthetic areas because there would be no sensory input.

Prolonged stimulation is necessary to be effective, e.g. 8 hours per day for a week, but 24 hours a day may be necessary. The patient may require the machine for 2–3 months.

Uses of TENS

1. Longstanding severe pain in a variety of conditions.

2. Post-herpetic neuralgia.
3. Causalgia.
4. Stump and phantom limb pain (see Chapter 16).
5. Trigeminal neuralgia.
6. Chronic neck, back or leg pain.
7. During labour (see Chapter 25).

Contraindications

Patients with pacemakers or cardiac arrhythmias. Area of carotid sinus and mouth.

Electromyographic (EMG) biofeedback

Biofeedback gives the patient immediate and accurate information on the state of selected muscles.

The patient is made aware of under- or over-exaggerated muscle activity through visual and/or auditory feedback which leads to a cortical response. The signal is triggered when the patient is (a) overusing the muscle being retrained or (b) uses the underactive muscle. As this becomes more automatic the patient becomes less dependent on 'cues' and less input is required to achieve the same results. The sensitivity of the machine can be increased as the patient's response improves. Two active electrodes are placed over the belly of the muscle and an indifferent electrode is placed conveniently to complete the circuit.

For biofeedback to be effective patient participation is essential.

Uses of biofeedback

It is useful to teach patients how to gain control over muscle activity.

1. To retrain under-active muscles, e.g. in peripheral nerve lesions.
2. To retrain function, e.g. heel strike in walking (with a pressure pad in the heel of the shoe).
3. To retrain overactive muscles in stroke patients.
4. To control weight bearing in walking, e.g. in partial-weight-bearing walking the amount of weight taken by the patient through the lower limbs can be controlled by a pressure pad.

Biofeedback should be used as an adjunct to, and not instead of, other forms of physiotherapy. Techniques to inhibit spasticity and facilitate muscle contraction should be used where appropriate.

Iontophoresis

Iontophoresis is the introduction of ions through the patient's skin into the body for therapeutic purposes, by means of a direct electrical current.

Negative ions are introduced under the cathode and positive ions are introduced under the anode because like charges repel. The ions produce a therapeutic response according to the nature of the ion (see Chapter 17).

References

Gifford, J. and Gifford, L. (1988) Connective tissue massage. In *Pain Management and Control in Pysiotherapy* (eds Wells, Frampton and Bowsher), Heinemann, London

Maitland, G. D. (1986) *Vertebral Manipulation* 5th ed. Butterworths, London

Melzack, R. and Wall, P. D. (1965) Pain mechanisms: A new theory. *Science*, **150**, 1–8.

Melzack, R. and Wall, P. D. (1982) *the Challenge of Pain*, Penguin Books, London

Appendix 2 – Orthopaedics and neurology

Hallux rigidus

This is a stiffness in the metatarsophalangeal joint of the great toe. It may be the result of inflammatory changes such as occur with rheumatoid arthritis, or it may be due to trauma.

Rest and relief of pressure may reduce the pain and muscle spasm. However, if severe pain persists, surgery may be required either by an arthrodesis or an operation such as Keller's procedure.

Hammer toe

This usually affects the second toe and results in dorsiflexion of the proximal phalanx, plantar flexion of the middle phalanx and either flexion or extension of the distal phalanx.

In a child it may be possible to correct this by manipulation and splinting combined with good footwear. If the deformity has become fixed and there is persistent pain, then surgery may be necessary.

Osteochondritis dissecans

This is a condition that is found in some synovial joints, in particular the knee and less commonly in the hip, ankle and elbow. A small portion of articular cartilage becomes separated from the rest of the cartilage. Sometimes sub-chondral bone may be attached to this portion and the separation may be partial or complete.

Most cases occur in children or young adults and particularly those engaged in fairly strenuous physical activity. This has led to the theory that the lesion is traumatic and this is supported by the pathological changes. However, some authorities suggest that it may be due to some abnormality of the cartilage or its nutritional supply.

Surgical intervention may be necessary to repair damage or to remove any loose fragments. Post-operative physiotherapy may be needed to restore normal function.

Osteomyelitis

This is an infection of bone caused by microorganisms. The condition may occur directly as the result of infection through an open wound, or indirectly via the circulation. The commonest organism causing this infection is *Staphylococcus pyogenes aureus* although there are other organisms that can lead to osteomyelitis.

The patient has a fever and there are local signs and symptoms over the infected bone. There is usually severe pain and if the bone is superficial there may be swelling. After a time the pus formed at the site of the infection may track to the surface through a sinus and this will form an abscess which will eventually burst.

Until the development of antibiotics the prognosis for this condition was poor. Antibiotics can now effectively cure the infection, provided the organism is sensitive to the particular drug used. Surgery may be required to remove any pus and dead bone.

Osteoporosis
Paget's disease (osteitis deformans)

Usually the age of onset of this disease is between the mid thirties and the fifties, although it may not become apparent until the patient is older.

There is a thickening and softening of bone which results in deformities according to the particular stresses on the affected bones. Later there is a recalcification and the bones become harder.

The skull and the bones of the lower limbs (pelvis, femur, tibia) are most commonly affected.

The clinical features vary, and the condition may present with pain and aching of the limbs, tenderness of muscle, or muscle cramps, or the first thing the patient may notice is the development of deformity such as bowing of the legs.

Fractures of the femur or tibia may occur as the result of fairly minor trauma.

Osteoarthritis may occur in the weight-bearing joints as a result of the altered mechanics and muscle weakness.

Physiotherapy

Treatment may be required to try to relieve the pain and tenderness in the muscles and to keep the patient mobile. More often patients are treated following fractures, or because of osteoarthritis developing in the hip or knee joints.

Periostitis

Traumatic periostitis caused by a blow on the bone is a fairly common injury, particularly in such vulnerable areas as the shaft of the tibia. Provided that there is no infection, the inflammation will clear up quite quickly although the bone may be a little thickened at the site of injury.

Pes cavus

This term is applied to a deformity of the foot in which there is an exaggeration of the longitudinal arch and a clawing of the toes. It may be a congenital or acquired deformity. As a congenital abnormality it may occur with talipes or other problems such as spina bifida. Pes cavus is often present in patients with Friedreich's ataxia or the peroneal type of muscular atrophy. The acquired form may be due to paralysis of the lumbricals and interossei.

Pott's disease

This is a tuberculosis of the spine and was first described by Sir Percival Pott. Most commonly it attacks the lower thoracic and upper lumbar region. The infection leads to a collapse of the affected vertebral body and may spread to other vertebrae. In some instances cold abscesses form, composed of the debris from the infection which may track to other areas of the body. Occasionally a cold abscess may pass to the vertebral canal and if it presses on the spinal cord it may cause a paralysis.

The collapse of one or more vertebral bodies is most marked in the thoracic spine because the normal curve is convex backwards. This gives an angular deformity and in severe cases the patient develops a hunch back.

The disease occurs more commonly in children than adults.

In recent years the advent of successful chemotherapy has decreased the incidence of this disease.

Rickets (rachitis)

Rickets is a disease of disordered calcium metabolism occurring in infants and young children, the most characteristic changes taking place in the bones. At one time it was a very common disease amongst the poor, and was particularly prevalent in large cities.

An adequate amount of calcium and vitamin D is essential during the growing period and a deficiency of either may cause rickets. Vitamin D is obtained from the diet or it is synthesized in the body by the action of ultraviolet light on 7-dehydrocholesterol in the skin. The chief action of vitamin D is to bring about absorption of calcium from the intestine, and if this is deficient then the calcium salts and phosphates in the body cannot be used to produce ossification of the bones.

Fortunately, rickets caused by the above deficiencies is now rare because of better social conditions. Some cases of rickets still occur because of primary metabolic abnormalities and these may be genetically determined.

Clinical features occurring as a result of this condition are general poor health, often with a slight fever. The muscles are hypotonic, weak and poorly developed. The nerves are hyperexcitable. Bone deformities develop as the result of the soft bone.

Sprengel's shoulder

This is a rare condition in which one scapula (or occasionally both) is in an abnormally high position on the thoracic wall.

Talipes

Talipes equinovarus is described in Chapter 7 but there are a number of similar foot deformities which are not described as they are not as common: talipes calcaneus, talipes calcaneo varus, talipes calcaneo valgus and talipes equino valgus.

Chondromalacia patellae

This is a diagnosis used to denote retro-patellar pain in patients who have no other obvious cause for the pain and are too young to be in the osteoarthritis age group. There is degeneration of the articular cartilage of the patella, particularly on the medial side.

Aetiology

Age group: 16–30 years.

Sex: Females are affected more than males.

Cause: This is unknown but sometimes can be related to an episode of trauma, change of footwear or change of lifestyle (e.g. leaving school and going to work).

Pathological changes

The articular cartilage softens, and fissures and erosions appear. Tags of cartilage and fibrous tissue are formed on the margins of the fissures (Smillie, 1978). There is some doubt as to whether these changes cause the pain because they have been seen in the cartilage of patients undergoing operation or investigation (arthroscopy) for other reasons (e.g. meniscus problems or fractured patella).

Clinical features

Pain – Deep aching in nature, behind the patella, aggravated by going up or down stairs or sporting activities involving weight-bearing knee flexion.

Crepitus – Compression and passive movement of the patella elicits a grating sound and sensation of roughness to the examiner.

Locking – Occasionally a locking sensation may be felt behind the patella which does not slide easily over the femoral condyles.

Muscle weakness

When the condition is unilateral, the quadriceps is weaker than on the other side. In bilateral cases the quadriceps may be weaker than the expected norm for the age, build and lifestyle of the patient. The vastus medialis is often wasted.

Posture

The patella or patellae may be directed medially (Figure A2.1).

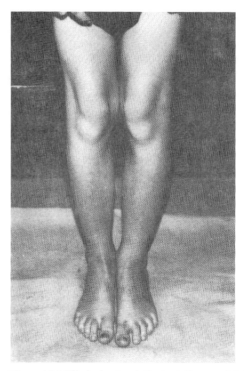

Figure A2.1 'Kissing' or 'squinting' patellae associated with chondromalacia patellae, tibial torsion and pronated feet

Physiotherapy

A helpful working hypothesis is to consider that the health of the articular cartilage is dependent on synovial sweep, which is created by intermittent compression. Lack of quadriceps power – the vastus medialis in particular – reduces the compression during everyday activities between the patella and femur, the cartilage loses nutrition and undergoes the changes described.

Techniques

Techniques that help are:

1. Mobilizations.
2. Strapping and bandaging.
3. Quadriceps strengthening.
4. Short-wave diathermy.

Mobilizations

Supero-inferior oscillations applied with compression to the patella reproduces 'grating' but not pain. Given over 3–4 treatment sessions this technique appears to help, in that the crepitus decreases and the patient reports less pain.

Strapping or bandaging

Strapping (Figure A2.2) is applied, bearing in mind the hypothesis that the medial side of the patella needs to be compressed; 2–3 bands are generally enough. These are applied from the lateral side of the patella as if to pull it medially, and then the strap is carried on to the medial side of the patella and up to the medial side of the femur. Fixing straps are required to stop the main bands rolling down. This may be applied for the patient who wants to compete in a sporting competition. It may be left *in situ* for 3–4 days and then reviewed.

Bandaging – A firm elastic bandage may be applied, again to produce compression on the patella. This may suit the patient better than strapping because he can be taught to apply it himself and the skin is less traumatized. Bandaging is not, however, a substitute for the strapping which can apply a more precise force.

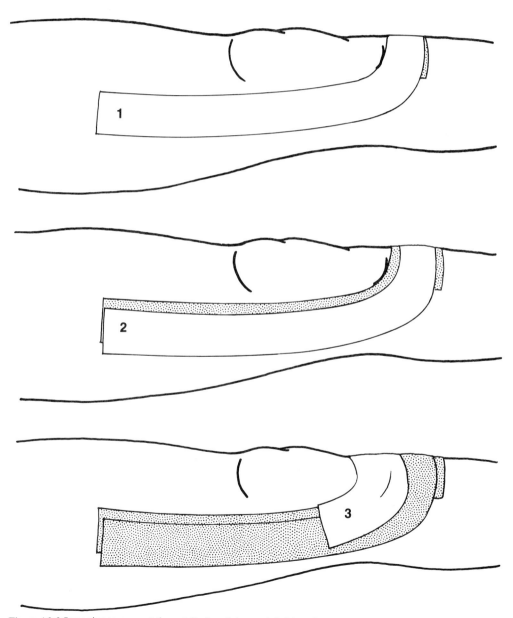

Figure A2.2 Strapping to support the patella (medial aspect, left knee)

Quadriceps strengthening

If the vastus medialis is weaker than the other three components it may be appropriate to apply a muscle stimulating current such as faradism. This is applied so that when the patient (in half lying) is asked to straighten the knee over a small pillow, the faradism is applied to boost the vastus medialis contraction.

PNF may be used in the flexion–adduction pattern of the leg, modified to include knee extension. If the patient sits with the knees flexed over the end of the plinth the physiotherapist can apply resistance to the foot, which is dorsiflexed and inverted, as well as to the quadriceps as the knee is straightened. The physiotherapist's other hand palpates the vastus medialis and she can instruct the patient to make the muscle work.

Once this has been successful, the patient should practise sitting with the ankles crossed and pushing the underneath ankle up against the resistance of the top one. He can be taught to feel the vastus medialis working and should practise this for 5 minutes every day.

Short-wave diathermy

Theoretically, if a co-planar technique is applied so that the field can increase the circulation to the synovium, nutrition to the cartilage will be improved. This is worth considering when the patient's pain is easily provoked, but should not feature in the treatment programme more than five or six times.

Long term

This condition usually develops insidiously and therefore takes some time to clear. The patient should therefore be treated until pain is diminished and the quadriceps is working fully. Then a review programme should be implemented, for example at 3–4 week intervals for up to 4 months.

If there is steady deterioration of function, an orthopaedic surgeon may contemplate scraping the cartilage or changing the mechanics of the quadriceps mechanism.

Neurology

Epilepsy

Epilepsy occurs as the result of abnormal electrical activity in the brain. The reaction of the patient to this depends on the cause and the area(s) affected.

Primary generalized or idiopathic epilepsy is familial and usually presents with grand mal or petit mal attacks. The abnormal activity starts in the upper brainstem and spreads to affect the cerebral hemispheres.

In a grand mal attack there is no warning and the patient suddenly stiffens and falls to the ground, losing consciousness (tonic phase – lasts about 40 seconds). This is followed by random disorganized movements (clonic phase – lasts from a few seconds up to 30 minutes). After the convulsive movements cease the patient is in a coma for a short period and then as consciousness returns feels confused and may be restless. Later the patient becomes drowsy and may feel tired for the next couple of days.

Petit mal as the name suggests is not nearly so dramatic. The patient becomes unaware of his surroundings for a few seconds and then recovers. It is very disconcerting both for the patient and anyone with him as there is a blank stare and loss of attention. Initially when it occurs it may be dismissed by observers, particularly if they are non-medicals, as 'day dreaming'.

Another cause of epilepsy is a neurological disorder, which could occur following a head injury, or be due to a disease. Usually this results in a focal epilepsy with the clinical features depending on the position and extent of the lesion.

Altered biochemistry due to drugs can result in epilepsy. It may be the reaction to drugs given to help a patient with another condition, for example following the use of anti-depressants. It may occur in patients undergoing withdrawal symptoms following drug addiction.

Management

This will depend on the cause and whether it can be dealt with. Primary generalized epilepsy will respond to anti-convulsants and it may be possible to keep the patient free from fits. This is very important as it allows the patient to lead a normal life at home, to be employed and to take part in leisure activities.

The physiotherapist is not concerned with treating epilepsy but it is important for her to know about the various forms of epilepsy and how to deal with a fit if it should occur. It is important to keep the airway clear and so the patient should be placed in a semisupine position if possible. During the clonic stage there is a danger of the patient injuring himself on any hard or sharp objects and so it is necessary to prevent this by moving any moveable objects or moving the patient. A patient having an attack should not be left unattended.

The physiotherapist should have information about any patients likely to have epileptic fits. If an unexpected attack occurs this must be reported to the doctor as it may be an indication of some abnormal pathology.

Patients who are known epileptics and whose condition is not under control with drugs may not be suitable to receive certain treatments as it could be dangerous – for example hydrotherapy, some forms of electrotherapy and possibly the use of gymnastic apparatus.

The physiotherapist should be aware of factors that can trigger an attack in some epileptics, for example flickering lights or short-wave diathermy.

Brachial plexus lesion

Trauma may cause an avulsion of one or more roots of the brachial plexus. If the lesion is total there will be a flaccid paralysis of the muscles of the arm and anaesthesia. It may be accompanied by Horner's syndrome.

Erb's palsy (Erb duchenne paralysis)

A fall on the shoulder or traction on the arm during birth may cause a lesion of the upper part of the brachial plexus involving the 5th and 6th cervical nerves.

Klumpke's paralysis

Forced abduction of the arm may cause injury to the 8th cervical and 1st thoracic nerve roots. The muscles supplied by these nerves will be paralysed, resulting in a claw hand, and there will be a loss of sensation in the area supplied by C8 and T1. There may be a sympathetic involvement indicated by Horner's syndrome.

Horner's syndrome

This is caused by the loss of sympathetic nerve supply to the eye. It may occur because of pre-ganglionic damage at the brainstem, cervical cord, anterior nerve roots of C8 and T1 or cervical sympathetic chain; or because of post-ganglionic damage due to internal carotid occlusion or middle fossa lesions. There is a ptosis whereby the affected eyelid tends to droop, and there is a constriction of the pupil.

Friedreich's ataxia

This is a progressive ataxia due to an inherited disorder which may occur as an autosomal recessive or autosomal dominant form. The pathological changes occur mainly in the thoracic region of the spinal cord with a degeneration and gliosis of the anterior and posterior spino-cerebellar tracts, corticospinal tracts and the posterior columns. There are some changes taking place in the cerebellum.

The onset happens in the first or second decade and affects both boys and girls.

Apart from the ataxia there are musculoskeletal abnormalities in most cases, particularly pes cavus and kyphoscoliosis, and many patients have a cardiac myopathy.

The prognosis is usually poor and death ensues within 10–20 years from cardiac failure or pulmonary complications.

Huntington's chorea

This is an inherited disorder with an autosomal gene. The pathology involves a loss of cells from the basal ganglia and the cerebral cortex.

The disease usually becomes evident in middle life with a progressive chorea and dementia exhibiting behavioural changes.

The prognosis is poor and death usually occurs in 10–15 years.

Myalgic encephalomyelitis

This condition seems to follow a viral infection. The patient is tired and listless and this may persist for months and even years. There may be muscular weakness and pain, which combined with the tiredness gives a reduced exercise tolerance. The reason why this condition should occur in some patients and not in others is still not clear although various theories have been suggested. It may be that certain people have impaired immunological response to a particular viral infection. Some authorities believe that it might be partly of wholly psychosomatic.

Physiotherapy is not often required as part of the management for these patients, but when there are muscular pains and weakness it may form a useful part of the rehabilitation programme.

Syringomyelia

This is a rare condition and seldom seen in a physiotherapy department. It is worth mentioning because of the contraindication to certain physiotherapy techniques.

The pathology involves the development of a cystic cavity within the spinal cord which becomes progressively larger. Usually it affects the lower cervical and upper thoracic segments.

The clinical features involve the loss of particular sensory modalities, especially those of pain and temperature. The upper limbs show signs of lower motor neuron lesions, the lower limbs may indicate an upper motor neuron lesion and sensory loss due to both descending and ascending tract involvement.

It is important that the physiotherapist appreciates the possible loss of pain and thermal sensation when assessing and deciding on a treatment programme.

Tabes dorsalis

This occurs in the tertiary stage of syphilis but is now rare due to effective treatment in the primary stage and to better education concerning the dangers of venereal disease.

Tabes dorsalis occurs due to a lesion affecting the posterior columns of the spinal cord and results in a proprioceptive sensory loss. This presents as an ataxia affecting mainly the lower limbs.

Frenkel's exercises (see Appendix 1, page 424) were specially designed to treat this condition.

Reference

Smillie, I. S. (1978) *Injuries of the Knee Joint,* 5th edn, Churchill Livingstone, London

Appendix 3 – Children's conditions

Respiratory

Cystic fibrosis – Chapter 13.
　　Asthma – Chapter 13.

Cardiac

Congenital disorders of the heart – Chapter 15.
　　Rheumatic fever – Chapter 15.

Neurology

Cerebral palsy – Chapter 22.
　　Spina bifida – Chapter 22.
　　Hydrocephalus – Chapter 22.

Orthopaedics and trauma – Chapters 3–6

Spinal deformities.
Talipes equino varus.
Congenital dislocation of the hip.
Coxa vara.
Genu valgum and varum.
Torticollis.
Greenstick fractures.

Rheumatology

Juvenile chronic polyarthritis – Chapter 9.

Skin

Burns – Chapter 18.

Appendix 4

Mobilizing exercises   *Strengthening exercises*

This appendix is designed to be a starting point for the inexperienced physiotherapist. The exercises are both specific for particular joint movements and muscle groups and general with a combination of joint and muscle groups. Specific exercises are used in the examination of a patient to test joint range and muscle strength. They are also used to help patients with problems that respond to mobilizing of joints and strengthening of muscles. The choice of exercise and method of application follow the principles indicated in Appendix 1. The effectiveness of an exercise is dependent on the teaching by the therapist and the performance by the patient together with correction by the therapist.

Mobilizing exercises

These are indicated where joint movement is limited by fibrous stiffness and should not be used in the presence of acute inflammation. Generally the exercises are performed within the pain-free range. The speed should be as near natural as possible, with emphasis at the limit of range. Important themes are frequent repetition, regular performance (e.g. 2–3 times per day) and good rhythm (often enhanced by music). The speed may need to be increased and a hold at the limit of movement may help to maintain the range gained.

Upper limb
Shoulder/shoulder girdle

Movements:

1. *Shoulder girdle* – Protraction, retraction, elevation, depression, medial and lateral rotation (combined with arm movements).

2. *Shoulder* – Flexion, extension, abduction, adduction, medial and lateral rotation, elevation.

1 Walk standing (one hand on forward knee)

(a) One arm swinging forward and back.
(b) One arm swinging out and in.

The effect is enhanced if a weight is held in the hand.

2 Stoop sitting (feet slightly apart)

Arms swinging forward and back.

3 Sitting or standing (arms by the side)

(a) Arms turning in and out.
(b) Elbows flexed to 90° – arms turning in and out.
(c) Arms raising forwards and upwards with turning in and out.
(d) Arms raise to one side and swing from side to side.
(e) Pass ball over head and back – pass ball behind back.
(f) Pass ball behind neck – place hands behind neck and behind back.
(g) Hands place one behind back one behind neck, change over.

4 Sitting with fingertips on shoulders

(a) Arms stretching forwards and back, upwards and back, sideways and back.
(b) Elbows circling.

5 Sitting or standing

(a) Punching into the air in different directions.
(b) Throwing ball underhand or overhand to partner or against a wall.

474

(c) Throwing a piece of cotton wool as high as possible against a wall.
(d) Elbows at right angles, shoulders abducted, arms turning up and down.
(e) Shoulder (girdles) raise, push down and relax.
(f) Shoulder girdle circling backwards.
(g) Shoulder girdles pulling forwards and backwards – may be enhanced by arms stretching forwards and elbows bending and pushing backwards.
(h) Alternate shoulder shrugging.
(i) Arms swinging forwards and backwards.

6 Lying

(a) Arms by the side back of hands on one bean bag each – arms raise sideways above head and down.
(b) Hands grasping a pole, arms raise above head and lower.
(c) Hands grasping a pole with shoulders abducted and elbows at right angles, arms turn to raise pole above head (lateral rotation) and lower (may be performed in sitting).

Elbow

Movements – flexion and extension.

1 Sitting

(a) Arm resting on a polished table or re-education board – elbow bending and stretching (a cloth under the forearm reduces friction).
(b) Position as above – polishing action at different speeds.
(c) Hands on shoulders – arms stretching in all directions (this may be progressed by making a punching action to increase the force and enhance the mobilizing effect).
(d) Grasping pole at shoulder level, arms stretch forwards and back, arms stretch up and back.

2 Standing

(a) Grasping ball – throw ball against wall with one hand or both (overarm).
(b) Grasping towel or rope – towelling action behind back.
(c) Placing the hand behind the neck and walking the fingers down the spine, placing the hand behind the back and walking the fingers up the spine (for elbow flexion).

Forearm

Movements – pronation and supination at the radioulnar joints.

1 Sitting

(a) Elbows flexed and held into the trunk – turn hands up and down.
(b) Same as above but the patient fixes one elbow with the opposite hand.
(c) Turning pages of a book.
(d) Practise screwing action holding pole, pencil or screwdriver in the hand.
(e) Balancing bean bag on back of hand – throw bean bag up, catch on palm and back of hand alternately.

2 Standing

(a) Grasping pole – swing pole through 180° and back.
(b) Bounce ball – catch with palm up and palm down alternately.

Wrist and hand

Movements:

(a) Wrist – flexion, extension, abduction (radial deviation) adduction (ulnar deviation).
(b) Hand – finger – flexion, extension, abduction adduction, opposition.
(c) Thumb – flexion, extension, adduction, abduction, medial and lateral rotation.
(d) Opposition – thumb flexion and medial rotation, finger flexion and lateral rotation.

1 Standing

Bouncing ball with forearm pronated, incorporating flexion and extension of the wrist.

2 Sitting

(a) Arms resting on a polished table – hand sliding from side to side (palms down for abduction and adduction).
(b) As above with forearm in midprone – wrist bending and stretching.
(c) As above pushing bean bag with back of hand to increase the force of extension.
(d) Squeezing soft foam rubber ball.
(e) Fingers stretching apart and closing.
(f) Palms down – tapping fingers as in typing to gain extension.
(g) Palms down – arching hand with fingers in extension (lumbrical action).
(h) Gathering a sock into the palm of the hand.
(i) Tying knots in rope, string, wool or thread.
(j) Doing up/undoing buttons.
(k) Picking up pieces of wood of varying thicknesses, pencil, paper, paper clips, pins, marbles.

Lower limb

Hip

Movements: flexion, extension, abduction, adduction, medial and lateral rotation.

1 Lying

(a) Slide leg sideways (leg on a blanket on a slippery floor).
(b) Bend knees to place feet on floor – bend one knee up on to chest (assist with hands round knee) lower and repeat with the other leg.
(c) Bend knees to place feet on floor – keep feet on floor and knees together – roll knees from side to side.
(d) Bend one knee on to chest pull with one hand round the knee – keep other leg flat on the floor (this hip is in extension).
(e) Side lying (underneath leg flexed) bicycling action with the top leg (ensure that the top leg hip abductors are strong enough to hold the leg horizontal).
(f) Side lying as above, top leg bending at the hip and knee and stretching back.
(g) Prone lying – bend one knee and lift this knee to extend the hip.
(h) Turn both legs inwards and outwards.

2 Sitting

(a) Turn trunk and pelvis from side to side.
(b) Keep feet and hips together, swing feet from side to side.
(c) Move feet apart and together.

3 Standing

(a) Hold bar or balance with one hand on a wall, stand on a low stool (or bottom step of stairs), swing one leg backwards and forwards.
(b) Hold on to bar (or another person) swing leg across in front and out to the side.
(c) Feet apart – step to one side and lunge to that side, recover and repeat to the other side.
(d) Turn feet in and out.
(e) Holding back of a chair – bend one knee up in front and stretch out behind. Repeat with other leg.

4 Prone kneeling

Bend one knee forwards and carrying back (keep the knee flexed for a short lever).

Knee

Movements: flexion, extension, medial and lateral rotation with the knee in flexion.

1 Lying

(a) Alternate knee bend and stretch (with heels sliding on a slippery surface).
(b) Prone lying – alternate knee bend and stretch.
(c) Side lying (underneath leg flexed, top leg on a re-education board) bend and stretch top knee.
(d) Bicycling action in the air with both legs.

2 Sitting

(a) On high plinth swing lower legs alternately backwards and forwards.
(b) On stool feet on floor, slide one foot backwards to gain flexion.
(c) Sitting on a blanket on a slippery floor – move forwards and backwards by bending and stretching the knees.

3 Prone kneeling

Keep hands steady and bend the hips and knees to sit back on the heels.

4 Standing

(a) Bend one knee and hip up in front and stretch out behind.
(b) Running on the spot kicking legs up behind.

Ankle and foot

Movements:

1. *Ankle* – Dorsiflexion, plantar flexion.
2. *Sub-talar and mid-tarsal joints* – Inversion, eversion.
3. *Toes* – Flexion, extension, abduction, adduction.

1 Lying or half-lying

(a) Alternate foot pulling up and pushing down.
(b) Foot circling.
(c) Feet turning in and out.

2 Sitting

(a) Alternate heel and toe tapping.
(b) Toes curling and stretching.
(c) Keeping lower leg steady – turn feet in and out.
(d) Crumpling paper or screwing up sock.
(e) Roll feet on to outer borders and then in to inner borders.
(f) Cross one leg over the other – top foot pulling up, pushing down and circling.

3 Standing

(a) Holding bar, standing on toes on the edge of a low stool – lower and raise heels (the same exercises may be performed using the lower rung of wall bars).

(b) Flicking bean bag in different directions with the foot.

(c) Walking up and down an inclined form forwards, backwards and sideways.

Trunk

The range of movement in the vertebral column as a whole is fairly large, although movement between individual vertebrae is very small.

Cervical spine

Movements:

(a) Atlanto-occipital joints, flexion, extension, small-range side-flexion.

(b) Atlanto-axial joints, principal movement is rotation.

(c) C2–C7 – flexion, extension, side-flexion, rotation.

1 Lying

(a) Head on blanket on slippery surface – bend head from side to side, turn head from side to side (keep chin tucked in and neck stretched throughout).

(b) Chin tucking in and neck stretching plus push shoulders down to the feet.

2 Sitting

(a) Head turning side to side.

(b) Head bending side to side.

(c) Head bending forwards (chin to chest) and stretching up.

(d) Head bending backwards (with chin tucked in).

(e) Head bending forwards and to the right then stretching up and to the left, repeat opposite way (oblique patterns).

(f) Pass bean bag over from hand to hand following movement with the head.

Thoracic spine

Movements: rotation, flexion, extension, side-flexion (in order of freedom).

1 Sitting

(a) Hands on opposite shoulders, trunk bending and stretching (localize the movement to the thoracic spine).

(b) Backs of hands on side of thorax – bend thoracic spine side to side.

(c) Trunk turning with arms swinging.

(d) Hands on opposite shoulders trunk turning side to side.

(e) Hands on opposite shoulders – arms stretching up and out with a deep breath in and arms lowering with breathing out.

2 Prone kneeling

(a) Trunk turning with one arm swinging.

(b) Walk hands round to one side and then the other (side flexion).

(c) Place hands sideways with elbows flexed – thoracic spine flexion and extension (Pluto sniff).

(d) Position as above – walk hands round to one side and then the other (side-flexion).

3 Lying

(a) Arms stretched sideways – trunk turning to clap hands.

(b) As above – slide right hand along left arm to fingertips and repeat to opposite side.

(c) Upper trunk on blanket on slippery surface – trunk bending side to side.

Lumbar spine

Movements: flexion, extension, side-flexion, rotation (in order of freedom).

1 Lying

(a) Pelvis and legs on blanket on slippery surface (arms stretched sideways) swing legs from side to side.

(b) As above – hitch one leg up and stretch down, repeat to opposite side (side-flexion).

(c) Side lying with pelvis and legs on a blanket on a slippery surface – swing legs and pelvis forwards and backwards.

(d) Bend knees on to chest, spread arms sideways and swing pelvis plus legs from side to side (keep knees and hips flexed throughout).

(e) Bend knees and place feet on floor, keep lumbar spine in contact with the floor and knees together – swing knees from side to side.

(f) Bend knees on to chest, put hands under the knees – rock knees to chest with hands helping.

2 Prone kneeling

(a) Swing pelvis from side to side.

(b) Hump and hollow the lumbar spine.

3 Sitting

(a) Place hands on hips and tilt the pelvis backwards and forwards.
(b) Place hands on hips – tilt the pelvis from side to side – rocking from one buttock to the other.
(c) Trunk turn from side to side swinging the arms.
(d) Trunk bend from side to side.

4 Standing

(a) Feet shoulder width apart – alternate hip updrawing.
(b) Feet shoulder width apart, knees in slight flexion and hands on hips – tilt the pelvis backwards and forwards.

Whole spine

1 Lying

(a) Arms stretched out to side – lift right leg (straight) turn to touch left hand with right foot – repeat to opposite side.
(b) Stretch arms above head and stretch legs and feet to give a longitudinal stretch to the spine.

2 Standing

(a) Feet apart, arms stretched above head – swing right arm down to touch left foot, stretch up and back. Repeat to the other side.
(b) Back to wall – turn to place hands flat on the wall first to one side then the other (feet must be kept steady).
(c) Bend left arm to point the elbow upwards, push the right arm downwards and bend the trunk to the right, repeat to the left.
(d) Hands clasped, stretch arms above head – bend forwards to touch the floor, in front of feet then to the right then to the left and stretch up (keep abdominal muscles contracted throughout).
(e) Stride standing, grasping ball – bounce ball in front, to the side and behind.

Strengthening exercises

These are indicated where muscles are weak and may be useful in strengthening muscles to the level of everyday function. They are also useful for maintaining strength up to a functional level. Muscles that are required to perform above-average tasks require a progressive resisted programme and each programme must be tailored to the patient's needs. These exercises should be performed slowly, smoothly and with control. Resistance (see Appendix 1) must be added to strengthen a muscle or muscle group progressively. A complete programme ensures that muscle groups work as agonists, antagonists, synergists and fixators.

Upper limb

Shoulder region

1 Lying

(a) With hands on shoulders – arms carry sideways.
(b) Arms carry sideways.
(c) Side-lying, top arm (hand on shoulder) raise and lower.
(d) Side-lying, top arm raise and lower.
(e) Hands on shoulders, stretch arms forwards and bend.
(f) Shoulder girdles raise, push down and rest.
(g) Hands on shoulders arms stretch above head and bend.

2 Sitting

(a) Clench fists and place one on top of the other, push up and down, hold and repeat with the hands the other way round.
(b) Clasp hands, keep clasped and try to pull apart, hold, push hands together and hold.
(c) Hands on shoulders: (i) arms raise sideways and lower, (ii) arms raise forwards and lower.
(d) Arms carry backwards, forwards, and rest.
(e) Arms carry sideways and lower.
(f) Elbows bend to place fingers on shoulders, stretch up, bend and lower.
(g) Hands on shoulders – raise arms sideways to a right angle – straighten right arm to the side and return, repeat with left arm.
(h) Hands on shoulders – stretch right arm up and left arm forward and return, change to left arm up and right arm forward.
(i) On the floor – place fists on floor, straighten arms to lift buttocks off the floor (the hands could be on blocks if the fists are uncomfortable).
(j) Turn arms outwards, pull scapulae down and together.
(k) Hold arms abducted, elbows at right angles forearms and hands pointing up – pull scapulae together, pull elbows forward to touch and stretch back.

3 Standing

(a) Place hands on wall, bend elbows and control body weight as chest moves towards the wall then push away.
(b) Place objects on shelves of different heights in front and at the side.
(c) Lift, carry and place down objects of different sizes, weights and shapes.

4 Prone kneeling

1. Keeping hands on the floor – elbows bend and stretch.

2. Stretch one arm forwards, bend to touch shoulder, stretch sideways bend and stretch towards feet, repeat with the other arm (this is important for the weight-bearing function of the arm).

Elbow

1 Lying

(a) Arms bend, stretch forwards, hold and lower.
(b) Prone on a bed or plinth with right upper arm supported and elbow flexed over the edge – elbow straighten, hold and bend.

2 Sitting

(a) Arms bending and stretching forwards, upwards and sideways.
(b) Forearms in supination elbows bend and stretch.
(c) Grasp ball (increasing the weight up to a medicine ball) arms stretch up, hold and bend.

3 Standing and prone kneeling

Exercises as for the shoulders above.

Note that most of these exercises can be progressed by the addition of strap-on weights round the wrists.

Forearm wrist and hand

1 Sitting

(a) Hands in warm water – squeeze cloth/sponge.
(b) As above – squeeze and wring cloth.
(c) Squeeze and release rubber ball (the ball can be kept in a pocket so that the patient can practise this exercise regularly every day).
(d) Crumple paper.
(e) Tear paper of different thicknesses.
(f) Use an elastic band to resist individual finger movements.
(g) Forearm resting on a table with the hand over the edge – hold weight in hand – lift and lower weight.
(h) Screw off lids or tops of jars, tins or bottles.
(i) Bounce a ball, catch, squeeze and bounce again.
(j) Hold pole in hand, keep elbow flexed and steady, turn pole from hand facing down to up.
(k) Lumbrical action on a table.
(l) Hold pencil/card between fingers, keep holding while object is pulled (either by the patient or the physiotherapist).
(m) As above, holding object between finger and thumb.
(n) Lift and carry objects of different weights.

Upper limb weight-bearing activities

1. Bunny jumps over an upturned form.
2. Bunny jumps on the floor.
3. Racing start, changing legs slowly at first then with a jump.
4. Lean on one hand on a table, slowly bend and stretch the elbow.
5. Sitting on a blanket or rug on a polished floor, push on hands to move body in different directions.
6. Pulling body weight up an inclined form (on a blanket).

Lower limb

Hip

1 Lying

(a) Knees flexed, feet on floor – pelvic raising and lowering.
(b) Start as above – bend alternate knees to chest.
(c) Start as above, bend one knee on to chest, pelvic raising and lowering – change legs (add passing ball under pelvis from side to side).
(d) Alternate straight leg raising and lowering.
(e) Prone lying – alternate leg raising and lowering.
(f) Side-lying, top leg raising and lowering.
(g) Side-lying, top leg positioned behind underneath one – underneath leg raising and lowering.

2 Prone kneeling

(a) Alternate leg lifting back (with knee in flexion).
(b) Alternate leg stretching back.
(c) Feet turning out and in to work the medial and lateral rotators.
(d) Stretch up to kneeling and back.

3 Kneeling

(a) Hands on opposite shoulders, sit back on to heels and return to kneeling.
(b) Lift one leg forwards to half-kneeling and return, repeat with other leg.

4 Sitting

(a) Swing both legs from side to side keeping feet together (to work the rotators).
(b) Keeping spine straight, trunk bend forwards and backwards.
(c) Stand up and sit down slowly.

5 Standing

(a) Stride (feet shoulder width apart) trunk bending forwards and stretching backwards.

(b) Trunk supported and hands grasping plinth, alternate leg lift and lower.
(c) One hand on wall, one leg carry sideways and lower; repeat with opposite leg.
(d) One hand on wall, heels raise, knees bend, knees stretch and heels lower.
(e) Step up and down using stools of different heights.
(f) Stand on one leg, pass bean bag round foot with toe of other leg.
(g) Stride jumping.
(h) Pas de bas.
(i) Marking time slowly.

Note: Strap-on weights can be placed round the ankle to progress the exercises.

Knee

1 Lying

(a) Quadriceps contractions.
(b) Knees flexed feet on floor – alternate knee stretching and bending.
(c) Prone, knees straightening (toes not tucked in at first then tucked in).
(d) Prone, alternate knee bend and stretch.
(e) Alternate straight leg raising and lowering.
(f) Knees flexed feet on floor, bend one knee on to chest straighten up, bend and lower to starting position (repeat other leg).
(g) One leg raise, knee bend, knee stretch, leg lower.
(h) Cycling action with both legs in the air (pelvis supported by hands).
(i) Side-lying, top leg lift to horizontal, knee bend stretch and leg lower (repeat other side).
(j) Side-lying bicycling action with top leg.

2 Sitting

(a) Alternate knee stretch and bend.
(b) Stand up sit down (may assist with arms).
(c) Arms crossed stand up sit down.
(d) As above on one leg only (other leg held out in front).
(e) As above with height of chair or stool made gradually lower.

3 Standing

(a) Holding fixed support, hips and knees bending and stretching (progress by increasing the range of bend to crouching).
(b) Facing a low stool or step – step up and down (progress by increasing the height of the stool).
(c) Stretch arms sideways – lunge to the right and recover, lunge to the left and recover.
(d) Stretch right arm forward, left arm back – lunge forward with right leg, recover, change arms and lunge with left leg.

Ankle and foot

1 Sitting

(a) Heels raising and lowering (progress by auto-resistance with hands on knees).
(b) Alternate heel and toe raising.
(c) Heels raising, then toes raising.
(d) Lumbrical action, at first with manual assistance to hold the toes in extension, progress to no assistance then have toes on a book to increase range then add manual resistance over the metatarsal heads (most patients need to be taught to stretch the toes passively prior to this exercise).
(e) Picking up a pencil/tissue paper/handkerchief/ string/elastic band with the toes (note that even if the object is not actually picked up the intrinsic foot muscles are worked well in the attempt).

2 Standing

1. Posture correction is essential so that the exercises are performed in a corrected position – patellae should face forward and lateral rotation of the hip by gluteus maximus will help to raise the medial borders of the feet.
2. Lumbrical action as in sitting.
3. Stand on right foot – point left toe forwards, bring heel back to right medial arch, repeat with toe pointing in different directions so that the foot moves through a quarter circle (repeat with left foot).
4. Hold on to a fixed object, alternate heels raising and lowering.
5. Stand on right foot – alternate heel and toe tapping with left foot (check posture of the right foot throughout the exercise), repeat, standing on left foot.

Lower limb activities

1. Stepping on and off a stool.
2. Heels raising knees bending, knees straightening and heels lowering (with or without holding on).
3. Arms crossed, sitting down and standing up on one leg.
4. Hopping, skipping, jumping, walking over uneven surfaces.

Trunk

Cervical spine

1 Lying

(a) Neck stretching and head pushing back, hold and rest.
(b) Head turn slowly from side to side.

(c) Prone lying, trunk supported on forearms, head raise, hold and lower slowly.

2 Sitting

(a) Hands clasped behind head, push head into hands, push elbows back and rest.
(b) Head turn slowly from side to side.
(c) Head bend slowly from side to side.

Thoracic and lumbar spine

1 Lying

(a) Knees flexed, feet on floor – tilt pelvis backwards and flatten the lumbar spine.
(b) As above, abdominal muscles contract to lift pelvis just off the floor/plinth (without contracting the glutei) hold and lower.
(c) As above, pelvis raise and lower.
(d) As above, pelvis raise – pass ball from hand to hand under the lumbar spine.
(e) As above, abdominal muscles contract, head and shoulders raise – stretch hands towards knees, hold and lower slowly (Figure A4.1).
(f) As above, knees roll slowly from side to side.
(g) As above, hands on shoulders – abdominal muscles contract, head and shoulders raise and

turn to touch right knee with left elbow, repeat to the opposite side.
(h) Prone lying – abdominal muscles contract to raise lumbar spine and lower.
(i) Prone lying – head and shoulders raise and lower (Figure A4.2).
(j) Prone lying, hands clasped behind head – head, shoulders and arms raise and lower.
(k) Side-lying with knees and hips flexed to a right angle – pelvis and legs raise and lower.
(l) Side-lying – head and shoulders raise slide upper arm down top leg and lower.

2 Prone kneeling

(a) Lumbar spine humping and hollowing.
(b) Right arm stretch forward, left leg stretch back hold and rest (keep abdominal muscles contracted throughout the exercise).
(c) Keep hands on the floor, change legs to take weight on feet, jump feet back to straighten knees and jump feet forward to starting position.
(d) As above, change feet alternately instead of together.

3 Sitting

(a) Pelvis tilt backwards and forwards.
(b) Alternate hip hitching.
(c) Abdominal muscles contract and hold – stretch tall.
(d) Fingers on shoulders, trunk turn from side to side.
(e) Arms stretched sideways, trunk turn from side to side.
(f) Trunk curl forwards and stretch up (Figure A4.3).

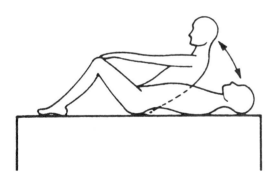

Figure A4.1 Crook lying: head and shoulder lifting with arms stretching forwards

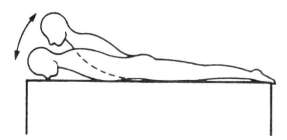

Figure A4.2 Prone lying: head and shoulder lifting and lowering

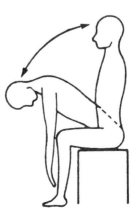

Figure A4.3 Sitting: trunk bending forward and stretching up

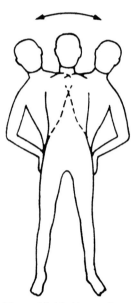

Figure A4.4 Stride standing: trunk bending to alternate sides

(g) Fingers on shoulders trunk bend side to side.
(h) Arms stretched above head, trunk bend side to side.

4 Standing

(a) Trunk bend from side to side, arms at the side (Figure A4.4), then repeat with fingers on shoulders, then arms out to side or stretched upwards.
(b) Trunk, hips and knees bend to curl forwards and stretch up tall with arms stretched up.
(c) Bend hips and knees (quarter to third way), pelvis tilt forward and back, pull abdominal muscles in and straighten up.
(d) Feet apart, alternate hip updrawing (progress by adding strap-on weights round the ankle).

Further reading

Chapter 2

Anderson, J. R. (ed) (1985) *Muir's Textbook of Pathology,* 12th edn, Edward Arnold, London

Davidson, S. (1981) *Principles and Practice of Medicine,* Churchill Livingstone, London

Thomson, A. D. and Cotton, R. E. (1983) *Lecture Notes on Pathology,* 3rd edn, Blackwell Scientific Publications, Oxford

Tighe, J. R. (1986) *Pathology,* 4th edn, Balliere Tindall, London

Walter, J. B. and Israel, M. S. (1979) *General Pathology,* 5th edn, Churchill Livingstone, Edinburgh

Williams, P. L. and Warwick, R. (eds) (1980) *Gray's Anatomy,* 36th edn, Longman, Edinburgh

Chapters 3–5

Adams, J. (1987) *Outline of Fractures,* 9th edn, Churchill Livingstone, London

Adams, J. (1986) *Outline of Orthopaedics,* 10th edn, Churchill Livingstone, London

Apley, A. G. (1985) *Systems of Orthopaedics and Fractures,* Butterworths, London

Downie, P. A. (ed) (1985) *Cash's Textbook of Orthopaedics and Rheumatology for Physiotherapists,* Faber & Faber, London

Duthie, R. B. and Ferguson, A. B. Jr. (1973) *Mercer's Orthopaedic Surgery,* Edward Arnold, London

Hadler, N. M. (1984) *Medical Management of the Regional Musculoskeletal Diseases,* Grune & Stratton, London

King, J. B. (1982a) Fractures – the upper limb 1. *British Journal of Hospital Medicine*

King, J. B. (1982b) Fractures – the upper limb 2. *British Journal of Hospital Medicine*

King, J. B. (1983a) Fractures – the axial skeleton. *British Journal of Hospital Medicine*

King, J. B. (1983b) Fractures – the lower limb 1. *British Journal of Hospital Medicine*

King, J. B. (1983c) Fractures – the lower limb 2. *British Journal of Hospital Medicine*

Wilson, N. J. (ed) (1982) *Watson–Jones Fractures and Joint Injuries,* 6th edn, Vols I and II, Churchill Livingstone, London

Chapter 6

Berry, G. (1989) Assessment and treatment of knee injuries with particular attention to hamstrings. *Physiotherapy,* **75**, 690

Bogduck, N. (1986) The anatomy and pathophysiology of whiplash. *Clinical Biomechanics,* **1**, 92–101

Brown, L. (1988) An introduction to the treatment and examination of the spine by combined movements. *Physiotherapy,* **74**, 347–353

Buckingham, L. and Hardie, S. (1986) The Roehampton approach to back fitness. *Physiotherapy,* **72**, 523–525

Dyson, M. and Suckling, J. (1978) Stimulation of tissue repair by ultrasound – a survey of the mechanisms involved. *Physiotherapy,* **64**, 105

Grieve, G. P. (ed) (1986) *Modern Manual Therapy of the Vertebral Column,* Churchill Livingstone, London

Grieve, G. P. (1979) Manipulation therapy for neck pain. *Physiotherapy,* **65**, 136–140

Grieve, G. P. (1984) *Common Vertebral Joint Problems,* Churchill Livingstone, London

Grisogono, V. (1984) *Sports Injuries, A Self Help Guide,* John Murray, Bristol

Hughston, G. (1988) Collars and corsets. *British Medical Journal,* **296**, 275

Hume-Kendall, P. and Jenkins, J. (1968) Lumbar isometric flexion exercises. *Physiotherapy,* **54**, 158–163

McDonald, R. (1988) *Taping/Strapping – A Practical Guide,* BDF Medical

Mealy, K., Brennan, H. and Fenelon, G. (1986) Early mobilisation of acute whiplash injuries. *British Medical Journal*, **292**, 656–657

Skinner, A. and Thomson, A. (1983) *Duffield's Exercises in Water*, Baillière Tindall, London

Wyke, B. (1979) Neurology of the cervical spinal joints. *Physiotherapy*, **65**, 71–76

Chapter 7

Adams, J. (1986) *Outline of Orthopaedics*, 10th edn, Churchill Livingstone, London

Apley, A. G. (1985) *Systems of Orthopaedics and Fractures*, Butterworths, London

Downie, P. A. (ed) (1985) *Cash's Textbook of Orthopaedics and Rheumatology for Physiotherapists*, Faber & Faber, London

Duthie, R. B. and Bentley, G. (eds) (1983) *Mercer's Orthopaedic Surgery*, 8th edn, Edward Arnold, London

Chapters 8–10

Barnwell, B. and Gall, B. (eds) (1988) *Physical Therapy Management of Arthritis*, Churchill Livingstone, London

Berry, H., Hamilton, E. and Goodwill, J. (1983) *Rheumatology and Rehabilitation*, Croom Helm, London

Clarke, A., Allard, L. and Braybrooks, B. (1987) *Rehabilitation in Rheumatology*, Dunitz, London

Downie, P. (ed.) (1984) *Cash's Textbook of Orthopaedics and Rheumatology for Physiotherapists*, Faber and Faber, London

Hart, F. D. (1983) *Practical Problems in Rheumatology*, Dunitz, London

Hickling, P. and Golding, J. (1984) *An Outline of Rheumatology*, Wright, Bristol

Hyde, S. A. (1980) *Physiotherapy in Rheumatology*, Blackwell Scientific Publications, Oxford

Moll, J. (ed.) (1980) *Ankylosing Spondylitis*, Churchill Livingstone, London

Moll, J. (1987) *Manual of Rheumatology*, Churchill Livingstone, London

Moskowitz, R. (1982) *Clinical Rheumatology*, 2nd edn., Lea and Febiger, Philadelphia

Skinner, A. and Thomson, A. (1983) *Duffield's Exercises in Water*, Baillière Tindall, London

Chapter 11

Butler, D. and Gifford, L. (1989) The concept of adverse mechanical tension in the nervous system. 1 & 2. *Physiotherapy*, **75**, 11, 622–636

Rose, F. C., Jones, R. and Vrbova, G. (1989) *Neuromuscular Stimulation; Basic Concepts and Clinical Implications*, Demos Publications, New York

Scott, O., Vrbova, G. and Dubowitz, V. (1984) *Effect of Nerve Stimulation on Normal and Diseased Muscle*, Raven Press, New York

Chapters 12–14

Anderson, C. and Goodchild, M. (1976) *Cystic Fibrosis. Manual of Diagnosis and Management*, Blackwell Scientific Publications, Oxford

Brewis, R. (1985) *Lecture Notes on Respiratory Disease*, 3rd edn., Blackwell Scientific Publications, Oxford

Clark, T. and Rees, J. (1985) *Practical Management of Asthma*, Dunitz, London

Collins, J. (1979) *A Synopsis of Chest Diseases*, Wright, Bristol

Downie, P. (ed.) (1983) *Cash's Textbook of Chest, Heart and Vascular Disorders for Physiotherapists*, 4th edn, Faber and Faber, London

Flenley, D. (1990) *Respiratory Medicine*, 2nd ed, Baillière Tindall, London

Milner, T. (1987) *Childhood Asthma, Diagnosis Treatment and Management*, Dunitz, London

Tinker, J. and Rapin, N. (1983) *Care of the Critically Ill Patient*, Springer Verlag, Berlin

Webber, B. (1988) *The Brompton Hospital Guide to Chest Physiotherapy*, 5th edn., Blackwell Scientific Publications, Oxford

West, J. (1985) *Respiratory Physiology. The Essentials*, 3rd edn., Williams and Wilkins, Baltimore

Chapter 15

Farrer-Brown, G. (1977) *A Colour Atlas of Cardiac Pathology*, Wolfe, London

Dercksen, M. (1976) Post-myocardial infarction rehabilitation. *South African Journal of Physiotherapy*, **32**, 3

Downie, P. A. (ed) (1987) *Cash's Textbook of Chest Heart and Vascular Disorders for Physiotherapists*, Faber & Faber, London

Fleming, A. and Baimbridge, B. (1974) *Lecture Notes on Cardiology*, 2nd edn, Blackwell Scientific Publications, London

Grant, N. I. (1975) Some longterm aspects of coronary rehabilitation in medically and surgically treated patients. *New Zealand Journal of Physiotherapy*, **5**, 2

Hampton, J. R. (ed) (1983) *Cardiovascular Disease*, Heinemann, London

Shephard, R. J. (1981) *Ischaemic Heart Disease and Exercise*, Croom Helm, London

Sturridge, M. F. and Treasure, T. (1985) *Belcher's Thoracic Surgical Management*, 5th edn, Biddles, Guildford, Surrey

Wilson, P. K., Fardy, P. S. and Froelicher, V. F. (1981) *Cardiac Rehabilitation, Adult Fitness and Exercise Testing*, Lea & Febiger, Philadelphia

Chapter 16

Downie, P. (ed.) (1987) *Cash's Textbook of Chest, Heart and Vascular Disorders for Physiotherapists*, 4th edn., Faber and Faber, London

Engstrom, B. and Van de Ven, C. (1985) *Physiotherapy for Amputees*, Churchill Livingstone, London

Hampton, J. (1983) *Cardiovascular Disease*, Heinemann, London

Horton, R. (1980) *Vascular Surgery*, Hodder and Stoughton, London

Mensch, G. and Ellis, P. (1987) *Physical Therapy Management of Lower Extremity Amputations*, Heinemann, London

Sanders, G. (1986) *Lower Limb Amputations. A Guide to Rehabilitation*, F. A. Davis, London

Vitali, M., Kingsley, P., Andrews, B. and Harris, E. (1986) *Amputations and Prostheses*, 2nd edn., Baillière Tindall, London

Chapter 17

Cotterill, J. A. (1980) Acne vulgaris and its management. *Physiotherapy*, **66**, 41

Grice, K. (1980) Hyperhidrosis and its treatment by iontophoresis *Physiotherapy*, **66**, 43

Kahn, J. (1987) *Principles and Practice of Electrotherapy*, Churchill Livingstone, London

Chapter 18

Boardman, A. and Walker, P. (1984) Plastic surgery. In *Cash's Textbook of General Medical and Surgical Conditions for Physiotherapists* (ed P. Downie), Faber & Faber, London

Burke, F. D. (1983) Microsurgery in the upper limb. *Physiotherapy*, **60**, 346

Burns, P. B. and Conin, T. A. (1987) The use of paraffin wax in the treatment of burns. *Physiotherapy*, **39**

Cason, J. S. (1981) *Treatment of Burns*, Chapman & Hall, London

Di Gregorio, V. R. (1984) *Rehabilitation of the Burn Patient*, Churchill Livingstone, London

Gilder, N. (1977) Treatment of burns in a General Hospital. *The South African Journal of Physiotherapy*, **33**

Hayne, C. R. (1984) Pulsed high frequency energy. *Physiotherapy*, **70**, 00–00

Keays, S. (1976) Burns – physiotherapy's challenge. *The South African Journal of Physiotherapy*, **32**

Kemble, J. V. H. and Lamb, B. E. (1984) *Plastic Surgical and Burns Nursing*, Baillière Tindall, London

Maxwell, H. F. (1976) Burns – the challenge of 1975. *The South African Journal of Physiotherapy*, **32**

Munster, A. M. (1980) *Burn Care for the House Officer*, Williams and Wilkins, London

Van der Spuy, A. (1977) The changing face of burns. *The South African Journal of Physiotherapy*, **33**

Wagner, M. M. (1981) *Care of the Burn-Injured Patient*, PSG Publishing, USA

Chapters 19–22

Bannister T. (1978) *Brain's Clinical Neurology,* 5th edn, Oxford University Press

Bobath, R. (1980) *A Neurological Basis for the Treatment of Cerebral Palsy,* CDM No. 75, Spastic International Medical Publishers, William Heinemann Medical Books, London

Bowsher, D. (1987) *Introduction to the Anatomy and Physiology of the Nervous System,* 5th edn,

Bromley I. (1976) *Tetraplegia and Paraplegia. Evaluation and Treatment,* 2nd edn, Churchill Livingstone, Edinburgh

Cotton, E. (1990) *Conductive Education and Cerebral Palsy,* The Spastics Society, London

Downie, P. A. (ed) (1986) *Cash's Textbook of Neurology for Physiotherapists,* 4th edn, Faber & Faber, London

Fitzgerald, M. J. T. (1985) *Neuro-anatomy, Basic and Applied,* Saunders, Philadelphia

Gillis Lynn (1980) *Human Behaviour in Illness Psychology and Interpersonal Relationships,* Faber & Faber, London

Guttman, L. (1976) *Spinal Cord Injuries,* 2nd edn, Blackwell Scientific Publications, Oxford

Levitt, S. (1984) *Treatment of Cerebral Palsy and Motor Delay,* 2nd edn, Blackwell Scientific Publications, Oxford

Lindsay, K. W., Bone, I. and Callander, R. (1986) *Neurology and Neurosurgery Illustrated,* Churchill Livingstone, London

Moffat, D. B. and Mottram, R. F. (1979) *Anatomy and Physiology for Physiotherapists,* Blackwell Scientific Publications, Oxford

Nixon Vickie, P. T. (1985) *Spinal Cord Injury,* Heinemann, London.

Scrutton, D. and Gilbertson, M. (1975) *Physiotherapy in Paediatric Practice,* Butterworths, London (out of print)

Wade, D. T. (1988) *Stroke – Practical Guides for General Practice 4.* Oxford University Press, Oxford

Walton, J. (1987) *Introduction to Clinical Neuroscience,* 2nd edn, Baillière Tindall, London

Wilkinson, I. M. S. (1988) *Essential Neurology,* Blackwell Scientific Publications, Oxford

Williams, P. L. and Warwick, R. (eds) (1980) *Gray's Anatomy,* 36th edn, Longman, Edinburgh

Wynn Parry, C. B. (1981) *Rehabilitation of the Hand,* 4th edn, Butterworths, London

Chapters 23 and 24

Downie, P. A. (ed) (1984) *Cash's Textbook of General Medical and Surgical Conditions for Physiotherapists,* Faber & Faber, London

486

Taylor, S. and Cotton, L. (1982) *A Short Textbook of Surgery,* Unibooks, Hodder and Stoughton, Sevenoaks

Macfarlane, D. A. and Thomas, L. P. (1984) *Textbook of Surgery,* 5th edn, Churchill Livingstone, London

Mann, C. V. and Rains, A. J. H. (eds) (1988) *Bailey and Love's Short Practice of Surgery,* 20th edn, H. K. Lewis Publications, London

Chapters 25 and 26

Haslett, S. and Jennings, H. (1984) *Hysterectomy and Vaginal Repair,* 2nd edn, Beaconsfield, England

Journal of the Chartered Society of Physiotherapy (1988) (Supplement), Incontinence

Laycock, J. (1987) Graded exercises for the pelvic floor muscles in the treatment of urinary incontinence. *Physiotherapy,* **73,** 371

Laycock, J. (1988) Interferential therapy in the treatment of incontinence. *Physiotherapy,* **74,** 161

Llewellyn-Jones, D. (1986) *Fundamentals of Obstetrics and Gynaecology,* 4th edn, Vol. II, Faber & Faber, London

McKenna, J. (1988) International perspectives. In *Physical Therapy,* Vol. 3, *Obstetrics and Gynaecology,* Churchill Livingstone, London

Mandlestam, D. (ed) (1986) *Incontinence and its Management,* 2nd edn, Croom Helm, London

Mitchell, L. (1987) *Simple Relaxation,* John Murray, London

Noble, E. (1982) *Essential Exercises for the Childbearing Year,* Houghton Miffen, Boston; John Murray, London

Whiteford, R. and Polden, M. (1988) *Postnatal Exercises,* 2nd edn, Century, London

Williams, M. and Booth, D. (1985) *Antenatal Education – Guidelines for Teachers,* 3rd edn, Churchill Livingstone, London

Chapter 27

Bradlow, A. (1983) Rheumatic disease in the elderly. Rehabilitation – a team effort. *Geriatric Medicine,* **13,** 811–813

Coakley, D. and Wagstaff, P. (1988) *Physiotherapy and the Elderly Patient (Therapy in Practice),* Croom Helm, London

Denham, M. J. (1983) *Care of the Long-stay Elderly Patient.* Croom Helm, London

Dougall, D. S. (1985) The effects of interferential therapy on incontinence and frequency of micturition. *Physiotherapy,* **71,** 135–136

Finn, A. M. (1986) Attitudes of physiotherapists towards geriatric care. *Physiotherapy,* **72,** 129–131

Frazer, F. W. (1979) Assessment of elderly patients. *Physiotherapy,* **65,** 212–213

Hawker, M. (1985) *The Older Patient and the Role of the Physiotherapist,* Faber & Faber, London

Jackson, O. L. (1983) *Physical Therapy of the Geriatric Patient,* Churchill Livingstone, London

Jackson, O. L. (1987) *Therapeutic Considerations for the Elderly,* Churchill Livingstone, London

Kinsman, R. and Smith, P. (1983) Exercise, advice and check-list. *Geriatric Medicine,* **13,** 817–820

Landsberger, B. H. (1985) *Long-Term Care for the Elderly. A Comparative View of Layers of Care,* Croom Helm, London

Muir Gray, J. A. (1982) Practising prevention in old age. *British Medical Journal,* **285,** 545–547

Oddy, R. J. (1987) Promoting mobility in patients with dementia, some suggested strategies for physiotherapists. *Physiotherapy Practice,* **3,** 18–28

Ransome, H. E. (1980) Role of the physiotherapist in homes for the elderly. *Physiotherapy,* **66,** 324–331

Squires, A. J. (1986) Physiotherapy assessment of the elderly patient. *Physiotherapy,* **72,** 617–620

Squires, A. J., Dolbear, R., Williams, R. and Smoker, S. (1987) Evaluation of physiotherapy in a day unit. *Physiotherapy,* **73,** 596–598

Squires, A. J. (1988) *Rehabilitation of the Older Patient (Therapy in Practice),* Croom Helm, London

Stedford, A. (1984) *Facing Death. Patients, Families and Professionals,* William Heinemann Medical Books, London

World Health Organization (1989) *Health of the Elderly,* WHO Technical Report Series 779, WHO, Geneva

Wright, W. B. (1983) The tired man. *Geriatric Medicine,* **13,** 782–783

Appendix 1

Basmajian, J. (1984) *Therapeutic Exercise*, 4th edn., Williams and Wilkins, London

Basmajian, J. (ed.) (1985) *Manipulation Traction and Massage*, 3rd edn., Williams and Wilkins, London

Basmajian, J. V. (ed) (1989) *Biofeedback Principles and Practice for Clinicians,* 3rd edn, Williams and Wilkins, Baltimore

Beaulieu, J. (1984) *Stretching for all Sports*, The Athletic Press, California

Blackman, J. and Pripp, K. (1988) *Mobilisation Technique*, Churchill Livingstone, London

Corrigan, B. and Maitland, G. (1983) *Practical Orthopaedic Medicine*, Butterworths, London

Cyriax, J. (1982) *Textbook of Orthopaedic Medicine,* Vol. 1, 8th edn., Baillière Tindall, London

Cyriax, J. (1984) *Textbook of Orthopaedic Medicine,* Vol. 2, 11th edn, Bailliere Tindall, London

Davis, B. and Harrison, R. (1988) *Hydrotherapy in Practice*, Churchill Livingstone, London

Dix, M. R. (1974) Treatment of vertigo. *Physiotherapy,* **60,** 380–384

Ebner, M. (1972) *Connective Tissue Massage, Theory and Therapeutic Application,* R. E. Krieger, New York

Ebner, M. (1978) Connective tissue massage. *Physiotherapy,* **64,** 208–210

Grieve, G. (1975) Manipulation. *Physiotherapy,* **61,** 11–18

Grieve, G. (1984) *Mobilisation of the Spine*, 4th edn., Churchill Livingstone, London

Grieve, G. (1989) Contraindications to spinal manipulations and allied treatment. *Physiotherapy, 75*, 445–453

Herdman, S. (1990) Treatment of benign paroxysmal positional vertigo. *Physical Therapy, 70*, 361–388

Hollis, M. (1987) *Massage for Therapists*, Blackwell Scientific Publications, Oxford

Holis, M. (1989) *Practical Exercise Therapy*, 3rd edn., Blackwell Scientific, Oxford

Janda, V. (1983) *Muscle Function Testing*, Butterworths, London

Kisner, C. and Colby, L. (1990) *Therapeutic Exercise. Foundations and Techniques*, 2nd edn., F. A. Davis, Philadelphia

Low, J. and Reed, A. (1990) *Electrotherapy Physical Agents. The Principles Explained*, Heinemann, London

McDonald, R. (1988) *Taping/Strapping. A Practical Guide,* BDF Medical, London

Mackenzie, R. (1981) *The Lumbar Spine*, Spinal Publications, New Zealand

Mackenzie, R. (1983) *Treat Your Own Neck*, Wright and Carman, New Zealand

Mackenzie, R. (1989) A perspective on manipulative therapy. *Physiotherapy, 75*, 440–444

Maitland, G. (1970) *Peripheral Manipulations*, 2nd edn., Butterworths, London

Maitland, G. D. (1986) *Vertebral Manipulation,* 5th edn, Butterworths, London

Michlovitz, S. (1986) *Thermal Agents and Rehabilitation*, F. A. Davis, Philadelphia

Nathan, P. (1976) The gate-control theory of pain. A critical review. *Brain, 99*, 123

O'Donoghue, C. E. (1983) Controlled trials of manipulation. *Manipulation Association of Chartered Physiotherapists Newsletter, 14*, 1–6

Savage, B. (1984) *Interferential Therapy*. Faber & Faber, London

Skinner, A. and Thomson, A. (1983) *Duffield's Exercise in Water*, 3rd edn., Baillière Tindall, London

Stoddard, A. (1969) *Manual of Osteopathic Practice,* Hutchinson, London

Stoddard, A. (1972) *Manual of Osteopathic Technique*, Hutchinson, London

Wadsworth, H. and Chanmugan, A. (1983) *Electrophysical Agents in Physiotherapy*, 2nd edn., Science Press, New York

Wells, P. E., Frampton, V. and Bowsher, D. (1988) *Pain, Management and Control in Physiotherapy,* Heinemann Medical Books, London

Wyke, B. D. (1985) Articular neurology and manipulative therapy. In *Aspects of Manipulative Therapy*, 2nd edn, (eds E. F. Glasgow, L. T. Turomey, E. R. Scull and A. M. Kleynhaus), Churchill Livingstone, Edinburgh

Index